Standard Beginning Steps

AT THE BEGINNING OF THE PROCEDURE:

All nurse assisting skills must include certain basic steps for the safety and well-being of the patient and the nursing assistant. To avoid repeating the same information in each procedure, the symbol is shown before "Complete Standard Beginning Steps" to remind you to:

1. Gather the necessary equipment.
2. Wash your hands.
3. Identify and greet the patient.
4. Identify yourself.
5. Tell the patient what you are going to do.
6. Provide privacy.
7. Raise the bed to a comfortable working height.
8. Lower the side rail on the side nearest to you if it was up.

The symbol ![hand symbol] reminds you to wear gloves during the procedure.

Standard Ending Steps

AFTER FINISHING THE PROCEDURE:

The symbol ◆ is shown before "Complete Standard Ending Steps" to remind you to:

1. Assist the patient to a comfortable position.
2. Place the signal light within reach.
3. Return the bed to its lowest position and ask if patient is comfortable.
4. Raise side rail if you lowered it.
5. Dispose of sharps according to facility policy.
6. Remove, clean, and store equipment used.
7. Remove and dispose of gloves if used.
8. Wash your hands.
9. Record the procedure.
10. Notify your charge nurse of any problems or abnormal observations.

Basic Nurse Assisting

Mary E. Stassi

Coordinator, Health Occupations
St. Charles Community College
St. Peters, Missouri

With 745 illustrations

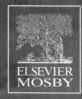

ELSEVIER
MOSBY

ELSEVIER
SAUNDERS

11830 Westline Industrial Drive
St. Louis, Missouri 63146

NOTICE

Health care is an ever changing field. Standard safety precautions must be followed, but as new research and clinical experience broaden our knowledge, changes in treatment or therapy may become necessary or appropriate. Readers are advised to check the most current information provided by the manufacturer of each piece of equipment to be used to verify the recommended usage, the correct method of application, and contraindications. It is the responsibility of the licensed prescriber, relying on experience and knowledge of the patient, to determine the best treatment for each individual patient. Neither the publisher nor the author assumes any responsibility for any liability or any injury and/or damage to persons or property arising from this publication.

International Standard Book Number 0-7216-91463-0

Executive Editor: Susan R. Epstein
Senior Developmental Editor: Robyn L. Brinks
Publishing Services Manager: John Rogers
Senior Project Manager: Beth Hayes
Senior Designer: Kathi Gosche

Printed in the United States of America

Last digit is the print number: 9 8 7 6 5 4 3 2 1

To my husband,
Chris,
for his unconditional love, support,
and willingness to do more than his fair share every day.

To my daughter,
Sarah,
for being the kind of daughter
every parent dreams about.

To my mother,
Bonnie,
who always believes in me.

To my father,
Tom,
for providing divine inspiration.

Mary E. Stassi is currently the health occupations coordinator at St. Charles Community College in St. Peters, Missouri. She is a well-known author, educator, and professional speaker, as well an advocate for nursing assistants and nursing assistant training. In addition to her position at the community college, she provides consulting services and works as a women's health educator for SSM St. Mary's Health Center in St. Louis, Missouri.

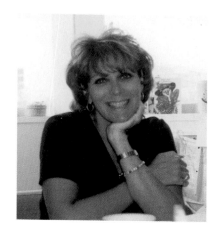

Mary was instrumental in the development and approval of the certified nursing assistant, certified medication technician, and restorative nursing assistant programs at St. Charles Community College and has taught in nursing assistant, certified medication technician, pharmacy technician, restorative nursing assistant, community health, and associate degree programs.

With more than 25 years of nursing experience, she has worked as a nursing assistant, staff nurse, charge nurse, infection control nurse, employee health nurse, nursing educator, and consultant in acute care, long-term care, and health information technology.

Ms. Stassi coordinated the revision of several textbooks, including *Nurse Assistant in a Long-Term Care Facility, Insulin Administration,* and *Level I Medication Aide,* for the Missouri Department of Health and Senior Services and the Instructional Materials Laboratory at the University of Missouri-Columbia College of Education. She served on the IV Therapy Task Force for the Missouri State Board of Nursing and was a contributing author for the 2003 revision of the textbook *Venous Access and Intravenous Infusion Treatment Modalities.* She is a contributing author to several nursing publications.

Ms. Stassi is a graduate of Lutheran Medical Center School of Nursing in St. Louis, Missouri and holds certification in gerontological nursing through the American Nurses Credentialing Center (ANCC). She is a past participant in the Geriatric Scholar Program at St. Louis University. She is a member of the St. Charles Community College Health Information Technology Advisory Committee and the Long Term Care Educators' Association (LTCEA) board of directors and served as president of the LTCEA in 2001 and 2002.

REVIEWERS

Renee Anderson
Director/Owner
Petra Allied Health
Springdale, Arizona

Gayle K. Campbell, RN, BSN, BAHS, BBA, MBA
Director of Care
Coordinator Health Sciences
President Consulting Firm
Oak Terrace Long Term Care
Georgian College of Applied Arts and Technology
Gayle Campbell and Associates
Ontario, Canada

Frances Garner, BSN
Allied Health Instructor
North Central Kansas Technical College
Hays, Kansas

Randall Gwin
Instructor
Minneapolis Community and Technical College
Minneapolis, Minnesota

Dorise Hughes, RN
CNA/CMT Instructor and Examiner
St. Charles Community College
St. Peters, Missouri

Rosie Miller, RN, MSN
CNA Instructor
Seneca High
Dwight, Illinois

Carolyn Ruppel, RN
Nursing Assistant Instructor
Red Rock Job Corps
Lopez, Pennsylvania

Jeanette Vilar, RN
Senior Nurse Instructor/Coordinator
Action for a Better Community Training Institute
Rochester, New York

ACKNOWLEDGMENTS

This book is the result of the creative efforts of many talented individuals. Special thanks to Denise Miller, health occupations instructor, who provided the inspiration for this project. I gratefully acknowledge all of the individuals who devoted their time and talents to make this book a reality.

This book could not have been completed without the dedication of the editorial staff. While it is impossible to list every individual at Elsevier who contributed to the success of this text, their efforts are both recognized and appreciated. I owe a special debt of gratitude to this team for their enthusiasm for the project, as well as their expertise and encouragement through the ups and downs of the developmental phase.

I am especially grateful and appreciative of the efforts by:

Suzi Epstein, executive editor at Elsevier, who gave me the opportunity to become involved with the project and believed in the need for a "user-friendly" text.

Robyn Brinks, senior developmental editor for nursing at Elsevier, who held my hand along the way and whose vision, attention to detail, and organizational skills kept the project on track. Without Robyn I would never have been able to keep all of the balls I had in the air at the same time.

Beth Hayes, senior project manager at Elsevier, for her guidance, insight, and careful management of the production process that resulted in an accurate and professional text.

Photographer Michael DeFilippo of St. Louis, who allowed me to give creative input and made the photography sessions fun.

The administration, staff, and residents at Lutheran Senior Services, Gables at Breeze Park, St. Charles, Missouri, for welcoming us into their facility and providing the photographic opportunities needed to complete the project. Special thanks to Bernice Bundren, director of nursing, longtime friend and colleague, for her support.

Diana Romans, nursing lab coordinator at St. Charles Community College, for graciously allowing us to use the nursing lab.

Francie Woods, occupational therapy assistant program coordinator at St. Charles Community College, for sharing her knowledge and resources.

Gail Schafers, readability specialist, who made suggestions that enhanced the text for students with limited English proficiency.

The artists at Graphic World, St. Louis, Missouri, for their efforts to turn my ideas into reality.

Bonnie Lask, Alice Bynum, Linda S. Ahart, Lois Unnerstall, Don MacPherson, Bernice Bundren, Dora Brante, Sheri L.

Clayton, Jennifer A. Lovelady, Haley Lovelady, Donnie Lovelady, Art Fuller, Ginny Tiller, DeQuette Harwell, Amanda Byrd, Denise Lammers, Ruth Moellering, Elsie Bredehoft, Dorothy M. Gerth, Evelyn Zorn, Virginia M. Niemeier, Lorene Prinster, Christine Hennemann, Marie Borgelt, Candy Johnson, Connie West, and Terry Etling, who willingly and cheerfully served as models for this text.

The professionals who gave their time to provide a thoughtful and candid review of the chapters.

My colleagues in the Long Term Care Educators' Association, who have provided ideas, inspiration, and friendship over the years.

Janis Levson and Susan Rhyne at the University of Missouri-Columbia, who have provided me with friendship, as well as literary guidance, on previous projects.

Special thanks to Mr. and Mrs. Sides, who shared their stories and allowed us to photograph them for this text. They are an inspiration.

I would like to extend my appreciation to the authors, publishers, and equipment companies who have granted us permission to use their illustrations and photographs in this text.

With warm regard I would like to recognize those very important individuals, the nursing assistants who continually strive for excellence in meeting the demands and challenges of the profession on a daily basis. Your patients appreciate all you do and so do I.

Finally, I thank my husband, Chris, and daughter, Sarah, for their unselfish love, endless patience, and quiet understanding that allowed me to devote such a large part of the last 2 years to the development of this text. Without their support this project would not have become a reality.

The goal of *Basic Nurse Assisting* is to provide a reliable source of information that instructors can use to teach nursing assistants how to provide high-quality care to many different types of patients. The content is designed to help students acquire the knowledge and skills necessary to permit them to become certified and function as skilled nursing assistants in hospitals, long-term care facilities, and home health agencies.

It was our goal to provide a text that is "user friendly" in both format and content that also meets the needs of students with various reading abilities, including English as a second language (ESL) students. Special consideration was given to assisting instructors with developing their instructional programs for the most efficient use of time and resources.

The nursing assistant is an important member of the health care team and makes valuable contributions during the care planning process. Nursing assistants must be helped to understand the vital role their observations, reporting skills, and attention to detail play in positive patient outcomes.

The text is divided into seven sections containing a total of 35 chapters. It is presented in a logical sequence, beginning with an introduction to health care and moving through caring for others, understanding the human body, and providing basic nursing care. Special emphasis is placed on the unique health care needs of children and older adults. Cultural considerations are included in the text as well. Each chapter is independent of the others, allowing the instructor flexibility when setting up a class schedule.

In addition to comprehensive content, key features of this text include:

- Specific measurable objectives open each chapter and are easily referenced in headings and subheadings.
- Key terms with definitions are listed at the beginning of the chapter and in **bold** print when they first appear in the chapter.
- Carefully reviewed and edited text ensures optimal reading level and comprehension, even for ESL students.
- More than 740 full-color photographs and illustrations provide an engaging and appealing instructional presentation.
- A helpful appendix provides key phrases and terms in Spanish.
- Boxes and tables list signs and symptoms, care guidelines, nursing measures, and other information to emphasize content.

- Omnibus Budget Reconciliation Act of 1987 (OBRA) and safety content are highlighted in the narrative.
- Streamlined procedures are written in a simple style giving step-by-step instructions. Special icons in procedures provide a visual cue to perform beginning and ending steps, which include infection control measures and communication guidelines.
- The NNAAP™ icon listed on the procedure page alerts students to those procedures that are part of the National Nurse Aide Assessment Program (NNAAP™).
- Special notes for age-specific and cultural considerations appear in the margin.
- Unique "How & Why" notes provide practical tips about performing specific procedures and give explanations behind nursing actions and patient responses.
- End-of-chapter review questions are helpful when reviewing the information contained in the chapter, as well as when studying for a test or competency evaluation.
- A comprehensive glossary contains every key term used in the text and provides simple definitions.
- The extensive index provides a reference to allow easy access to information contained in the book.

Extensive Teaching/Learning Package

A complete teaching package includes:
- Instructor's guide with teaching tips and tools, video suggestions, critical thinking exercises, and test bank.
- Computerized test bank in ExamView.
- Comprehensive student workbook reinforces the text content and includes a variety of questions, interesting exercises and puzzles, and checklists for procedures in the text. A certification review section and flash cards are also included in the student workbook.
- Unique instructor's book provides each page from the student text reduced in size to allow for marginal notes to guide the instructor, including teaching strategies and activities.
- More than 50 dynamic transparency acetates to enhance your classroom presentation.

I hope that this book provides you and your students with the information needed to build a solid foundation for providing quality patient care and that you will enjoy using this text as much as I have enjoyed participating in its development.

Mary

Welcome to the exciting world of health care! This book was designed to help you learn the skills and information needed for certification and employment as a nursing assistant. As a nursing assistant you are an important member of the health care team. Nursing assistants are vital to the operation of hospitals, long-term care facilities, and home health care agencies.

The information contained in each chapter provides you with a foundation on which to build future knowledge and skills. The book is written in a style that speaks directly to you, the reader.

Special features that make learning easier include:

- Clearly stated objectives list what will be covered in each chapter. These objectives are used in the workbook, as well as the textbook.
- Key terms with definitions are listed at the beginning of the chapter and in **bold** print when they first appear in the chapter.
- Simple language accommodates students at various reading levels.
- Generous use of color photographs and illustrations help you to better understand the written material.
- Boxes and tables stress important information and are helpful when studying.
- Safety alerts direct your attention to safety concerns.
- Easy-to-follow procedures are written in a simple style giving step-by-step instructions. Beginning and ending step icons remind you to follow important steps when beginning or ending care.
- The NNAAP™ icon listed on the procedure page alerts you to procedures that are part of the National Nurse Aide Assessment Program (NNAAP™). Your instructor will provide you with information regarding your state's requirements and participation in the NNAAP™ exam.
- Omnibus Budget Reconciliation Act of 1987 (OBRA) and safety content is highlighted in color to remind you to pay special attention to these important guidelines.
- Notes in the margins on culture, older adults, and children provide information helpful when caring for each group of people.
- The "How & Why" sections provide practical tips about performing a task or give an explanation about certain actions or patient responses.
- Review questions are helpful when reviewing the information contained in the chapter, as well as when studying for a test or competency evaluation.

- The glossary contains all of the vocabulary words or key terms used in the text and provides simple definitions.
- An appendix provides key phrases and terms in Spanish.
- The index provides a reference to allow easy access of information contained in the book.

How to Use This Book

Each student has a different style of learning and studying. Some students learn best by reading; others learn better by hearing the information, such as during a lecture in class. Still other students learn best through the use of pictures, illustrations, videos, or hands-on activities. This book and the accompanying workbook provide opportunities for students to learn using their preferred style or combination of styles.

Before the beginning of each class, read over the objectives and key terms listed at the beginning of the chapter. This will help you to be familiar with the main idea of what will be presented in class and help you learn new terms. Some instructors will ask that you read the entire chapter before attending class. This allows you to be prepared to discuss the material. Other instructors prefer that you read the chapter after the information is presented in class. While you are reading the information in the chapter, pay special attention to boxes, tables, and special considerations. Some students benefit by underlining or highlighting important information. When you have finished reading the chapter, answer the review questions and check your answers. This will tell you how much of what you read you remember and understand. You may need to re-read some areas of the chapter in order to answer the questions. Some instructors will assign the review questions as homework. Other instructors may ask you to complete the review questions as a classroom assignment. Remember, this book was written with you, the student, in mind!

Health care is never boring! The field of health care is dynamic and always changing. Keeping your skills current and up-to-date means that you will be a lifelong learner. Your instructor will provide you with new information as it becomes available. Never be afraid to ask questions. Remember that as a nursing assistant you are making a difference in the lives of your patients and their families each day.

A Note About Word Choice

The term *patient* is used throughout this text. The term used to describe the person being cared for in a health care facility varies from facility to facility and even region to region. Generally we refer to the person receiving care as a *patient* when the person is cared for in a hospital, doctor's office, or clinic. *Resident* is used to describe the person who is admitted to a long-term care or rehabilitation facility. The term *client* is commonly used in mental health and other outpatient settings. There are even some facilities that refer to the person receiving care as a *guest*. Your instructor or nursing supervisor can tell you which term is appropriate for the area in which you are working or performing your clinical hours.

Happy Learning!

STUDY TIPS

This text was created to assist you in achieving the objectives of each chapter and establishing a solid base of knowledge in nurse assisting. Regardless of reading level or native language, these hints will help you study.

Ask Questions!

There are no stupid questions. If you do not know something or are not sure, you need to find out. Other people may be wondering the same thing but may be too shy to ask. The answer could mean life or death to your patient. That is certainly more important than feeling embarrassed about asking a question.

Chapter Objectives

At the beginning of each chapter in the textbook are objectives that you should have mastered when you finish studying that chapter. Write these objectives in your notebook, leaving a blank space after each. Fill in the answers as you find them while reading the chapter. Review to make sure your answers are correct and complete. Use these answers when you study for tests. This should also be done for separate course objectives that your instructor has listed in your class syllabus.

Key Terms

At the beginning of each chapter in the textbook are key terms that you will encounter as you read the chapter. Text page number references are provided for easy reference and review, and the key terms are in **bold** print the first time they appear in the chapter. It is hoped that a more general competency in the understanding and use of medical and scientific language may result.

Reading Hints

When reading each chapter in the textbook, look at the subject headings to learn what each section is about. Read first for the general meaning. Then re-read parts you did not understand. It may help to read those parts aloud. Carefully read the information given in each table, and study each figure and its caption.

Concepts

While studying, put difficult concepts into your own words to see if you understand them. Check this understanding with another student or the instructor. Write these in your notebook.

Class Notes

When taking lecture notes in class, leave a large margin on the left side of each notebook page, and write only on right-hand pages, leaving all left-hand pages blank. Look over your lecture notes soon after each class, while your memory is fresh. Fill in missing words, complete sentences and ideas, and underline key phrases, definitions, and concepts. At the top of each page, write the topic of that page. In the left margin, write the key word for that part of your notes. On the opposite left-hand page, write a summary or outline that combines material from both the textbook and the lecture. These can be your study notes for review.

Study Groups

Form a study group with some other students so you can help one another. Practice speaking and reading aloud. Ask questions about material you are not sure about. Work together to find answers.

References for Improving Study Skills

Good study skills are essential for achieving your goals in nursing. Time management, efficient use of study time, and a consistent approach to studying are all beneficial. There are various study methods for reading a textbook and for taking class notes. Some methods that have proven helpful can be found in *Saunders Student Nurse Planner: A Guide to Success in Nursing School.* This book contains helpful information on test taking and preparing for clinical experiences. It includes an example of a "time map" for planning study time and a blank form that the student can use to formulate a personal time map.

Vocabulary

If you find a non-technical word you do not know (for example, *drowsy*), try to guess its meaning from the sentence (for example, "Some medicines may make the patient feel tired or drowsy"). If you are not sure of the meaning, or if it seems particularly important, look it up in the dictionary.

First-Language Buddy

English as a second language (ESL) students should find a first-language buddy—another student who is a native speaker of English and who is willing to answer questions about word meanings, pronunciations, and culture. Maybe your buddy would like to learn about your language and culture as well. This could help in your buddy's nursing experience.

Vocabulary Notebook

Keep a small alphabetized notebook or address book in your pocket or purse. Write down new non-technical words you read or hear, along with their meanings and pronunciations. Write each word under its initial letter so you can find it easily, as in a dictionary. For words you do not know or for words that have a different meaning in nursing, write down how they are used and sound. Look up their meanings in a dictionary, or ask your instructor or first-language buddy. Then write the different meanings or usages that you have found in your book, including the nursing meaning. Continue to add new words as you discover them. For example:

PRIMARY
- Of most importance; main: *the primary problem or disease*
- The first one; elementary: *primary school*

SECONDARY
- Of less importance; resulting from another problem or disease: *a secondary symptom*
- The second one: *secondary school (in the United States, high school)*

CONTENTS

Section 3

Basic Nursing Skills

Section 5

Therapeutic and Technical Skills

Section 6

Special Care Needs

Section 7

Professional Skills

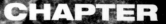

Working in Health Care

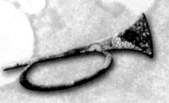

What you will learn

- The different types of health care workplaces
- Members of the health care team and their jobs
- How health care is paid for

KEY TERMS

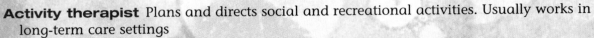

Activity therapist Plans and directs social and recreational activities. Usually works in long-term care settings

Acute care Care provided during a short-term illness or injury

Inpatient care Care provided to the patient who is in the hospital and stays there overnight

Licensed practical nurse (LPN)/licensed vocational nurse (LVN) Licensed nurse who gives patient care, drugs, and treatments. Works under the supervision of a registered nurse

Managed care Ways insurance companies try to control health care costs

Medicaid State-managed health care plan that covers health care services for people with low income. Sometimes covers older, blind, and disabled people

Medicare Federal government health care plan that pays for health care services for people over age 65

Nursing assistant Person who gives hands-on patient care such as bathing and feeding. Works under the supervision of a registered nurse and in some states a licensed practical nurse/licensed vocational nurse

Occupational therapist (OT)/occupational therapy assistant (OTA) Helps patients to learn the skills they need to resume activities of daily living such as dressing and grooming. Focuses on small (fine) motor skills

Outpatient care Health care services for a person who is not hospitalized

Pharmacist Fills prescription orders. Teaches and advises patients, caregivers, and health care team members about drugs

Physical therapist (PT)/physical therapy assistant (PTA) Helps patients relearn skills such as getting out of bed and using things such as crutches and walkers. Focuses on improving large-muscle skills

Private health insurance A plan that pays for the cost of health care. Each insurance plan has its own rules. Not paid for by state or federal money

Registered dietitian (RD) Looks at a patient's nutritional needs. Supervises meal planning and preparation. Teaches patients and caregivers about nutrition and diets

Registered nurse (RN) Licensed nurse who plans, coordinates, and supervises patient care and carries out doctors' orders. Supervises LPNs/LVNs and nursing assistants

Rehabilitation Health care to help people maintain or return to their highest level of normal activity after an illness or injury. Also known as **Restorative** care

Respiratory therapist Performs breathing treatments and procedures

Social worker Helps organize services to provide patient care, especially after a patient leaves the hospital or nursing home. Plans transfers to other facilities for patients who cannot return home

Speech language pathologist/speech therapist Assists patients who have speaking and swallowing disorders

Working in a Health Care Setting

Welcome to the exciting world of health care! During your training you will learn the right way to perform many basic nursing procedures. **Nursing assistants** work in many different settings. Some of these settings include:

Doctor's offices/clinics—Many people receive care from their family doctor in an office or clinic setting. They see the doctor for minor illnesses and general health care. One or more doctors often work together in the same office or clinic. This type of setting is called **outpatient care**. The term *outpatient* means that the patient is not admitted to the office or clinic and leaves after the scheduled visit (Figure 1-1).

Hospitals—The hospital provides care for a person who needs surgery or has a serious illness or injury. Hospitals are sometimes called **acute care** facilities. Hospitals differ in size from small rural hospitals to large medical centers. All hospitals provide **inpatient** care. This means that the patient is admitted to the hospital and remains there overnight. Many hospitals also have outpatient care such as emergency department care (Figure 1-2).

Nursing homes and rehabilitation facilities—These settings are called long-term care (LTC) centers. They give 24-hour care to people who are sick or disabled and cannot care for themselves. Specially trained staff members provide physical, occupational, and speech therapy to help patients return to their highest level of wellness and ability. The LTC setting may provide temporary care for a person who gets better and is able to return home. The LTC center may also serve as a permanent home for the person who is unable to return

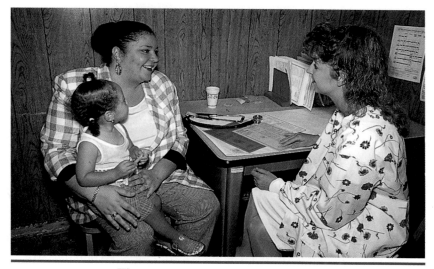

***Figure* 1-1**   Doctor's office/clinic.

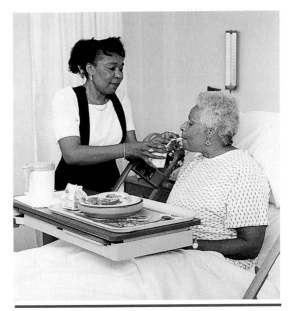

Figure **1-2**　A patient in the hospital.

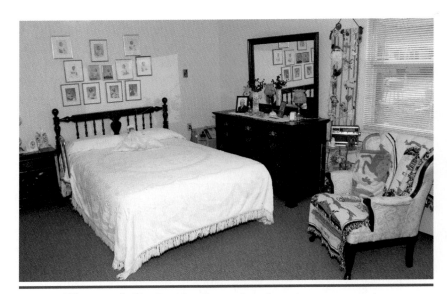

Figure **1-3**　Resident room in a long-term care center.

home. Many residents of LTC centers are elderly, but LTC is
for people of all ages (Figure 1-3).

Home care—This is care for people in their own homes. Often
people who are recovering from an illness or operation recover more quickly in a familiar setting than in a hospital or
nursing home. Home care is usually less expensive than
acute or long-term care (Figure 1-4).

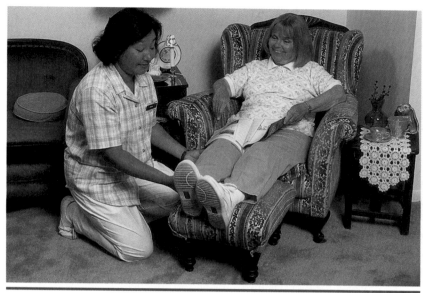

***Figure* 1-4**   Care being provided to a patient in her home.

Becoming a Member of the Health Care Team

The health care team includes many different people (Table 1-1). Each person on the team provides a different service to the patient. Some services are provided in only one type of setting. As a nursing assistant, you will have more direct contact with patients than the other members of the health care team. The health care team members you will work with most closely are the RN and LPN/LVN. Together you form a nursing care team that works to meet the physical, emotional, social, and spiritual needs of your patients. Together the members of the team look at the patient's needs. The team plans how to provide the care and services needed. The most important members of the health care team are the patient and the patient's family. All of the services provided by the members of the team revolve around patients and their needs (Figure 1-5).

Nursing assistants receive their patient care assignments from a team leader or charge nurse. The team leader or charge nurse may be an RN or an LPN, depending on the setting. The charge nurse reports to the next person in the chain of command, usually a supervisor or the assistant director of nursing. The director of nursing is responsible for supervising all members of the nursing department. Health care facilities vary in the number of levels in their chain of command.

Table 1-1

MEMBERS OF THE HEALTH CARE TEAM

Title	Job description
Activities director/ Activity staff	Works in long-term care centers. Plans and carries out activities for residents
Audiologist	Tests hearing and prescribes hearing aids
Clergy/Pastoral care	Works in all health care settings. Helps patients to meet their spiritual needs. Includes priests, ministers, rabbis, deacons, nuns, and laypeople
Dentist	Prevents and treats disorders of the gums, mouth, and teeth
Dietitian/Dietary staff	Plans and prepares meals for patients. Teaches patients and families about special diets
Doctor	Diagnoses patient, orders medications and treatments
Health information technician/ Medical records technician	Maintains medical records for all patients
Nurse (RN or LPN/LVN)	Plans and provides care for patients. Supervises other nursing staff such as nursing assistants and medication technicians
Nursing assistant	Provides hands-on care to patients under the supervision of a nurse
Medication technician/ Medication aide	Administers medications to residents in long-term care centers
Occupational therapist/ Occupational therapy assistant	Assists patients with learning skills needed to perform activities of daily living after an illness or injury
Pharmacist	Fills medication and prescription orders. Consults with doctors and nurses about patient medications
Physical therapist/ Physical therapy assistant	Assists people with musculoskeletal problems to regain function after an injury or illness
Podiatrist	Specializes in treating disorders of the feet and lower legs
Respiratory therapist	Assists with treating disorders of the lungs, gives oxygen and respiratory treatments as ordered by the doctor
Social worker/ Social services designee	Helps patients and families deal with the effects of illness. Services include providing referrals to community services
Speech language pathologist/ Speech therapist	Works with patients who have disorders of speech or swallowing

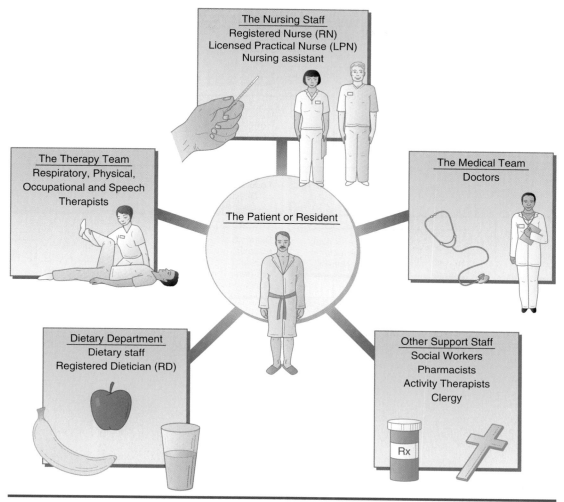

Figure **1-5** All of the services provided by the members of the team revolve around patients and their needs.

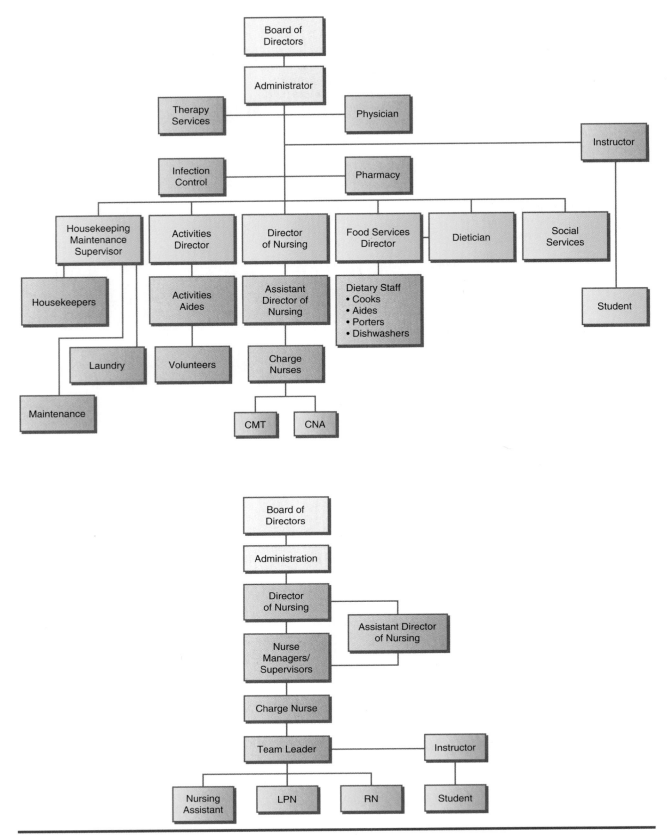

***Figure* 1-6** The chain of command in a long-term care center and in a hospital.

As a student, you report to your instructor or the person designated as your supervisor. Figure 1-6 shows examples of the chain of command in a long-term care center and a hospital. It is important that you learn the chain of command for your facility.

The Cost of Health Care

Health care in America is big business. Americans want to receive high-quality health care. This kind of care is very expensive. There are three ways that most health care is paid for in the United States.

In 1965 the federal government created a health insurance plan called **Medicare.** Most people covered by Medicare are over age 65. The federal government supervises the Medicare program. Each state oversees **Medicaid.** Medicaid is a program that uses state and federal money to pay for health care for people with low incomes. Some people who are older, blind, or disabled also receive Medicaid benefits. The money to pay for Medicare and Medicaid comes from the taxes you pay. Many Americans have **private health insurance.** Some companies pay the cost of health insurance. Some companies pay part of the cost of health insurance, and the employee pays the rest. There are many people who do not have private insurance and are not eligible for Medicare or Medicaid.

Since the late 1980s the health care industry has tried to keep medical care costs low. One way they have done this is through **managed care.** With managed care, insurance companies arrange with health care providers to give care at a lower cost. With managed care the patients in the hospital are usually sicker. Patients leave the hospital and go home sooner than in the past. For example, a woman who had a baby in the 1950s or 1960s stayed in the hospital for 5 to 7 days. Most new mothers now go home 24 to 48 hours after delivery.

As a nursing assistant, you will have many different jobs to choose from. The field of health care is always changing. This course will prepare you to become a valuable member of the health care team.

CHAPTER REVIEW

1. List the 4 most common types of health care settings.

2. The hospital has discharged Ms. Trask, and she will be admitted to another health care facility after her stroke. She will need physical, occupational, and speech therapy services. What type of a setting do you think she will be moved to?

3. Ms. Trask's family members plan to take care of her when she is ready to go home. Which type of health care agency will best help Ms. Trask's family learn how to take care of her at home?

4. Who are the most important members of the health care team?

5. What are the 3 ways most health care is paid for in the United States?

Circle the one BEST response.

6. Which health care provider will help coordinate Ms. Trask's care after her discharge?
   a. Activity director
   b. Dietitian
   c. LPN/LVN
   d. Social worker

7. Which health care provider supervises the patient's care?
   a. RN
   b. LPN/LVN
   c. Nursing assistant
   d. Patient care assistant

Answers are on page 703.

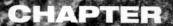

CHAPTER 2

Your Role as a Nursing Assistant

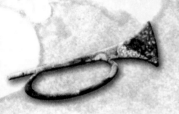

What you will learn

- The role of the nursing assistant
- State and federal laws that affect nursing assistants
- Tasks you may and may not perform as a nursing assistant
- Qualities of a professional caregiver
- Ethical and legal aspects of caring for others
- Reporting abuse and neglect

11

KEY TERMS

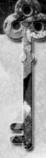

Abuse Hurting a person physically, emotionally, or financially

Consent Giving permission for care or treatment

Emotional neglect Not giving care and attention

Ethics A person's beliefs about what is right and wrong

Lawsuit Legal charges by people who say they were injured or hurt by another person

Malpractice Professionals, such as a nurse, doctor, or dentist, not doing something that they are responsible for so that the patient is hurt

Neglect Not giving food, clothing, personal care, or medical care and treatment

Negligence An action that harms a person because of someone not being careful

Nursing assistant registry Record of information about nursing assistants licensed or certified in a state

Omnibus Budget Reconciliation Act of 1987 (OBRA) Laws passed by Congress to improve the quality of care for nursing home residents

The Role of the Nursing Assistant

Nursing assistants are an important part of the nursing care team. Nursing assistants can have many different titles. Nurse's aide and certified nurse assistant are just two of the titles. As a nursing assistant, you will perform the tasks given to you by the nurse. After you finish your training program, you will be able to perform the following hands-on patient care procedures with supervision:

- Give basic daily care, including bathing, feeding, and dressing
- Take a person's temperature, pulse, respirations, and blood pressure
- Give range-of-motion exercises
- Measure height and weight
- Admit, transfer, and discharge patients
- Apply heat and cold treatments
- Collect specimens
- Assist with oxygen therapy
- Prepare a patient for surgery
- Care for a dying person
- Care for new mothers and their babies
- Lift and transfer patients

In the 1970s and 1980s only a few states had formal nursing aide training programs. Many people learned on-the-job.

In 1987 the federal government passed the **Omnibus Budget Reconciliation Act.** This law is called **OBRA.** The goal of the OBRA law is to improve the care given to nursing home residents. The law includes rules for the training and certification of nursing assistants. Since then, each state has developed training programs that follow these rules.

OBRA

State and Federal Laws That Affect Nursing Assistants

Each state has laws that control what RNs and LPNs/LVNs may and may not do in that state. To give patient care, a nurse must be licensed in the state in which the nurse works. The purpose of these laws is to protect the patient. Some of these laws also affect nursing assistants. Like a nurse, you must be certified or licensed in the state in which you are working as a nursing assistant.

The beginning of the chapter talked about the Omnibus Budget Reconciliation Act of 1987, or OBRA. Many states apply these same standards to nursing assistants working in other health care settings as well.

OBRA requires each state to have a nursing assistant training program. OBRA also established rules for nursing assistant training. These rules include:
- Length of the training program
- Material taught during the program
- Instructor qualifications
- Competency evaluation program
- Nursing assistant registry
- Ongoing in-service education

OBRA

Your instructor will share these guidelines with you during class. You will also learn about the laws that affect your work as a nursing assistant in your own state. It is important that you understand what you are learning and why. The OBRA requirements are discussed below.

Length of the Training Program

OBRA requires that a nursing assistant training program be at least 75 hours long. The nursing assistant must spend 16 of those hours giving nursing care to another person. A qualified RN or LPN/LVN must supervise the clinical training (Figure 2-1).

OBRA

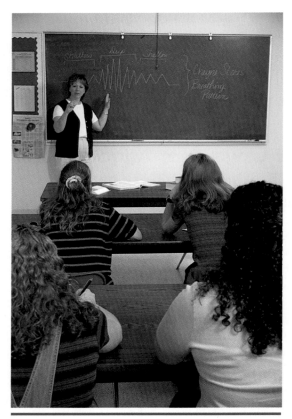

Figure **2-1   A,** Nursing assistant students in a classroom.

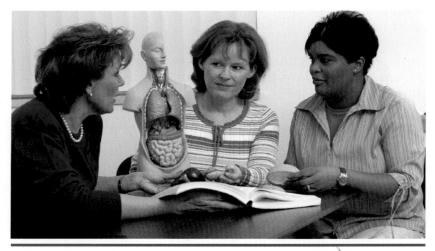

Figure **2-1   B,** Nursing assistant students practice skills in a lab setting.

Material Taught During the Program

The training program teaches basic nursing care. It must include:

- Communication
- Residents' rights
- Infection control
- Safety and emergency procedures
- Basic nursing skills
- Personal care skills, including skin care and dressing
- Feeding techniques
- Toileting procedures
- Turning, positioning, ambulation, and transfer techniques
- Range-of-motion exercises
- Signs and symptoms of common diseases and conditions
- Caring for patients who have problems with thinking and memory

OBRA

Many states have a training program that is longer than 75 hours. States may also require more supervised clinical practice. Your instructor will share with you the requirements of the state in which you are working.

Instructor Qualifications

Each state decides what qualifications nursing assistant instructors need. Your instructors will tell you about their education and experience.

Competency Evaluation

Competency evaluation of nursing assistant skills has two parts. You will take a written test and a skills test. You take both tests after completing the training program. Each state decides what the student must do to pass the tests.

The written test is usually multiple choice. During the skills portion of the test you will be asked to perform nursing care skills that you learned in your training program. Your instructor will tell you which skills will be tested during your competency evaluation exam. If you do not pass the exams, you can retest. OBRA allows three opportunities to pass both parts of the competency evaluation exams.

Some states use written and skills exams that the National Nurse Aide Assessment Program (NNAAP™) developed. You will fill out a test application. After you pick a test date, you will send in the application and the testing fee. Your instructor will help you through this process.

Figure 2-2 gives you an outline of the topics for the written and demonstration parts of the test.

NATIONAL NURSE AIDE ASSESSMENT PROGRAM (NNAAP™) WRITTEN EXAMINATION CONTENT OUTLINE

The NNAAP Written Examination is comprised of seventy (70) multiple choice questions. Ten (10) of these questions are pre-test (non-scored) questions on which statistical information will be collected.

I. Physical Care Skills

A. Activities of Daily Living . . . 7% of exam
  1. Hygiene
  2. Dressing and Grooming
  3. Nutrition and Hydration
  4. Elimination
  5. Rest/Sleep/Comfort
B. Basic Nursing Skills . . . . . . 37% of exam
  1. Infection Control
  2. Safety/Emergency
  3. Therapeutic/Technical Procedures
  4. Data Collection and Reporting
C. Restorative Skills . . . . 4% of exam
  1. Prevention
  2. Self Care/Independence

II. Psychosocial Care Skills

A. Emotional and Mental Health
  Needs. . . . . 10% of exam
B. Spiritual and Cultural
  Needs. . . . . 3% of exam

III. Role of the Nurse Aide

A. Communication. . . . . 10% of exam
B. Client Rights. . . . . 15% of exam
C. Legal and Ethical Behavior . . 3% of exam
D. Member of the Health Care
  Team . . . . 9% of exam

NATIONAL NURSE AIDE ASSESSMENT PROGRAM (NNAAP™) SKILLS EVALUATION†

List of Skills

1. Washes hands
2. Measures and records weight of ambulatory client
3. Provides mouth care
4. Dresses client with affected right arm
5. Transfers client from bed to wheelchair
6. Assists client to ambulate
7. Cleans and stores dentures
8. Performs passive range-of-motion on one shoulder
9. Performs passive range-of-motion on one knee and one ankle
10. Measures and records urinary output
11. Assists clients with use of bedpan
12. Provides perineal care for incontinent client
13. Provides catheter care
14. Takes and records oral temperature
15. Takes and records radial pulse and counts and records respirations
16. Takes and records client's blood pressure (one-step procedure)
17. Takes and records client's blood pressure (two-step procedure)
18. Puts one knee-high elastic stocking on client
19. Makes an occupied bed
20. Provides foot care
21. Provides fingernail care
22. Feeds client who cannot feed self
23. Positions client on side
24. Gives modified bed bath (face, and one arm, hand, and underarm)
25. Shampoos client's hair in bed

Reprinted with permission of the National Council of State Boards of Nursing, Chicago, Ill. Copyright © November, 2001 by Promissor, Inc. Reproduced from the candidate handbook and the Promissor Website Copyright, © 2002, with the permission of Promissor, Inc.
†All states do not participate in the program. Such states have other arrangements for nurse aide competency and evaluation program.
The NNAAP™ skills identified in this textbook may be evaluated in part, or in full, on the NNAAP™ Skills Evaluation. The above materials are not endorsed by Promissor, Inc.

Figure 2-2 National Nurse Aide Assessment Program (NNAAP™) Written Exam Content Outline and Skills Evaluation.

Nursing Assistant Registry

OBRA requires each state to have a **nursing assistant registry**. The registry is a record of everyone who is licensed or certified in that state. The registry includes the following information about each nursing assistant:

- Full name, including maiden name, married name, and other names used
- Home address
- Date of birth
- License/certificate registration number and expiration date
- Date competency evaluation taken and passed
- Last known employer, date of hire, and date employment ended
- Information about findings of abuse, neglect, or dishonest use of property

All of this information remains in the registry for at least 5 years. Registry information is a public record, and any agency can request to see it.

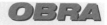

Ongoing In-Service Education

OBRA requires nursing care facilities to offer educational programs for nursing assistants on a regular basis.

This policy helps you to learn new information and skills so you will provide up-to-date care. While you are working, the nurse manager of your unit usually evaluates your job skills as a nursing assistant (Figure 2-3).

HOW & WHY

Nurse managers have watched you give patient care. They have also seen how well you work with others.

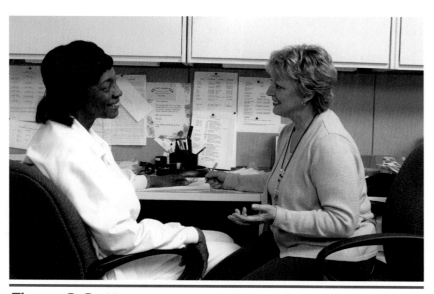

Figure 2-3 Nurse manager reviewing a performance evaluation with a nursing assistant.

If you have not worked as a nursing assistant for 2 years (24 months), OBRA requires you to re-take the competency evaluation before you give patient care again. Your state may also require you to complete more training. This makes sure that your skills and knowledge are current and competent.

Tasks You May and May Not Perform as a Nursing Assistant

In general, you will work under the supervision of an RN (Figure 2-4). In some states, LPNs/LVNs supervise nursing assistants. Your role is to provide direct care to patients as described in a patient care plan. Sometimes you will help a nurse to provide care. Other times you will provide care without the nurse in a patient's room. You must be familiar with the procedures and tasks your state laws allow you to perform as a nursing assistant. Before performing a task you should ask yourself:

1. Does the state law allow a nursing assistant to perform the procedure?
2. Is the procedure in my job description?
3. Have I been taught how to perform the procedure?
4. Is a nurse available for supervision and questions?

If the answer to any of these questions is "No," do not perform the procedure and discuss the situation with your supervising nurse.

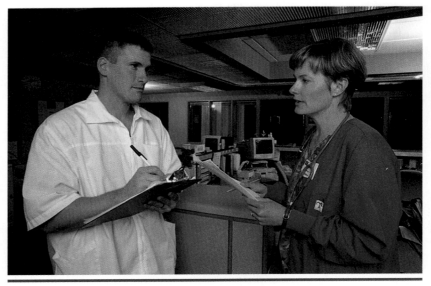

Figure 2-4 Nursing assistant receiving a patient care assignment from the charge nurse.

Job Descriptions

A job description will give you guidelines for what you are expected and able to do (Figure 2-5). When you apply for a job, ask for a copy of the job description for that position. Carefully review the tasks you will be expected to perform. Tell the employer about any tasks you have not been trained to do. Also, talk to the employer about any tasks that you are not comfortable performing because of moral or religious reasons.

Remember that before you take a job, and when you are on the job, no one can force you to perform a task that is not within the legal limits of what your state allows you to do. You cannot refuse to perform a task just because you do not like or want to do the task.

Once you accept a task, you are responsible for doing the task safely and correctly. The licensed nurse is also responsible for supervising the care you provide.

POSITION DESCRIPTION/PERFORMANCE EVALUATION

Job Title:　Certified Nursing Assistant (CNA),　　　　Supervised by: Licensed Nurse
　　　　　　Skilled Nursing Facility

Prepared by: _____　Date: _____　Approved by: _____　Date: _____

Job Summary: Provides direct and indirect resident care activities under the direction of an RN or LPN/LVN. Assists residents with activities of daily living, provides for personal care and comfort, and assists in the maintenance of a safe and clean environment for an assigned group of residents.

DUTIES AND RESPONSIBILITIES:

E=Exceeds the Standard　　M=Meets the Standard　　NI=Needs Improvement

Demonstrates Competency in the Following Areas:	E	M	NI
Assists in the preparation for admission of residents.	2	1	0
Assists in and accompanies residents in the admission, transfer, and discharge procedures.	2	1	0
Provides morning care, which may include bed bath, shower or whirlpool, oral hygiene, combing hair, back care, dressing residents, changing bed linen, cleaning overbed table and bedside stand, straightening room, and other general care as necessary throughout the day.	2	1	0
Provides evening care, which includes hands/face washing as needed, oral hygiene, back rubs, peri-care, freshening linen, cleaning overbed tables, straightening room, and other general care as needed.	2	1	0
Notifies appropriate licensed personnel when resident complains of pain.	2	1	0

Figure 2-5　Certified nursing assistant job description and performance evaluation form.　　　　　　　　　　　　　　　　　　　　　　　　*Continued*

POSITION DESCRIPTION/PERFORMANCE EVALUATION—cont'd

Provides post-mortem care and assists in transporting bodies to the morgue.	2	1	0
Assists nurses in treatment procedures.	2	1	0
Provides general nursing care such as positioning residents, lifting and turning residents, applying/utilizing special equipment, assisting in use of bedpan or commode, and ambulating the residents.	2	1	0
Performs all aspects of resident care in an environment that optimizes resident safety and reduces the likelihood of medical/health care errors.	2	1	0
Takes and records temperature, pulse, respiration, weight, blood pressure, and intake-output.	2	1	0
Makes rounds with outgoing shift. Knows whereabouts of assigned residents.	2	1	0
Makes rounds with oncoming shift to ensure the unit is left in good condition.	2	1	0
Adheres to policies and procedures of the facility and the Department of Nursing.	2	1	0
Participates in socialization activities on the unit.	2	1	0
Turns and positions residents as ordered and/or as needed, making sure no rough surfaces are in direct contact with the body. Lifts and turns with proper and safe body mechanics and with available resources.	2	1	0
Checks for reddened areas or skin breakdown and reports to RN or LPN/LVN.	2	1	0
Ensures residents are dressed properly and assists, as necessary. Ensures that clothing is properly stored in bedside stand or on hangers in closet. Ensures that all residents are clean and dry at all times.	2	1	0
Checks unit for adequate linen. Cleans linen cart. Provides clean linen and clothing. Makes beds.	2	1	0
Treats residents and their families with respect and dignity.	2	1	0
Accompanies residents to appointments as directed.	2	1	0
Follows center policies and procedures when caring for persons who are restrained.	2	1	0
Provides reality orientation in daily care.	2	1	0
Prepares residents for meals. Serves and removes food trays. Assists with meals or feeds residents, if necessary.	2	1	0
Distributes drinking water and other nourishments to residents.	2	1	0
Performs general care activities for residents in isolation.	2	1	0
Answers residents' signal lights promptly. Anticipates residents' needs, and makes rounds to assigned residents.	2	1	0
Assists residents with handling and care of clothing and other personal property (including dentures, glasses, contact lenses, hearing aids, and prosthetic devices).	2	1	0
Transports residents to and from various departments, as requested.	2	1	0
Reports and, when appropriate, records any changes observed in condition or behavior of residents and unusual incidents.	2	1	0
Participates in and contributes to Resident Care Conferences.	2	1	0
Follows directions, both oral and written, and works cooperatively with other staff members.	2	1	0
Establishes and maintains interpersonal relationships with residents, family members, and other facility personnel while assuring confidentiality of resident information.	2	1	0
Must have the ability to acquire knowledge of and develop skills in basic nursing procedures and simple charting.	2	1	0
Attends inservice education programs, as assigned, to learn new treatments, procedures, skills, etc.	2	1	0
Maintains personal health in order to prevent absence from work due to health problems.	2	1	0

Figure 2-5, cont'd Certified nursing assistant job description and performance evaluation form.

POSITION DESCRIPTION/PERFORMANCE EVALUATION—cont'd

Professional Requirements:	E	M	NI
Meets dress code standards. Appearance is neat and clean.	2	1	0
Completes annual education requirements.	2	1	0
Maintains regulatory requirements.	2	1	0
Meets center's standards for attendance.	2	1	0
Consistently completes and maintains assigned duties.	2	1	0
Wears identification while on duty.	2	1	0
Practices careful, efficient, and nonwasteful use of supplies and linen. Follows established charge procedure for resident charge items.	2	1	0
Attends annual review and department inservices, as scheduled.	2	1	0
Attends at least 75% of staff meetings. Reads and returns all monthly staff meeting minutes.	2	1	0
Represents the organization in a positive and professional manner.	2	1	0
Actively participates in the Continuous Quality Improvement (CQI) activities.	2	1	0
Complies with all organizational policies regarding ethical business practices.	2	1	0
Communicates the mission, ethics, and goals of the facility, as well as the focus statement of the department.	2	1	0
Possesses a genuine interest and concern for older and disabled persons.	2	1	0
TOTAL POINTS	___	___	___

Regulatory Requirements:

- High School graduate or equivalent

- Current Certified Nursing Assistant (CNA) certification in State of _____ for Long-Term Care Facilities

- Current Basic Cardiac Life Support for Healthcare Providers certification within three (3) months of hire date

Language Skills:

- Ability to read and communicate effectively in English

- Additional languages preferred

Skills:

- Basic computer knowledge

Physical Demands:

- For physical demands of position, including vision, hearing, repetitive motion, and environment, see following description

  Reasonable accommodations may be made to enable individuals with disabilities to perform the essential functions of the position without compromising care.

I have received, read, and understand the Position Description/Performance Evaluation above.

_____   _____
Name/Signature   Date Signed

Figure 2-5, cont'd   Certified nursing assistant job description and performance evaluation form.

Qualities of a Professional Caregiver

As a nursing assistant, patients, families, employers and co-workers think of you as a professional. During your training program you will learn patient care skills, and you will also learn how to talk to patients, their families, and other health care team members.

What does being "professional" look like and sound like? Professional behavior means your appearance, habits, and behavior in the workplace. These are skills that you can learn and practice every day when you give patient care and work with other team members. Soon these skills and habits become part of who you are. Professional behavior also helps patients and their families feel less stress and worry less.

Table 2-1 identifies behaviors and skills that a professional demonstrates.

Table 2-1

PROFESSIONAL BEHAVIORS AND SKILLS	
Category	**Behavior, skill, or habit**
Personal health, hygiene, and appearance	• Practice habits that promote good physical and mental health—healthy diet; enough exercise, rest, and sleep; avoiding use of illegal and unhealthy substances such as drugs or alcohol; stress management and relaxation. • Bathe regularly; avoid use of strong scents; keep hair, nails, and clothing neat and clean. • Dress and wear jewelry appropriate for the setting. Most facilities have dress codes for employees (Figure 2-6, *A*).

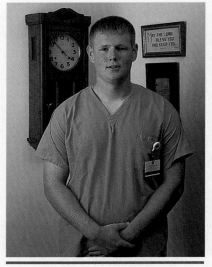

***Figure* 2-6** **A,** The nursing assistant is well groomed.

Continued

Table 2-1, cont'd

PROFESSIONAL BEHAVIORS AND SKILLS	
Category	Behavior, skill, or habit

Attendance
- Maintain regular attendance and be on time (Figure 2-6, *B*).

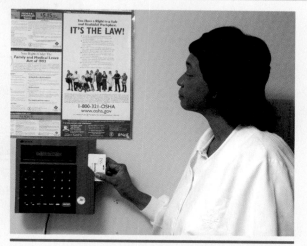

Figure 2-6 **B,** The nursing assistant arrives at work on time and clocks in.

Work habits
- Plan, organize, and complete assigned tasks on time, following standards of safety and quality.
- Follow personal health and safety practices—for example, use of good body mechanics.
- Take the initiative to identify and complete tasks that need to be done; show enthusiasm and interest in your work.
- Take responsibility for your decisions and actions; be honest.
- Practice good communication skills with patients, families, and team members.
- Show respect for patients, families, and co-workers by showing care, concern, and courtesy (Figure 2-6, *C*).

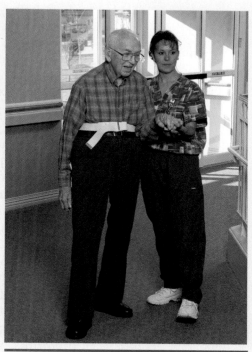

Figure 2-6 **C,** Nursing assistants are pleasant and show respect for their patients.

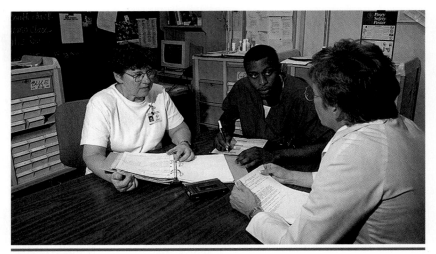

Figure 2-7   Good communication skills help the team to work together more efficiently.

As a nursing assistant, you will work with people who may have different life-styles, experiences, values, and ways of behaving than your own. Good teamwork and communication skills help you to "tune in" and be sensitive to other people's needs. This helps create a positive work and care environment (Figure 2-7).

Skills that demonstrate good teamwork and communication include:

- Work well with others
- Showing respect and flexibility in team situations
- Identifying and using strengths of each team member to give quality patient care
- Using problem-solving skills
- Recognizing and respecting personal and cultural differences
- Speaking clearly; listening attentively
- Giving and receiving feedback in a positive manner

The next chapter will discuss more features of good communication skills.

When you become a nursing assistant, you become a lifelong learner. You have a responsibility to yourself, your patients, and employers to keep your skills and knowledge up-to-date. You can keep your skills current by attending continuing education programs. Your employer will give you information about programs you should attend. You can also read nursing magazines, look up information on the Internet, and learn new skills from other health care team members (Figure 2-8, *A*). Some states re-

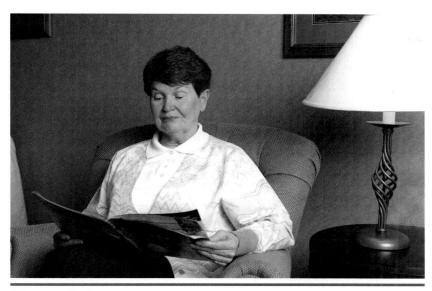

Figure 2-8 **A,** Nursing assistants keep their skills and knowledge up-to-date. Nursing assistant reading a professional journal.

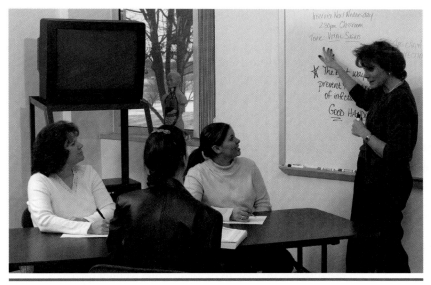

Figure 2-8 **B,** Nursing assistants attending a continuing education program/in-service.

quire health care professionals to attend a certain number of continuing education programs to keep their certificates active (Figure 2-8, *B*). Federal regulations require that all certified nursing assistants attend at least 12 hours of in-service training each year.

Ethical and Legal Aspects of Caring for Others

Ethics are formed by a person's values, beliefs, and morals. A person's experiences, culture, family, and spiritual beliefs help form the person's values. In health care, ethics deals with what is "right" and "wrong" when planning and giving care.

Ethical conduct and behavior includes:
- Respect for each person as an individual
- Caring for others without prejudice or bias
- Avoiding judging others by your own values and standards
- Not performing any task or procedure for which you have not been trained or that is not allowed in your state
- Keeping patient information confidential

There are legal aspects to think about when giving care. Laws are rules created by federal, state, and local governments. Health care–related laws are made to protect people from harm. If people feel that a health care provider has injured them, they can file a **lawsuit** against the provider. Two common types of lawsuits filed against health care providers are **negligence** and **malpractice** suits. The term *negligence* is used to describe an action that harmed a person because someone was not being careful. The term *malpractice* refers to a negligent act by a professional, such as a nurse, doctor, or dentist. Negligence and malpractice are considered unintentional, which means that the caregiver did not harm the patient on purpose.

Table 2-2 gives examples of negligence and malpractice that could occur in a health care setting.

Table 2-2

EXAMPLES OF NEGLIGENCE AND MALPRACTICE		
	Action	**Example**
Negligence	• A caregiver did not mean to cause harm or injury. • The caregiver did not act in a reasonable and careful manner, and a person was injured.	• A caregiver leaves a side rail down on a bed where a patient is recovering from general anesthesia. The patient then falls out of bed and breaks a hip. • A caregiver does not answer a signal light in a timely manner. The patient tries to get out of bed without help and falls, breaking an arm. • A caregiver is cleaning a patient's glasses. The caregiver drops the glasses, and they break. • A postoperative patient who just had the spleen removed complains of severe abdominal pain and cramping. The caregiver does not report the symptoms to the nurse. The patient goes into shock and then dies.
Malpractice	• Malpractice is negligence by professionals, such as nurses, doctors, and dentists.	• A patient is given a drug to which the patient is known to be allergic. The patient goes into shock and dies.

Sometimes a caregiver does something on purpose to harm a person or a person's property. Examples of intentional acts that can occur in a health care setting are described in Table 2-3.

How can you protect yourself and your patients? How can you guard their privacy and rights? How can you prevent injury and harm? These guidelines will help you provide safe, respectful care:

- Perform only tasks and procedures that you are trained to do.
- Perform only tasks that are in your job description and within the legal limits of practice.
- Remember that even though a nurse is your supervisor, you are responsible for your own actions when providing patient care.
- You have a duty to question any task you are worried about performing.
- Keep all patient information confidential.
- Discuss patient care only with your supervising nurse.

Table 2-3

EXAMPLES OF INTENTIONAL HARMFUL ACTS

	Description	Example
Assault	Intentionally trying to or threatening to touch a person without the person's permission	• Threatening to restrain an uncooperative patient
Battery	Touching a person's body without the person's permission	• Performing a procedure, such as taking a blood pressure, without the patient's permission
False imprisonment	Threat of and/or unlawful restriction of a person's freedom of movement	• Leaving a helpless patient in a room with the door closed and no signal light within reach
Fraud	Saying or doing something to deceive, trick, or fool another person	• Nursing assistants telling a patient they are a nurse
Invasion of privacy	Making public a person's name, photograph, or private business without the person's **consent**	• Opening and reading a patient's mail without the patient's consent • Telling a patient's roommate or visitor the patient's medical information without the patient's consent
Libel	Writing false statements about a person	• Writing something about a patient in the patient's medical record that is not true
Slander	Saying false statements about a person	• Telling an untrue statement about a patient to another person

Abuse and Neglect

Abuse and neglect are legal considerations with which you must be familiar. **Abuse** is hurting a person physically, emotionally, or financially. Abuse is a crime. The law requires health care providers to report abuse or neglect. **Neglect** involves not giving a person food, clothing, personal care, or needed medical care and treatment. Abused or neglected individuals are often ill, weak, old, or dependent. Caregivers or family members sometimes abuse children or elderly persons. All patients, including those who are unconscious or in a coma, must be protected from abuse.

Table 2-4 describes the different types of abuse and neglect.

Signs and symptoms of abuse or neglect may be visible or difficult to identify. Any time you see possible signs and symptoms of abuse or neglect, report your observations to your charge nurse. If you are worried about the safety and well-being of your patient, report and discuss your concerns immediately with your supervising nurse. Your supervising nurse will then follow up with a report to a state agency. Some states require that anyone who witnesses abuse or neglect report it to the state agency. It is important for you to know the rules in your state. Your instructor will talk to you about the regulations in your state and how to report your observations.

Signs and symptoms of abuse may include:

- The person and/or the person's clothing are dirty and unkempt.
- The person has lost weight and/or is dehydrated.

Table 2-4

TYPES OF ABUSE AND NEGLECT	
Type of abuse	**Description**
Physical abuse	• Includes hitting, kicking, striking, or beating a person.
Physical neglect	• Includes not giving a person care or things to meet basic needs. Examples of physical neglect in a health care setting include not answering a signal light or not cleaning a patient who has been incontinent of urine or stool in a timely way.
Verbal abuse	• Use of verbal or written words or gestures to criticize another person.
Financial abuse	• Using a person's money or belongings without the person's consent.
Involuntary seclusion	• Confining and isolating a person to a certain area or room.
Emotional abuse	• Making someone feel ashamed and stupid, or threatening someone again and again with physical harm, or taking away something a person needs.
Emotional neglect	• Not giving attention and affection to a person.
Sexual abuse	• Attacking, or threatening to attack a person sexually.

- Medications are not given properly, or the person is over-medicated.
- The person has many injuries that are hard to explain.
- The person has many visits to the emergency department.
- The person has unexplained fractures or broken bones.
- The person has new and old bruises.
- The person has unexplained marks on the body such as welts, bite marks, or burns.
- The person is nervous and upset, afraid, anxious, or very quiet and refuses to talk or answer questions.
- The person lives in dirty, unsafe living conditions.
- The person is kept alone in a small space for long periods of time.
- Caregivers do not allow the patient to have a private conversation with another person.
- The person may not have a doctor or may see many doctors.
- The person has bleeding or bruising of the genitals.
- The person has blood or stains on underwear.

Dealing with abuse and neglect issues may be one of the more difficult situations you have as a nursing assistant. Timely reporting of your concerns can be lifesaving. Your supervising nurse can offer support as you work together to make decisions to do something about these difficult issues.

CHAPTER REVIEW

1. List 5 patient care procedures you will be able to perform when you finish the nursing assistant training program.

2. What are main parts of the OBRA laws?

3. What is the nursing assistant registry?

4. List 5 signs or symptoms of abuse.

5. What should you do if you think that someone has abused or neglected your patient?

Circle the one BEST response.

6. What was the goal behind the laws passed in the Omnibus Budget Reconciliation Act of 1987 (OBRA)?
   a. Regulating medical care provided by doctors
   b. Regulating care provided by physical and occupational therapists
   c. Improving quality of care for nursing home residents
   d. Improving quality of care for hospitalized intensive care patients

7. When should you refuse to perform a task that an RN has assigned to you?
   a. When you are not allowed to perform the task by state law
   b. When you have not been trained how to perform the task
   c. When the task is not in your job description
   d. All of the above

8. Which of these is an example of professional behavior?
   a. Arriving at work when you feel like it
   b. Arriving at work on time
   c. Wearing the same dirty scrubs you have worn for the past 2 days
   d. Applying your favorite, strong-smelling cologne just before arriving at your workplace

9. Which of these behaviors demonstrates professional work habits?
   a. Sharing confidential patient information with friends and family
   b. Carrying out assigned tasks on time
   c. Ignoring patient and family concerns
   d. Blaming co-workers for tasks that were not completed during your shift

CHAPTER REVIEW

10. Which of these actions is an example of good teamwork?
- a. Respecting others' personal and cultural differences
- b. Refusing to work with other members of the team that you do not like
- c. Turning away when a co-worker offers you feedback about the care you are providing
- d. All of the above

11. How can you keep your skills and knowledge up-to-date?
- a. Read nursing magazines
- b. Research current topics on the Internet
- c. Attend continuing education programs
- d. All of the above

12. Which of the following is an example of ethical conduct and behavior?
- a. Judge others by your own values and standards.
- b. Share confidential patient information with others.
- c. Do any task or procedure you feel you can perform.
- d. Respect each person as an individual.

13. Which is an example of negligence by a nursing assistant?
- a. Dropping and breaking a patient's glasses while cleaning them
- b. Making sure both side rails are raised on the bed of a patient who is recovering from anesthesia
- c. Placing a signal light near the person after personal care is completed
- d. None of the above

14. Which is an example of slander?
- a. Reporting a patient's behavior to the charge nurse
- b. Making false statements about a person verbally
- c. Sharing a person's medical information with a visitor
- d. All of the above

15. What is abuse?
- a. Physical, emotional, or financial harm
- b. Withholding food, clothing, personal care, and necessary medical care and treatment
- c. Both of the above
- d. None of the above

Answers are on pages 703 to 704.

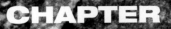

Communication

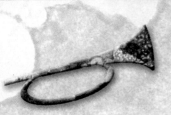

What you will learn

- How to use verbal and nonverbal communication
- Active listening skills
- How to deal with conflict and harassment
- Confidentiality rules
- How to use the care plan
- Charting in health care
- How to observe and report information
- How to record patient information
- Correct use of medical terms and abbreviations

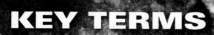

KEY TERMS

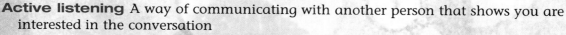

Active listening A way of communicating with another person that shows you are interested in the conversation

Care plan The directions for the care needed by a patient

Communication Sending and receiving information between two or more people

Confidential Keeping patient information private

Conflict A disagreement or a difference of opinions

Goal Outcome or result that a patient and the patient's caregivers want

Harassment Action, statement, or behavior that offends another person

Health Insurance Portability and Accountability Act of 1996 (HIPAA) A law that protects people who might suffer discrimination in health coverage based on a factor that relates to a person's health

Medical record (chart) Written record containing medical information about a patient

Minimum data set (MDS) Patient assessment and screening tool used in long-term care. Required by the Omnibus Budget Reconciliation Act of 1987 (OBRA)

Nonverbal communication Type of communication that uses gestures, posture, facial expressions, and eye contact

Nursing process The process of getting information, identifying problems, planning care, giving care, and evaluating the care given

Objective information Observations you make about things that you can see, hear, feel, or smell

Observation Information you obtain by using your eyes, ears, nose, and sense of touch

Report Process by which patient information and care needs are given to the nurse or the next shift of caregivers

Resident assessment protocols (RAPs) Guidelines that help nurses develop a care plan for a long-term care resident. Required by OBRA

Subjective information (symptoms) Information patients tell you about how they feel

Verbal communication Type of communication that uses words, tone of voice, and rate of speech

OBRA

Verbal and Nonverbal Communication

Communication is sending and receiving information between two or more people (Figure 3-1). In health care you will use verbal and written communication. Communicating with patients, families, and health care team members is an important skill.

Verbal communication uses words to send a message. Choose words carefully so that other people understand what you are trying to tell them.

The words you use and your tone of voice affect the meaning of what you say. To understand how this works, try this exercise. Work with a partner, and take turns saying the simple statement "That sounds like fun." Change your tone of voice each time you say the sentence. Ask your partner if the meaning of the sentence changed based on how you said the words.

The OBRA guidelines require that long-term care centers permit residents to communicate in a language they understand. This may mean that a family member or an interpreter will help you to communicate with a resident who does not speak or understand English.

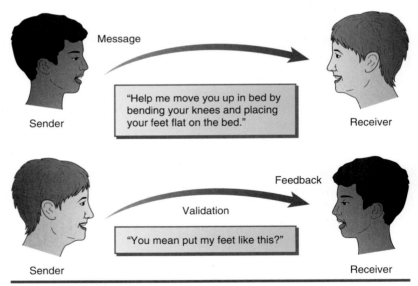

Figure **3-1**   Communication is sending and receiving information.

Another kind of communication is **nonverbal communication**. Nonverbal communication includes gestures, posture, facial expression, and eye contact to send a message (Figure 3-2). If the nonverbal and verbal communication "match," the person will believe what you are saying. If the cues do not match, the person may not believe that what you are saying is true.

Try this exercise to see the power of nonverbal communication. Again, work with a partner, and take turns saying the statement "This sounds like fun." This time, use different gestures, posture, and facial expression each time you say the statement. Ask your partner if the meaning of the sentence changed based on your nonverbal communication.

Table 3-1 outlines tips that will help you build good communication skills that you can use with patients, families, and team members.

NOTES ON
☯ Culture

Certain verbal or nonverbal cues may be considered impolite by some cultures. Speaking too loudly, standing close to the other person, looking the person in the eye, or pointing may offend some people.

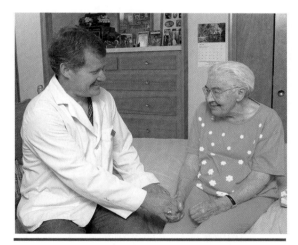

Figure 3-2 Nonverbal communication shows that the nursing assistant is interested in the patient and what she is saying.

Table 3-1

TIPS FOR EFFECTIVE VERBAL AND NONVERBAL COMMUNICATION	
Type of communication	Example
Verbal Communication	
Word choice	• Use terms that patients and families can easily understand. • Do not use too many medical terms.
Tone of voice	• Use a pleasant, friendly, interested tone. • Do not use words such as "Honey" or "Dear." • Do not sound bored or sarcastic.
Rate of speech	• Speak at a moderate pace. • Avoid very fast or very slow speeds. • Speak clearly.
Nonverbal Communication	
Gestures	• Use hand gestures and movements of arms and legs to send your message. • Do not use excessive movements, which can be confusing.
Posture	• Face a person, look at a person, and lean forward a little to show interest in a conversation. • Do not use gestures that show a lack of interest, such as crossing your arms, looking away from a person, turning away from a person, or standing far away from the person.
Eye contact	• Make eye contact with a person during the conversation; this shows interest. • Do not look at other objects or look beyond or beside a person. This shows a lack of interest.
Facial expression	• Smiling shows interest in a conversation. • Do not frown, look bored, or have a neutral expression. This shows a lack of interest.

HOW&*WHY*

Effective communication = Verbal messages + nonverbal messages + active listening

Listening Skills

Listening is another important part of communication. What is the purpose of talking to people if we do not listen to their answer? We need to listen in order for communication to take place. **Active listening** shows the speaker that you are interested in the conversation. Active listening also uses both verbal and nonverbal messages (Figure 3-3). Table 3-2 gives examples of active listening techniques.

Even the person with good communication skills will sometimes have a hard time getting a message across. If you have questions about communicating with a person of a different culture or age-group than your own, your charge nurse can give you suggestions.

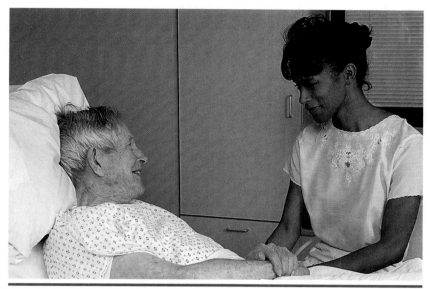

Figure 3-3   Active listening shows the other person that you are interested.

Table 3-2

EFFECTIVE ACTIVE LISTENING TECHNIQUES	
Type of communication	Example
Verbal Techniques	
Clarifying a statement	"Can you tell me again. . . . ?" "Can you tell me more about. . . . ?"
Restating	"So, you're telling me that. . . ." "So, what you are saying is. . . ."
Nonverbal Techniques	
Gestures	Using hand gestures, drawings, or pictures to clarify communication.
Posture	Leaning forward slightly and facing a person shows interest in the conversation.
Eye contact	Looking at the person shows interest.
Facial expression	Smiling and having an interested expression on your face shows interest.

Dealing With Conflict

Conflict is a disagreement or a difference of opinions (Figure 3-4). Conflict is all around us. Conflict occurs at home and in the workplace. Causes of conflict involve two people having different ideas, values, or beliefs about a situation or event. Examples of conflicts that happen in a work setting include differences of opinion over work schedules or how patient care should be managed. The most important thing to learn is to identify the conflict and find a way to resolve the situation in a positive, professional manner. Using good communication skills shows that you have a sincere desire to work through a problem. Other tips for helping resolve conflict in a positive way are listed in Box 3-1.

Harassment is an action, statement, or behavior that upsets or offends another person. Harassment can be verbal, physical, or sexual. Verbal harassment includes saying things about a person's age, ethnic background, spiritual beliefs, gender, or disability that will make the person upset or angry. Even if you are joking with your co-workers, a comment you make might make them upset. It is important that you think about what you are saying and think about how other people will feel about what you say. Physical harassment includes touching another person without the person's permission. Sexual harassment ranges from making offensive statements about a person's sexuality or gender to sexual touching or sexual acts. **Harassment in the workplace is illegal** (Figure 3-5).

A first step in dealing with harassment is to ask the other person to stop the offending behavior. For example, co-workers are

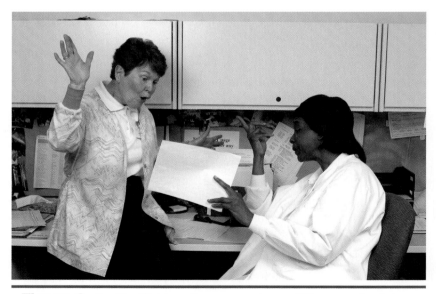

Figure 3-4 Conflict is a disagreement or a difference of opinions.

telling a joke about people of different ethnic backgrounds. They may not think that the joke is offensive, but you do and ask them to stop telling the joke. They should respect your request to stop. If the individuals do not stop the behavior, leave the area. If the individuals repeat or continue harassing behaviors, tell your supervising nurse immediately. The nurse will follow through with the steps outlined in your facility's policy for handling harassment issues.

Another way to prevent harassment is by being a role model yourself. Treat all patients, families, and co-workers with dignity and respect—both in what you say and what you do.

Box 3-1

GUIDELINES FOR POSITIVE CONFLICT RESOLUTION

- Approach the person with whom you have a conflict in a positive, calm, polite manner. Ask to speak with the person privately. Explain the situation as factually as possible.
- If you need additional support or feedback, ask to speak with your supervising nurse privately and explain the situation.
- When explaining the problem, focus on the facts. Avoid talking about feelings and emotions.
- Be open to the other person's ideas and suggestions when working toward a solution.
- Discuss and agree on a solution that is agreeable to both people involved.
- Thank the person for listening and helping to solve the problem.

HOW&*WHY*
Conflict resolution tip: Focus on the problem, not the person.

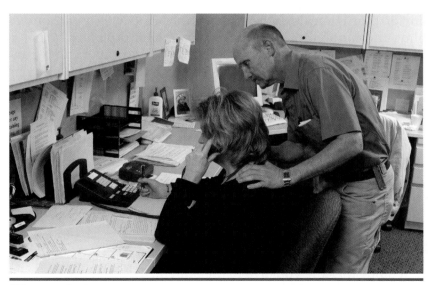

***Figure* 3-5** Harassment is an action, statement, or behavior that upsets or offends another person. Harassment in the workplace is illegal.

Box 3-2

SAFEGUARDS FOR MAINTAINING CONFIDENTIALITY

- Discuss patient information only with health care team members directly involved in the patient's care.
- Never talk with other patients, co-workers, families, visitors, or your own friends and family about a patient's care.
- Never talk about a patient or a patient's care in public areas such as the cafeteria.
- Do not listen to others' conversations about a patient.
- Do not take written patient records or charts away from the nursing station area.
- Close written records or charts containing patient information when you are not reading them.

Confidentiality

Information about a patient's health, medical conditions, and treatment is confidential. The term **confidential** means to keep information private. In health care settings, the people directly involved in the patient's care share information about a patient. In fact, patients have a legal right to have their health care information kept private.

OBRA guarantees that residents of a long-term care center have a right to have their information kept confidential.

The **Health Insurance Portability and Accountability Act of 1996 (HIPAA)** was signed into law on August 21, 1996. This law protects millions of working Americans and their families who might suffer discrimination in health coverage based on a factor that relates to a person's health. HIPPA also guarantees that information in a medical record is kept private.

How can you make sure that patient information stays confidential and private? Follow the safeguards in Box 3-2 in your daily work and communication with others to avoid violating confidentiality.

All health care providers work hard to keep information about patients private and confidential. Violating confidentiality of patient information is a reason for termination of employment by many employers.

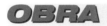

NOTES ON
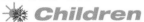 **Children**

When caring for minor children (under the age of 18), the parent has the right to information about the child and makes the decisions for the child.

NOTES ON
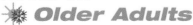 **Older Adults**

In some situations an adult child, spouse, or legal representative will have written permission to obtain information about the patient and to make decisions for the elderly person.

Using the Care Plan

As a member of the nursing care team, the nursing care plan will guide the care you give to the patient. The **care plan** is simply the directions for the care a patient needs. When a patient is admitted to a facility, information about the patient's condition is gathered. The charge nurse usually talks to the patient and asks a series of questions to help the nurse decide what kind of care the patient needs. The nurse may ask you to help get part of this information by taking the patient's vital signs, height, and weight. After the nurse has gotten all of the information needed, the nurse will identify the patient's most important problems, called a nursing diagnosis (Appendix B, p. 675). After a nursing diagnosis is identified, the nurse will develop a plan to help the patient reach the patient's goal.

A goal is the result that patients and their caregivers can work toward. A goal helps the patient work toward their highest level of function, independence, or rehabilitation possible.

Many different team members provide the care in the care plan. For example, the dietary department provides high-protein shakes for a patient who has a problem with wound healing. The physical therapist provides help with walking and a walker for the patient who is recovering from hip surgery. As the care is provided, members of the team shares their thoughts and observations about the way the patient is responding. It is important to know if the care is helping the patient to get better or if the patient is getting worse. Periodically the team comes together and discusses the care plan and makes changes. This process of gathering information, identifying problems, planning care, giving care, and evaluating the care given is called the **nursing process.**

Nurses use the nursing process to plan and give care for patients of all ages in all types of health care settings. Because you spend more time with your patients than any other member of the health care team, your input into the care plan is very important. In some health care settings the care plan is called a clinical pathway or a critical pathway. The purpose of a clinical or critical pathway is the same as the care plan, to help the patient to reach his goals.

OBRA requires long-term care centers to use interdisciplinary care planning (ICP). The ICP is a care planning conference that includes team members from areas outside of nursing such as dietary, therapy, and pharmacy.   **OBRA**

Figure 3-6 shows part of a sample nursing care plan.

As a nursing assistant, you would be involved in most of the nursing actions this patient needs to help avoid skin breakdown. When the patient is discharged, the nurse indicates on the care plan that the goal has been achieved—that is, the patient's skin remained intact throughout his hospitalization.

As a nursing assistant and nursing team member, your care and observations are very important in helping to reach the goals listed in the care plan.

Problem (Nursing Diagnosis)	Goal	Nursing Actions
Risk for skin breakdown/ Impaired skin integrity	Patient's skin will remain intact throughout hospital stay.	• Turn and reposition patient every 2 hours • Check skin, especially over bony prominences, when turning and repositioning patient; report any redness, skin color changes, or blistered or open areas immediately to nurse • Use pressure relief mattress • Use pillows and other devices to prevent pressure on bony prominences • Promptly cleanse patient's skin following episodes of incontinence • Use draw sheet and overbed trapeze to decrease shearing and friction when turning and repositioning patient • Apply lotion to dry skin and over bony prominences as needed

Figure **3-6**   Part of a sample nursing care plan.

Charting in Health Care

Medical information about patients, their health problems, and their care are contained in a **medical record.** The medical record is also called a **chart.** A medical record is a legal document and is kept and stored for a number of years after it is completed. There are many different parts of a medical record. A medical record may include:

- Admission sheet
- Medical history and physical exam
- Doctors' orders
- Doctors' progress notes
- Consultation reports
- Surgery and anesthesia reports
- Nursing assessment and history
- Multidisciplinary progress notes (for nursing and other health care team members)
- Graphic record for height, weight, and vital signs
- Medication record
- Intravenous (IV) therapy record
- Respiratory therapy record
- Radiology (x-ray) reports
- Lab reports

- Other reports (for example, physical therapy, occupational therapy, speech pathology)
- Advance directives forms
- Consent forms

The forms contained in a patient's medical record depend on the type of care the facility gives. Each page of the patient's medical record is usually stamped with identifying information about that patient. Facilities have written policies and guidelines about how to complete forms. Remember that all patient information is private and confidential and that only caregivers directly involved in a patient's care can see the patient's medical record.

Following are brief descriptions and examples of the medical record documents that you will read and use most frequently.

Admission Sheet

This form is completed when a patient is admitted to a facility. It contains the information about a patient's birth date, address, religion, insurance and employment information, emergency contacts, medical diagnoses, doctor information, and date and time of admission. The first section of Figure 3-7 shows an example of an admission sheet.

Nursing Assessment and History

An RN or LPN/LVN completes this form when a patient is admitted to a facility. The nurse may ask you to get some of the information, such as vital signs. The nursing assessment is used to help identify patient problems and develop the nursing care plan. Review this information to help you learn more about your patient. Figure 3-8 provides an example of a nursing assessment and history used in a hospital setting.

Multidisciplinary Progress Notes

This is a form used by health care team members other than doctors to record patient response to care measures, patient progress toward goals, new assessment information, and updated plans for care. Depending on your facility guidelines, you may or may not document observations about the care you provided in these progress notes. Figure 3-9 is an example of a multidisciplinary progress note.

OBRA requires that summaries of care be written at least every 3 months.

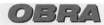

Text continued on p. 50

ADMISSION RESIDENT ASSESSMENT

ADMISSION NOTE: _____

Date of admission: _____ Time: _____ Transported by: _____ Accompanied by: _____

1st Day: T _____ P _____ R _____ B/P _____ Age _____ Sex _____

2nd Day: T _____ P _____ (Reg. _____ Irreg. _____) R _____ B/P _____ Weight _____ Height ___ Ft. __ In.

Orders verified by physician: ☐ Yes ☐ No   Time: _____ am/pm Date: _____

Diagnoses: _____

_____ Resident aware of Dx: ☐ Yes ☐ No

Date of last chest x-ray or PPD _____ Results for TB: Pos. _____ Neg. _____ Unknown _____

ALLERGIES: Medications _____

Food _____ Other _____

SKIN CONDITION: Indicate below all body marks such as old or recent scars (surgical and other), bruises, discolorations, abrasions, pressure ulcers or any questionable markings. Indicate size, depth (in cms), color and drainage.

RIGHT   LEFT   LEFT   RIGHT

DESCRIPTION:

_____
_____
_____
_____
_____

SPECIAL TREATMENTS & PROCEDURES:

_____
_____
_____
_____
_____

CURRENT STATUS

1. GENERAL SKIN CONDITION: Ashen ☐ Cold ☐ Cyanotic ☐ Dry ☐ Jaundiced ☐ Moist ☐ Oily ☐ Pale ☐ Reddened ☐
Warm ☐   Edema ☐ Site of Edema _____ Pedal pulses present LT _____   RT _____

2. PHYSICAL STATUS: (Describe)
 a. Paralysis/paresis-site _____
 b. Contracture(s)-site _____
 c. Fracture-site _____
 d. Brace _____ Splint _____ Cast _____ Immobilizer _____

3. FUNCTIONAL STATUS:
 a. Transfers-able to transfer
  ☐ Independently
  ☐ 1 person assist
  ☐ 2 person assist
  ☐ Total assist
 b. Ambulation able to ambulate
  ☐ Independently
  ☐ 1 person assist
  ☐ 2 person assist
  ☐ With device
   Type _____
  ☐ Wheel Chair only
  ☐ Wheel Chair/propels self
  ☐ Bedrest

 c. Weight bearing - able to bear
  ☐ Full weight
  ☐ Partial weight
  ☐ Non-weight bearing
 d. Supportive Devices Used
  Abductor pillow ☐
  Air Mattress ☐ Bed Cradle ☐
  Eggcrate ☐ Elastic hose ☐
  Footboard ☐ Hand rolls ☐
  Sling ☐ Trapeze ☐
  Other _____
 e. Restraints ordered ☐ Yes ☐ No
  Type _____
  If yes, complete Restraint Assessment
  Form

4. DRUG THERAPY:
Psychotropics ☐ Yes ☐ No

 Diagnosis _____

 Drug _____ Freq. _____

Antibiotics ☐ Yes ☐ No

 Diagnosis _____

 Drug _____ Freq. _____

I.V. ☐ Yes ☐ No

 Site _____

 Peripheral _____

 Central Line _____

NAME - LAST	FIRST	MIDDLE	ATTENDING PHYSICIAN	ROOM NO.

Figure 3-7 Sample nursing admission sheet.

5. **HEARING:**   Right   Left

    Adequate   ☐   ☐
    Adequate w/aid   ☐   ☐
    Poor   ☐   ☐
    Deaf   ☐   ☐

6. **VISION:**   Right   Left

    Adequate   ☐   ☐
    Adequate w/glasses   ☐   ☐
    Poor   ☐   ☐
    Blind   ☐   ☐
    Reading _____ at all times _____

7. **ORAL ASSESSMENT:**

    Own Teeth: ☐ Yes   ☐ No
    Dentures: _____
    Upper-Complete ☐   Partial ☐
    Lower-Complete ☐   Partial ☐
    Do dentures fit: ☐ Yes   ☐ No
    Condition of teeth:_____
    _____

8. **EATING/NUTRITION:**

    Dependent ☐ Independent ☐ Needs Assist ☐
    Dysphagic ☐ Reason: _____
    Adaptive equipment:_____
    Type/consistency of diet: _____
    Tube Feeder: ☐ Yes   ☐ No
    Type of Tube: _____
    Type of Feeding: _____
    Rate: _____

9. **PERSONAL HYGIENE/GROOMING:**

	Indep.	Assist.	Dependent
Tub	☐	☐	☐
Shower	☐	☐	☐
Bed Bath	☐	☐	☐
Time Preferred _____ AM _____ PM			
Oral Hygiene	☐	☐	☐
Shave	☐	☐	☐
Grooming	☐	☐	☐
Dressing	☐	☐	☐
Shampoo	☐	☐	☐

10. **SLEEPING.**

    Usual bed time   _____ am / pm
    Usual arising time   _____ am / pm
    Nap time   _____ am / pm

11. **BOWEL & BLADDER EVALUATION:**

    Uses: Toilet ☐ Urinal ☐ Bedpan ☐
           Bedside Commode ☐
    BOWEL HABITS: Continent: ☐ Yes   ☐ No
    Constipated: ☐ Yes   ☐ No
    Colostomy: ☐ Yes   ☐ No
    Laxative Used: ☐ Yes   ☐ No
    Bowel Sounds Present: ☐ Yes   ☐ No
    Enemas Used: ☐ Yes   ☐ No
    Last bowel movement?_____
    BLADDER HABITS: Continent: ☐ Yes   ☐ No
    Dribbles: _____ Catheter (Type):_____
    Diagnosis:_____
    Urine Color: _____ Consistency: _____
    Time of last voiding:_____

12. **RESPIRATORY STATUS:**

    Lung sounds: Clear ☐ Congested ☐   Other _____
    O_2 ☐ Yes ☐ No   Flow Rate _____
    Canula ☐ Mask ☐ Trach ☐

13. **COMMUNICATION:**

    Aphasic ☐ Clear ☐ Dysphasic ☐
    Language(s) spoken   _____

14. **PSYCHOSOCIAL ASPECTS:**

    FAMILY RELATIONSHIPS:
    Members visit   _____
    Closest relationship with   _____
    _____
    WHICH WORDS DESCRIBE PATIENT?
    Alert ☐ Angry ☐ Combative ☐ Cooperative ☐ Fearful ☐
    Friendly ☐ Noisy ☐ Lethargic ☐ Non-questioning ☐
    ANSWERS QUESTIONS:
    Readily ☐ Reluctantly ☐ Inappropriately ☐
    Does not respond ☐
    MOOD: Elated ☐ Depressed ☐ Homesick ☐
    Hyperactive ☐ Passive ☐ Questioning ☐ Quiet ☐
    Secure ☐ Talkative ☐ Wanders mentally ☐
    COMPREHENSION: Slow ☐ Quick ☐
    Unable to understand ☐
    ORIENTED: Yes ☐ No ☐
    DISORIENTED: Time ☐ Place ☐ Person ☐
    Pt Participated in Assessment: Yes ☐ No ☐
    Family Participated in Assessment: Yes ☐ No ☐
    PERSONAL HABITS: Smokes: Yes ☐ No ☐
    Uses Alcohol: Yes ☐ No ☐

15. **DISCHARGE EVALUATION**

    Prior living arrangements:
    Where: _____
    With whom: _____
    Still available: Yes ☐ No ☐
    Family plans: _____
    _____
    Short term care: _____
    Long term care w/dischg.poss. _____
    Long term care no dischg.poss. _____

16. **ORIENTATION TO FACILITY:**

    Activities ☐ Bathroom ☐ Business Office ☐ Call light ☐
    Facility ☐ Lighting ☐ Meal time ☐ Side rails ☐
    Smoking Rules ☐ Staff ☐ Storage ☐ Visiting hours ☐
    UNABLE TO ORIENT (Reason)   _____
    _____
    _____

Signature _____

Title_____ Date _____

               Review   9   DGE007-1993

Figure 3-7, cont'd Sample nursing admission sheet.

ADMISSION DATE & TIME:	PRIMARY LANGUAGE IF NOT ENGLISH	ADMITTED FROM: ☐ED ☐ECF ☐HOME ☐DIRECT_____ ☐OTHER_____	HT. IN.	WT. ☐STANDING	REASON FOR DEFERRED WT.
ROOM NUMBER:	☐SIGN LANGUAGE	MODE OF TRANSFER: ☐ W/C ☐BED ☐GUERNEY ☐AMBULATED	☐STATED ☐MEASURED	☐BED SCALE ☐CHAIR SCALE	

Patient Statement / Complaint:

VITAL SIGNS

T   R   / min.
R   L
P   BP

Instruction of Routines and Services to Patient/Family
☐ Nurse call system / Intercom
☐ Bed controls
☐ Side Rails
☐ Telephone/TV
☐ Pastoral Care
☐ Visiting policy / Cellular Phone Use
☐ Smoking policy
☐ Identiband
SIGNATURE & TITLE

The valuables/personal effects policy has been explained, and, I understand that Marian Medical Center does not assume responsibility for valuables (money, jewelry, or other personal effects) not secured in the Marian Medical Center safe.

_____ Signature
Patient or Responsible Person

La poliza tocante objetos de valor ha sido explicada, y yo entiendo que Marian Medical Center no asume responsibilidad for estos objetos (alhajas, dinero, etc.) o cualquier otra prenda personal que no sea asegurada en la caja fuerte de Marian Medical Center.

_____ Firma
Paciente o persona responsible por el paciente

MEDICAL HISTORY

	YES	NO		Any other Medical/Surgical Conditions:	COMMENTS:
Diabetes	☐	☐			
Asthma	☐	☐			
Epilepsy	☐	☐			
Family Bleeding Tend.	☐	☐			
Glaucoma	☐	☐			
Cardiac	☐	☐			

PHARMACY

CURRENT MEDICATIONS: (Prescribed and non-prescribed)

DISPOSITION OF MEDICATIONS: ☐ Home ☐ To Pharmacy
Medications sent to Pharmacy noted on Administrative Data Screen.

Medication	Dosage	Frequency	Last Dose	Medication	Dosage	Frequency	Last Dose

Do you take any supplements or herbal remedies? ☐ No ☐ Yes List:_____

☐ NO KNOWN ALLERGIES
MEDICATIONS / FOODS   Type of Reaction

ALLERGIES

ADHESIVE TAPE:	YES ☐	NO ☐		
IODINE SKIN PREP:	YES ☐	NO ☐		
LATEX:	YES ☐	NO ☐		

PAGE 1   PATIENT ADDRESSOGRAPH

Marian Medical Center
✳ CHW
1400 East Church Street
Santa Maria, CA 93454

L.V.N. Signature:_____

R.N. Signature:_____

PATIENT ADMISSION ASSESSMENT

460062

Figure 3-8   Sample of hospital nursing assessment form.

			N	Normal
	PUPIL SIZE CHART		S	Sluggish
			NR	Non-Reactive

NEUROLOGICAL STATUS

LEVEL OF CONSCIOUSNESS: ☐ ALERT ☐ ORIENTED
☐ Confused ☐ Slow to respond/Comprehend
☐ Disoriented ☐ Lethargic ☐ Vertigo
☐ Pupils: Size & reaction: Right:_____ Left:_____
SENSORY LIMITATIONS: ☐ WNL Glasses
☐ Taste ☐ Speech ☐ Sight Contact Lenses ☐ R ☐ L
☐ Touch ☐ Smell ☐ Hearing Hearing Aid ☐ R ☐ L

If Pt. Uses / If with Patient (columns)

DESCRIBE ABNORMAL FINDINGS

FUNCTIONAL STATUS (LEVEL OF SELF CARE)

MOBILITY: ☐ WNL ☐ Decreased mobility over last month
Limitations: If Pt Uses   If with Patient
☐ Walking ☐ Stairs
☐ Transfer ☐ Standing   Cane/Crutches/Walker ☐ ☐
☐ Turning in bed ☐ Generalized Weakness   Artificial Limbs ☐ R ☐ L ☐ ☐
       Brace ☐ ☐
WEAKNESS PARALYSIS/TRAUMA/ SURGERY: _____
MOTOR FUNCTION
RUE→ ☐ WNL ☐ Weak ☐ Absent
RLE→ ☐ WNL ☐ Weak ☐ Absent   ASSISTANCE REQUIRED:
LUE→ ☐ WNL ☐ Weak ☐ Absent   ☐ Hygiene/Grooming ☐ Dressing ☐ Meals ☐ Other
LLE→ ☐ WNL ☐ Weak ☐ Absent

☐Request Rehab. Services consult from M.D. for changes in mobility within the last month.

SAFETY RISK

☐ Patient Not oriented to person, place or time
☐ Patient has no recent memory
☐ Patient unable to respond/follow instructions
☐ Previous falls
☐ Recent change in mobility
☐ Mobility assessed as unsteady or unable to ambulate without assistance
☐ Medications: sedatives/narcotics/diuretics/muscle relaxants
☐ **Safety risk criteria not met**

☐ Patients who meet two or more criteria are at risk
☐ Initiate Safety risk protocol

RESPIRATORY

☐ NORMAL BREATH SOUNDS RATE WNL
☐ Accessory Muscles ☐ Secretions ☐ Nasal Flaring
☐ Dyspnea ☐ Tracheostomy ☐ Orthopnea
☐ Abnormal Breath Sounds ☐ Tachypenea ☐ Cough
☐ Oxygen ☐ _____

CARDIO VASCULAR

☐ REGULAR RHYTHM, RATE WNL
☐ Abnormal Pulses ☐ Abnormal Heart Sounds ☐ Pedal Edema
   Apical/Radial/Pedal ☐ Jugular Vein Distension ☐ Pacemaker

GASTRO INTESTINAL

☐ WNL   ☐ INCONTINENT OF BOWEL
☐ NAUSEA/VOMITING   ☐ OCCASIONAL ☐ FREQUENT
☐ TUBES   ☐ BOWEL SOUNDS
   ☐ N/G ☐ G/T ☐ J/T   ☐ NORMAL ☐ HYPO ☐ HYPER ☐ ABSENT
☐ OTHER_____   ☐ CONSTIPATION ☐ DIARRHEA
☐ BLOODY STOOL   ☐ ABDOMINAL EXTENSION
☐ LAST BOWEL MOVEMENT: _____   ☐ ABDOMINAL TENDERNESS/PAIN
☐ OSTOMY/ELIMINATION AIDS   LOCATION _____
   ☐ OTHER_____

Genitourinary /GYN

☐ Anuric ☐ WNL
☐ Nocturia ☐ Other:_____
☐ Burning ☐ Catheter
☐ Urgency   Date Placed_____
☐ Urinary Incontinence
☐ Urinary Frequency
☐ Stress Incontinence

GYN
☐ Not Applicable
☐ Vaginal Discharge
   _____
☐ Unusual Bleeding
   Pad Count_____
☐ Pregnant
☐ LMP_____

☐ If pregnant and over 20 weeks, complete OB Assessment.

PAGE 2

Figure 3-8, cont'd   Sample of hospital nursing assessment form.

SKIN

- ☐ TURGOR, TEMPERATURE & COLOR WNL
- ☐ INTACT, MOIST MUCOUS MEMBRANES WNL
- ☐ Edema
- ☐ Dry
- ☐ Diaphoretic
- ☐ Scaly
- ☐ Poor skin turgor
- ☐ Cool
- ☐ Cyanotic
- ☐ Flushed
- ☐ Pale
- ☐ Jaundiced
- ☐ Mottled
- ☐ Hot

SKIN ASSESSMENT CODE
B – Bruises
D – Decubitus
  Grade I II III IV (circle)
L – Lacerations
S – Scar
R – Rash
A – Abrasions
Bu – Burn
St – Stoma
V - Vascular access

POTENTIAL FOR SKIN BREAK DOWN
- ☐ Poor General Health
- ☐ Diminished mental status
- ☐ Decreased oral/fluid intake
- ☐ Incontinence
- ☐ Decreased activity
- ☐ Immobility
- ☐ "At risk for skin breakdown" Criteria not met

- ☐ Patient who meet four or more criteria are **"at risk for breakdown"** Initiate integumentary care plan
- ☐ Request ET consult if Patient has stage IV decubitus

NUTRITION

- ☐ DIAGNOSIS OF MALNUTRITION
- ☐ POOR INTAKE/NPO> 4 DAYS
- ☐ TPN
- ☐ SWALLOWING DIFFICULTY
- ☐ OTHER CONCERNS:
- ☐ NEW ONSET DIABETES
- ☐ UNPLANNED WEIGHT LOSS > 10 LBS IN 1 MONTH
- ☐ TUBE FEEDINGS

_____

| DENTURES | ☐ UPPER | ☐ LOWER | ☐ PARTIAL |
| WITH PT: | ☐ | ☐ | ☐ |

- ☐ Request dietician Consult if any boxes are checked

PERSONAL HABITS

	DENIES USE	Type/Amount per day
Caffeine Beverages	☐	_____
Alcohol	☐	_____
Tobacco	☐	_____
Other	☐	_____

PAIN

- ☐ 0 – 10 Pain Rating Scale explained validated

Do you have pain   yes ☐ no ☐
Where is your pain_____
Using the pain scale what # do you rate your pain_____
Onset _____
Duration: ☐ constant ☐ intermittent ☐ sharp ☐ radiating
☐ aching ☐ burning ☐ numbness ☐ dull ☐ other_____
What relieves your pain _____

PEDIATRICS

Is your child: ☐ Breast fed ☐ Bottle fed ☐ Uses a spoon ☐ Uses cup ☐ Feeds self ☐ Feeds self with help
Are immunizations up to date? ☐ YES ☐ NO   Explain:_____
Any exposure to communicable diseases: ☐ YES ☐ NO Explain: _____
(when & where) _____
Name of Pediatrician:_____
Growth/Development: ☐ Appropriate for age ☐ Other:_____
Head circumference_____ Fontanel: ☐ Soft ☐ Flat ☐ Sunken ☐ Bulging ☐ NA
Does your child know why he or she is being admitted to the hospital? ☐ YES ☐ NO
Does your child have a favorite toy or security item? _____
Any other information/routine we need to know to make this hospital easier?_____

PAGE 3

EDUCATION

Anticipated learning needs: ☐ Diet ☐ Meds ☐ Lifestyle Changes ☐ Pain Management
☐ Diagnosis / Illness
Other:_____

Anticipated barriers to learning:
- ☐ Cultural
- ☐ Motivation
- ☐ Religious
- ☐ Language
- ☐ Emotional
- ☐ Cognitive
- ☐ Financial
- ☐ None Identified

- ☐ Plan of Care reviewed and agreed upon

Figure 3-8, cont'd Sample of hospital nursing assessment form.

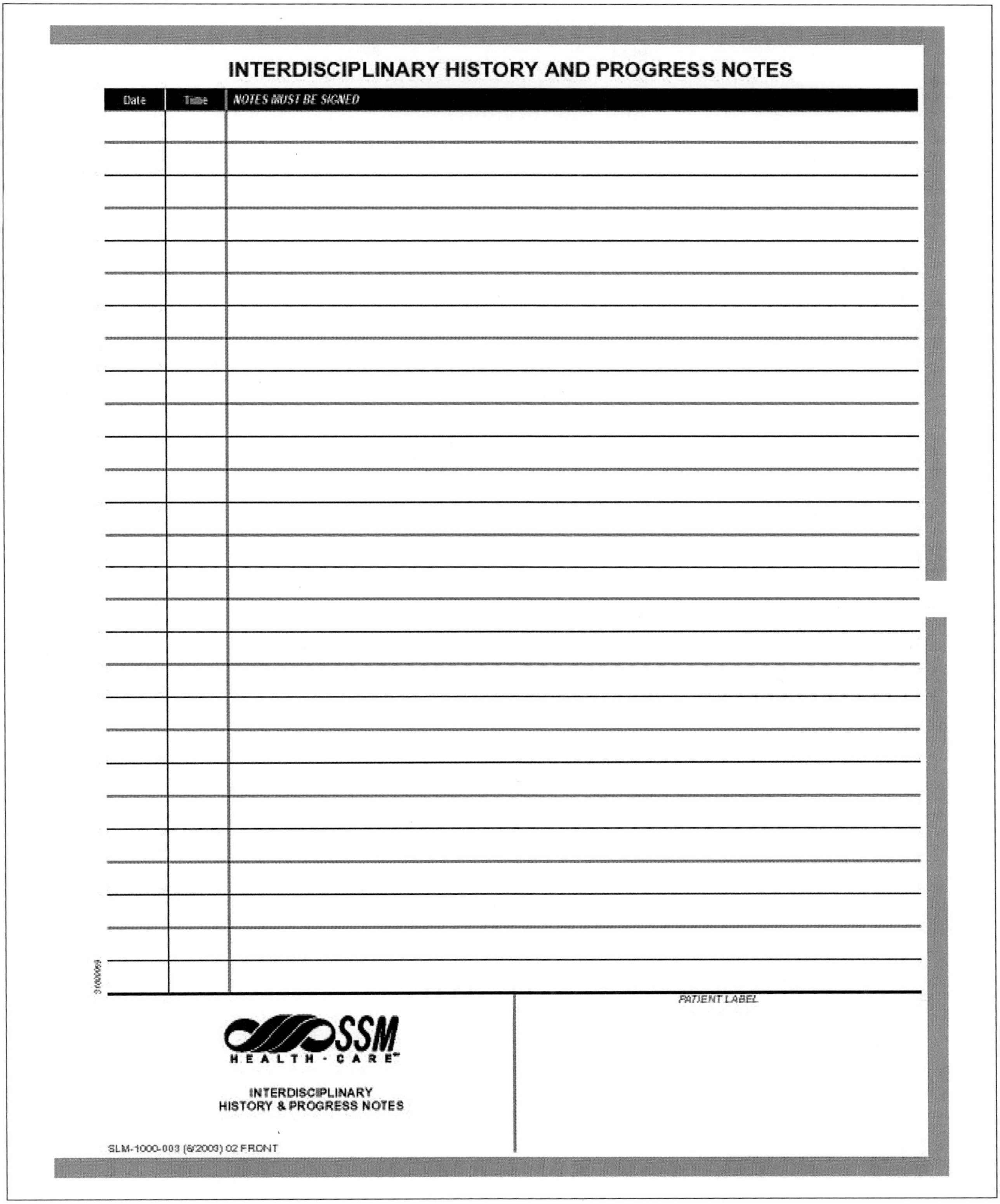

INTERDISCIPLINARY HISTORY AND PROGRESS NOTES

Date	Time	NOTES MUST BE SIGNED

SSM
HEALTH·CARE

INTERDISCIPLINARY
HISTORY & PROGRESS NOTES

SLM-1000-003 (6/2003) 02 FRONT

PATIENT LABEL

Figure 3-9 Sample of a multidisciplinary progress note.

Graphic Records

Graphic records indicate measurements such as vital signs, intake and output, and other routine care measures. Many graphic records are designed so that you record observations and care measures performed during your shift. Figure 3-10 shows examples of vital signs, intake and output, and activities of daily living records.

Other Forms

Other forms contained in the patient's medical record will give you more information about a patient's health problems, plans for medical care, specific treatments, and response to care. This information helps focus and guide the care that you and other members of the health care team provide.

Documentation and Long-Term Care

Documentation for residents in long-term care centers includes additional assessment and care planning forms.

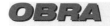

OBRA requires that an assessment and screening tool called a **minimum data set (MDS)** be completed for every resident admitted to a long-term care center.

The MDS is used to develop the nursing care plan for a patient. This tool is updated at least once a year or whenever a patient's condition changes. Figure 3-11 shows the first page of an MDS.

The other steps in the long-term care planning process are the use of **RAPs**, or **resident assessment protocols**, and interdisciplinary planning conferences (Appendix A, p. 673-674). RAPs are guidelines, also known as triggers, that help the nurse develop a nursing care plan. Information shared by health care team members is used to develop a care plan, which takes place in an interdisciplinary care planning (ICP) conference.

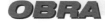

The RAPS and ICP are also required by OBRA.

Text continued on p. 56

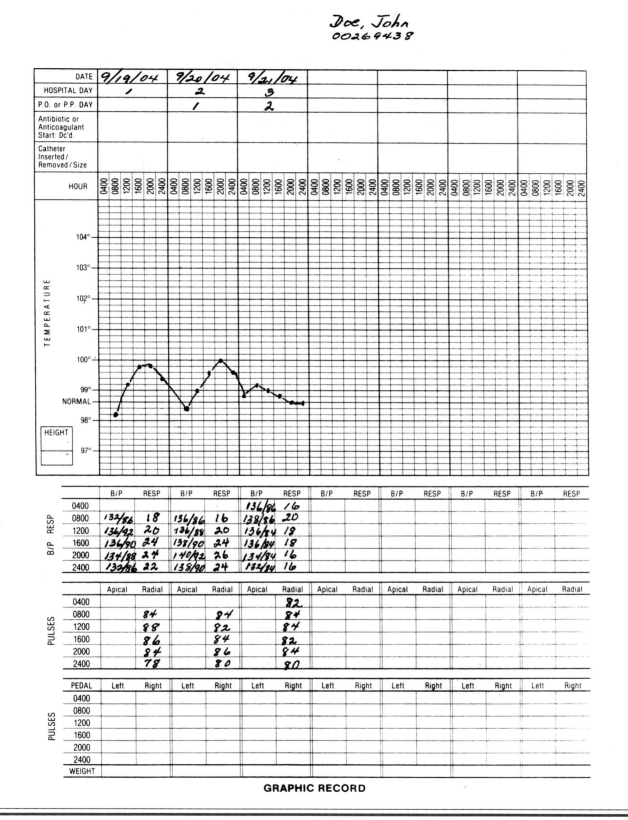

Doe, John
00269438

DATE	9/19/04	9/20/04	9/21/04				
HOSPITAL DAY	1	2	3				
P.O. or P.P. DAY		1	2				
Antibiotic or Anticoagulant Start: Dc'd.							
Catheter Inserted / Removed / Size							

	B/P	RESP	B/P	RESP	B/P	RESP	B/P	RESP	B/P	RESP	B/P	RESP	B/P	RESP
0400					136/86	16								
0800	132/86	18	136/86	16	138/86	20								
1200	136/92	20	136/88	20	136/84	18								
1600	136/90	24	138/90	24	136/84	18								
2000	134/88	24	140/92	26	134/84	16								
2400	132/86	22	138/90	24	132/84	16								

	Apical	Radial	Apical	Radial	Apical	Radial	Apical	Radial	Apical	Radial	Apical	Radial	Apical	Radial
0400						82								
0800		84		84		84								
1200		88		82		84								
1600		86		84		82								
2000		84		86		84								
2400		78		80		80								

PEDAL	Left	Right	Left	Right	Left	Right	Left	Right	Left	Right	Left	Right	Left	Right
0400														
0800														
1200														
1600														
2000														
2400														
WEIGHT														

GRAPHIC RECORD

Figure **3-10** **A,** Sample of a vital sign record.

Continued

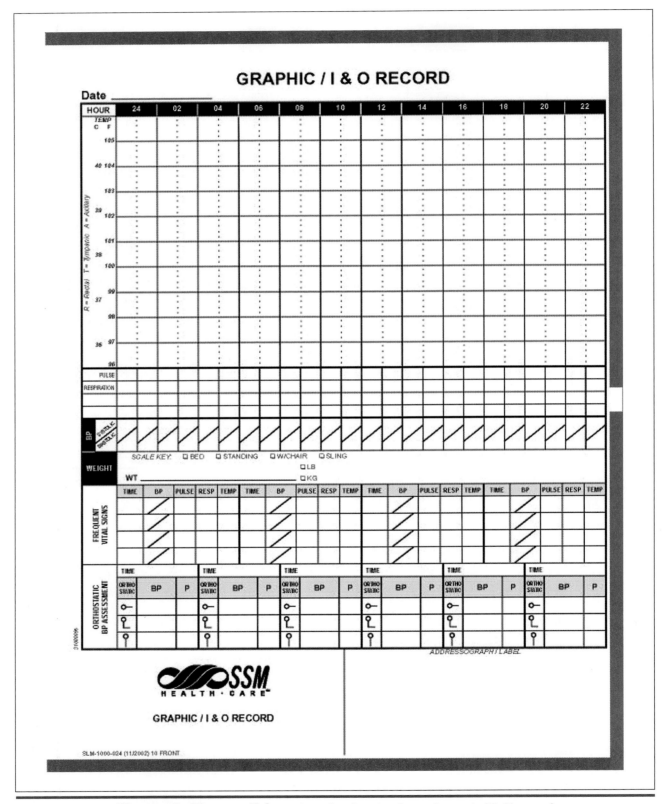

***Figure* 3-10, *cont'd* B**, Sample of an intake and output (I&O) record.

GRAPHIC I & O RECORD

Date _____ **INTAKE**   KEY: Continent / Incontinent   **OUTPUT**

	Parenteral				Oral / Tube Feedings			Urine		Other				
Type:					Oral	TF	Flush							BM
To Count:					Amt	Amt	Amt	Amt	Amt	Amt	Amt	Amt	Amt	Amt/Freq
2300														
2400														
0100														
0200														
0300														
0400														
0500														
0600														

8 hr Sub Totals ___ ___ ___ ___ ___ ___ ___   8 hr Sub Totals ___ ___ ___ ___ ___ ___ ___

8 hr Total Parenteral _____   8 hr total Oral/tube _____

To Count:					8 hr Shift Intake				8 hr Shift Output					
0700														
0800														
0900														
1000														
1100														
1200														
1300														
1400														

8 hr Sub Totals ___ ___ ___ ___ ___ ___ ___   8 hr Sub Totals ___ ___ ___ ___ ___ ___ ___

8 hr Total Parenteral _____   8 hr total Oral/tube _____

To Count:					8 hr Shift Intake				8 hr Shift Output					
1500														
1600														
1700														
1800														
1900														
2000														
2100														
2200														

8 hr Sub Totals ___ ___ ___ ___ ___ ___ ___   8 hr Sub Totals ___ ___ ___ ___ ___ ___ ___

8 hr Total Parenteral _____   8 hr total Oral/tube _____

8 hr Shift Intake   8 hr Shift Output

Twenty-four hour Total   **Twenty-four hour Total**

FLUID EQUIVALENTS
1 oz	30cc	8 oz (1 cup)	240cc
4 oz (1/2 cup)	120cc	12 oz (soda-1 can)	360cc
6 oz (3/4 cup)	180cc		

ADDRESSOGRAPH / LABEL

SSM
HEALTH · CARE™

GRAPHIC I & O RECORD

SLM-1000-024 (11/2002) 10 BACK

Figure **3-10,** *cont'd* **B,** Sample of an intake and output (I&O) record.

Continued

DATE: 7/22/04

	NIGHTS NOTES TIME	DAYS NOTES TIME	EVENINGS NOTES TIME
DIET			
TYPE OF DIET TAKEN & AMOUNT	NONE ☑	BREAKFAST 2/3 LUNCH 1/2	DINNER 2/3
DIETARY SUPPLEMENTS AND SNACKS	NONE ☑ TYPE ____	NONE ☑ TYPE ____	NONE ☑ TYPE ____
FOOD TAKEN PER	SELF ☐ ASSIST ☐ FED ☐	SELF ☑ ASSIST ☐ FED ☐	SELF ☑ ASSIST ☐ FED ☐
TUBE FEEDING (Indicate Solution + Rate)	NA ☑ SOLUTION ____ RATE ____	NA ☑ SOLUTION ____ RATE ____	NA ☑ SOLUTION ____ RATE ____
FLUIDS	NA ☑ ENCOURAGED ☐ RESTRICTED ☐	NA ☐ ENCOURAGED ☑ RESTRICTED ☐	NA ☐ ENCOURAGED ☑ RESTRICTED ☐
SKIN HYGIENE			
BED BATH, TUB, SHOWER, SITZ (CIRCLE)	SELF ☐ ASSIST ☐ COMPLETE ☐	SELF ☐ ASSIST ☑ COMPLETE ☐	SELF ☐ ASSIST ☐ COMPLETE ☐
SHIFT CARE	HS ☐ SHAVE ☐	AM ☑ SHAVE ☐	PM ☑ HS ☐ SHAVE ☐
ORAL CARE	NA ☑ SELF ☐ ASSIST ☐ COMPLETE ☐	NA ☐ SELF ☑ ASSIST ☐ COMPLETE ☐	NA ☐ SELF ☑ ASSIST ☐ COMPLETE ☐
PERI CARE	NA ☑ SELF ☐ ASSIST ☐ COMPLETE ☐	NA ☐ SELF ☑ ASSIST ☐ COMPLETE ☐	NA ☑ SELF ☐ ASSIST ☐ COMPLETE ☐
SKIN CARE	NA ☑ SELF ☐ ASSIST ☐ COMPLETE ☐	NA ☐ SELF ☐ ASSIST ☑ COMPLETE ☐	NA ☐ SELF ☑ ASSIST ☐ COMPLETE ☐
CONDITION	WARM ☑ COLD ☐ DIAPHORETIC ☐ DRY ☑ CLAMMY ☐	WARM ☑ COLD ☐ DIAPHORETIC ☐ DRY ☑ CLAMMY ☐	WARM ☑ COLD ☐ DIAPHORETIC ☐ DRY ☑ CLAMMY ☐
ABRASIONS/RASH (Location)	NA ☑	NA ☑	NA ☑
EDEMA (Location, Extent)	NO ☑ YES ☐	NO ☑ YES ☐	NO ☑ YES ☐
ACTIVITY			
EQUIPMENT	NA ☐ EGGCRATE ☑ CLINITRON ☐ OTHER ____	NA ☐ EGGCRATE ☑ CLINITRON ☐ OTHER ____	NA ☐ EGGCRATE ☑ CLINITRON ☐ OTHER ____
TYPE OF ACTIVITY	BED ☑ CHAIR ☐ AMB ☐ BSC ☐ DANGLE ☐ BRP ☐ ROM ☐	BED ☑ CHAIR ☑ AMB ☑ BSC ☐ DANGLE ☐ BRP ☑ ROM ☑	BED ☐ CHAIR ☑ AMB ☑ BSC ☐ DANGLE ☐ BRP ☐ ROM ☐
HOW ACCOMPLISHED	SELF ☐ ASSIST ☐ P.T. ☐	SELF ☐ ASSIST ☑ P.T. ☑	SELF ☐ ASSIST ☑ P.T. ☐
LENGTH OF TIME, DISTANCE TOLERANCE		Amb in hall & back x 3 3 problem	
DEEP BREATHE AND COUGH	NA ☑ Q2H ASSISTED ☐ Q2H SELF ☐	NA ☐ Q2H ASSISTED ☐ Q2H SELF ☑	NA ☐ Q2H ASSISTED ☐ Q2H SELF ☑
REPOSITION	NA ☐ Q2H ASSISTED ☑ Q2H SELF ☐	NA ☐ Q2H ASSISTED ☑ Q2H SELF ☐	NA ☐ Q2H ASSISTED ☑ Q2H SELF ☐
SAFETY			
EQUIPMENT	NA ☐ K-PAD ☐ PAS HOSE ☐ TEDS ☑ TIME OFF ____ TIME ON ____	NA ☐ K-PAD ☐ PAS HOSE ☐ TEDS ☑ TIME OFF ____ TIME ON ____	NA ☐ K-PAD ☐ PAS HOSE ☐ TEDS ☐ TIME OFF ____ TIME ON ____
SIDERAILS UP	HEAD ↑☑ ↓☐ FOOT ↑☑ ↓☐	HEAD ↑☑ ↓☐ FOOT ↑☐ ↓☑	HEAD ↑☑ ↓☐ FOOT ↑☑ ↓☐
BED IN LOW POSITION	YES ☑ NO ☐	YES ☑ NO ☐	YES ☑ NO ☐
CALL BUTTON WITHIN REACH	YES ☑ NO ☐ OTHER ____	YES ☑ NO ☐ OTHER ____	YES ☑ NO ☐ OTHER ____
SEIZURE PRECAUTIONS	NA ☑ NO ☐ YES ☐	NA ☑ NO ☐ YES ☐	NA ☑ NO ☐ YES ☐
RESTRAINTS (On / Off)	NA ☑ POSEY ☐ WRIST ☐ ANKLE ☐ TIME ON ____ TIME OFF ____	NA ☑ POSEY ☐ WRIST ☐ ANKLE ☐ TIME ON ____ TIME OFF ____	NA ☑ POSEY ☐ WRIST ☐ ANKLE ☐ TIME ON ____ TIME OFF ____
ISOLATION	NA ☑ TYPE ____	NA ☑ TYPE ____	NA ☑ TYPE ____
PAIN			
LOCATION & INTENSITY	NA ☐ Abdominal "3"	NA ☐ Abdominal "6"	NA ☑
MEDICATION GIVEN	NA ☐ YES ☑	NA ☐ YES ☑	NA ☑ YES ☐
RESULTS	RELIEF ☑ NO RELIEF ☐ ACTION TAKEN ____	RELIEF ☑ NO RELIEF ☐ ACTION TAKEN ____	RELIEF ☐ NO RELIEF ☐ ACTION TAKEN ____
OB			
FUNDUS	FIRM ☐ OTHER ☐	FIRM ☐ OTHER ☐	FIRM ☐ OTHER ☐
LOCHIA	LIGHT ☐ MODERATE ☐ HEAVY ☐	LIGHT ☐ MODERATE ☐ HEAVY ☐	LIGHT ☐ MODERATE ☐ HEAVY ☐
BREASTS	SOFT ☐ FILLING ☐ OTHER ☐	SOFT ☐ FILLING ☐ OTHER ☐	SOFT ☐ FILLING ☐ OTHER ☐

Figure 3-10, cont'd C, Sample of a daily assessment/activity flow sheet.

Numeric Identifier_____

MINIMUM DATA SET (MDS) — *VERSION 2.0*
FOR NURSING HOME RESIDENT ASSESSMENT AND CARE SCREENING

BASIC ASSESSMENT TRACKING FORM

SECTION AA. IDENTIFICATION INFORMATION

O	**a.** (First) **b.** (Middle Initial) **c.** (Last) **d.** (Jr/Sr)
O	

1. American Indian/Alaskan Native   4. Hispanic
2. Asian/Pacific Islander   5. White, not of
3. Black, not of Hispanic origin   Hispanic origin

5. **SOCIAL SECURITY⊙ AND MEDICARE NUMBERS⊙** [C in 1st box if non med. no.]
 a. Social Security Number
 b. Medicare number (or comparable railroad insurance number)

6. **FACILITY PROVIDER NO.⊙**
 a. State No.
 b. Federal No.

7.

---

9. **Signatures of Persons who Completed a Portion of the Accompanying Assessment or Tracking Form**

I certify that the accompanying information accurately reflects resident assessment or tracking information for this resident and that I collected or coordinated collection of this information on the dates specified. To the best of my knowledge, this information was collected in accordance with applicable Medicare and Medicaid requirements. I understand that this information is used as a basis for ensuring that residents receive appropriate and quality care, and as a basis for payment from federal funds. I further understand that payment of such federal funds and continued participation in the government-funded health care programs is conditioned on the accuracy and truthfulness of this information, and that I may be personally subject to or may subject my organization to substantial criminal, civil, and/or administrative penalties for submitting false information. I also certify that I am authorized to submit this information by this facility on its behalf.

Signature and Title	Sections	Date
a.		
b.		
c.		
d.		
e.		
f.		
g.		
h.		
i.		
j.		
k.		
l.		

GENERAL INSTRUCTIONS

Complete this information for submission with all full and quarterly assessments (Admission, Annual, Significant Change, State or Medicare required assessments, or Quarterly Reviews, etc.)

⊙ = Key items for computerized resident tracking

☐ = When box blank, must enter number or letter   [a.] = When letter in box, check if condition applies

MDS 2.0 September, 2000

***Figure* 3-11**   The first page of minimum data set (MDS) used for nursing home resident assessment and care.

How to Observe and Report Information

An **observation** is information you obtain by using your eyes, ears, nose, and sense of touch. Because you will spend more time with the patient than any other member of the health care team, your observations are very important. As you provide care, you will observe the patient's response. You will also look for signs and symptoms related to patient problems. You will tell the nurse about your findings. In some settings you will also record your findings in the medical record. You should report changes in the patient's condition or abnormal signs and symptoms immediately. Your observations will include things patients tell you about how they feel, called **subjective information.** An example of subjective information is patients telling you they have a headache or feel dizzy. You cannot actually see, hear, feel, or smell the patient's symptoms. The other type of observation you make involves things that you can see, hear, feel, or smell, called **objective information.** An example of objective information is the patient's vital signs.

When you verbally report information to the nurse, include:
- Patient's name
- Patient's room and bed number
- Time that care was provided or observations were made
- Description of care or observations

Information about a patient's condition and care needs are passed on from shift to shift during a process called **report** (Figure 3-12). Depending on where you work, you may participate in and listen to report at the beginning and/or end of the shift. At the end of the shift, the nurse in charge will give a report to the next shift. This process provides for continuity of care.

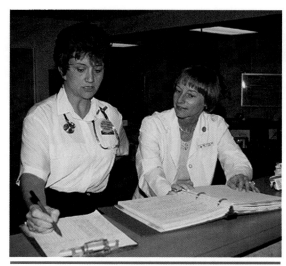

***Figure* 3-12**   Information about a patient's condition and care needs are passed on from shift to shift during a process called report.

Recording Patient Information

The medical record is a permanent record of a patient's medical and nursing care. It is a legal document and can be used as evidence in court. The information in the medical record must be accurate and complete.

Health professionals use specific guidelines for writing and recording patient information. Follow the guidelines listed in Box 3-3 to help you record information.

HOW&*WHY*

Check the policies and procedures in your own facility for any additional written documentation guidelines.

Box 3-3

GUIDELINES FOR WRITTEN DOCUMENTATION

- Always use a black ink pen.
- Include the date and time for each entry. Your facility may have you write times in AM/PM format or in military time (Figure 3-13).

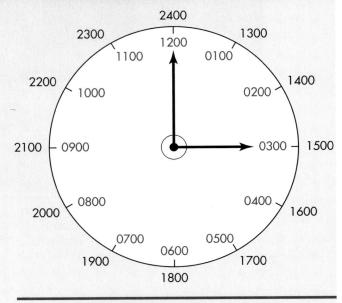

Figure 3-13 Military time.

- Sign all entries with your first initial, last name, and title (Figure 3-14, *A*).
- Use only abbreviations on your facility's lists of approved abbreviations.
- Do not erase or use correction fluid to cover an entry. If you make an error, draw a single line through the mistake. Write "mistaken entry" and your initials above the entry (Figure 3-14, *B*). Some agencies have a policy that requires that an error be corrected by writing the word "error" above the incorrect entry (Figure 3-14, *C*).
- Do not skip lines. If a line is only partially filled in, draw a single line through the remainder of the line. This prevents others from adding to entries that you have made and signed (Figure 3-14, *D*).
- Record only information and care that you have observed or performed.
- Record care **after** it has been completed.
- Be factual and accurate. Use a patient's exact words, written within quotation marks, when possible. Do not record your opinions or feelings (Figure 3-14, *E*).
- When recording changes from normal, also write down the time that you notified the nurse of your findings (Figure 3-14, *F*).

Box 3-3

GUIDELINES FOR WRITTEN DOCUMENTATION—cont'd

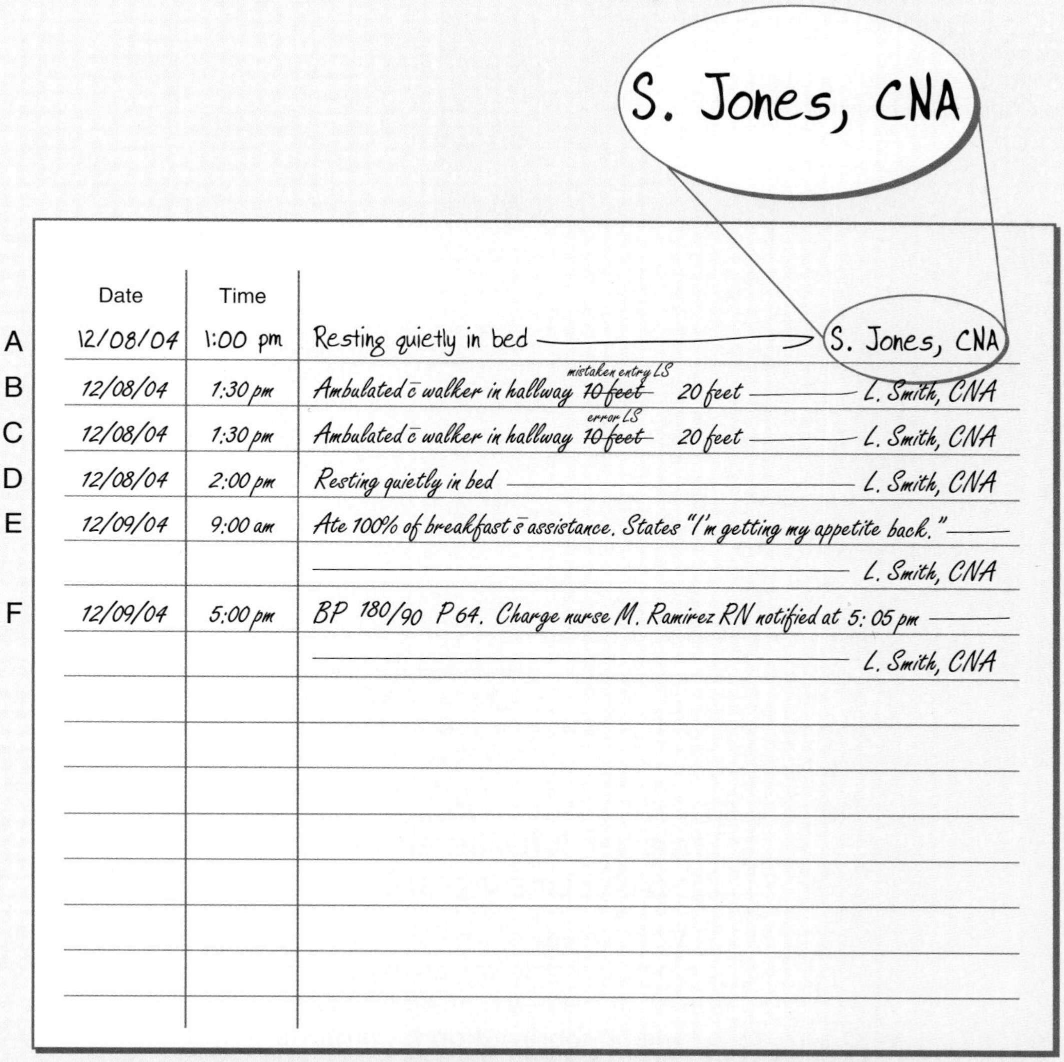

	Date	Time	
A	12/08/04	1:00 pm	Resting quietly in bed —————————→ S. Jones, CNA
B	12/08/04	1:30 pm	Ambulated c̄ walker in hallway ~~10 feet~~ *mistaken entry LS* 20 feet ————— L. Smith, CNA
C	12/08/04	1:30 pm	Ambulated c̄ walker in hallway ~~10 feet~~ *error LS* 20 feet ————— L. Smith, CNA
D	12/08/04	2:00 pm	Resting quietly in bed ————————————— L. Smith, CNA
E	12/09/04	9:00 am	Ate 100% of breakfast c̄ assistance. States "I'm getting my appetite back." ——— ————————————————————— L. Smith, CNA
F	12/09/04	5:00 pm	BP 180/90 P 64. Charge nurse M. Ramirez RN notified at 5:05 pm ———— ————————————————————— L. Smith, CNA

***Figure* 3-14** **A,** Sign all entries with your first initial, last name, and title. **B,** If you make an error, draw a single line through the mistake. Write "mistaken entry" and your initials above the entry. **C,** Some facilities have a policy that requires that an error be corrected by writing the word "error" above the incorrect entry rather than "mistaken entry." **D,** Do not skip lines. If a line is only partially filled in, draw a single line through the remainder of the line. This prevents others from adding to entries that you have made and signed. **E,** Use a patient's exact words, written within quotation marks, when possible. **F,** When recording changes from normal, also indicate that you have notified the nurse of your findings, as well as the time of notification.

Continued

Box 3-3

GUIDELINES FOR WRITTEN DOCUMENTATION—cont'd

- Make sure that each form you write on contains the patient's identifying information (Figure 3-15).
- Write or print neatly.
- Use correct spelling and punctuation.
- Use correct medical terminology.

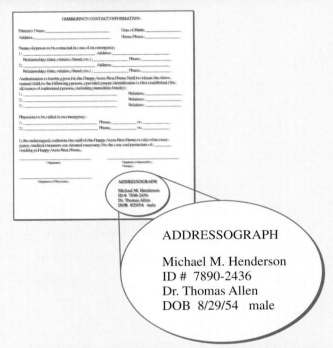

ADDRESSOGRAPH

Michael M. Henderson
ID # 7890-2436
Dr. Thomas Allen
DOB 8/29/54   male

Figure 3-15   Each form should contain the patient's identifying information.

Use of Medical Terms and Abbreviations

HOW&**WHY**
The abbreviation for magnetic resonance imaging is MRI.

Many medical terms come from the Latin and Greek languages. Other terms are named after people who discovered an illness or created a procedure or treatment. Even other terms are a type of abbreviation for a group of words.

You will learn some medical terminology as you complete your nursing assistant training program. You will also learn terms as you work with other health professionals. Medical terminology courses can be taken at vocational education schools and community colleges.

Medical abbreviations are used frequently in documentation. An abbreviation can be a shorter form of a word or phrase. It can also represent numbers, times, and measurements. Use of abbreviations saves time and space when you are writing information. Your facility will have a list of approved abbreviations that you may use. Some of the most commonly used medical abbreviations are listed in Box 3-4.

Box 3-4

MOST COMMONLY USED MEDICAL ABBREVIATIONS

$\bar{a}$	before	MRSA	methicillin-resistant *Staphylococcus aureus*
abd	abdomen		
$\overline{ac}$	before meals	N/A	not applicable
ADL	activities of daily living	NAS	no added salt
ad lib	as desired	NCS	no concentrated sweets
AIDS	acquired immunodeficiency syndrome	NG	nasogastric
		NKA	no known allergies
a.m.	morning	NPO	nothing by mouth
AMA	against medical advice	O_2 or O2	oxygen
amb. or amb	ambulatory	OOB	out of bed
amt. or amt	amount	OT	occupational therapy
AROM	active range of motion	$\bar{p}$	after
B&B	bowel and bladder	$\overline{pc}$	after meals
b.i.d., bid, or BID	twice a day	p.m.	afternoon
BM	bowel movement	PO	by mouth
BP	blood pressure	prn	whenever necessary
BRP	bathroom privileges	PROM	passive range of motion
BSC	bedside commode	PT	physical therapy
$\bar{c}$	with	PUD	peptic ulcer disease
CA	cancer	PVD	peripheral vascular disease
cath. or cath	catheter	PWB	partial weight bearing
CHF	congestive heart failure	$\bar{q}$	every (for example, q1h—every 1 hour, q2h—every 2 hours)
c/o or C/O	complains of		
CVA	cerebrovascular accident	q.i.d, qid, or QID	four times daily
D/C	discontinue	R or ®	right
DJD	degenerative joint disease	RAI	resident assessment instrument
DNR	do not resuscitate	R/O	rule out
dx	diagnosis	R.O.M. or ROM	range of motion
ECG, EKG	electrocardiogram	$\bar{s}$	without
FF	frequent fluids	SLP	speech language pathologist
Fx	fracture	SOB	shortness of breath
G/C	Geri-chair	SR	side rail
GI	gastrointestinal	Stat, STAT, or stat	immediately
G-tube or g-tube	gastrostomy tube	STD	sexually transmitted disease
GU	genitourinary	TB	tuberculosis
H or hr	hour	Tbsp	tablespoon
H_2O	water	TIA	transient ischemic attack
HBV	hepatitis B virus	t.i.d, tid, or TID	three times daily
HIV	human immunodeficiency virus	TPR	temperature, pulse, respiration
		tsp	teaspoon
H.O.B. or HOB	head of bed	tx	treatment or traction
HOH	hard of hearing	URI	upper respiratory infection
ht	height	UTI	urinary tract infection
I&O	intake and output	VRE	vancomycin-resistant enterococci
IV	intravenously	VS	vital signs
L or Ⓛ	left	W/C	wheelchair
l	liter	wt	weight
liq. or liq	liquid	↑	up, elevate, or increase (Be careful when using this symbol. Draw the arrow precisely in an upward direction.)
LTC	long-term care		
MDS	minimum data set		
meds	medications	↓	down or decrease (Be careful when using this symbol. Draw the arrow precisely in a downward direction.)
MI	myocardial infarction		
mL	milliliter		

CHAPTER REVIEW

1. What is communication?

2. List 4 non-verbal ways that you can show that you are actively listening to what another person is saying.

3. What is a care plan?

4. What is a "goal" on the care plan?

5. List 3 items required by OBRA when planning care for residents of long-term care centers.

6. How do you know which abbreviations are approved by your facility for use in the medical record?

7. Sign your name as you will when you complete the certification process.

Circle the one BEST response.

8. John is using hand gestures, facial expressions, and drawings to communicate with Mr. Garcia. What type of communication is this?
a. Nonverbal communication
b. Passive listening
c. Verbal communication
d. All of the above

9. Jane is upset that she has been scheduled to work both Christmas and New Year's holidays. Which method listed below is the best way to talk with the charge nurse who wrote the schedule?
a. Insist loudly and firmly that she will work on only one of the holidays
b. Tell the nurse that he is being unfair
c. Ask the nurse if she could speak with him privately, then state her concerns factually, using a calm voice
d. Threaten to quit if the nurse does not change the schedule

10. Making negative comments about a person's age and appearance is which type of harassment?
a. Physical
b. Sexual
c. Verbal
d. All of the above

CHAPTER REVIEW

11. Two nursing assistants are talking about a patient's medical problems in a crowded hospital elevator. Which legal right is being violated?
a. Confidentiality
b. Freedom of information
c. Free speech
d. All of the above

12. The nurse asks you to take Mr. Simone's blood pressure and pulse. What kind of information is this?
a. Hypothesis
b. Nursing diagnosis
c. Objective data
d. Subjective data

13. Mr. Simone tells you, "My muscles ache all over, and I'm freezing cold." What kind of information is this?
a. Hypothesis
b. Nursing diagnosis
c. Objective data
d. Subjective data

14. Where are vital signs recorded in the medical record?
a. Admission sheet
b. Graphic record
c. Medication record
d. Nursing care plan

15. You are documenting a patient's symptoms on a progress note, and you make a spelling error. How do you correct your error?
a. Use correction fluid to cover the error, then write over the area.
b. Completely darken through the misspelled word, then rewrite the word correctly.
c. Draw one line through the misspelling. Write "mistaken entry" and your initials above the mistake, then rewrite the word correctly.
d. Any of these methods is correct.

Answers are on page 704.

CHAPTER 4

Understanding Basic Human Needs

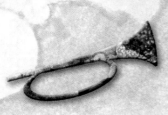

What you will learn

- Caring for the "whole" person
- Basic human needs and Maslow's hierarchy of needs
- Cultural and spiritual beliefs
- Working with families and visitors
- Patient rights

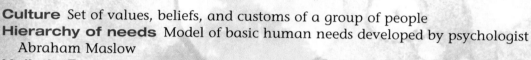

KEY TERMS

Culture Set of values, beliefs, and customs of a group of people
Hierarchy of needs Model of basic human needs developed by psychologist Abraham Maslow
Holistic Term meaning "whole"
Need Something that is required for a person's survival or well-being
Self-actualization Term that relates to people's need to be creative and fulfill their potential
Self-esteem What people think about themselves

Caring for the "Whole" Person

Nurses care for patients using a **holistic** approach. The word *holistic* means whole. A whole person has physical, social, emotional, and spiritual needs. These needs are related to each other. Nursing care helps to meet these needs. The following example shows how a nurse provides care in a holistic way.

Ms. Schmidt is in the hospital with pneumonia. She is a single parent with two young children. She is very worried about being away from her children. She also wonders when she can return to work. The nurse plans care to help Ms. Schmidt recover from her medical problem. The nurse also knows that Ms. Schmidt's worries can slow her recovery. The nurse offers emotional support and asks social services to see Ms. Schmidt. In this example the nurse works to meet the physical, social, and emotional needs of the patient.

Basic Human Needs

A **need** is something that is required for people to live or for their well-being. That "something" can range from the need for food and water to the need to be creative and artistic. Psychologist Abraham Maslow created a model called the **hierarchy of needs** that places basic human needs in five main categories or levels. Figure 4-1 shows a picture of the model.

Maslow listed the needs in their level of importance. So people can survive, they must meet their physical and safety needs. You can see in the picture that Maslow placed these needs at the bottom, or foundation, of the pyramid. When people meet these

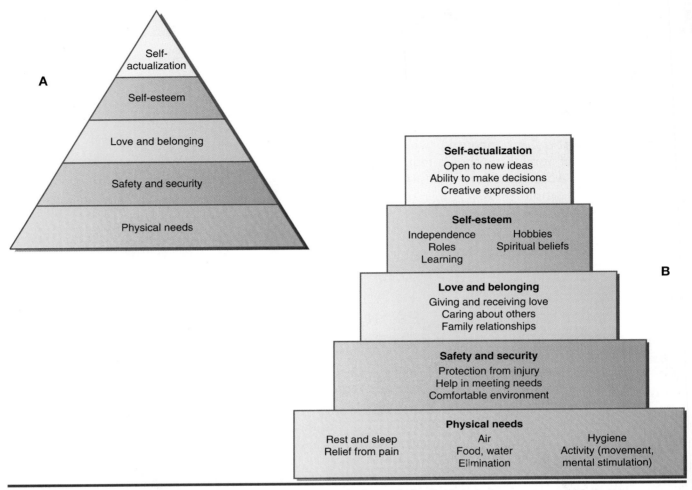

Figure 4-1 **A,** Maslow's hierarchy of needs. **B,** Understanding Maslow's ideas helps you to provide better care based on the person's level of need.

lower level needs, they can pay attention to higher level needs. These higher level needs are the categories of love and belonging, self-esteem, and self-actualization. These needs relate to people's well-being and happiness.

Adults normally meet their own basic needs. When they are ill, they may need help to meet their needs. When people cannot do things by themselves, they may feel frustration, fear, anxiety, or anger. A nurse's role is to figure out how to help patients meet their basic needs. Nurses also help the patients deal with and adjust to stresses caused by illness.

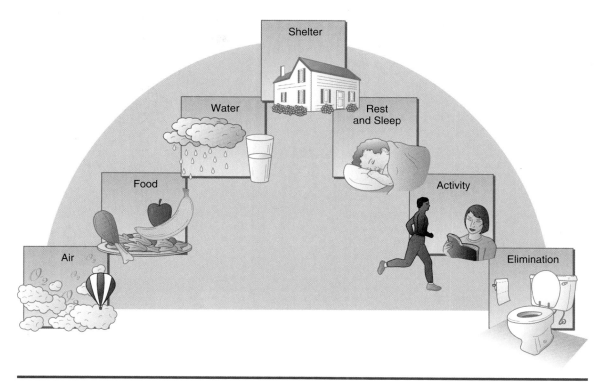

Figure 4-2   Physical needs include air, food, water, shelter, rest and sleep, activity, and elimination.

Physical Needs

Physical needs are the most basic survival needs. They include air, water, food, shelter, rest and sleep, and elimination (Figure 4-2). These needs must be met before all others. When they are met, a person can focus on other concerns.

Safety and Security Needs

Meeting safety and security needs helps protect us from harm and helps us to feel safe. Examples of these needs include the security of a home and family, having a safe place to live, and having the comfort of spiritual beliefs. People need to feel safe and secure before they can think about the higher level needs.

The Need for Love and Belonging

People need to feel that others love and accept them. They need to feel that someone cares about them and have close, meaningful relationships. They also have a desire to belong to groups. Examples of groups include clubs, work groups, religious groups, and families.

Self-Esteem

Self-esteem is what people think about themselves. People with healthy or good self-esteem feel that they are a valuable, good person. They also feel that other people value them. Self-esteem can be affected by illness or injury.

Self-Actualization

Self-actualization relates to people's need to be creative and fulfill their potential. This is the highest level need in Maslow's hierarchy. A person can spend time and energy in creative and satisfying activities when other needs are met. Ways to meet this need include learning more and spending time in artistic, musical, or dance activities.

Cultural and Spiritual Beliefs

As a nursing assistant, you will care for people who have many different cultural and spiritual beliefs. Learning about and developing respect for these different points of view is an important part of becoming a professional caregiver.

Culture is a set of values, beliefs, and customs of a group of people. Cultural practices are passed on from family to family, and generation to generation. People's culture affect their views about health care. Different cultures have their own health care practices and views about the cause and treatment for illnesses. They also may have particular beliefs and customs about death and dying. Box 4-1 gives examples of certain health care beliefs and practices of different cultures. Keep in mind that *not all people* within a culture will follow the cultural beliefs.

A person's spiritual beliefs can also affect health care practices. Religious beliefs and practices may affect a person's views toward health, illness, use of medicine, birth control, dietary habits, and lifestyle choices. When a person is ill, spiritual beliefs can give comfort and support. Patients often ask for a visit from their pastor or spiritual advisor. When a priest, minister, or rabbi visits, the nursing assistant should provide privacy for the patient and the visitor. Box 4-2 gives examples of some religious beliefs that affect health care practices.

Care planning for patients includes thinking about a person's cultural and spiritual needs. Understanding each individual's needs helps you provide care for a patient. Helping patients meet these needs may also help them recover from illness more quickly.

NOTES ON
☯ Culture

Keep in mind that people may choose not to follow a specific custom usually practiced by their culture. Avoid stereotyping by treating each person as an individual.

Box 4-1

CULTURAL HEALTH CARE BELIEFS AND PRACTICES

- Some **Hispanic** cultures may use folk healers to help prevent or cure illness. Families may seek the help of a *jerbero,* who uses herbs and spices, or a *curandera* to help treat physical and mental illness. A *bruja* (witch), who uses magic, may even be consulted.
- Some **Hispanic** and **Asian** cultures view illness as an imbalance between the "hot" and "cold" forces in the body and the environment. Examples of "hot" conditions are fever, infection, ulcers, diarrhea, and constipation. "Cold" conditions include colds, cancer, paralysis, headaches, menstrual periods, and ear disorders. To restore balance in the body, a "hot" disorder is treated with cold foods and medicine. Similarly, a "cold" disorder is treated with hot foods and medicine.
- Certain **Asian** cultures believe that a person's soul and spirit are in the area of the head and shoulders. So it is considered disrespectful to touch a person's head and shoulders excessively. These individuals may also believe that taking pictures of a person may harm or "take away" the person's spirit.

Box 4-2

RELIGIOUS BELIEFS AFFECTING HEALTH CARE PRACTICES

- Certain **Jewish** groups follow specific dietary and food preparation practices. This is called "keeping kosher."
- **Jehovah's Witness** beliefs prohibit a person of that faith from receiving blood or blood products.
- **Latter Day Saints (Mormon)** groups teach members to avoid use of caffeine, alcohol, and tobacco products.
- The **Catholic** faith teaches that only "natural" forms of birth control are permitted.

Working With Families and Visitors

Family members and visitors often provide a valuable support and caregiving role for ill or injured patients. Family and visitors also help meet needs that people cannot meet themselves. For example, Mr. Garcia is a patient in a skilled nursing facility. He is recovering from a stroke. His wife visits daily and helps the nursing assistant with his personal care and position changes. She also helps during meals, encouraging Mr. Garcia to eat soft foods and drink liquids. She reassures him when he becomes upset or depressed. Ms. Garcia is helping meet Mr. Garcia's physical and security needs and his need for love and belonging and self-esteem. She plays an important role in helping Mr. Garcia get better. The nursing staff also recognizes the importance of her role. They include Ms. Garcia in care conferences. The charge nurse updates her daily about plans for Mr. Garcia's care and rehabilitation. Ms. Garcia is a valuable member of the caregiving team. She will continue to assist with her husband's care when he returns home. She will support his needs until he is able to manage independently.

When family or friends visit, staff should allow for private, uninterrupted conversation. OBRA guarantees residents of long-term care centers the right to meet privately with visitors.

If an interruption is necessary or if you need to provide care, politely ask the visitors to leave the room and show them to a waiting area. When you have completed your care, tell the visitors promptly that they may return to the patient's room. The patient has the right to receive care in privacy.

Sometimes, a patient will want a family member to remain in the room while care is provided (Figure 4-3). If you are providing care in this situation, explain what you are going to do. Perform the care, exposing only the part of the body that is necessary.

Another part of patient privacy to consider relates to patient information. Family and friends are often worried and upset about the illness and condition of a patient. They may ask you questions about a person's diagnosis or treatment. **You may not answer these questions. Refer them to the supervising nurse.**

Sometimes visits from family or friends may tire or upset a patient. If you observe this, report your concerns to the nurse. The nurse will then talk with the visitors about the patient's need for rest.

Patient Rights

Over the years patients began wanting more information and more involvement in the kind of health care decisions and treatment they were receiving. They also wanted to receive

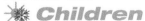
OBRA

HOW & WHY

Do not expose a person's body in front of visitors. This violates a person's right to privacy.

NOTES ON
❊ **Children**

Children may want a family member to remain in the room for support and comfort while procedures or treatments are being done.

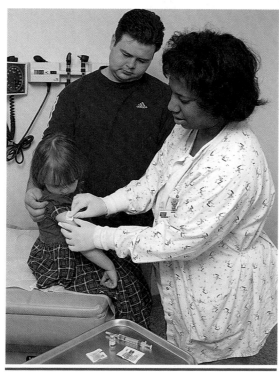

***Figure* 4-3**   Allowing a parent to remain with the child while a procedure is performed helps the child to be more comfortable and less afraid.

higher quality care. Each patient admitted to your facility has rights. These rights are guaranteed under federal and state laws. When patients are admitted to a facility or before they receive medical treatment or consultation, patients must be informed of their rights verbally. Patients must also receive a written copy of their rights.

The purpose of patient or resident rights is to guide ethical and legal decisions about patient care. These rights originally were about the care the doctors and nurses provide. But these rights also apply to care provided by all health care team members and facilities.

The resident's rights must be given orally and in writing in the language used and understood by the resident or legal representative.

The main points of patient rights are listed in Box 4-3.

Resident rights are an important part of the Omnibus Budget Reconciliation Act (OBRA) passed in 1987. OBRA requires that all long-term care centers provide care in a manner and setting that enhances each person's quality of life.

OBRA

OBRA

Box 4-3

PATIENT RIGHTS

The Right to Confidentiality

- Patient information is confidential.

The Right to Privacy

- The patient's body, care, medical record, and personal matters are private. This right continues even after a patient dies.
- The patient has the right to meet with visitors in a private area.
- The patient has the right to receive and send mail unopened.

The Right to Consideration and Respect

- Each person has the right to be treated as an individual and receive kind and respectful care.
- Personal and cultural values and beliefs are respected and included in plans for care.
- Each person has the right to receive care that promotes dignity and well-being.
- Each person has the right to be free from abuse, mistreatment, or neglect.
- Each person has the right to be free from restraints.

The Right to Continuing Care

- The patient is informed about plans for care after discharge from a facility.

The Right to Professional Services

- The patient may expect that a health care facility can provide necessary services. When emergency needs are met, a patient can be transferred to another facility that can best meet the patient's medical needs. The patient has a right to be informed of this plan, as well as any care alternatives.

The Right to Information

- The doctor must inform the patient about diagnosis, treatment, and prognosis in understandable terms. An interpreter must be provided if a patient does not speak or understand English.

The Right to Information on Research and Human Experimentation

- A patient must be given information and explanations about any proposed research conducted as part of the patient's care. The patient must give informed consent.
- A patient has the right to refuse to participate in the research.

The Right to Informed Consent

- The doctor gives the patient information and explanations about any treatments or procedures. This includes the purpose, risks, alternatives, and probable length of recovery for a treatment. The doctor also explains who will perform the treatment.

The Right to Know Institutional Rules and Regulations

- The patient and family are given verbal and written rules and regulations.

The Right to the Patient's Bill

- The patient has the right to examine the bill and get explanations about the bill. The patient has this right even if an insurance company or government agency is paying the bill.

The Right to Refuse Treatment

- The patient may refuse treatment.
- The patient does not have to consent to each treatment or procedure recommended by the doctor.
- The doctor must inform the patient of the health risks involved in refusing a treatment.

The Right to Personal Choice

- The patient has the right to select a doctor and to take part in planning care and activities.
- The patient has the right to state complaints or concerns without fear of punishment.

CHAPTER REVIEW

1. What is a "need"?

2. What does the term *culture* mean?

3. A visitor asks you what a patient's medical diagnosis and prognosis are. What should you do?

Circle the one BEST response.

4. Ms. Lamb's care plan addresses her physical, emotional, spiritual, and social needs. What is this approach called?
   a. Focused
   b. Holistic
   c. Individualized
   d. Needs-based

5. Examples of this type of need are food, air, and water.
   a. Love and belonging
   b. Physical
   c. Safety and security
   d. Self-esteem

6. Having a family and a place to live are examples of this type of need.
   a. Love and belonging
   b. Physical
   c. Safety and security
   d. Self-esteem

7. Mr. Wong tells you that his diet needs to include hot foods to treat his cold. This is an example of which type of practice?
   a. Cultural
   b. Ethical
   c. Moral
   d. Spiritual

8. You are caring for a 6-year-old who cries every time a hospital staff member enters his room. His mother asks if she can remain in the room while you provide care. How should you respond?
   a. "I'm sorry, but you will have to leave the room while I am doing this procedure."
   b. "You are welcome to stay. Children need their parents when they feel scared."
   c. "I'll have to check with the doctor before I can allow you to remain in the room."
   d. "Hospital rules require that all patient care be provided in complete privacy."

9. A doctor explains a procedure to a patient. The patient then refuses to go ahead with the procedure. Which patient right is honored in this situation?
   a. The right to informed consent
   b. The right to information
   c. The right to information on research and human experimentation
   d. The right to refuse treatment

Answers are on page 704.

CHAPTER 5

Understanding Human Growth and Development

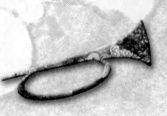

What you will learn

- Basic principles of growth and development
- Physical changes that occur as a person ages
- Erik Erikson's theory of human development

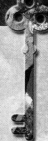

KEY TERMS

Development Changes in psychological and social functioning; how people act or behave at different ages of their life

Developmental task Also known as a **conflict** or **identity crisis.** Set of behaviors or actions a person is able to do during a stage of life

Growth Series of physical changes that occur as a person ages

8 Stages of psychosocial development Theory described by psychologist Erik Erikson about how a person grows and develops throughout life

Basic Principles of Growth and Development

In Chapter 4, you learned about basic human needs and how you can help meet these needs in your patients. Another way to help you better understand how people act and behave throughout their life is by learning about the stages of human growth and development.

Growth is the series of physical changes that occur as a person ages. We measure growth by using height and weight and observing body changes and functions throughout a person's life.

Development is the change in psychological and social functioning. We measure development by observing how a person behaves and acts at certain ages.

Changes in growth and development do not always happen at the same time. For example, children increase in height and weight between their twelfth and thirteenth birthdays but may not change the way they behave. It is also true that children may become more mature in the way they behave without a change in their physical growth.

As you read in Chapter 4, nursing care deals with the whole patient, that is, the physical, social, emotional, and spiritual aspects of a person. One theory about how people grow and develop throughout their life talks about these aspects. The model was developed by Erik Erikson, a well-known psychologist. Nurses have used this theory for many years to help better understand human behavior.

About Erikson's Theory

Erikson's theory is called the **8 stages of psychosocial development.** Erikson explains that people's personality development is influenced by other people around them and by history and culture.

The theory divides human development into eight separate stages. Each stage describes a set of developmental tasks that a person must work through. If a person is not able to successfully work through a **developmental task** at a particular stage, Erikson says that the person will continue to struggle with the task later in life.

As you learn about the developmental tasks people work through as they grow and age, you will begin to identify behaviors and developmental tasks that go along with these stages and levels of maturity as you care for your patients.

Table 5-1 provides a brief summary of the eight stages. Following the summary is more information about each stage.

Growth and Development Throughout Life

Because nursing care is for the whole patient, we look at not just a person's physical changes, but the person's emotional and social development also. Growth and development are connected. Both usually take place in a predictable pattern. Both can occur at a steady or uneven pace. The following summaries describe physical growth and developmental changes that happen during the eight stages of the life span.

NOTES ON
Culture

Different cultures may view the tasks of each stage of life a little bit differently. It is important to respect each person's belief even if it is different from your own.

Table 5-1

SUMMARY OF ERIKSON'S 8 STAGES OF PSYCHOSOCIAL DEVELOPMENT				
Stage	**Ages**	**Important task**	**Summary**	
1. Oral-sensory	Birth to 12-18 months	Feeding	Infant must form a loving, trusting relationship with the caregiver.	
2. Muscular-anal	18 months to 3 years	Toilet training	Child develops physical skills, including walking and bowel control.	
3. Locomotor	3 to 6 years	Independence	Child becomes more confident and takes more initiative.	
4. Latency	6 to 12 years	School	Child learns what must be done to learn new skills, especially in school.	

Continued

Table 5-1

SUMMARY OF ERIKSON'S 8 STAGES OF PSYCHOSOCIAL DEVELOPMENT—cont'd				
Stage	Ages	Important task	Summary	
5. Adolescence	12 to 18 years	Peer relationships	Teenager achieves a sense of identity.	
6. Young adulthood	19 to 40 years	Love relationships	Young adult develops intimate relationships.	
7. Middle adulthood	40 to 65 years	Parenting	Adult cares for and supports the next generation.	
8. Maturity (late adulthood)	65 years to death	Reflection on and acceptance of one's life	Older adults review and reflect on their life. Develop sense of fulfillment and acceptance of their life experiences.	

Infancy

Infancy is a busy stage of life (Figure 5-1). Growth and development is rapid. Most full-term newborns weigh 7 to 9 pounds at birth and are 19 to 21 inches long. By 6 months, a baby's weight usually doubles, then triples by 12 months. Length may range from 22 to 30 inches by 12 months. Physical changes progress from uncoordinated muscle movements at birth to being able to hold the head up steadily by 3 months. At 4 months, most infants can roll over. An infant can hold objects at 5 months, sit up at 6 months, and begin to stand with support at 8 months. Between 8 months and a year, babies progress from standing to crawling to cruising (moving around while holding on to objects for support) to walking. Eyesight improves from blurred vision at birth to focused, clear vision by 2 to 3 months. Vocalizing progresses from crying and random sounds to speaking a few words. One-year-old children can feed themselves finger foods and has progressed from breast milk or formula to solid foods.

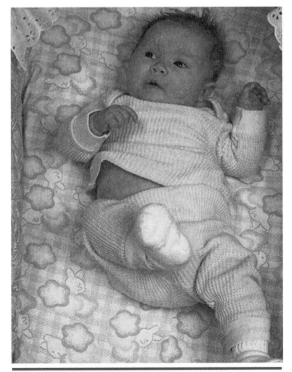

***Figure* 5-1**   Infancy is a time of growth and change.

Developmentally, the most important task is centered on feeding. An infant depends on a caregiver for food, comfort, and care. If these needs are regularly and lovingly met, the infant develops a bond and trusting relationship with the caregiver. If basic caregiving needs are not met, a baby may become fearful, less cooperative, and mistrusting of others.

Toddlers

The toddler stage is from 1 to 3 years (Figure 5-2). Physical growth is still rapid. Toddlers learn to run, jump, climb, walk up and down stairs, and ride tricycles. Their hand coordination improves. They begin to feed themselves independently, and they play with easy-to-hold toys, blocks, crayons and markers, and books. Language skills grow. They can understand many words, and they learn to speak in short sentences. They spend a lot of time playing but do not share well with others. Often, the child has temper tantrums and says "no" because the child wants to become more independent.

Self-control and self-confidence develop during these years. The important developmental task is toilet training and the children's bowel and bladder control. If children can dress themselves, feed themselves, and use the bathroom indepen-

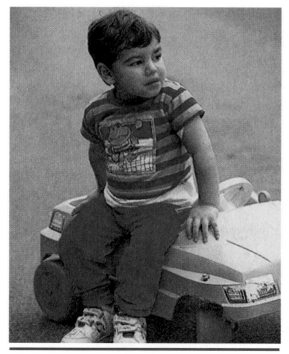

***Figure* 5-2**   The toddler develops physical skills, including walking and bowel control.

dently, they will be confident and have a sense of control. Toddlers who cannot master these skills may feel unsure about their ability to function in the world.

Preschool

Preschool is from 3 to 6 years (Figure 5-3). Preschool children continue to become more independent and self-reliant. Their physical coordination improves, and they are full of energy. They learn to write and color with more control and handle small objects more easily. Speech is fluent, and vocabulary grows. Preschoolers are social and learn to play and share with others. Children this age learn the concepts of time and gender differences. They are curious and ask many questions. They like to help and imitate others.

Independence is the main developmental task for these years. If the people around children encourage them to become self-reliant and use their energy, social skills, and creativity in positive ways, these children continue on to the next developmental stage. If the people around children do not encourage them to be responsible and do things on their own, a sense of guilt may develop. They may feel that they cannot do anything correctly.

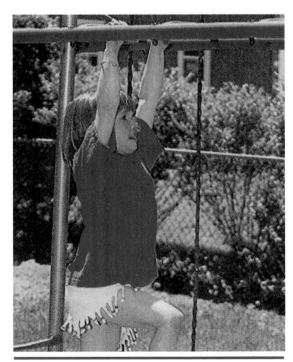

***Figure* 5-3** A preschool child continues to become more independent and self-reliant.

Childhood

Middle childhood is from 6 to 9 years, and late childhood, or preadolescence, is from 9 to 12 years of age (Figure 5-4). Children's life is now centered around school. They are very physically active. Large muscle and fine motor coordination continues to improve. Strength, balance, and flexibility increase. Children grow $\frac{1}{2}$ to 1 inch a year, and girls grow up to 2 inches a year during preadolescence. At this time children are social and prefer friends of the same gender and group activities. Some children, especially girls, begin puberty between ages 10 and 12.

Children this age enjoy doing work on their own. They need to be productive and successful. Experiences in school and with their friends help them reach this goal. Difficulty in school or with family and friends may cause children to feel inferior or unsuccessful as they grow older.

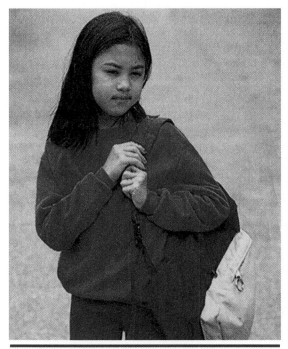

***Figure* 5-4** During childhood, life is focused and centered around school.

Adolescence

The teen years are filled with physical and emotional changes (Figure 5-5). Adolescents go through puberty. For girls, physical changes include breast development, the beginning of menstrual periods, growth of underarm and pubic hair, and increases in height and weight. Most girls reach their adult height during their teens. Physical changes in boys include change in voice and growth of facial, underarm, and pubic hair. Their sex organs mature, and height, weight, and muscle mass increase. Most boys reach adult height in their late teen years.

Adolescents are searching for an identity. They are looking for the answer to "Who am I?" They make decisions about education, job and career, sexual orientation, and spiritual beliefs. They also begin to separate physically and emotionally from their parents. Young people who are not able to develop a secure sense of identity during these years may have difficulty with relationships, decisions, and choices as adults.

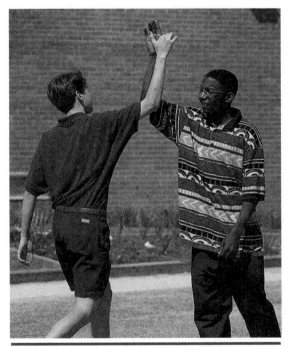

***Figure* 5-5** The teen years are filled with physical and emotional changes.

Young Adulthood

Young adulthood is from 19 to 40 years (Figure 5-6). Physical growth is complete. Young adults devote time and energy to school and jobs. They build lives separate from their parents and work toward financial independence and security. During these years the most important events focus on intimate relationships. Many people choose to marry or live with a partner. Most choose to have children. Adults develop communication and parenting skills; they learn to help others physically and emotionally. Young adults who are not able to develop close, personal relationships may become emotionally separated from others.

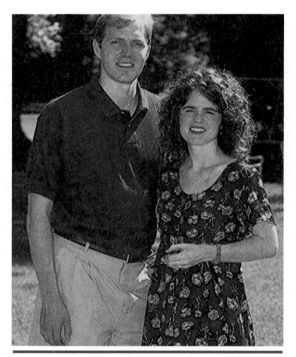

Figure 5-6   For young adults the most important events focus on intimate relationships.

Middle Adulthood

Middle adulthood is from 40 to 65 (Figure 5-7). Physical changes include gradual decreases in energy, endurance, and strength. Weight gain is common as metabolism slows. Signs of aging appear, such as gray hair, wrinkles, and the need for reading glasses. Women go through menopause. During these years, health problems and chronic illnesses are more likely to develop.

For most adults, this is a more stable financial time. Middle-age adults have more free time to do activities they enjoy. Children are usually older and have become independent or moved away.

This age has also been called the "sandwich generation." Many middle-age adults may have started their families when they were in their 30s or 40s. So at the same time that they are caring for young children, they need to help care for their own aging parents

Middle-age adults think about the growth and success of future generations. They wish to raise children who are mature, responsible adults. They may spend time in community service or volunteer activities.

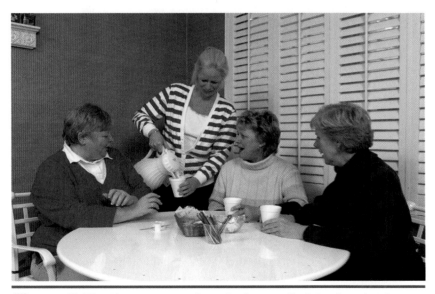

Figure 5-7   This age range has also been called the "sandwich generation."

Late Adulthood

Maturity, or late adulthood, is from age 65 to a person's death (Figure 5-8). Physical health declines as body systems and functions age. Illness and health problems become more frequent. A person may need help with daily living and personal care and may not be able to live alone. Emotional and social changes may include retirement, a smaller income, and death of partners and friends.

Older adults spend time thinking about past events in their life. If they feel positive about themselves and what they have done in life, they feel a sense of satisfaction. This also helps them to accept their eventual death. Older adults who are not satisfied about things in the past may feel hopeless and fearful.

Chapter 6 explores the physical, emotional, and social changes of an older adult in more detail.

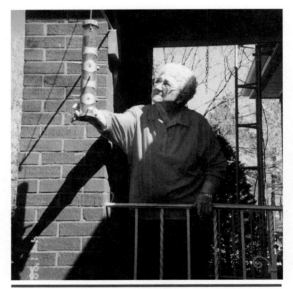

***Figure* 5-8** Emotional and social changes during late adulthood may include retirement, reduced income, and death of partners and friends.

CHAPTER REVIEW

1. What are the physical changes that occur as a person ages called?

2. What word refers to changes in psychological and social functioning?

Circle the one BEST response.

3. An infant develops these skills during the first year of life.
   a. Walking
   b. Speaking a few words
   c. Beginning to feed himself
   d. All of the above

4. Which developmental task is most important for toddlers?
   a. Feeding himself
   b. Climbing and running
   c. Toilet training
   d. Learning to play well with others

5. Preschoolers work toward which developmental goal?
   a. Playing by themselves
   b. Toilet training
   c. Independence and self-reliance
   d. Dependence on caregivers

6. What stage of life is centered around school?
   a. Toddlers
   b. Preschool
   c. Childhood
   d. Adolescence

7. Young people go through puberty during this time period.
   a. Childhood
   b. Adolescence
   c. Young adulthood
   d. Middle adulthood

8. Which developmental task is most important for an adolescent?
   a. Sense of independence
   b. Productivity
   c. Sense of identity
   d. Intimacy

9. Developing close relationships with partners and children occurs during which stage of life?
   a. Adolescence
   b. Young adulthood
   c. Middle adulthood
   d. Late adulthood

10. What age range often must care for children and aging parents?
   a. Adolescence
   b. Young adulthood
   c. Middle adulthood
   d. Late adulthood

11. People in which stage think about their life and accomplishments?
   a. Adolescence
   b. Young adulthood
   c. Middle adulthood
   d. Late adulthood

Answers are on page 704.

Caring for Older Adults

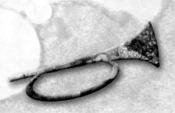

What you will learn

- The physical changes of aging
- Social, emotional, and cognitive changes of aging
- OBRA guidelines that help long-term care residents have a good quality of life

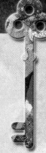

KEY TERMS

Cognitive The intellectual (thinking) functions of the brain

Confusion A mental state in which people do not know who the people around them are, where they are, or what time period they are in. Both memory and thinking are affected

Dementia Confusion caused by an injury to the brain or a long-term lack of blood flow to the brain; the confusion starts slowly, gets worse over time, and is permanent

Geriatrics Health care specialty for the care of older adults

Gerontology Study of the changes that occur with aging

Late Adulthood

Americans are living longer each year. Today 1 of every 8 Americans is age 65 or older. Older Americans are generally healthier and more active than in the past. During your career as a nursing assistant, you will likely care for many older adults. This special area of health care is called **geriatrics.**

Late adulthood extends from age 65 until a person's death. The older person has many physical, social, mental, and emotional changes during these years. This chapter will help you better understand the changes that can affect an older person's health and quality of life.

NOTES ON
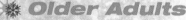 **Older Adults**

Study of the changes that occur with aging is called **gerontology.**

Physical Changes of Aging

Aging is a normal, expected part of life. Most physical changes of aging are gradual. This allows people to make changes in his lifestyle and health practices. That way, they can stay as active and healthy as possible as the years go by.

Table 6-1 describes the most common physical changes that occur in the body systems. As you read, think about the care measures you might use to prevent additional problems or complications related to that body system.

HOW & WHY

Keep in mind that aging is a normal life process.

Table 6-1

PHYSICAL CHANGES OF AGING	
Body system	**Physical changes**
Integumentary (skin)	• Skin becomes thinner, more dry, less elastic. • Wrinkles and age spots appear. • Less nerves, blood vessels, and fatty tissue. Less sensitive to pain. More sensitive to heat and cold. • Skin bruises easily and is easily injured. Healing takes longer. • Decreased sweating and oil gland production. • Hair color fades or becomes gray; hair loss and thinning. • Nails become thick and dry.
Musculoskeletal	• Energy level, ability to move and bend, and strength decreased. • Decreased amount of muscle tissue and cartilage. • Decreased bone mass. Bones break more easily. • Joints stiff and painful. • Decreased height.
Nervous	• Decreased function of senses. Hard of hearing. Decreased vision and sense of taste, smell, and touch. • Reduced blood flow to brain and loss of brain cells. • Memory loss, confusion, forgetfulness, slowed response time, change in sleep patterns. • Dizziness.
Cardiovascular (circulatory)	• Arteries narrowed and less elastic. • Blood pressure increases. • Heart muscle has to work harder, but pumps with less force and strength. • Reduced circulation and feeling in extremities, especially hands, lower legs, and feet.
Respiratory	• Lung tissue less elastic. • Breathing muscles weaker, leading to shortness of breath, weaker cough.
Digestive	• Decreased production of saliva and digestive juices. • Slower digestion, leading to constipation. • Decreased appetite; weight loss. • Indigestion; harder to digest fatty foods. • Difficulty swallowing; possible loss of teeth.
Urinary and reproductive	• Decreased blood flow to kidneys leads to reduced kidney function. • Urinary frequency, urgency, incontinence; need to urinate at night frequently. Decreased bladder capacity. • Enlarged prostate gland. • Slower sexual response.
Endocrine	• Reduced ability of the body to process sugars. • Decreased production of hormones, including testosterone, estrogen, progesterone. • Decreased total body water.
Immune	• Reduced ability of the body to fight infection.

Social and Emotional Changes

One of the biggest lifestyle changes older adults experience is retirement from a job or career. Most adults have worked for many years and look forward to retiring. They look forward to having more time to relax (Figure 6-1). They may also want to have the chance to travel, spend more time with family and friends, and have hobbies. Age at retirement varies (Figure 6-2). Most people retire between the ages of 58 and 70.

Retirement brings many changes. For many, the workplace is a social environment and source of friends. Work can also give people a good feeling about what they do. If people have few friends outside of work, retirement may make them feel lonely and isolated. If people have not developed other hobbies and interests, they may feel they are not doing anything important (Figures 6-3 and 6-4).

Retirement also brings income changes. The income of people who retire is often about half of their work earnings. Daily living expenses are not always smaller. Insurance benefits may be less, and the person may be spending more on health care expenses.

Social changes in late adulthood are often related to loss. Children grow up and may move away. Older and same-age friends and family may become ill, move away, or die. These kinds of separation and loss can lead to loneliness and depression. Loneliness can be increased if people are living alone or are trying to stay independent in their own home.

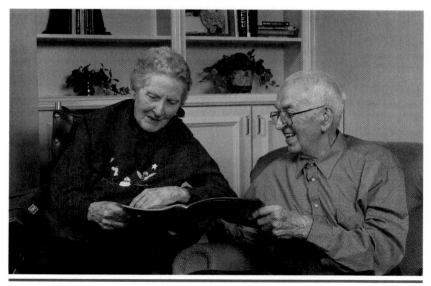

***Figure* 6-1**   A retired couple enjoying time together.

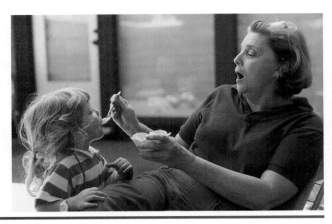

Figure 6-2 **A,** Many retired people remain active. **B,** The retired person enjoys many activities.

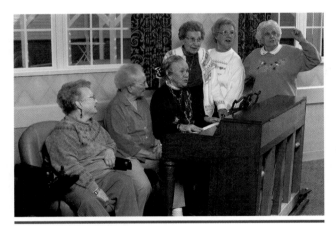

Figure 6-3 Exercise and activity help the older adult stay healthier.

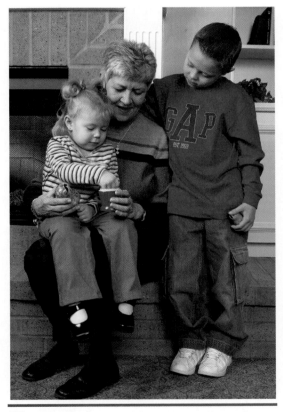

Figure 6-4 An older woman enjoys her grandchildren.

Death of a partner often occurs in late adulthood. Living with the loss of a partner is a big change. If people have had a healthy relationship with their partner, they have a better chance of adjusting to the loss in a positive way. The help of family and friends after the death also helps the person to deal with the loss. Problems in the relationship or lack of support in the grieving period can lead to serious physical and mental health problems.

Older adults may gradually need to get help from family and friends in carrying out daily activities (Figure 6-5).

As physical limitations increase, people may no longer be able to live alone.

Older adults may need to move to a place where they can get help with activities of daily living and personal care. If someone has to depend on family members for care, it can cause stress in family relationships. If people have to move away from their own home, they may feel angry, depressed, or helpless.

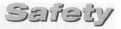

NOTES ON
☯ Culture

The way people deal with the physical, social, and emotional changes that occur with aging may be determined by their cultural background. In many cultures the older person is considered the most important member of the family and expects to be given special treatment. In some cultures it is expected that older people will move in with their children or grandchildren.

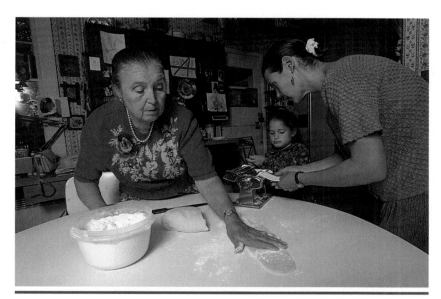

Figure 6-5   Family relationships play an important role in the life of the older person.

Cognitive Changes

Cognitive changes also affect an older person's quality of life and health. The term **cognitive** relates to the intellectual functions the brain carries out. These functions include thinking, memory, judgment, reasoning, and problem solving.

Cognitive effects of aging include the following:

- Memory loss, especially short-term memory loss
- Forgetfulness or having a hard time remembering things
- Slower response and thinking time. This affects judgment and problem-solving skills.
- **Confusion** or being mixed up
- Dizziness and impaired balance
- Personality changes
- A change in sleep patterns such as difficulty sleeping or sleeping more
- **Dementia** or inability of the brain to think or understand in normal ways

Not every older person has these symptoms of cognitive impairment. In fact, memory for events that happened a long time ago is sometimes very good. Research studies have shown that negative cognitive changes can be reduced if a person is physically and mentally active throughout life.

HOW & WHY

As we age, brain cells die. The total mass of brain tissue decreases. As blood vessels become narrowed and less elastic, blood flow to brain tissue decreases. A smaller amount of oxygen affects all brain functions.

OBRA Guidelines for Residents Living in Long-Term Care Settings

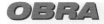

The Omnibus Budget Reconciliation Act of 1987 (OBRA) included guidelines and requirements for long-term care settings. These guidelines focus on improving the quality of life, health, and safety of residents in these centers. State and federal laws require nursing care centers to follow these guidelines. The guidelines protect and promote resident rights. Key resident rights are described in Box 6-1.

OBRA additionally has some very specific requirements about actions that keep a resident's dignity and privacy. These measures are so important that when state surveyors evaluate the care given in a center, they check to make sure that these actions are done for each resident. Box 6-2 details these care measures, which are listed under four main categories.

Box 6-1

OBRA REQUIREMENTS—RESIDENT RIGHTS

- Nursing care centers must tell residents their rights orally and in writing. The center must present this information before or during admission to the center, and the center must present it in a language that the person understands.
- Residents must be able to exercise their rights without interference from the center.

Information

- Residents and their legal representative have the right to see to all records about the resident. Information must be available within 24 hours of the request.
- Residents and their legal representative have the right to be told about the residents' medical conditions and their doctors.

Refusing Treatment

- Residents have the right to refuse treatment and/or take part in medical research.

Privacy and Confidentiality

- Residents have the right to personal privacy. Staff must obtain permission from the residents before persons not directly involved in the patient's care may observe any treatments or procedures.
- Residents have the right to talk with visitors or talk on the phone in private.
- Residents have the right to send and receive mail. Mail may not be opened by other people without the residents' permission.
- All information about the resident's care, treatment, and diagnoses is confidential. Information about money is also confidential.

Personal Choice

- Residents can choose their own doctor and can take part in the care planning and treatment process.
- Residents have the right to choose activities, schedules, and care according to what they prefer.

Disputes and Grievances

- Residents have the right to ask questions about care that they are receiving. The center must answer questions promptly about the concerns. Residents cannot be treated badly in any way for asking questions.

Work

- Residents are not required to work or perform services for the center. However, they may choose to do some work or service for the center as part of their care plan.

Participation in Resident and Family Groups

- Residents have the right to form and participate in resident and family groups.

Care and Security of Personal Possessions

- Residents have the right to keep and use the things they own. These items are to be treated with care and respect by caregivers.
- The center must try to make sure to not damage the person's property.

Freedom From Abuse, Mistreatment, and Neglect

- Residents have the right to be free from verbal, physical, sexual, and mental abuse. (These rights were explained in detail in Chapter 2.)
- Centers cannot employ persons who have been convicted of abusing, neglecting, or mistreating other people.

Freedom From Restraints

- Residents have the right to not have their body movements restricted. Restraints cannot be used for convenience of caregivers or as punishment.

Activities

- Centers must offer activity programs that meet the interests and physical and psychosocial needs of each resident. The residents may choose the activities they want to participate in.

Environment

- OBRA also outlines specific requirements concerning space, equipment, and features in the resident's environment that help keep the resident comfortable and safe.

Box 6-2

Courteous and Dignified Care to Residents

- Respect resident's private space and property.
- Assist with ambulation and transfers without limiting independence.
- Assist with bathing and personal hygiene without limiting independence. Care for hair, beard, and nails following resident preference. Appearance should be neat and clean.
- Help resident use glasses, hearing aids, dentures, and other prosthetic devices correctly.
- Assist with dressing in appropriate clothing of resident's choice that is neat and clean. Clothing and shoes are properly applied, fitted, and fastened.
- Help residents keep their dignity and independence while eating meals.

Courteous and Dignified Interactions With Residents

- Use proper name and title when talking to resident.
- Use appropriate tone of voice and eye contact during interactions.
- Stand or sit close to resident as appropriate. Touch resident only if the resident gives permission.
- Get residents' attention before speaking to them. Respect their social status, and listen with interest.
- Do not yell at, criticize, or embarrass the resident.

Maintain Personal Choice and Independence

- Involve and encourage residents to make decisions about their care planning, preferences, level of independence, room and roommate change, and scheduling and participation in activities.
- The resident may smoke in designated areas.

Privacy and Self-Determination of Residents

- Knock on resident's door before entering; wait to be asked in.
- Close door to resident's room, and use screens or curtains when performing personal care or procedures.
- Keep the resident's body covered when performing care and during doctor's examinations to avoid body exposure and embarrassment.
- Close bathroom door when resident is using bathroom.

CHAPTER REVIEW

1. What is the medical specialty concerned with the care of older adults.

2. What changes can occur in the immune system in older adults?

3. What changes may older adults face after retirement?

4. What is the focus of the OBRA guidelines concerning resident rights?

Circle the one BEST response.

5. Which change in the skin occurs with aging?
   a. Increased fatty tissue
   b. Improved circulation
   c. Increased sweating
   d. Thinner, more fragile tissue

6. How is the musculoskeletal system affected by aging?
   a. Less bone and muscle mass
   b. More bone and muscle mass
   c. Increased joint flexibility
   d. Improved endurance

7. Which factor is most responsible for changes in brain function as people age?
   a. Increased oxygen levels in the brain
   b. Increased blood flow to the brain
   c. Reduced blood flow to the brain
   d. Increased number of neurons

8. How is cardiovascular function affected as we age?
   a. Arteries are narrowed and stiff; circulation decreases.
   b. Arteries are enlarged and stiff; heart muscle function strengthens.
   c. No changes occur with aging.
   d. Overall blood flow increases throughout the body.

9. What happens to lung capacity as a person ages?
   a. Capacity is increased.
   b. Capacity is decreased.
   c. Capacity stays the same.
   d. Capacity doubles.

10. Which changes in digestive function occur with aging?
    a. Decreased production of saliva and digestive juices
    b. Decreased appetite and weight loss
    c. Difficulty swallowing and indigestion
    d. All of the above

CHAPTER REVIEW

11. What are symptoms of altered cognitive function in older adults?
   a. Memory loss and faster response time
   b. Memory loss and slower response time
   c. Memory improvement and improved judgment
   d. Changes in sleep patterns and improved judgment

12. Mr. Salazar is a resident in a long-term care center. He has a visitor and asks that he be able to talk in private with his friend. Which resident right relates to this request?
   a. Information
   b. Personal choice
   c. Privacy and confidentiality
   d. Activities

13. After you help Mr. Salazar shower, you ask him how he would like his hair styled. Which OBRA-required care measure are you following?
   a. Courteous and dignified care to residents
   b. Courteous and dignified interactions with residents
   c. Maintain personal choice
   d. Privacy and self-determination of residents

Answers are on pages 704 to 705.

CHAPTER 7

Body Structure and Function

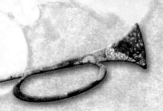

What you will learn

- How the human body is organized
- The organs and purpose of each body system:
  - Integumentary system
  - Musculoskeletal system
  - Nervous/sensory system
  - Cardiovascular (circulatory) system
  - Respiratory system
  - Digestive system
  - Urinary system
  - Reproductive system
  - Endocrine system
  - Immune system
- Normal changes that occur in the body as we age

KEY TERMS

Adipose tissue Fat tissue

Body systems Organs that work together to perform a specific function

Cell The basic unit of body structure

Cerumen Earwax

Ceruminous gland Specialized sweat gland in the ear that secretes cerumen

Dermis The layer of tissue under the epidermis

Epidermis The outer layer of the skin

Expiration The act of breathing out

Hormones Substances secreted by the endocrine glands into the bloodstream

Inspiration The act of breathing in

Joint The union where two or more bones come together

Organs Group of tissues that perform a specialized function, such as the lungs

Pathogens Disease-causing organisms

Perspiration Sweat

Respiration The cycle of breathing in and out

Saliva Liquid in the mouth secreted by the salivary glands, sometimes called "spit"

Subcutaneous Tissue beneath the dermis that contains the fat layer

Sutures A type of immovable joint in between the bones in the skull

Tissue Groups of cells that perform a specialized function

Understanding the Human Body

The human body has millions of parts that work together to keep you going. The basic unit of body structure is the **cell.** Cells are so small they can only be seen with a microscope. Each cell has the same basic structure, but the way cells work, their size, and their shape may be different. Cells need food, water, and oxygen to live and do their jobs well. Cells are the building blocks of the body.

Groups of cells that are similar make up **tissues.** Tissues are groups of cells that work together to perform the same task. Skin and muscles are two types of tissues. Groups of tissues that perform a specific function are called **organs.** The heart, stomach, and brain are all examples of organs. Organs that work together to perform a specific function make up **body systems.** The digestive system is an example of a body system (Figure 7-1).

The body is divided into 10 major body systems. Each body system helps the total body to function. It is important to understand the normal functioning of the human body so that you understand how normal aging and illness affect the body.

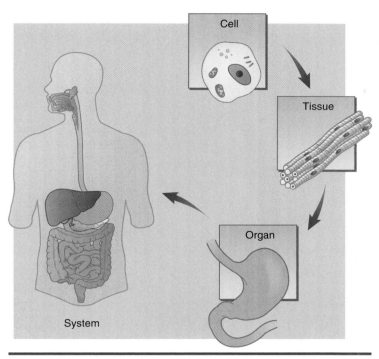

***Figure* 7-1**   How the body is organized.

The Body Systems

Integumentary System

The integumentary system is the largest system of the body (Figure 7-2). The skin, hair, and nails make up the integumentary system. It covers the body and protects the internal organs and helps regulate body temperature and eliminate waste through **perspiration** (sweat). Nerve endings in the skin allow you to feel cold, heat, pain, pressure, and other sensations. The skin protects the body and contains both dead and living cells. Dead cells constantly fall off and are replaced by new cells.

The skin has two different layers, the **epidermis** (outer layer) and the **dermis** (inner layer). Under the dermis is the **subcutaneous** layer. This layer is not really part of the skin. The subcutaneous layer has connective tissue and **adipose** (fat) tissue. The subcutaneous layer insulates the body and connects the skin to what is under it.

Hair is a part of the integumentary system too. Hair covers the entire body except for the nipples, parts of the external reproductive organs, the palms of the hands, and the soles of the feet. Nails protect the tips of the fingers and toes.

Hair shaft — Pore

Stratum corneum

Epidermis

Touch receptors

Stratum germinativum

Free nerve endings

Sebaceous gland

Nerve ending

Dermis

Pressure receptor

Subcutaneous layer

Artery

Nerve (pain)

Vein

Sweat gland

Adipose tissue

Connective tissue

Figure 7-2 The skin.

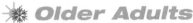
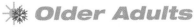
The skin contains oil and sweat glands. Oil glands are located near the hair shaft. They make an oily substance near the hair shaft that goes up to the surface of the skin. The oil keeps the skin moist. Sweat glands are in all areas of the skin with many on the bottom of the feet and palms of the hands. You have approximately 3 million sweat glands in your body. Sweat glands respond to emotional stress and secrete more sweat when you become frightened or upset. Another type of sweat gland is the **ceruminous gland.** The ceruminous glands are in the ear canal and make **cerumen,** or earwax.

Musculoskeletal System

The parts of the musculoskeletal system are the bones, joints, cartilage, ligaments, and muscles (Figures 7-3 and 7-4). The bones support the weight of the body and protect internal organs. With the help of the muscles and joints the bones allow us to move around. Bones store important minerals such as calcium and make red blood cells. Muscle movement produces heat, which helps to control body temperature.

Bones are actually living tissue. The human body has 206 bones. The place where two or more bones meet is called a **joint.** Joints keep the bones together and allow us to move. Without joints we would be stiff and unable to move around. But there are some joints that are immovable, which means

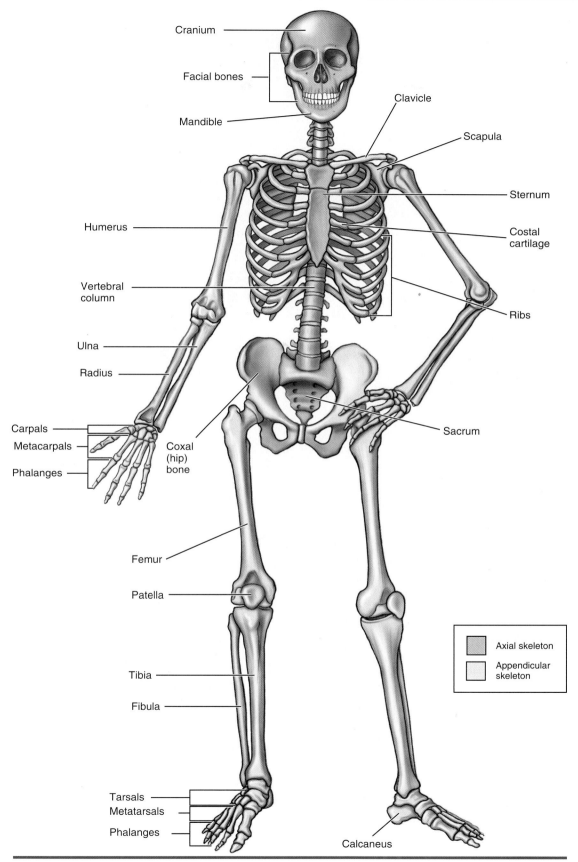

Cranium

Facial bones

Mandible

Clavicle

Scapula

Sternum

Humerus

Costal cartilage

Vertebral column

Ribs

Ulna

Radius

Carpals

Metacarpals

Phalanges

Coxal (hip) bone

Sacrum

Femur

Patella

Tibia

Fibula

Tarsals

Metatarsals

Phalanges

Calcaneus

Axial skeleton

Appendicular skeleton

Figure 7-3   The skeleton.

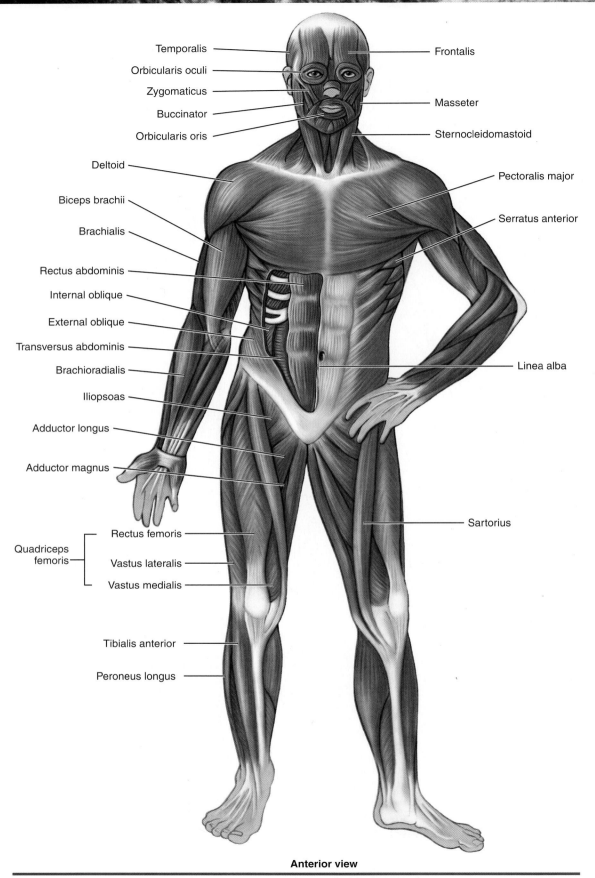

Temporalis
Orbicularis oculi
Zygomaticus
Buccinator
Orbicularis oris

Frontalis
Masseter
Sternocleidomastoid

Deltoid
Biceps brachii
Brachialis
Rectus abdominis
Internal oblique
External oblique
Transversus abdominis
Brachioradialis
Iliopsoas
Adductor longus
Adductor magnus

Pectoralis major
Serratus anterior
Linea alba

Quadriceps femoris
{ Rectus femoris
Vastus lateralis
Vastus medialis }

Sartorius

Tibialis anterior
Peroneus longus

Anterior view

Figure 7-4 **A,** Major muscles of the body. *Continued*

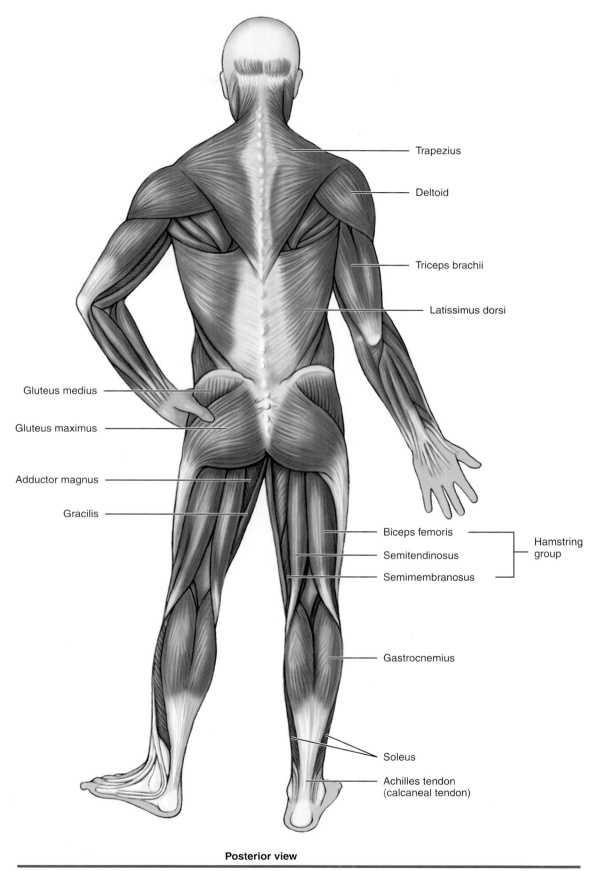

Trapezius

Deltoid

Triceps brachii

Latissimus dorsi

Gluteus medius

Gluteus maximus

Adductor magnus

Gracilis

Biceps femoris

Semitendinosus

Semimembranosus

Hamstring group

Gastrocnemius

Soleus

Achilles tendon (calcaneal tendon)

Posterior view

Figure 7-4, cont'd **B,** Major muscles of the body.

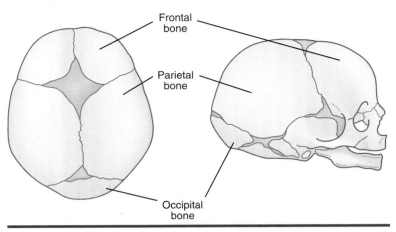

Figure 7-5 The joints in the skull where the bones come together are called sutures and are considered an immovable joint.

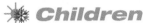
that they do not move. The joints in the skull where the bones come together are called **sutures** and are an immovable joint (Figure 7-5).

A disk of cartilage connects the bones in the spine. The spinal column has slightly movable joints (Figure 7-6).

Freely movable joints allow you to move around more than the other two types of joints. There are three main types of freely movable joints.

1. A hinge joint allows movement like a hinge on a door. Elbows, knees, and fingers are examples of hinge joints.
2. A ball-and-socket joint is formed when the ball-shaped end of one bone fits into the cup-shaped socket on another bone. This type of joint allows you to move in many different directions. The shoulder and hip are examples of ball-and-socket joints.
3. A pivot joint allows for rotation. An example of this motion would be the side-to-side movement of your head when you shake your head no. Where the first bone in the neck pivots on the second bone in the neck is this type of joint (Figure 7-7).

The human body has more than 500 muscles. Some muscles are voluntary, which means that you can control them. The muscles in your arms or legs are voluntary muscles. Involuntary muscles work automatically and cannot be consciously controlled. The muscles in the stomach and heart are involuntary and do their job whether you are thinking about them or not.

Tough connective tissues called tendons connect the muscles to the bones. When the muscles shorten (contract), the tendons at each end of the muscle make the bone move. When muscles

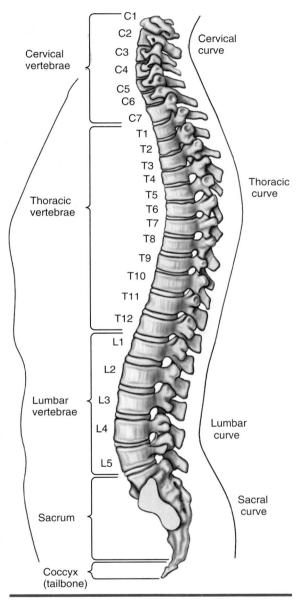

Cervical
vertebrae

C1
C2
C3
C4
C5
C6
C7

Cervical
curve

Thoracic
vertebrae

T1
T2
T3
T4
T5
T6
T7
T8
T9
T10
T11
T12

Thoracic
curve

Lumbar
vertebrae

L1
L2
L3
L4
L5

Lumbar
curve

Sacrum

Coccyx
(tailbone)

Sacral
curve

Figure 7-6   A disk of cartilage connects the
bones in the spine. The spinal column has
slightly movable joints.

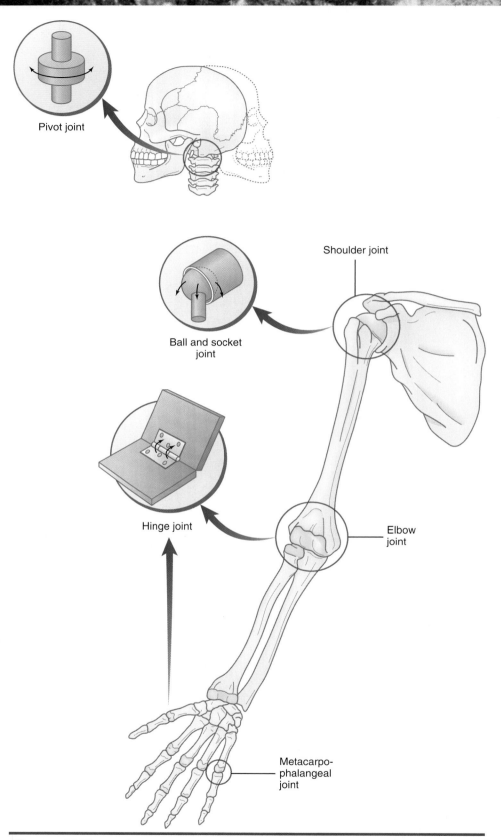

Pivot joint

Shoulder joint

Ball and socket
joint

Hinge joint

Elbow
joint

Metacarpo-
phalangeal
joint

Figure 7-7 Freely movable joints allow you to move more freely than the other two types of joints. Hinge joints, ball-and-socket joints, and pivot joints are freely movable joints.

move, they produce heat. The more you move, the more heat you produce. An example of this is a person who is cold doing a few jumping jacks to warm up.

Nervous System/Sensory System

The nervous system is the mechanical control system of the body and is made up of the brain, the spinal cord, and the nerves (Figure 7-8). Messages are carried from the brain to all parts of the body and back again through the nerves. The brain and spinal cord make up the central nervous system. The

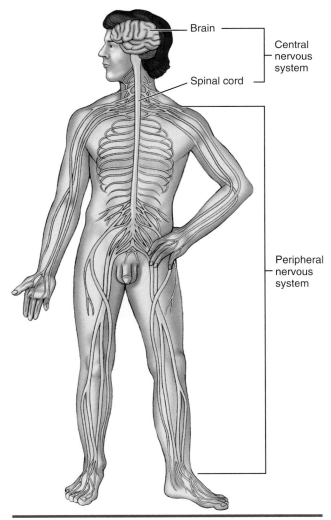

Brain

Central nervous system

Spinal cord

Peripheral nervous system

Figure 7-8   The brain and spinal cord make up the central nervous system. The nerves that connect the brain and spinal cord to the rest of the body are called the peripheral nervous system.

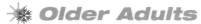
nerves that connect the brain and spinal cord to the rest of the body are called the peripheral nervous system.

The brain is inside the skull, and each section of the brain controls a different part of the body. The right side of the brain controls the left side of the body, and the left side of the brain controls the right side of the body. In the brain there are different parts to control movement, speech, memory, and other activities.

Your 5 senses gather information about what you see, hear, taste, smell, and feel (Figure 7-9). The information is sent to your brain, where it is processed. Your eyes are your organ of sight or vision (Figure 7-10). When you look around the room, you see

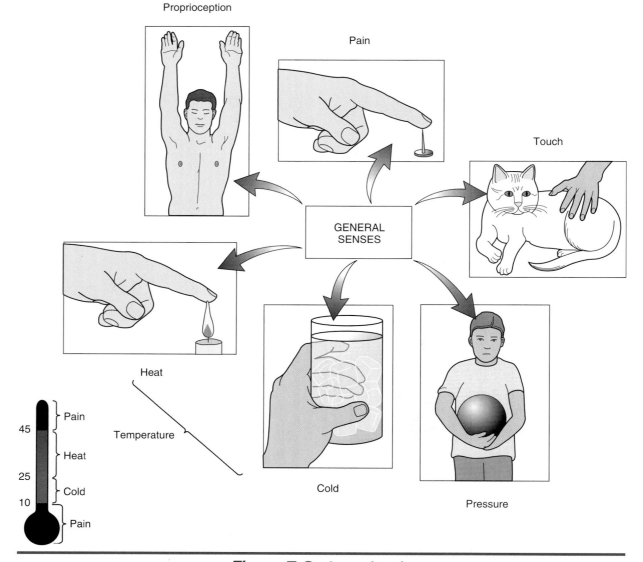

Figure 7-9   Sense of touch.

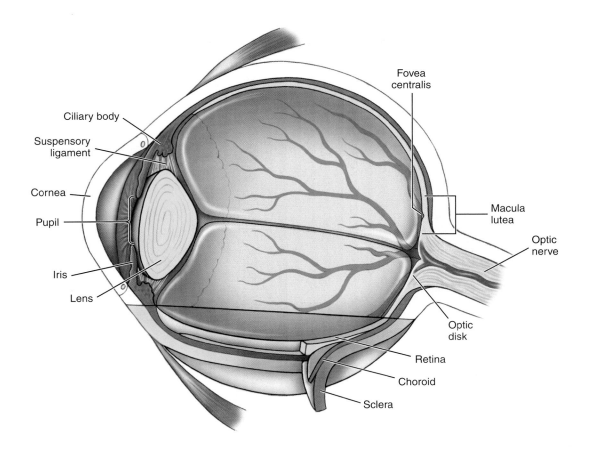

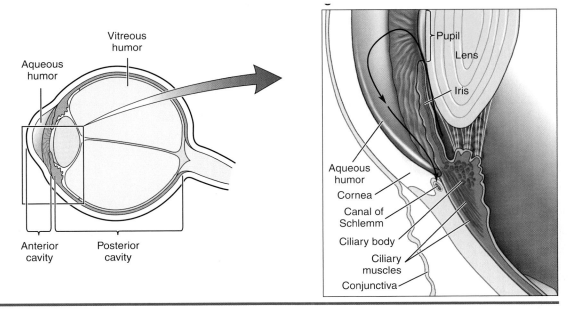

Figure 7-10   Structure of the eyeball.

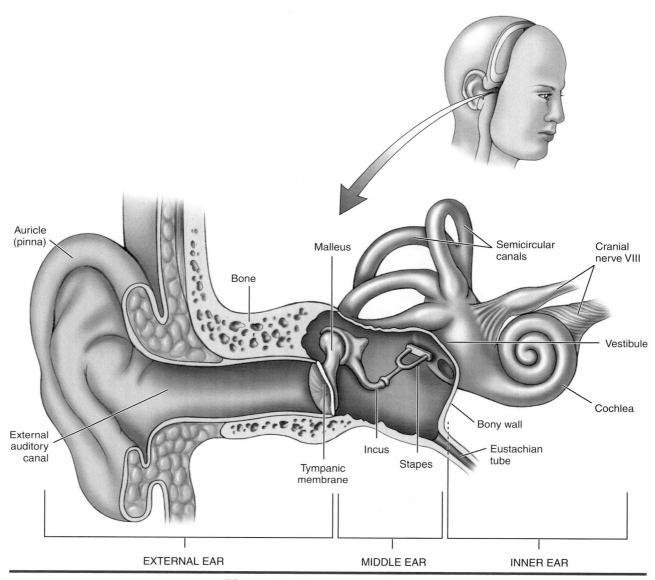

Auricle
(pinna)

Bone

Malleus

Semicircular
canals

Cranial
nerve VIII

Vestibule

Cochlea

Bony wall

Eustachian
tube

Stapes

Incus

Tympanic
membrane

External
auditory
canal

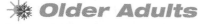

EXTERNAL EAR   MIDDLE EAR   INNER EAR

Figure 7-11   Structure of the ear.

NOTES ON
✳ *Older Adults*

It is normal for vision and hearing to decrease slightly with aging. It becomes more difficult to read small print and hard to hear high- and low-pitched sounds. The sense of taste and sense of smell get weaker.

the pictures on the wall and the person sitting next to you. Your ears are the organ of hearing and balance (Figure 7-11). When a dog barks or the radio is on, the information is sent to your brain through the ears.

Your sense of taste is found in your tongue, which has receptors that are called taste buds (Figure 7-12). When you take a bite of chocolate or drink lemonade, the message about the taste is sent to your brain. Your nose provides you with your

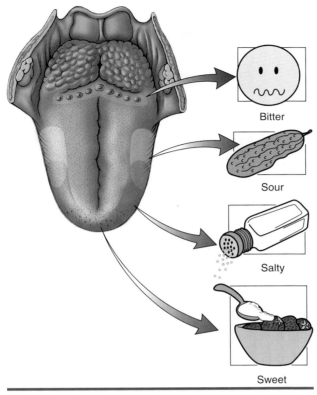

Bitter

Sour

Salty

Sweet

Figure 7-12   Sense of taste; four sensations: bitter, sour, salty, and sweet.

sense of smell (Figure 7-13). If someone is smoking a cigar, your nose picks up on the odor and sends a message to your brain.

The skin has the ability to "feel." Sharp, dull, hot, cold, smooth, and rough are just a few of sensations your skin can feel. As your senses gather information, it is sent to the brain to be processed. The brain puts all of the information together and sends out a message to the muscles causing you to move or to take some action. For example, imagine that you are holding a small puppy in your arms. Your eyes can see the puppy and send a message to your brain about the color and size of the animal. If the puppy is barking, your ears will also send that message to the brain. Let's say that this puppy just had a bath and smells fresh and feels warm and soft. All these messages are being sent to the brain at the same time. The brain tells your muscles that this is a pleasant experience and you give the puppy a gentle hug. This is an example of 4 of your senses working together with your brain. Your sense of taste was not used at this time. If you were given a taste of

NOTES ON
☯ *Culture*

People's culture or background can determine what they think is a "good" smell or a "bad" smell.

HOW & WHY

If young people touch a hot stove, they will immediately pull their hand away. If elderly people touch the same hot stove, it takes longer for the message to get from the hand to the brain that the stove is hot and longer for the message to get back to the hand telling them to move their hand. Because of this, the older person is more likely to be burned.

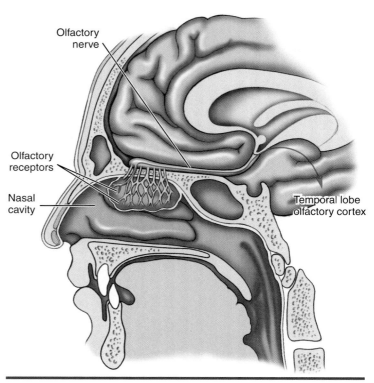

***Figure* 7-13** Sense of smell.

HOW & WHY

Because both taste and smell are important in our enjoyment of foods, some older people do not eat as well as they did when they were younger or may add more sugar or salt to the meals.

NOTES ON
❄ Older Adults

As we age, the heart muscle becomes slightly weaker and may not do a good job of circulating the blood.

NOTES ON
❄ Children

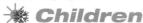

The heart rate of a child at birth is normally between 120 and 160 beats per minute. As the child ages, the heart rate gradually slows, and by the time a child has reached adulthood, between the ages of 18 and 20, the normal heart rate is only 60 to 110 beats per minute.

something, you would be able to tell if it was something sweet, salty, sour, or bitter. For example, you could tell if a liquid you tasted was vinegar or lemon-lime soda, even though they look very much alike.

Problems with memory and thinking are not normal parts of the aging process and will be discussed in Chapter 8.

The Cardiovascular System

The cardiovascular system, sometimes called the circulatory system, is made up of the heart, blood vessels, and blood. The heart is a strong hollow muscle that pumps blood to all parts of the body through the blood vessels (veins, arteries, and capillaries) (Figure 7-14). The heart pumps an average of 72 times per minute, which means that your heart will beat more than 3 billion times if you live to be 75 years old. The heart is about the size of your closed fist and is in the chest between your lungs (Figure 7-15). The blood takes oxygen and nutrients to the cells and takes away waste products from the cells (Figure 7-16). The blood and blood vessels also help to control your body temperature.

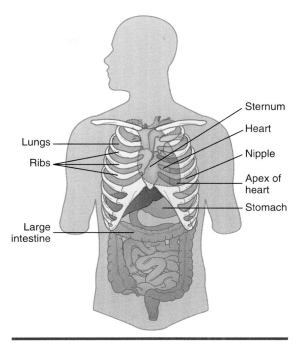

***Figure* 7-14**   Location of the heart in the chest cavity.

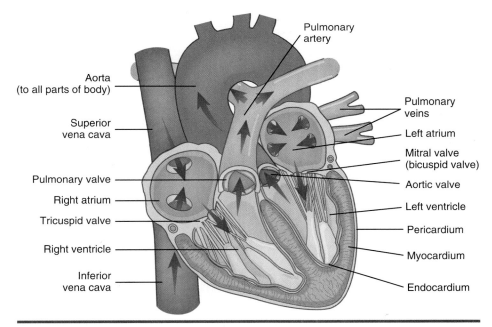

***Figure* 7-15**   Structures of the heart.

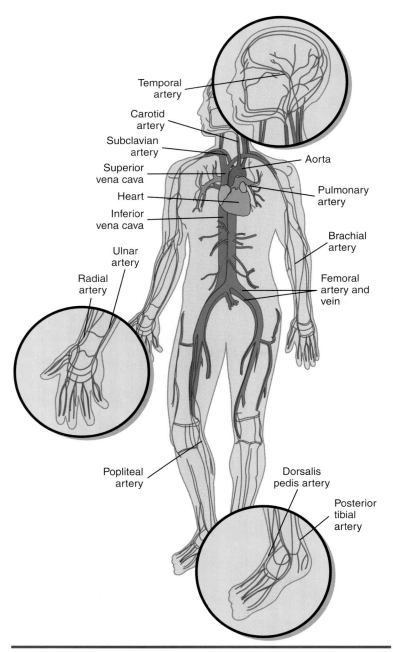

Figure 7-16 Arterial system.

HOW_&WHY

HOW&WHY

When the body is hot, the blood vessels dilate (open up) to help cool the body. When your cheeks become pink after you have been in a warm room, this is an example of the blood vessels dilating to allow the heat to leave the body. The blood vessels constrict (close up) to help keep heat in the body. If you go outside on a cold day without your gloves, the blood vessels in your hands will constrict and your fingers may become pale or turn slightly blue if you stay outside too long. This is your body's way of retaining as much heat as possible.

Sometimes fat deposits build up on the inside of the walls of the blood vessels. This causes the blood pressure to go up. Diseases of the cardiovascular system will be covered in Chapter 8.

When taking a person's pulse or blood pressure, you are using information from the cardiovascular system about your patient's health. Both pulse and blood pressure will be discussed in Chapter 13.

Respiratory System

The respiratory system contains the upper and lower respiratory tracts (Figure 7-17). The upper respiratory tract contains the organs located outside of the chest: the nose, pharynx, larynx, and upper part of the trachea. The lower respiratory tract is made up of the organs inside of the chest: the lower trachea and the lungs. Inside of the lungs the air passage is called the bronchial tree. The bronchial tree contains the bronchi, bronchioles, and alveoli (Figure 7-18). The respiratory system brings oxygen-rich air into the lungs during **inspiration** (breathing in). During **expiration** (breathing out), air, carbon dioxide, and other waste products leave the lungs. The cycle of breathing in and out is called **respiration.**

As you breathe in, air passes through the nose and mouth, where it is warmed and moistened. The lining of the nose traps dust and other small particles. This cleans the air when you inhale. Air passes through the pharynx into the larynx. The larynx is also called the voice box. The larynx produces your voice and does not let food and liquids go into your lungs. The trachea, also known as the windpipe, is a 4- to 5-inch–long tube that connects the larynx with the bronchial tree in the lungs. As air enters the lungs, it goes into either the right or the left lung through the bronchi. The bronchi break down into smaller passages called the bronchioles. The bronchioles control the flow of air into the alveoli, which are very small air sacs at the end of the respiratory passages. Oxygen passes across the very thin walls of the alveoli into the bloodstream. Carbon dioxide and other waste products pass from the bloodstream into the alveoli and are exhaled as you breathe out.

The lungs themselves occupy most of the chest cavity (Figure 7-19). Healthy lungs expand like balloons when you breathe in.

Diseases of the respiratory system such as emphysema affect the lung's ability to expand and the amount of oxygen that moves into the bloodstream each time a person breathes. Diseases of the respiratory system will be discussed in Chapter 8.

NOTES ON
❄ *Older Adults*

As we age, the lungs become less elastic and are not able to inflate as well.

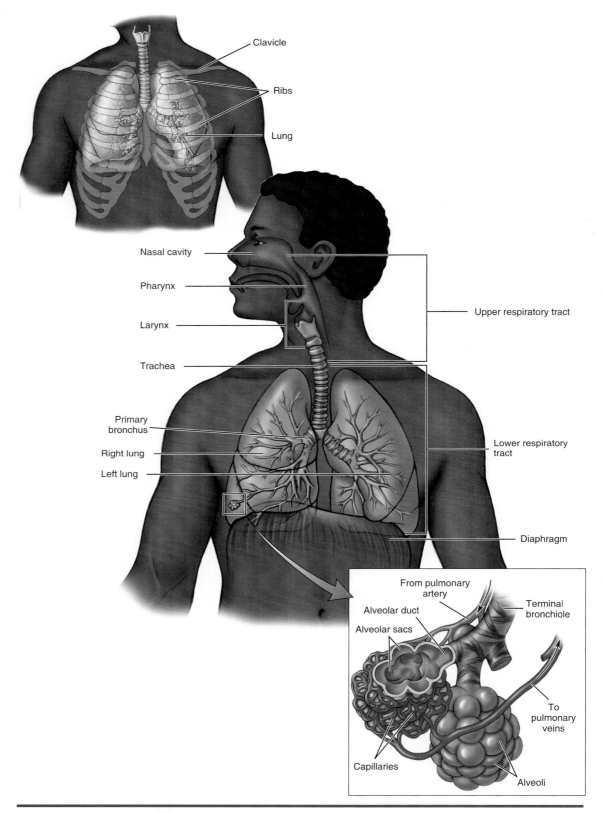

Figure 7-17 Organs of the respiratory system.

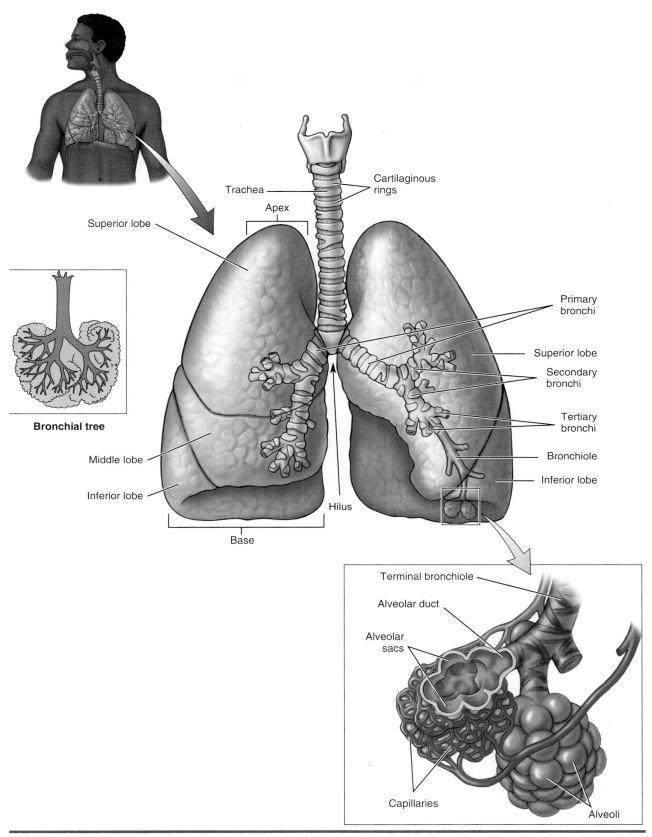

Bronchial tree

Trachea

Cartilaginous rings

Apex

Superior lobe

Primary bronchi

Superior lobe

Secondary bronchi

Tertiary bronchi

Bronchiole

Inferior lobe

Middle lobe

Inferior lobe

Hilus

Base

Terminal bronchiole

Alveolar duct

Alveolar sacs

Capillaries

Alveoli

***Figure* 7-18**   The bronchial tree contains the bronchi, bronchioles, and alveoli.

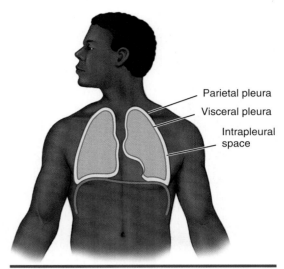

Figure **7-19** The lungs occupy most of the chest cavity.

Digestive System

Every cell of the body must have food to work properly. The digestive system breaks down the food you eat into particles small enough to be absorbed. The 3 purposes of the digestive system are the ingestion (taking in) of food, digestion (breaking down) of food, and the elimination of waste products (Figure 7-20). The digestive system begins at the mouth, where the teeth chew the food and the salivary glands produce **saliva** to moisten it. The food then travels down the pharynx into the esophagus, which is a long hollow tube that moves it into the stomach. In the stomach, the liver and pancreas make chemicals and enzymes. These mix with the food and help break it down. Then the food moves into the intestines, where the nutrients and water are absorbed from the food. The waste products that are left move through the rectum and exit the body through the anus in the form of stool, or feces.

There are actually 2 types of digestion in the digestive system. The first is called mechanical digestion. Mechanical digestion is the breakdown of the large food pieces into smaller pieces through chewing. The teeth, tongue, and muscles of the face and mouth all work together to make this happen. The second type of digestion is called chemical digestion. As food moves through your digestive system, saliva and other digestive enzymes are added to the food to help break it down.

In a healthy person with a well-balanced diet, the digestive process works well. As we age, the muscles of the digestive sys-

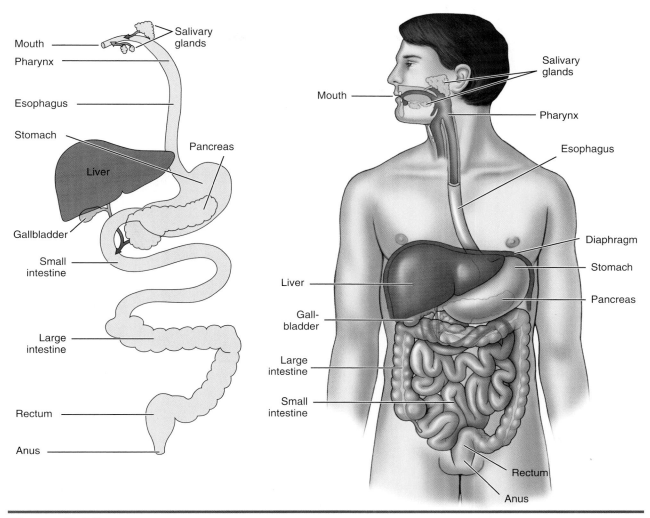

Figure 7-20 The digestive system begins at the mouth. The food then travels down the pharynx into the esophagus, which is a long hollow tube that moves it into the stomach. From the stomach, food moves into the intestines, where the nutrients and water are absorbed from the food. The waste products that are left move through the rectum and exit the body through the anus in the form of stool, or feces.

tem slow down and food moves through the system more slowly. The intestines reabsorb more water so the stool is drier, which can lead to constipation. The salivary glands may produce less saliva, so chewing can be more difficult. If the older person has lost some or all of his teeth, mechanical digestion is affected. Diseases and abnormal conditions of the digestive tract will be covered in Chapter 8 and nutrition in Chapter 19.

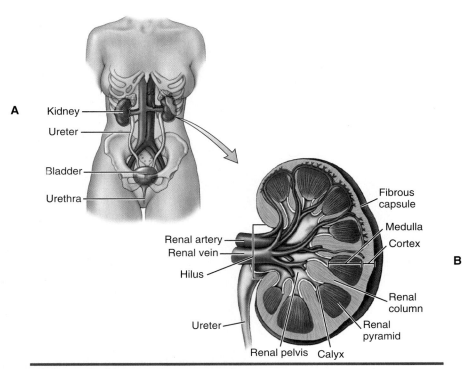

Figure 7-21　**A,** Organs of the urinary system. **B,** Internal structure of the kidney.

NOTES ON
✳ *Older Adults*

As people age, the ability of the kidneys to concentrate urine decreases. By the time you are 70 to 80 years of age, almost 50% of your filtering cells are gone.

NOTES ON
✳ *Older Adults*

Because of the decreased ability to concentrate urine, older people have to urinate more frequently. The aging bladder shrinks and becomes less able to contract and relax. This also means the older person has to urinate more frequently. Frequent urination in older men may be the result of an enlarged prostate gland, which will be discussed with the reproductive system.

NOTES ON
✳ *Children*

Some children also have difficulty concentrating their urine. This may cause bed-wetting even in children who have been potty trained.

Urinary System

The purpose of the urinary system is to remove waste from the body, to keep a stable balance of water and chemicals in the body, and to make urine. The urinary system is made up of the 2 kidneys, 2 ureters, the urinary bladder, and the urethra (Figure 7-21).

Your kidneys are located on either side of your spine above the level of your waist. Each bean-shaped kidney is about 4 inches long, 2 inches wide, and 1 inch thick. Blood flows into the kidney, where waste products and extra fluids are removed. These waste products and extra fluids make up urine. The urine moves through the kidneys into the ureters, where it goes to the bladder for storage. The bladder is a muscular sac that can hold up to 1000 ml or a little bit more than 4 cups of urine. When the bladder has about 200 ml or a little less than a cup of urine, you will feel the urge to urinate. The muscles of the bladder work together to move the urine through the urethra and out of the body. Male and female urethras differ in length. In women the urethra is short, about 1½ inches long. In men the urethra is about 8 inches long.

Urine is made of 95% water. Normal urine is clear and light yellow or straw colored. The average adult who drinks enough fluids each day will make an average of 1500 ml or around 7 cups of urine every 24 hours.

A

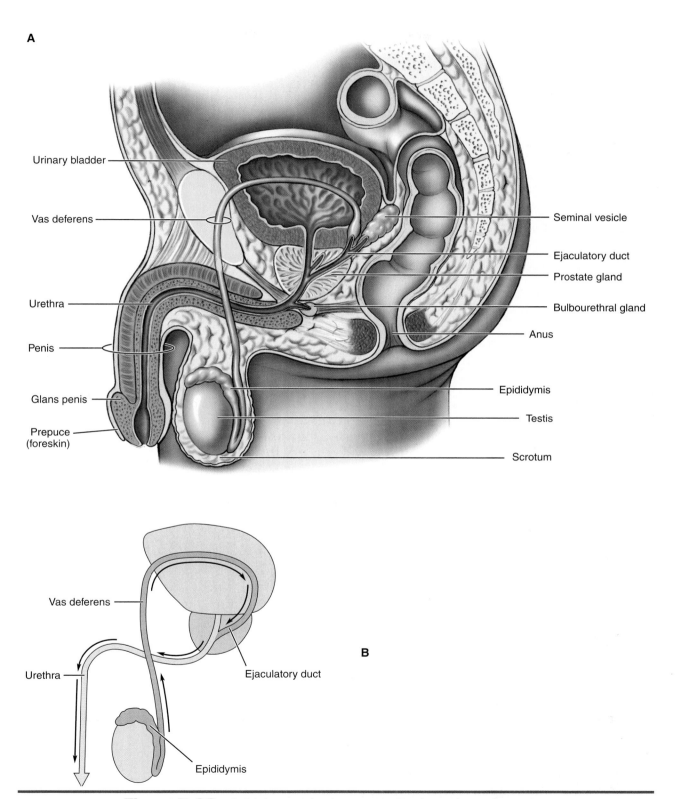

Urinary bladder

Vas deferens

Urethra

Penis

Glans penis

Prepuce
(foreskin)

Seminal vesicle

Ejaculatory duct

Prostate gland

Bulbourethral gland

Anus

Epididymis

Testis

Scrotum

Vas deferens

Urethra

B

Ejaculatory duct

Epididymis

Figure 7-22 **A,** Male reproductive organs. **B,** The pathway for semen.

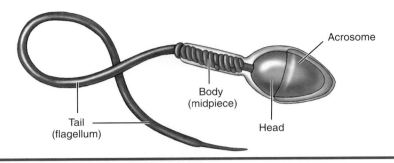

Figure 7-23 A sperm looks like a tadpole.

Reproductive System

The reproductive system has 2 functions. First it produces, nurtures, and transports the reproductive cells, ova (eggs) and sperm. Secondly it makes hormones. The male and female reproductive systems are similar in function but different in their structures.

The male reproductive system is made up of the testes, the penis, the prostate and other glands, and the urethra (Figure 7-22). You may remember that the urethra is also part of the urinary system. The testes are located in a sac between the thighs called the scrotum. Each day an adult male makes millions of sperm in his testes. Each sperm will contain 23 chromosomes, which carry the traits of the man. A sperm looks like a tadpole (Figure 7-23). Sperm and secretions from the male glands make up semen. The secretions nourish the sperm, help it to be transported, and lubricate the reproductive tract. Ejaculation is the movement of semen from the urethra to the outside and is controlled by the nervous system. Also, the testes produce the male hormone testosterone. When a boy reaches age 10 to 13, the production of testosterone increases rapidly. This development is called puberty. Men need testosterone to make sperm. Testosterone also causes development of secondary sex characteristics such as hair growth (especially on the face), deepening of the voice, increased activity of oil and sweat glands, and increased musculoskeletal growth.

The female reproductive system is made up of the ovaries, the fallopian tubes, the uterus, and the vagina (Figure 7-24). The 2 almond-shaped ovaries are located in the abdominal cavity on either side of the uterus. Women do not continue to produce eggs. At birth the female infant has approximately 2 million immature eggs. By puberty that number has decreased to about 400,000. Throughout her lifetime only about 400 eggs fully mature because a woman usually only releases one egg per month between puberty and menopause. Beginning at puberty, it is normal for one egg to mature fully and be released from the ovary during a process called ovulation. The egg contains 23 chromosomes, which carry the traits of the woman. The egg travels into 1 of the 2 fallopian tubes. If a sperm fertilizes the egg in the fallopian tube, the egg will normally continue into the uterus, where it will implant and grow into a baby. This journey through the fallopian tubes takes about 4 to 5 days. If fertilization does not occur, the egg deteriorates and is excreted from the body in the menstrual flow. The uterus is shaped like an upside-down pear and is located between the urinary bladder and the rectum. The primary function of the uterus is to provide a safe and nurturing place for a growing baby. The ovaries produce the female hormones estrogen and progesterone. These female hormones are important in the maturation of eggs. They are also responsible for the female secondary sex characteristics such as breast development, onset of the menstrual cycle, and fat deposits in the thighs, breasts, and buttocks. In the female, puberty is marked by the first period of menstrual bleeding, somewhere between the ages of 9 and 16. Menstrual periods normally continue regularly until the woman is in her late 40s or early 50s, when they become irregular and gradually stop. This phase is called menopause.

For reproduction to occur, the sperm and the egg must come together in a process called fertilization. The sperm and the egg each give 23 chromosomes for a total of 46. Each cell of the developing baby then contains half of its traits from its mother and half from its father. The fertilized egg implants itself into the uterine lining, where it will develop into a baby. It takes an average of 38 to 42 weeks for a baby to develop fully.

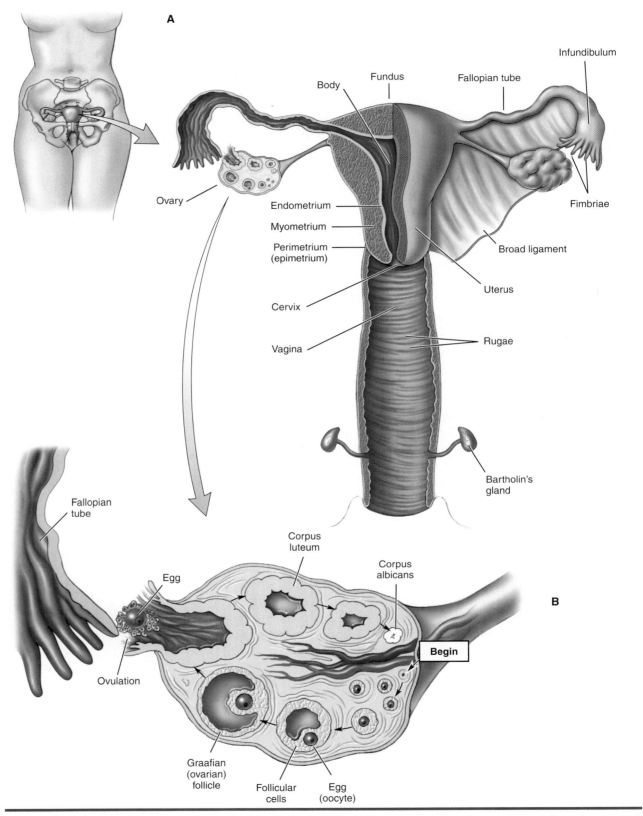

A

Infundibulum

Body

Fundus

Fallopian tube

Ovary

Endometrium

Myometrium

Perimetrium
(epimetrium)

Cervix

Vagina

Fimbriae

Broad ligament

Uterus

Rugae

Bartholin's
gland

Fallopian
tube

Corpus
luteum

Corpus
albicans

Egg

Begin

Ovulation

B

Graafian
(ovarian)
follicle

Follicular
cells

Egg
(oocyte)

Figure 7-24 **A,** Female reproductive organs. **B,** Beginning at puberty, one egg normally fully matures and is released from the ovary during a process called ovulation.

As women age, their ovaries shrink and menstrual periods stop. There is a decrease in estrogen production, which causes thinner tissue in the vagina and a decrease in secretions. This makes older women more likely to have vaginal infections. By the age of 50 the uterus has decreased in size by 50%, and supporting muscles and ligaments are weaker. The uterus may drop down or "sag." As men age, there is a decrease in testosterone and decrease in sperm count. Despite these changes, many men continue to father children into their 80s and 90s.

Endocrine System

If the nervous system is the mechanical control center for the body, the endocrine system can be considered the chemical control system (Figure 7-25). The endocrine system is made up of endocrine glands that make **hormones.** The hormones control

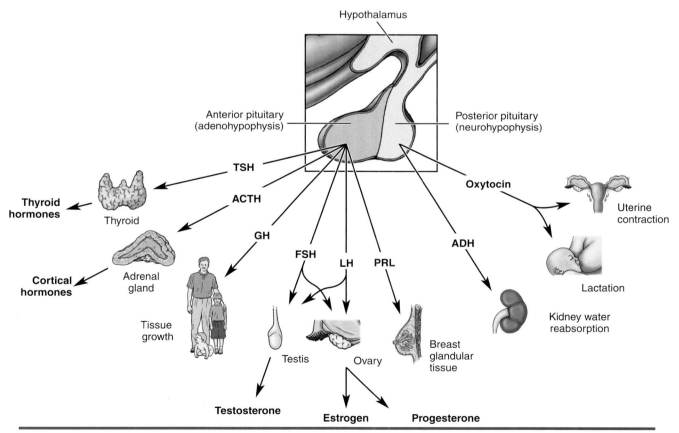

Figure 7-25 The pituitary gland is located in the brain and stimulates many of the other glands to do their jobs.

NOTES ON
❄ *Older Adults*

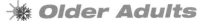

As we age, there is a decrease in most of our hormones. In most cases this does not cause illness, but the body systems and metabolic rate slow down.

many processes in the body. Hormones are important for growth and development, as discussed in the section on the reproductive system.

The pituitary gland is in the brain. Basically this gland makes many of the other glands become active. It also stimulates the growth of bone and soft tissue.

The thyroid gland is located in the neck just below the larynx (Figure 7-26). The thyroid gland controls metabolism, growth, and development. The parathyroid glands are on the back side of the thyroid gland. The parathyroid glands control the calcium levels in the body (Figure 7-27). The two small glands located above the kidneys are called the adrenal glands. The adrenal glands make hormones that help the body to respond to stress and inflammation and to control salt and sugar levels (Figure 7-28). They also make very small amounts of male and female sex hormones. The pancreas in the abdomen is also considered a part of the digestive system. The pancreas makes insulin and glucagon to control blood sugar levels (Figure 7-29). The ovaries and the testes are considered gonads and are part of the endocrine system, as well as the reproductive system. The thymus gland is in the chest behind the breastbone. The thymus gland makes a hormone important to the immune system. The pineal gland is located in the brain. It makes a hormone that controls sexual maturation. Many believe it plays a role in the sleep/wake cycle.

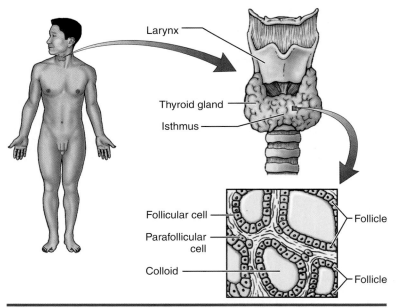

Figure 7-26   The thyroid gland is located in the neck just below the larynx.

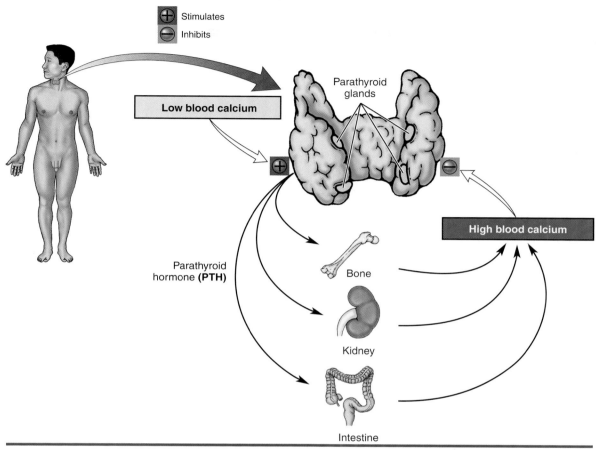

Figure 7-27   The parathyroid glands are on the back side of the thyroid gland and control the calcium levels in the body.

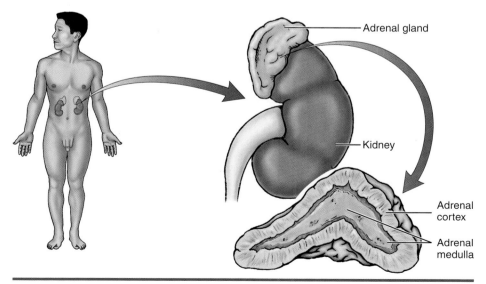

Figure 7-28   The adrenal glands are located above the kidneys. They secrete hormones that help the body to respond to stress and inflammation and to control salt and sugar levels.

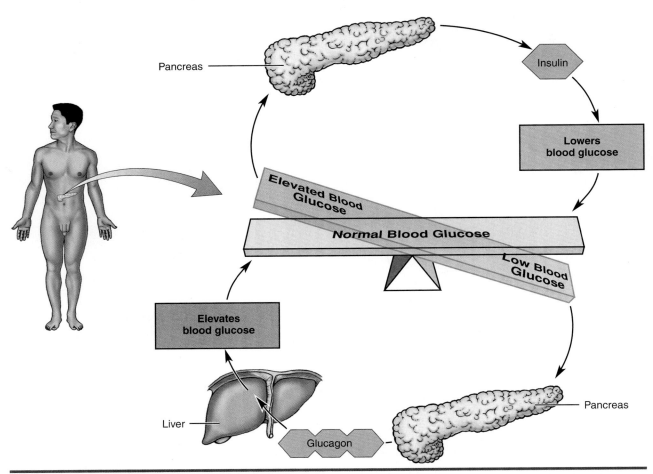

Figure 7-29 The pancreas makes insulin and glucagon to control blood sugar levels.

Immune System

Each day an army of germs (**pathogens**) attack your body and try to find a way into your body (Figure 7-30). Most of these attackers are turned away. This defense is called your immune system. The purpose of the immune system is to protect your body from disease and illness. The first line of defense includes mechanical barriers such as your skin and mucous membranes. When these barriers are intact, germs cannot enter the body. In addition, chemical barriers or secretions such as tears and

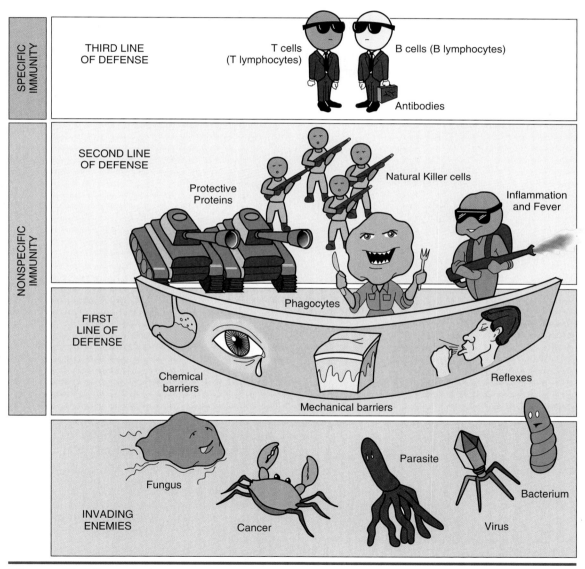

Figure 7-30   Each day your body is attacked by an army of germs, or pathogens, trying to find a way into your body. Most of these attackers are turned away. This defense is called your immune system. The immune system has three lines of defense (read from bottom to top).

saliva wash away germs before they can enter the body. Reflexes such as sneezing and coughing help to remove germs from your respiratory tract.

The second line of defense is needed if germs enter your body. Your white blood cells (phagocytes) ingest the harmful germs. When you are ill and have a fever, your body tries to kill the germs using your body's own temperature (fever and inflammation). The body also produces chemicals called protective proteins that help to fight the invading germs. Your third line of defense comes from special cells called T cells and B cells that have the ability to fight specific invaders. Your tonsils, spleen, and lymph nodes are all part of the immune system and help you to fight off disease.

There are 2 types of immunity. When you get a disease such as the measles, your body builds up a resistance to the disease so that you cannot get it again. Infants are born with this type of immunity, which lasts for about 6 months. The second type of immunity occurs when you are given a vaccination against a disease such as a polio vaccine. You do not have to actually get the disease to be resistant to it with this type of immunity.

NOTES ON
❄ *Older Adults*

As we age, our immune systems are not as effective and we are more likely to get infections. Many medications given to older people can affect their immune systems as well.

CHAPTER REVIEW

1. What type of a joint is the hip?

2. What connects muscles to bones?

3. Mr. Johnson has an inflammation of the bronchi. Which body system is affected?

4. Which body system is responsible for the ingestion of food?

5. Which body system makes hormones that regulate many processes in the body?

6. Which organ secretes insulin?

Circle the one BEST response.

7. The basic unit of body structure is a(n):
   a. Cell
   b. Tissue
   c. Organ
   d. Body system

8. Which body system do the skin, hair, and nails belong to?
   a. Integumentary
   b. Musculoskeletal
   c. Immune
   d. Digestive

9. Which body system do the bones, joints, and ligaments belong to?
   a. Immune
   b. Nervous
   c. Reproductive
   d. Musculoskeletal

10. Which body system is considered the mechanical control center for the body?
    a. Nervous system
    b. Immune system
    c. Endocrine system
    d. Musculoskeletal system

11. Which body system contains the heart, blood vessels, and blood?
    a. Respiratory system
    b. Digestive system
    c. Cardiovascular system
    d. Immune system

12. Which body system removes wastes from the body and maintains a stable balance of water and chemicals in the body?
    a. Urinary system
    b. Reproductive system
    c. Immune system
    d. Nervous system

CHAPTER REVIEW

13. Which body system is very different in structure in men and women?
a. Nervous system
b. Digestive system
c. Immune system
d. Reproductive system

14. Which body system protects you from illness or disease?
a. Respiratory system
b. Digestive system
c. Reproductive system
d. Immune system

15. How does the integumentary system change as people age?
a. The skin becomes drier and more fragile.
b. The subcutaneous layer of the skin becomes thicker.
c. The oil and sweat glands are more active.
d. There is an increase in hair growth.

16. How does aging affect the urinary system?
a. The number of filtering cells increases.
b. Older people urinate less frequently.
c. The urine is less concentrated.
d. The aging bladder stretches and becomes larger.

Answers are on page 705.

CHAPTER 8

Common Health Problems

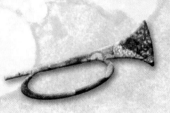

What you will learn

- Common health problems of each body system:
  - Integumentary system
  - Musculoskeletal system
  - Nervous system
  - Sensory system
  - Cardiovascular (circulatory) system
  - Respiratory system
  - Digestive system
  - Urinary system
  - Reproductive system
  - Endocrine system
- Communicable diseases
- How communicable diseases are spread
- Immune system

KEY TERMS

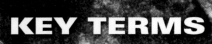
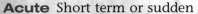

Acute Short term or sudden

Ascites A buildup of fluid in the abdomen

Bacteria Very small living things, some of which cause illness or disease; germs

Bronchitis Inflammation of the bronchi

Chronic Long-lasting or ongoing

Contagious Refers to a disease that can be spread from one person to another, such as a cold or the flu

Gangrene A condition in which the tissue dies

Hemiplegia Paralysis on one side of the body

Hepatitis Inflammation of the liver

Hyperglycemia High blood sugar

Hypoglycemia Low blood sugar

Incontinence Inability to control bowel and/or bladder functions

Jaundice A yellowish discoloration of the skin

Metastasize To spread

Paralysis (paralyzed) Inability to move

Paraplegia Paralysis from the waist down

Quadriplegia Total paralysis from the neck down

Seizure (convulsion) Sudden uncontrolled muscle contraction resulting from abnormal brain activity

It is important to understand the normal function and structure of the body systems talked about in Chapter 7. This will help you to understand the common health problems that affect each system. As you read the information in this chapter, you may find it helpful to refer back to Chapter 7. It is also important for you to know that the normal changes that occur in each system as we get older are not the same as illnesses or diseases. As a nursing assistant, you will spend more time with the patient than any other member of the health care team. If you are caring for a patient who has a disease that you do not know about, your charge nurse will tell you about the disease and its effect on the body. By knowing about common health problems, you can give better care to your patients.

Integumentary System

The skin performs many functions. It protects, acts as a barrier, controls temperature, detects touch, makes vitamin D, and gets rid of waste. Problems of this system include:

Acne

Acne is a condition of the skin in which the oil glands produce too much oil (Figure 8-1). The oil and dead skin cells block the pores, causing blackheads and whiteheads. A pimple is formed when the blocked pore becomes infected.

Athlete's Foot

Athlete's foot is an infection of the skin caused by a fungus. The skin itches, cracks, and is painful. This infection is most common on the feet and toes but can also affect the fingers, palm, and groin areas.

Dermatitis

Dermatitis is an inflammation of the skin caused by contact with something that is irritating, such as a chemical or plant (Figure 8-2). The skin becomes red and may develop bumps or blisters, which can become crusty and scabbed. Poison ivy is an example of dermatitis.

NOTES ON
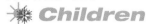 **Children**

While there are some forms of acne that affect adults, adolescents and teenagers most commonly get acne.

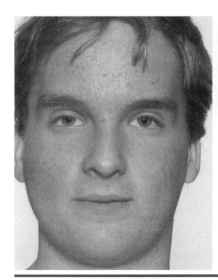 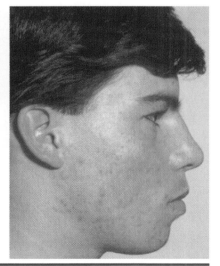

Figure **8-1**   Acne.

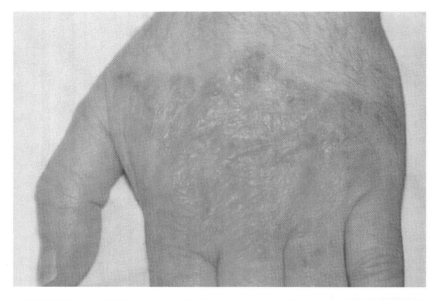

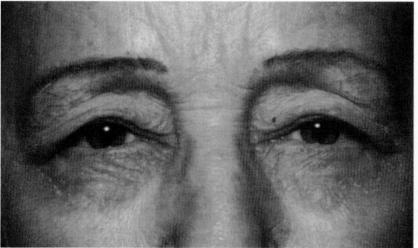

Figure 8-2 Dermatitis.

Eczema

Eczema is also an inflammation of the skin. In the early stage it causes redness and itching, and liquid comes out of the skin. In later stages the skin becomes dry and scaly. The cause of eczema is not known.

Hives

Hives are red patches and bumps on the skin that itch. Hives are due to an allergic reaction and may be caused by drugs, food, insect bites, or emotional stress.

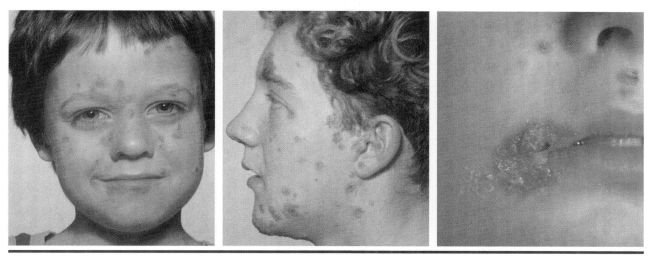

***Figure* 8-3** Impetigo.

Impetigo

Impetigo is a **contagious**, or spreadable, infection of the skin caused by **bacteria** (germs) (Figure 8-3). The skin is red and blistered and becomes crusted as the blisters break open.

Pressure Ulcers

Pressure ulcers are open areas on the skin caused by poor circulation. Additional information on pressure ulcers can be found in Chapter 23.

Psoriasis

Psoriasis is a chronic condition of the skin in which the skin becomes red with raised areas covered by silvery dry skin (Figure 8-4).

Skin Cancer

Skin cancer is one of the most common forms of cancer (Figure 8-5). Skin cancer may look like red, raised, hardened areas on the skin. Some skin cancers are open areas that scab but do not heal. Skin cancer may be caused by too much time in the sun.

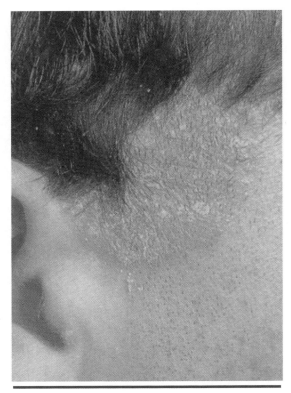

Figure **8-4**   Psoriasis.

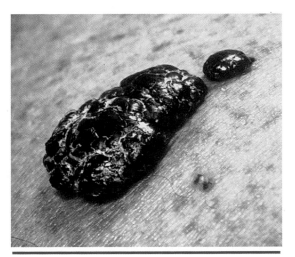

Figure **8-5**   Skin cancer is one of the most common forms of cancer. Skin cancer may look like red, raised, hardened areas on the skin.

Musculoskeletal System

Because the musculoskeletal system helps us to move, conditions of this body system usually limit a person's ability to move around freely. Problems of this system include:

Amputation

Amputation is the surgical removal of an extremity such as a hand or a foot (Figure 8-6). People may have a part of their body amputated after a severe injury or because of complications of a disease such as **gangrene** (tissue death) (Figure 8-7) or cancer.

Arthritis

Arthritis is an inflammation of a joint that is painful and usually swollen. There are many forms of arthritis. Osteoarthritis is the most common form and is caused by wear and tear on the joints (Figure 8-8). Rheumatoid arthritis is another kind of arthritis that affects primarily the joints. Gout is a form of arthritis caused by uric acid crystals in the joints (Figure 8-9).

NOTES ON
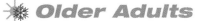 **Older Adults**

Osteoarthritis is frequently seen in older people. It commonly affects the hips, knees, spine, fingers, and thumbs.

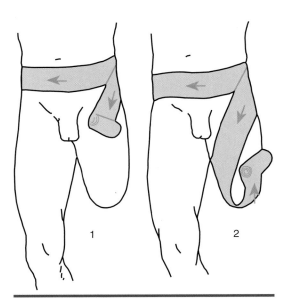

***Figure* 8-6** Midthigh amputation is bandaged to shape and shrink the stump.

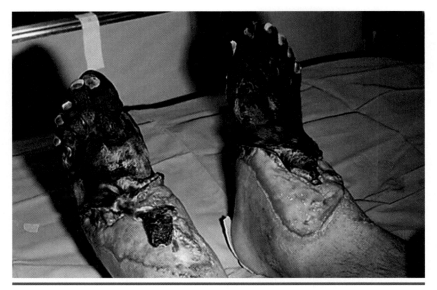

***Figure* 8-7**   Gangrene.

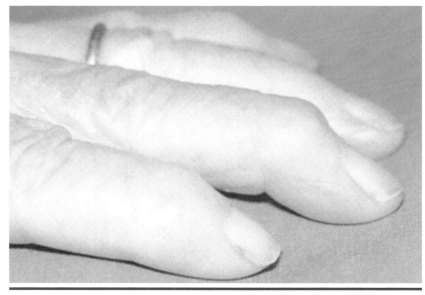

***Figure* 8-8**   Osteoarthritis.

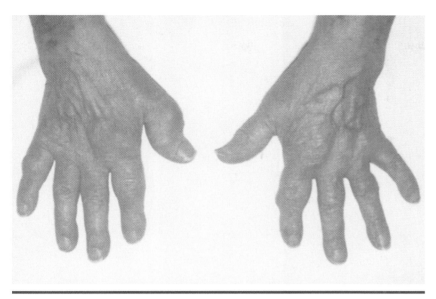

***Figure* 8-9**   Rheumatoid arthritis.

Atrophy

Atrophy is a wasting away of the muscle tissue. The muscles become smaller and weaker. Patients who are unable to move, such as those who have had a stroke or spinal cord injury may have atrophy. Additional information on atrophy can be found in Chapter 12.

Carpal Tunnel Syndrome

Carpal tunnel syndrome is an injury of the tendons and nerves that pass from the wrist into the hand. Not feeling anything or feeling a tingling in a hand are the most common symptoms. It is caused by repeated twisting and turning of the wrist.

Fracture

A fracture is a break in the bone. If the broken bones remain together and do not come through the skin, it is called a closed fracture. If the bones come through the skin, it is called an open fracture (Figure 8-10). Fractures can be due to an injury such as a fall. Fractures are also common in patients with osteoporosis.

NOTES ON
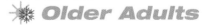
Older Adults

Hip fractures in the elderly are often the reason for admission to a nursing home. If there are complications from a hip fracture and surgery to repair the fracture, the patient may die.

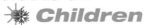
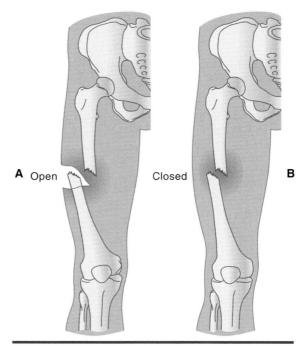

Figure 8-10 **A,** Open fracture. **B,** Closed fracture.

Osteoporosis

Osteoporosis is a bone disorder in which the bones become brittle and break easily. The spine, hips, and wrists are commonly affected. Osteoporosis occurs more frequently in the elderly and is more common in women than in men.

Nervous System

The brain is responsible for controlling the entire body, and diseases of the brain and nervous system can affect the entire body.

Alzheimer's Disease

Alzheimer's disease is a degenerative disease of the brain that usually affects older people. People with Alzheimer's disease have memory loss, which gets worse over time. Additional information on Alzheimer's disease and dementia can be found in Chapter 30.

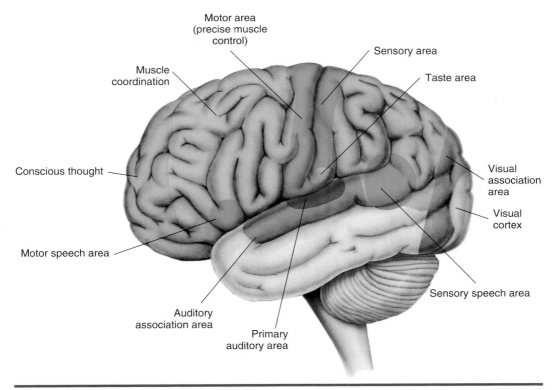

Motor area
(precise muscle
control)

Sensory area

Muscle
coordination

Taste area

Conscious thought

Visual
association
area

Visual
cortex

Motor speech area

Sensory speech area

Auditory
association area

Primary
auditory area

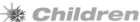

Figure **8-11**   Functions lost from a stroke depend on the area of brain damage.

Amyotrophic Lateral Sclerosis

Amyotrophic lateral sclerosis (ALS) is also called Lou Gehrig's disease. The patient loses strength, and the muscles become weaker. About half of persons with this disease die within 2 to 5 years.

Cerebral Palsy

Cerebral palsy (CP) is a condition caused by injury to an infant's brain before, during, or after birth. Lack of oxygen to the brain is the most common cause. Muscles and speech are affected.

Cerebrovascular Accident

Cerebrovascular accident (CVA) is also known as a "stroke." A CVA is caused by not enough oxygen getting to the brain because of a blood clot or bleeding in the brain. The brain cells die, and functions controlled by that part of the brain are affected (Figure 8-11). Patients who have had a stroke may have

NOTES ON
✳ Children

Children who are high risk for cerebral palsy include premature infants, babies with a low birth weight, and those who sustain head injuries such as falls or child abuse.

Box 8-1

WARNING SIGNS OF STROKE

Sudden numbness or weakness of the face, arm, or leg, especially on one side of the body
Sudden confusion, trouble speaking or understanding
Sudden trouble walking, dizziness, or loss of balance or coordination
Sudden trouble seeing in one or both eyes
Sudden, severe headaches with no known cause

NOTES ON
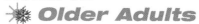 *Older Adults*

Strokes are the leading cause of disability in older adults and the third leading cause of death in the United States.

loss of body control, changing emotions, problems with vision or speech, memory loss, and **incontinence** (inability to control bowel and/or bladder functions). Patients who have had a CVA may also have **hemiplegia**, or **paralysis** (inability to move) on one side of the body. Warning signs of a stroke are listed in Box 8-1.

Epilepsy

Epilepsy is a seizure disorder in which the patient has chronic seizures. A **seizure** or **convulsion** is a violent and sudden contraction or shaking of muscle groups caused by changes in the brain's electrical function. The cause of epilepsy is not known.

Multiple Sclerosis

Multiple sclerosis is a chronic disease that affects the covering of the nerves. Eventually the person becomes disabled and must use a wheelchair. It is more common in white women between the ages of 20 and 40.

Parkinson's Disease

Parkinson's disease is a nervous system disorder that affects the person's coordination and causes tremors (shaking) and stiffness (Figure 8-12). The cause of this condition is not known. It is more common in white men over the age of 50.

Spinal Cord/Head Injuries

Spinal cord/head injuries are commonly caused by automobile accidents, falls, sports injuries, and stab or bullet wounds. These injuries can cause permanent damage to the nervous system. The problems the patient will have depend on the area that is injured.

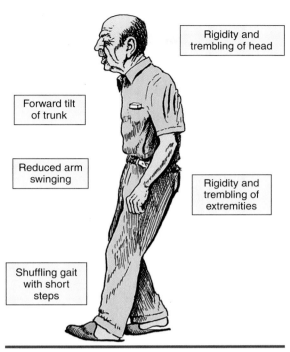

Rigidity and trembling of head

Forward tilt of trunk

Reduced arm swinging

Rigidity and trembling of extremities

Shuffling gait with short steps

***Figure* 8-12**   Signs of Parkinson's disease.

Total paralysis from the neck down is called **quadriplegia**. These patients have injuries to the neck and upper spine. **Paraplegia** is paralysis from the waist down (Figure 8-13). These patients have spinal cord injuries below the area of the neck and upper spine.

Sensory System

Common problems of the sensory system include diseases that affect the person's ability to see, hear, smell, or feel.

Cataract

Cataract is a disorder in which the lens of the eye becomes cloudy (Figure 8-14). The vision becomes blurred, and the person is sensitive to light and glare.

Glaucoma

Glaucoma is a buildup of pressure inside the eye that damages the nerve and eventually causes blindness (Figure 8-15).

NOTES ON
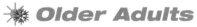 *Older Adults*

Aging is the most common cause of cataracts.

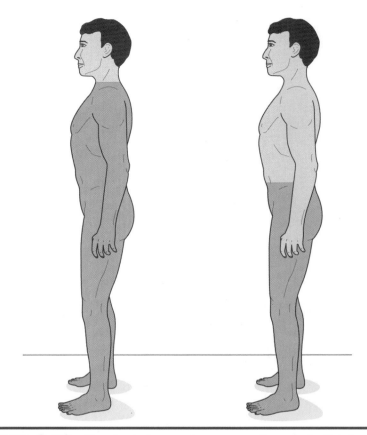

Figure 8-13   The shaded areas show areas of paralysis. Total paralysis from the neck down is called quadriplegia. Paraplegia is paralysis from the waist down.

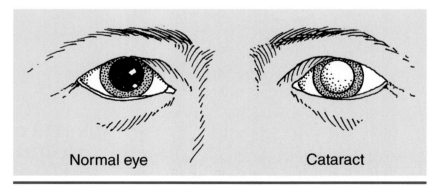

Normal eye   Cataract

Figure 8-14   In this drawing the right eye is normal, and the left eye has a cataract.

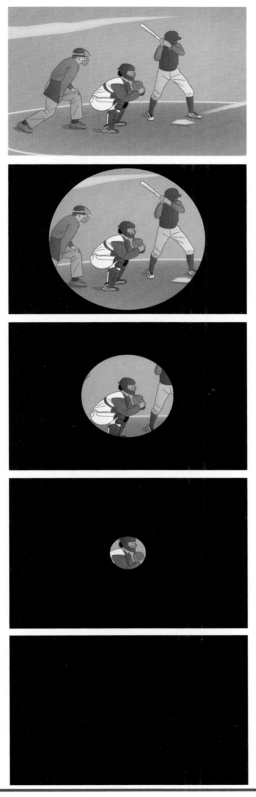

***Figure* 8-15**   The patient with glaucoma gradually loses his vision
with eventual blindness.

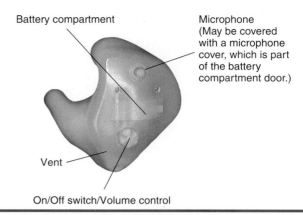

Battery compartment

Microphone
(May be covered
with a microphone
cover, which is part
of the battery
compartment door.)

Vent

On/Off switch/Volume control

***Figure* 8-16** A hearing aid.

Hearing Loss

Hearing loss can be caused by damage to the ear, wax buildup, or nerve damage. Hearing loss can be very mild or can be complete deafness or inability to hear any sounds. Some people with hearing loss can use a hearing aid to make sounds louder (Figure 8-16). A hearing aid does not correct the hearing problem.

Macular Degeneration

Macular degeneration is a loss of people's ability to see things that are directly in front of them.

Cardiovascular System

When blood is pumped throughout the body, oxygen and nutrients are supplied to all of the cells. Diseases of the cardiovascular system include:

Anemia

Anemia is a condition in which the number of red blood cells or the amount of iron in the blood is too low. There are many types and causes of anemia. The person with anemia may be pale, feel tired, or have a hard time breathing.

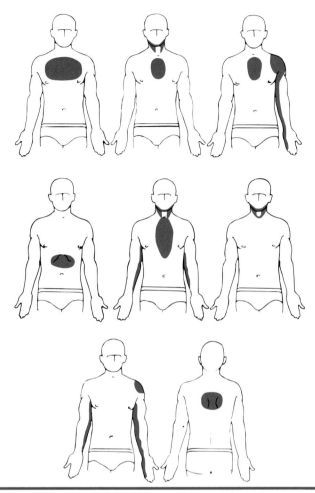

Figure 8-17 Anginal pain may be felt in areas other than the chest as shown by the shaded areas.

Angina

Angina is chest pain caused by not enough oxygen getting to the heart muscle. Some patients have pain in the jaw, neck, and down one or both arms (Figure 8-17). Exercise or emotional stress can cause angina. The person may be pale, feel faint, and sweat.

Arteriosclerosis

Arteriosclerosis is sometimes called "hardening of the arteries." Blood pressure usually goes up with this disease.

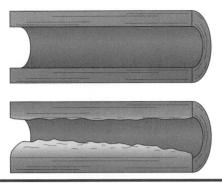

***Figure* 8-18**   Normal artery and artery showing the narrowed opening due to fatty deposits in a person with atherosclerosis.

Atherosclerosis

Atherosclerosis is a narrowing of the arteries that slows the flow of blood (Figure 8-18). People with diabetes are likely to have this disease, which can cause toe, foot, and leg amputations (surgical removal of the body part).

Congestive Heart Failure

Congestive heart failure (CHF) occurs when the heart cannot pump blood normally. The blood backs up into the tissues. A damaged or weakened heart usually causes CHF. A person with CHF may have swelling of the legs and feet or a buildup of fluid in the lungs that makes it hard for the person to breathe.

Hypertension

Hypertension is blood pressure that is too high. Narrowed blood vessels are a common cause of high blood pressure. Hypertension can lead to stroke, heart attack, heart failure, and kidney failure. A person with high blood pressure may not have any symptoms. Risk factors for hypertension are listed in Box 8-2.

Myocardial Infarction

Myocardial infarction (MI) is also known as a heart attack (Figure 8-19). A heart attack occurs when there is not enough blood and oxygen getting to the heart muscle, and the heart muscle starts to die. Signs and symptoms of a heart attack are listed in Box 8-3.

Box 8-2

RISK FACTORS IN HYPERTENSION

Age—men over 45 or women over 55
Being overweight
Family history of hypertension
No exercise
Race—African-Americans at greater risk than whites
Sex—men at greater risk than women
Smoking
Stress
Too much alcohol
Too much salt in the diet

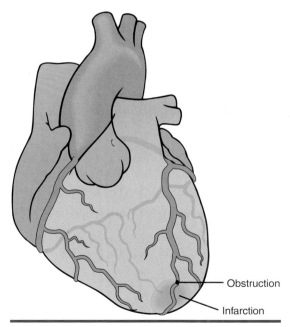

— Obstruction

— Infarction

Figure 8-19   A heart attack occurs when there is not enough blood and oxygen getting to the heart muscle because of an obstruction and the heart muscle starts to die (infarct).

Box 8-3

SYMPTOMS OF A HEART ATTACK

Cold skin
Confusion
Cyanosis—bluish discoloration of the skin
Dizziness
Feeling of doom
Dyspnea
Fear
Indigestion
Low blood pressure
Nausea
Pain in left side of chest that does not stop with rest
Pain in other places such as shoulder, neck, arm, and jaw
Paleness
Severe pain
Sudden pain
Sweating
Unsteadiness
Weak pulse

Phlebitis

Phlebitis is an inflammation of a vein that is painful and swollen (Figure 8-20).

Thrombophlebitis

Thrombophlebitis is a blood clot in a vein (Figure 8-21).

Varicose Veins

Varicose veins are veins that become large and twisted. Varicose veins are usually found in the legs but can affect other areas of the body as well (Figure 8-22). Varicose veins in the legs can cause the legs to hurt.

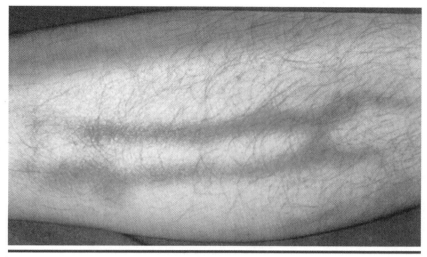

Figure 8-20   Phlebitis.

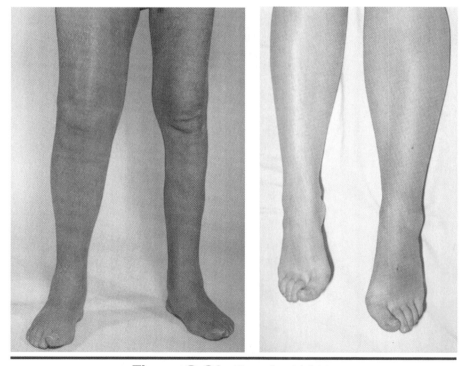

Figure 8-21   Thrombophlebitis.

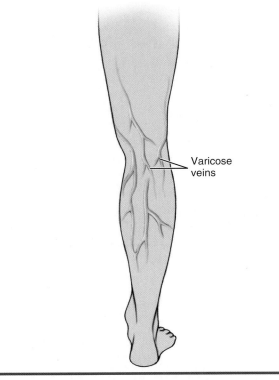

***Figure* 8-22**   Varicose veins are veins that become large and twisted. They are frequently found in the legs.

Respiratory System

Breathing brings oxygen into the body and removes carbon dioxide and wastes. Diseases of the respiratory system include:

Asthma

Asthma is a narrowing of the breathing passages due to breathing in something the person is allergic to. Asthma can also be triggered by exercise.

Cancer

Lung cancer usually affects people who are smokers (Figure 8-23). As the tumor grows, it becomes harder to breathe. Lung cancer often **metastasizes** or spreads to other parts of the body.

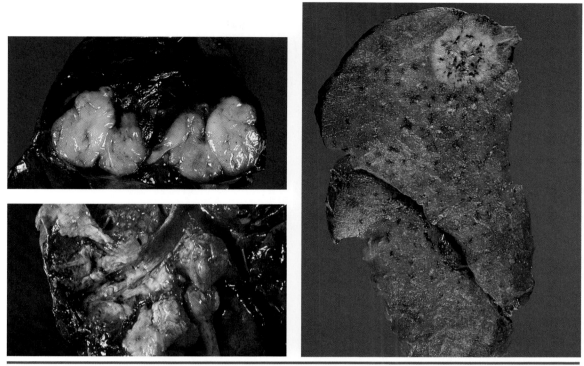

***Figure* 8-23**   Three forms of lung cancer.

Chronic Obstructive Pulmonary Disease

Chronic obstructive pulmonary disease (COPD) describes several diseases of the lungs that interfere with breathing. Emphysema (Figure 8-24) and chronic **bronchitis** (inflammation of the bronchi) are examples of COPD. Infection, air pollution, and industrial dust can cause COPD, but smoking is the main cause.

Influenza

Influenza is also call the "flu." A virus that attacks the respiratory tract causes the flu. Influenza can turn into pneumonia, especially in older people and children.

Pneumonia

Pneumonia is an infection/inflammation of the lungs. The alveoli (air sacs) fill up with fluid. It is very difficult and sometimes painful for the person with pneumonia to breathe. Some forms of pneumonia are contagious and can be spread from one person to another.

HOW&WHY

Influenza is considered a contagious or communicable disease and is also covered under communicable diseases and in Chapter 9.

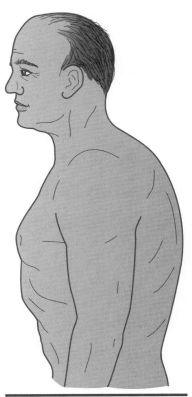

Figure **8-24** One form of COPD, called emphysema, causes air to become trapped in the lungs, and the person develops a barrel-shaped chest.

Digestive System

The digestive system breaks down food for our bodies and eliminates waste. Diseases of the digestive system include:

Anorexia

Anorexia is a loss of appetite. Being upset, diseases, or medicines can cause anorexia (Figure 8-25).

Cirrhosis

Cirrhosis is a disease that causes the tissue in the liver to be scarred. It is often caused by long-term alcohol abuse, some medicines, and **hepatitis** (inflammation of the liver).

The person with cirrhosis may develop **jaundice** (a yellowish discoloration of the skin).

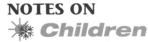

NOTES ON
Children

Severe anorexia and weight loss is more commonly seen in adolescent and teenage girls and can result in serious health problems leading to death.

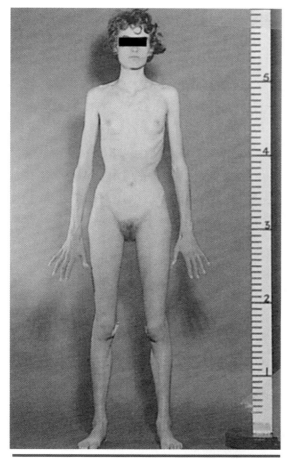

Figure 8-25   Patient with anorexia.

Diverticulitis

Diverticulitis is an inflammation of the diverticula (pouches) on the lining of the intestine (Figure 8-26).

Gallstones

Gallstones are small stonelike deposits that can block the bile ducts so that the bile, a fluid the liver makes, backs up. The person with gallstones develops jaundice (a yellowish discoloration of the skin) (Figure 8-27).

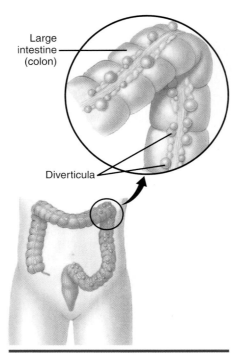

Large intestine (colon)

Diverticula

Figure 8-26 Diverticulitis.

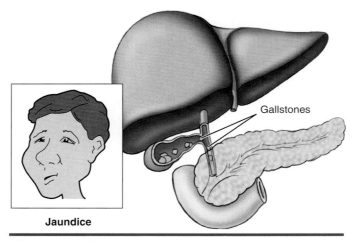

Gallstones

Jaundice

Figure 8-27 Gallstones can block the bile ducts so that the bile backs up, causing the person to develop jaundice.

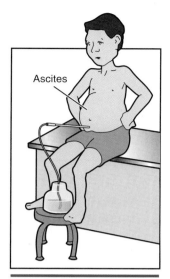

***Figure* 8-28**   People with hepatitis may develop jaundice and ascites. In severe cases the fluid is removed from the abdomen.

Hepatitis

Hepatitis is an inflammation of the liver usually caused by a virus. There are several types of hepatitis. All types of hepatitis cause damage to the liver cells and are serious diseases. People with hepatitis may develop jaundice and ascites (a buildup of fluid in the abdomen) (Figure 8-28).

Hiatal Hernia

Hiatal hernia is a bulging of the top of the stomach through the diaphragm muscle (Figure 8-29). A person with a hiatal hernia may have upper abdominal or chest pain or pressure.

Pancreatitis

Pancreatitis is an inflammation of the pancreas. It is a painful condition and may cause death (Figure 8-30).

Ulcers

Ulcers are open sores that can occur anywhere in the gastrointestinal tract. They are common in the stomach (Figure 8-31).

HOW & WHY

Some types of hepatitis are contagious and are discussed in the section on communicable diseases and in Chapter 9.

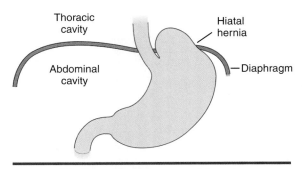

Figure 8-29   Hiatal hernia.

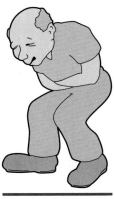

Figure 8-30
Pancreatitis is
a painful
condition.

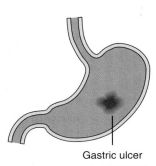

Gastric ulcer

Figure 8-31   Ulcers
are common in the
stomach.

Urinary System

The urinary system cleans waste products from the blood.
The urinary system also controls fluid and chemical levels in
the body.

Renal Calculi

Renal calculi are also known as kidney stones. Symptoms can
include back or abdominal pain, fever and chills, difficulty urinating, bloody urine, foul-smelling urine, and frequent urination. Patients on bedrest or with a poor fluid intake are at risk
for developing stones.

NOTES ON
☯ Culture

White men between the ages of 20
and 40 are at greatest risk of getting kidney stones.

Box 8-4

SYMPTOMS OF CHRONIC RENAL FAILURE

Abnormal breathing	Headaches
Bad breath	High blood pressure
Bleeding	Inflammation of the mouth
Bruises	Irregular pulse
Burning in feet and legs	Itchy skin
Coma	Leg cramps at night
Confusion	Less urine output
Congestive heart failure	Loss of appetite
Constipation	Nausea
Convulsions	Sleep disorders
Diarrhea	Susceptibility to infection
Dry skin	Thin skin
Fatigue	Twitching muscles
Gastric ulcers	Weight loss
Gastrointestinal bleeding	Yellow skin

Renal Failure

Renal failure can be an **acute** (short term or sudden) or **chronic** (long lasting) condition of the kidney. In people with renal failure, their kidneys are unable to filter wastes and control the fluid and chemical levels in the body. Renal failure can occur because of other diseases such as diabetes. Heart failure and hypertension easily result from renal failure. The buildup of waste affects every system in the body, and death can occur. Signs and symptoms of chronic renal failure are listed in Box 8-4.

Urinary Tract Infections

Urinary tract infections (UTIs) are infections that affect the bladder (cystitis) or kidneys (pyelonephritis). Symptoms of a UTI can include fever, chills, pain or burning when urinating, foul-smelling urine, bloody or cloudy urine, frequent urination, and abdominal or back pain. In severe cases, the patient may also have nausea and vomiting. Bacteria found in the intestine are a common cause of urinary tract infections.

HOW&WHY

Women get UTIs more often than men because the female urethra is shorter than the length of the urethra in men, and the female urethral opening is close to the rectum.

NOTES ON
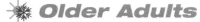
Older Adults

The first symptom of a UTI in an elderly person may be confusion.

Reproductive System

Benign Prostatic Hypertrophy

Benign prostatic hypertrophy (BPH) is a non-cancerous enlargement of the prostate gland that commonly affects men over the age of 50. Men with BPH may have difficulty urinating.

Cancer

Cancer of the reproductive organs can occur in both men and women.

Pelvic Inflammatory Disease

HOW & WHY

PID may be caused by sexually transmitted diseases, which are considered contagious or communicable diseases.

Pelvic inflammatory disease (PID) is a general term to describe an infection of the female reproductive organs. PID can cause infertility in women.

Sexually Transmitted Diseases

HOW & WHY

Sexually transmitted diseases are considered contagious or communicable diseases.

Sexually transmitted diseases (STDs) may also be called venereal diseases. STDs often occur in the genital and rectal areas and are spread by sexual contact. Some STDs can be spread by saliva, open areas on the skin, or by contaminated needles or syringes. Herpes, genital warts, syphilis, gonorrhea, hepatitis B, and human immunodeficiency virus (HIV) are all examples of STDs (Figure 8-32). Some people with STDs do not have symptoms and are unaware of the infection. Other people know they have the disease but are embarrassed or afraid to get treatment.

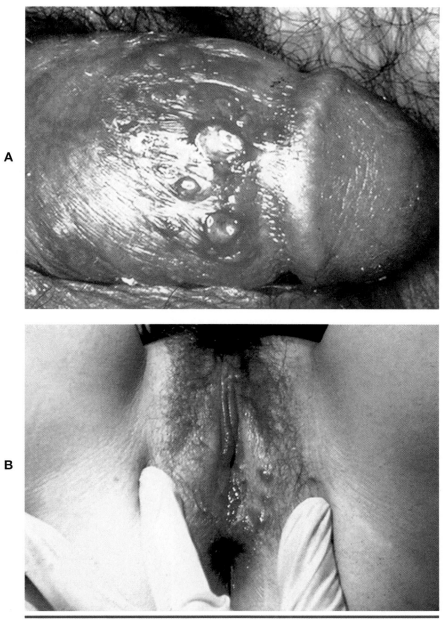

Figure 8-32   **A,** Herpes sores on the penis. **B,** Herpes sores on the female perineum.

Endocrine System

Diabetes

Diabetes occurs when the body cannot produce enough insulin to metabolize the food that the person eats. It is the most common endocrine disorder. There are 3 types of diabetes.

- Type 1 occurs most often in children and young adults. The pancreas produces little or no insulin.
- Type 2 occurs in adults, usually over the age of 40. The pancreas produces insulin, but the body does not use it well.
- Gestational diabetes occurs during pregnancy.

All types of diabetes must be controlled. A combination of medications, healthy eating, and exercise is used. If diabetes is not controlled, blindness, renal failure, nerve damage, hypertension, stroke, heart attack, and slow wound healing can occur. Both **hypoglycemia** (low blood sugar) and **hyperglycemia** (high blood sugar) are complications of diabetes and can lead to death if untreated. Box 8-5 lists the symptoms of both.

NOTES ON *Culture*

African-Americans, Native Americans, Hispanics, and Asian and Pacific Islander Americans are at higher risk for type 2 diabetes. Whites are at greater risk than non-whites of developing type 1 diabetes.

Box 8-5

SYMPTOMS OF HYPERGLYCEMIA AND HYPOGLYCEMIA

Hyperglycemia	Hypoglycemia
Blurred eyesight	Cold skin
Coma	Confusion
Cramps in legs	Dizziness
Dry skin	Emotional changes
Fast heartbeat	Eyesight changes
Fatigue	Fainting
Flushed face	Fast breathing
Frequent urination	Fast heartbeat
Headaches	Fatigue
Hunger and thirst	Headaches
Low blood pressure	Hunger
Slow, difficult breathing	Low blood pressure
Sweet breath	Shakes
Vomiting	Sweats
Weak heartbeat	Unclear speech
Weakness	Unconsciousness
	Weakness

Graves' Disease

Graves' disease is a secretion of too much thyroid hormone (Figure 8-33). The person with Graves' disease has an abnormally fast metabolism, and a severe episode can cause the heart to fail.

Hypothyroidism

Hypothyroidism is a deficiency of the hormone that controls metabolism (Figure 8-34). The person with hypothyroidism has a metabolism that is too slow and may feel tired.

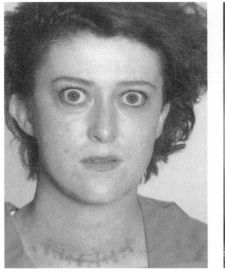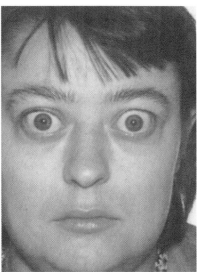

***Figure* 8-33**   Graves' disease.

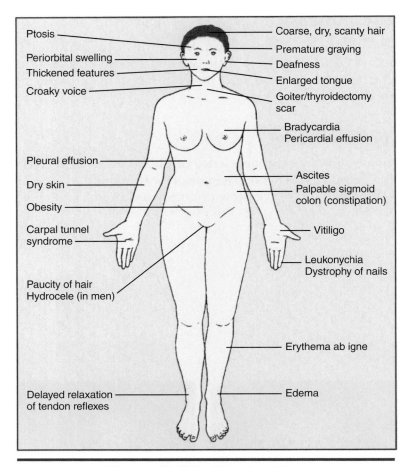

Figure **8-34**   Hypothyroidism.

Communicable Diseases

Communicable diseases are contagious and can spread from person to person. Chapter 9 discusses the appropriate things to do to prevent the spread of communicable diseases in health care settings. To better understand how to control communicable diseases, you will need to understand the ways that diseases can be spread. Some diseases can be spread by more than one route.

- *Direct:* Spread from person to person by direct contact such as touching the other person. Impetigo is an example of an infection that can be spread through direct contact.
- *Indirect:* Spread by contact with an item the infected person used, such as sharing a drinking glass or sharing needles. The common cold and hepatitis C can be spread through indirect contact.

Box 8-6

SYMPTOMS OF AIDS

Blurry vision
Confusion
Cough
Dementia
Diarrhea
Difficult and painful swallowing
Fatigue
Fever
Forgetfulness
Headache
Loss of appetite
Night sweats
Purple blotches that do not disappear
Shortness of breath
Sore throat
Sores in the mouth and on the tongue
Swollen glands in the neck, underarms, and groin
Weight loss

- *Airborne:* Spread through coughing or sneezing. Influenza is considered an airborne disease.
- *Vehicle:* Spread through eating or drinking something that has the germs on it. Hepatitis A is spread by eating food contaminated with the hepatitis A virus.
- *Vector:* Spread by animals or insects, such as West Nile virus

There are many diseases that are contagious. Some contagious diseases have already been discussed under the body system that they affect. Listed are just a few of the more commonly seen communicable diseases.

Acquired Immunodeficiency Syndrome

Acquired immunodeficiency syndrome (AIDS) is an infection caused by the virus HIV. It attacks the immune system. The most common symptoms are weight loss, fever, and being tired. It is spread by contact with blood or body fluids and can be spread sexually. Some people infected with HIV are symptom free for many years but are still able to spread the virus to others. Symptoms of AIDS are listed in Box 8-6.

HOW & WHY

The virus that causes chickenpox is the same virus that causes shingles. If a person has had chickenpox, the virus is dormant in his body, but can re-appear as shingles at a later time.

Chickenpox

Chickenpox is also known as varicella. This disease is most common in children and is usually seen in the winter and spring months. Patients with chickenpox have an itchy rash that develops scabs as it heals (Figure 8-35). It is an airborne disease.

Hepatitis

There are several forms of hepatitis.
- Hepatitis A is spread by the oral/fecal route. The virus enters the body when eating or drinking food or water that has been contaminated with feces (stool).
- Hepatitis B (HBV) is spread by contact with blood or body fluids such as saliva, semen, or vaginal secretions carrying the virus. It can be spread through sexual contact, contaminated blood, or needles.
- Hepatitis C is usually spread by contact with infected blood. A person can have the virus but not have symptoms for many years. Serious liver disease may develop later in life. Hepatitis C can also be spread by contaminated needles and sexual contact.

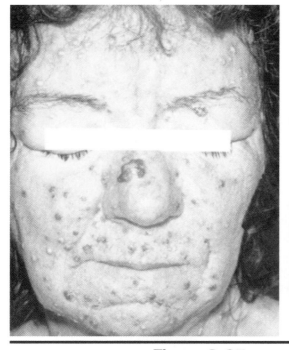

A

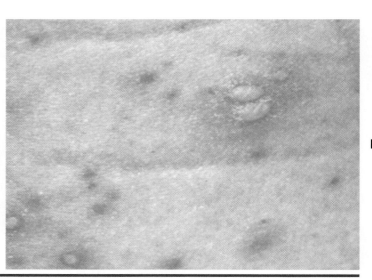

B

Figure 8-35 **A,** Patient with chickenpox. **B,** Chickenpox.

- Hepatitis D and Hepatitis E. Hepatitis D occurs in people infected with Hepatitis B and is spread in the same manner. Hepatitis E is seen in countries where the water supply is contaminated with feces.

Influenza

Influenza is a respiratory infection that can be spread through airborne, direct, or indirect contact.

Measles

Measles (rubeola) is a highly contagious disease. Patients usually have a fever and a rash. It is spread through respiratory droplets that are in the air. German measles (rubella) is similar in appearance but not as contagious (Figure 8-36).

Mumps

Mumps is a contagious virus spread by respiratory droplets and saliva. Neck glands are swollen, and the patient complains of a headache, fever, and earache.

NOTES ON
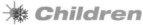 *Children*

Severe cases of influenza in small children and the frail elderly can result in death.

NOTES ON
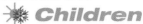 *Children*

Measles is most common in school-age children.

NOTES ON
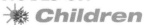 *Children*

Measles, mumps, and rubella vaccinations are required for school-age children in most states in the United States.

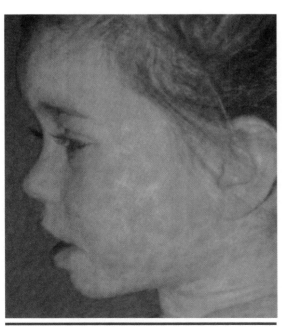

Figure 8-36 Measles.

Strep Throat

Strep throat is also called streptococcal pharyngitis. This disease is considered airborne.

HOW&*WHY*

People who have frequent contact with a person infected with TB are at greatest risk. Most health care facilities require annual TB testing for all employees, and some long-term care settings test residents on admission.

Tuberculosis

Tuberculosis (TB) is a contagious respiratory disease spread through the air by coughing and sneezing. Sometimes the bacteria do not cause illness for many years.

CHAPTER REVIEW

1. What is diabetes?

2. What are the 5 ways bacteria and diseases are spread?

Circle the one BEST response.

3. Mr. Long is complaining of itching on the soles of his feet. The skin is cracked and painful. He most likely has
   a. Acne
   b. Athlete's foot
   c. Dermatitis
   d. Hives

4. The form of arthritis cause by uric acid crystals in the joints is called
   a. Gout
   b. Lupus
   c. Osteoarthritis
   d. Rheumatoid arthritis

5. Ms. Green is having blurred vision. She also tells you that she is sensitive to light and glare. What type of vision problem do you think she has?
   a. Cataract
   b. Epilepsy
   c. Glaucoma
   d. Macular degeneration

6. The medical term for abnormally high blood pressure is
   a. Angina
   b. Hypertension
   c. Myocardial infarction
   d. Phlebitis

7. Mr. Lee has been diagnosed with pneumonia. Which of the following statements describes his condition?
   a. It is a tumor in the lung that makes it hard to breathe.
   b. It is a narrowing of the air passages because of an allergy.
   c. It is a type of COPD.
   d. It is an infection/inflammation of the lungs.

8. Which condition of the gastrointestinal system commonly causes jaundice?
   a. Anorexia
   b. Diverticulitis
   c. Gallstones
   d. Hiatal hernia

9. Which of the following statements is true regarding urinary tract infections (UTIs)?
   a. They are more common in women than in men.
   b. They usually affect white men between the ages of 20 and 40.
   c. They are the same as kidney stones.
   d. They cause renal failure in most people.

CHAPTER REVIEW

10. Which of the following is a sexually transmitted disease?
a. BPH
b. Cancer
c. Gonorrhea
d. Pyelonephritis

11. A person with Graves' disease has
a. A deficiency of the body to produce enough insulin
b. An abnormally fast metabolism
c. A deficiency of the hormone that controls metabolism
d. An abnormally slow metabolism

12. Which of the following contagious diseases is commonly seen in school-age children?
a. AIDS
b. Hepatitis
c. Influenza
d. Measles

Answers are on page 705.

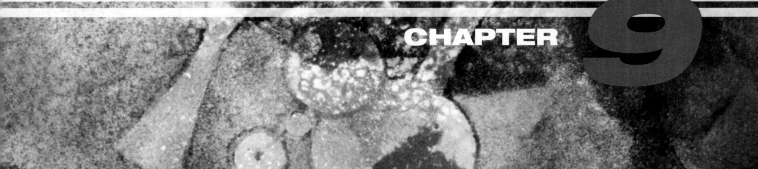

CHAPTER **9**

Infection Control

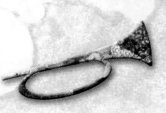

What you will learn

- What causes an infection
- Signs and symptoms of an infection
- The purposes of an infection control program
- The chain of infection
- How, when, and why to wash your hands
- How to use Standard Precautions/Universal Precautions
- How to use Isolation Precautions/Transmission-Based Precautions
- How to put on and remove gloves, gown, and mask and goggles

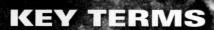
KEY TERMS
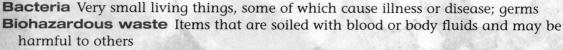

Bacteria Very small living things, some of which cause illness or disease; germs

Biohazardous waste Items that are soiled with blood or body fluids and may be harmful to others

Immune system The body system that protects us from infections

Infection An illness that occurs when a disease-producing germ enters the body

Infection control A facility program that helps you to avoid spreading infections

Microorganisms Tiny living objects, sometimes called germs

Nosocomial infection An infection people get while they are a patient in the hospital or resident in a nursing home

Standard Precautions Precautions that protect you from patients with known infections and from patients who have infections that they are not aware of

Universal Precautions Precautions designed to protect health care workers from diseases carried in the blood such as human immunodeficiency virus (HIV), acquired immunodeficiency syndrome (AIDS), and hepatitis

Virus One-celled microorganism that is much smaller than a bacterium

What Causes Infections?

Infections are caused by **microorganisms**. Microorganisms are tiny living objects, sometimes called germs. Microorganisms are on all surfaces and inside everything around us, including the human body. An **infection** occurs when a disease-producing microorganism enters the body. The body's natural **immune system** usually protects us. The two most common kinds of microorganisms that cause illness in humans are **bacteria** and **viruses**. A bacterium is a small one-celled microorganism that grows best in a warm, dark, moist environment. Bacteria grow well in food and waste products. Antibiotics kill most bacteria. If you have ever had "strep throat," you had a bacterial infection. The microorganism grew well in your throat because it is warm, dark, and moist. Your doctor probably gave you antibiotics to kill the "strep" bacteria. Not all bacteria are bad. Many bacteria live in your body, but they do not make you sick. The body needs these "good" germs to work correctly. For example, the bacteria in your intestines help to break down waste products.

A virus is also a one-celled microorganism, but it is much smaller than bacteria (Figure 9-1). Viruses cannot live outside of the body and are harder to kill than bacteria. The common cold is an example of a viral infection. Antibiotics do not kill viruses.

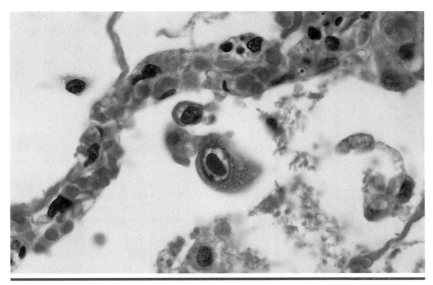

***Figure* 9-1**   A view of a virus through a microscope.

Signs and Symptoms of an Infection

When disease-causing microorganisms enter your body, they release waste products that make you sick. Your immune system tries to fight off the infection. The signs and symptoms that an infection is present include:

- Fever or chills
- Pain
- Redness
- Swelling
- Drainage
- Fatigue
- Nausea
- Disorientation

NOTES ON
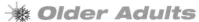
Older Adults

A person with an infection may have 1 or more of these symptoms. Disorientation is more commonly seen in the elderly patient.

The Purposes of an Infection Control Program

Infection control is an important part of keeping your patients safe. Every facility has an infection control program to help you to avoid spreading infections. Your employer will review the infection control program with you every year.

The infection control program protects staff, patients, and visitors from getting an infection from someone else. It also keeps patients from getting an infection a second or third time. The goal of the infection control program is to keep the facility as germ-free as possible.

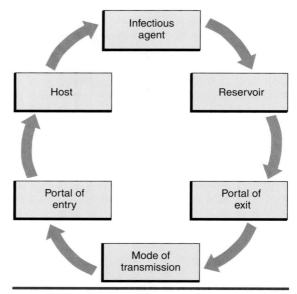

Figure 9-2 The chain of infection.

The Chain of Infection

To prevent the spread of infections, you must first understand the chain of infection (Figure 9-2). The chain of infection is the manner in which infections can live and be spread. In order for an infection to occur, there must be:

- A disease-causing organism
- A place where the germs can grow and multiply (sometimes called a reservoir)
- A way for the germs to exit the place where they have been growing
- A way to be transmitted from person to person (See "Communicable Diseases," p. 168, in Chapter 8 for additional information on modes of transmission.)
- A way for the germs to enter the body of another person
- An individual who cannot fight off the infection

It is sometimes easier to understand the chain of infection if you think about an illness you or a member of your family may have had recently. A good example is the common cold. Consider the following:

Susan, your co-worker, has a cold. In this situation the disease-producing organism is the cold virus. Susan is the reservoir where the virus grows and multiplies. When Susan coughs or sneezes, the virus leaves her body on droplets and travels through the air. When you breathe in the droplets, the virus enters your body. If you have not already had this virus, a couple of days later you will have the same cold symptoms as Susan. You have now become the reservoir where the virus is growing. When you cough or sneeze, the virus leaves your body on droplets and travels through the air. Your co-worker Bill breathes in the droplets, and if he has not already had the virus, within a couple of days he starts to have the same cold symptoms as both you and Susan.

This chain of infection continues until someone or something breaks the chain. In this situation, if Susan had covered her mouth and nose with a tissue when she coughed or sneezed, the chain could have been broken.

As you may recall, Chapter 8 discussed the ways that diseases can be spread. You learned that the 5 ways microorganisms are transmitted are direct contact, indirect contact, airborne transmission, vehicle transmission, and vector transmission. Figure 9-3 shows a diagram of these modes of transmission.

One of the most common ways that diseases spread from one person to another is by touching. This can happen when you shake hands with people who have disease-causing germs on their hands. Germs can also spread when someone touches something, such as the faucets on the sink, after someone with dirty hands touched them.

People can develop infections while they are patients in health care settings. These infections that are acquired after the person is admitted to the facility are called **nosocomial infections**. The most common types of nosocomial infections are:

- Urinary tract infections
- Respiratory infections
- Wound infections

While it is impossible to prevent 100% of infections in health care settings, using proper infection control techniques decreases the spread of microorganisms.

Another part of your facility's infection control program is the separation of "clean" and "dirty" items. Many of the supplies that you use are disposable, and you throw them away after they are used. These items include bedpans, drinking cups, and wash basins. They are labeled with the patient's name and room number. They are never "borrowed" for use by another patient. When the person is discharged, the items are thrown away. Larger items and expensive equipment are cleaned and re-used. Each facility has its own policy about cleaning reusable supplies and equipment. In some places the items are sent to a central supply room for cleaning, and then they are returned to your unit (Figure 9-4).

NOTES ON
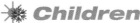
Children

Small children have a harder time fighting off infection. It is up to the health care team to prevent the spread of germs before they can cause illness.

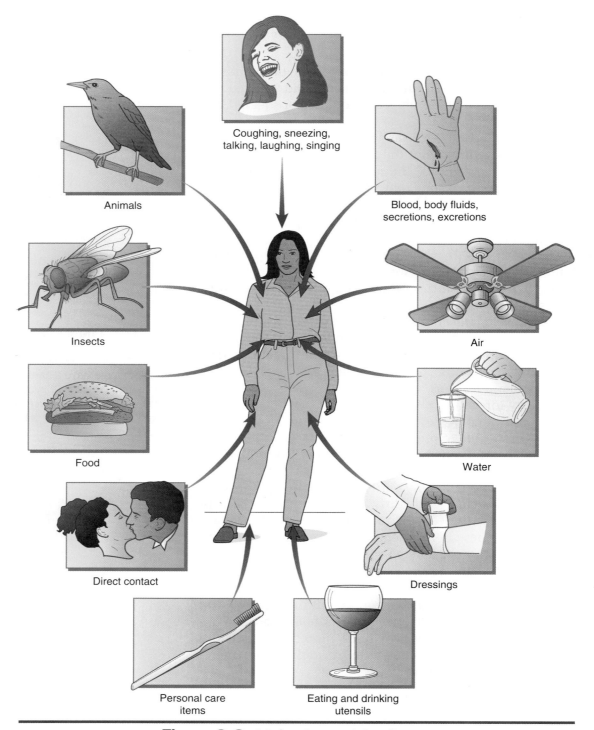

Coughing, sneezing, talking, laughing, singing

Animals

Blood, body fluids, secretions, excretions

Insects

Air

Food

Water

Direct contact

Dressings

Personal care items

Eating and drinking utensils

***Figure* 9-3** Modes of transmitting diseases.

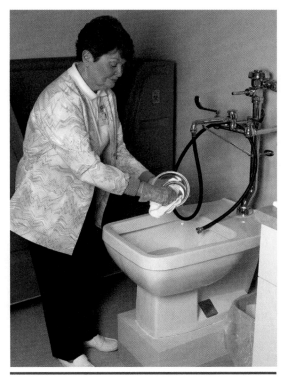

***Figure* 9-4** Items being cleaned in a central supply room.

Your facility will have 2 different areas for "clean items" and "dirty items." Clean items include things such as new water pitchers, bedpans, urinals, toothbrushes, wash basins, and other new supplies. Re-usable equipment that has been properly cleaned and is ready to be used would also be stored in the "clean" utility room. Items that have not been used by a patient are "clean."

"Dirty" items would include things that you are throwing away such as used bedpans, drinking cups, or wash basins. Equipment that has not been cleaned and is not ready to be used is kept in the "dirty" utility room (Figure 9-5).

Think about it: you use your hands in almost every task you perform. The best and easiest way to prevent the spread of infection and to break the chain is to ***wash your hands before and after giving care or handling dirty equipment!***

Safety

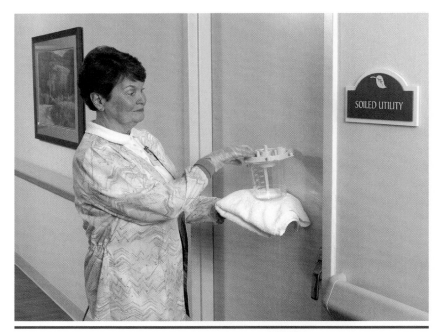

***Figure* 9-5** The nursing assistant holds dirty equipment away from her uniform to avoid contaminating her clothing with germs from the equipment.

How and When to Wash Your Hands

As a nursing assistant, you will touch many people and things that can cause infection each day. When you wash your hands, you decrease the risk of spreading an infection from person to person. It is also the best way to avoid taking infections home to your family. Hands should be washed:

- Before beginning your shift
- Before and after contact with a patient, even if gloves were worn
- Before handling food or food trays
- After using the bathroom
- After coughing, sneezing, or blowing your nose
- Before and after your break or meal time
- After having contact with soiled linens
- Before leaving the facility at the end of your shift

Procedure
HAND WASHING

EQUIPMENT

- **Water**
- **Soap**
- **Paper towels**
- **Wastebasket**

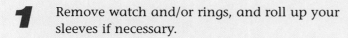

1 Remove watch and/or rings, and roll up your sleeves if necessary.

2 Turn the water on to a comfortably warm temperature. *NOTE:* Do not touch the faucet again during the procedure.

3 Wet hands and areas above the wrists thoroughly with warm water. Hold hands with fingers pointed downward and hands lower than elbows (Figure 9-6).

4 Apply a generous amount of soap to the hands.

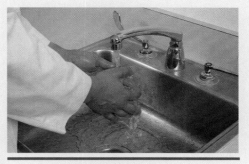

Figure 9-6 Step 3.

5 Scrub the hands for at least 15 seconds. Wash the palms and back of the hands in a circular motion. Wash in between the fingers (Figure 9-7). Wash the wrists in a circular motion.

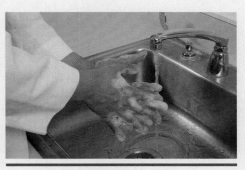

Figure 9-7 Step 5.

Continued

Procedure
HAND WASHING—cont'd

6 Rinse the hands and wrists well beginning at the wrist and working toward the fingers. Remember to keep the fingers down and the hands lower than the elbows (Figure 9-8).

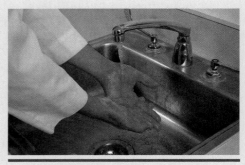

Figure 9-8 Step 6.

7 Dry hands using a clean paper towel for each hand (Figure 9-9). If necessary, repeat with an additional clean paper towel.

8 Throw away used paper towel(s) in wastebasket.

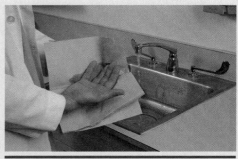

Figure 9-9 Step 7.

9 Turn off the faucet using a clean, dry paper towel (Figure 9-10).

10 Throw away the used paper towel in the wastebasket.

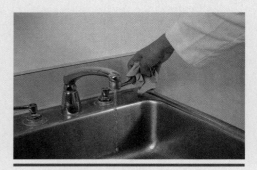

Figure 9-10 Step 9.

How to Use Standard Precautions/ Universal Precautions

To prevent the spread of infection, the Centers for Disease Control and Prevention (CDC) has developed guidelines for health care workers called **Standard Precautions.** Standard Precautions protect you from patients with known infections and patients who have infections that they are not aware of. When using Standard Precautions you will wear gloves any time you are in contact with:

- Blood
- All body fluids except for sweat
- Non-intact skin or open areas
- Mucous membranes

Body fluids refers to any fluid coming out of the body and includes urine, tears, saliva, amniotic fluid (from around a baby), emesis or vomit, and liquid stool. If it is a liquid and it comes from the body, it has the potential to carry infection. Examples of non-intact skin would include surgical incisions, pressure ulcers, cuts, and scrapes and puncture wounds. If the skin is open, even if no bleeding is present, there is a potential for infection. Mucous membranes line the mouth, nose, vagina, eyes, and rectum. If you are going to have contact with these areas, you must wear gloves. Contact with mucous membranes also has the possibility to spread infection.

A branch of the federal government called OSHA enforces **Universal Precautions.** OSHA is the Occupational Safety and Health Administration. Universal Precautions are designed to protect health care workers from diseases carried in the blood such as HIV, AIDS, and hepatitis. Universal Precautions are only for blood and body fluids that contain blood. If you are using Standard Precautions, you are also using Universal Precautions.

How to Use Isolation Precautions/ Transmission-Based Precautions

Isolation or transmission-based precautions are used in addition to Standard/Universal Precautions when the patient has an infectious disease. The type of precaution used depends on the way the disease is spread.

Airborne precautions are used to prevent the spread of diseases by air currents. These germs are so small and light that they can be suspended on dust particles in the air. Airborne diseases include tuberculosis (TB), chickenpox, and measles.

HOW & WHY

The protective equipment you wear may frighten patients who are placed on Transmission-Based Precautions/Isolation. They may also feel lonely or "dirty" because of their infection and limited inter-action with staff. Make sure to take time to talk with the patients so they will not feel frightened.

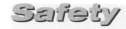

Droplet Precautions are used to prevent the spread of diseases such as influenza. Sneezing, coughing, and talking can spread the droplets up to 3 feet.

Contact Precautions are used with infections that are spread by coming in contact with germs from the patient's wound or an item heavily infected with germs, such as a dressing. Contact Precautions would be used with infected wounds, impetigo, and conjunctivitis ("pink eye").

Protective or Reverse Precautions protect the patient who has a decreased ability to resist disease. Patient with burns or leukemia and some chemotherapy patients are placed on Protective Precautions.

The charge nurse will instruct you on the type of precautions to use for each patient (Table 9-1).

A notice will be placed on the door so that all staff and visitors are aware of the need to use special precautions.

Following the correct type of precautions with each patient protects you, your co-workers, visitors, and other patients from the infection.

Table 9-1

USING APPROPRIATE PRECAUTIONS

Precaution	Standard Precautions	Gown	Mask	Other
Airborne Precautions (TB, chickenpox, measles)	Yes	No, only if soiling is likely	Yes	Private room with door closed
Droplet Precautions (influenza)	Yes	No, only if soiling is likely	Yes	Door open if bed is more than 3 feet from door
Contact Precautions (wound infection, scabies, gastroenteritis)	Yes	Yes	No, only if risk of splashing	Do not move patient care items (for example, blood pressure cuff) to other rooms
Protective/Reverse Precautions	Yes	Yes	Yes	Door closed

How to Put on Gloves, Gown, and Mask

Gloves protect your skin from contact with infection. It is important that you wash your hands before you put on gloves and after you remove gloves. You do not need to wear gloves when there is no risk of infection.

Procedure
PUTTING ON AND REMOVING NON-STERILE GLOVES

EQUIPMENT
- **Water**
- **Soap**
- **Paper Towels**
- **Wastebasket**
- **Non-sterile gloves**

Putting Gloves On

1 Wash your hands.

2 Remove gloves from box one at a time.

3 Place one hand through the opening of the glove, and pull the glove up and over the wrist.

4 Repeat step 3 with the second glove.

5 Adjust gloves to cover the wrist or cuffs of the gown if wearing a gown (Figure 9-11).
Note: Do not touch any part of your body with your gloved hand.

6 Complete patient care.

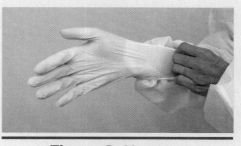

Figure 9-11   Step 5.

Removing Gloves

7 Grasp one glove at the inside of the wrist $1/2$ inch below the band of the dirty side of the glove without touching your skin (Figure 9-12).

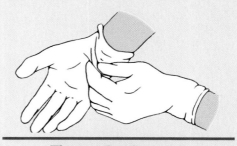

Figure 9-12   Step 7.

Continued

Procedure
PUTTING ON AND REMOVING NON-STERILE GLOVES—cont'd

8 Pull glove down, turning it inside out, and pull it off your hand. Hold the glove in the still-gloved hand.

9 Insert fingers of ungloved hand inside the cuff of the glove on the other hand (Figure 9-13).

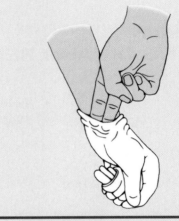

Figure 9-13 Step 9.

10 Pull glove down until it is inside out, drawing it over the first glove.

11 Place both gloves in the wastebasket according to your facility's policy (Figure 9-14).

12 Wash your hands.

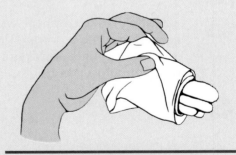

Figure 9-14 Step 11.

Gowns protect your uniform from soiling. Some facilities use fabric gowns that are washed and re-used. Other facilities use disposable paper gowns. The gown must cover your uniform entirely to provide protection.

Procedure

PUTTING ON AND REMOVING A NON-STERILE GOWN

EQUIPMENT

- **Water**
- **Soap**
- **Paper towels**
- **Gown**
- **Gloves if being used**
- **Mask if being used**

Putting on Gown

1 Wash your hands.

2 If needed for procedure, put on mask according to procedure.

3 Unfold gown with opening at the back (Figure 9-15).

4 Put on gown, slipping arms into sleeves and adjusting the gown over your shoulders.

5 Tie neck tie, or fasten strips at back of neck.

6 Reach behind and overlap the edges of the gown.

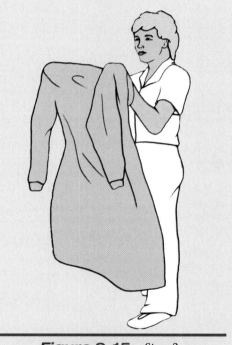

Figure 9-15   Step 3.

Continued

Procedure

PUTTING ON AND REMOVING A NON-STERILE GOWN—cont'd

7 Bring waist ties to the back and tie. If they are long enough to come around to the front, they may be tied in the front (Figure 9-16).

8 Put on gloves according to procedure.

9 Complete patient care.

Removing Gown

10 Untie waist tie.

11 Remove gloves according to procedure, and dispose of according to facility policy.

12 Turn on water faucet with clean, dry paper towel.

13 Wash and dry hands according to procedure.

14 If wearing a mask, hold by ties/elastic and discard according to facility policy.

15 Untie ties or fasteners at neck of gown and loosen.

16 Slip fingers of one hand inside the cuff of the other arm. NOTE: Do not touch the outside of the gown.

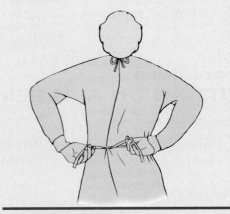

Figure 9-16   Step 7.

Continued

Procedure

PUTTING ON AND REMOVING A NON-STERILE GOWN—cont'd

17 Pull gown down over your hand (Figure 9-17).

18 With gown-covered hand, pull gown down over other hand.

19 Fold gown away from your body with the contaminated side inward.

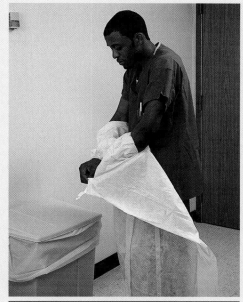

Figure 9-17 Step 17.

20 Roll the gown into a ball, and dispose of according to your facility policy (Figure 9-18).

21 Turn on faucet with a clean paper towel.

22 Wash your hands.

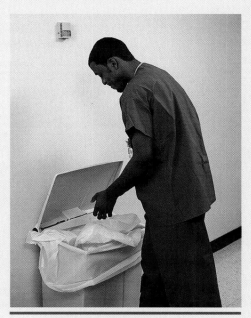

Figure 9-18 Step 20.

Procedure
PUTTING ON AND REMOVING A MASK

EQUIPMENT
- Water
- Soap
- Paper towels
- Mask

Putting on Mask

1 Wash your hands.

2 Pick up mask.

3 Adjust mask over your mouth and nose.

4 Tie top string behind head, or adjust elastic band around ears (Figure 9-19).

5 Tie lower string behind neck.

6 Complete patient care. *NOTE:* Replace mask if it becomes wet or soiled.

Removing Mask

7 Wash hands according to procedure. If wearing gloves, remove them before washing hands.

8 Untie bottom tie, or remove elastic band from behind ears (Figure 9-20).

9 Untie top string.

10 Remove mask, holding it by the top strings.

11 Discard mask by dropping it into the waste-basket according to facility policy.

12 Wash your hands.

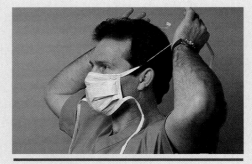

Figure 9-19   Step 4.

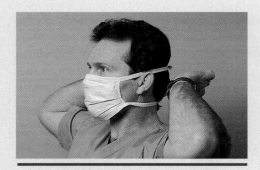

Figure 9-20   Step 8.

Masks are used once and thrown away. A mask is only effective for about 30 minutes due to the moisture in normal respirations. If a mask becomes wet or soiled, change it. Never allow a mask to hang around your neck. Always make certain your hands are clean before putting a mask on or taking it off.

Protective eyewear or goggles are used to protect the mucous membranes of your eyes from being infected through splashing (Figure 9-21). Some masks have an attached face shield that protects the eyes. Other facilities provide goggles that fit snuggly against the face and protect the eyes from the sides, top, and bottom, as well as from the front.

Regular eyeglasses do not give enough protection from splashing.

The symbol in Figure 9-22 is called the *BIOHAZARD* symbol. When you see this symbol on a dirty utility room door or trash container, you know that the items in that area have the potential to spread infection. These items are called **biohazardous waste** and could be harmful. Any item that has blood, body fluids, secretions, or excretions on it (such as urine or stool) is considered biohazardous waste.

HOW&*WHY*

Goggles are used when there is a risk of splashing, such as when assisting the nurse in cleaning an infected wound.

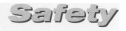

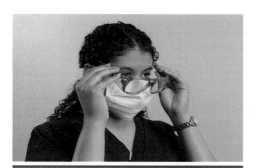

Figure 9-21   Protective eyewear or goggles are used to protect the mucous membranes of your eyes from being infected through splashing.

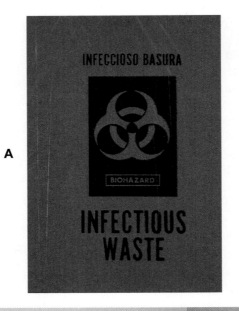

A

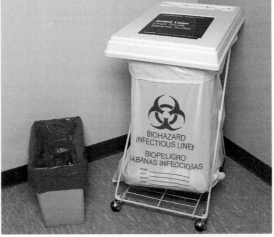

B

Figure 9-22 **A**, Biohazard symbol. **B**, Bio-hazard symbol on a linen container.

Dressings removed from a person's wound are a biohazardous waste. The dressings that have blood on them are potentially harmful and can spread infection. The dirty dressings are disposed of in a biohazard bag or container where other people do not have to touch them. Another example of biohazardous waste is linens soiled with stool or urine. The dirty linens are placed in a special plastic bag that melts in the hot water in the washing machine. Once the dirty linens are in the sealed bag, no one has to touch them until after they have been washed. It is important that you know your facility's policy for handing contaminated trash and linens and follow it.

Occasionally the outside of a trash or linen bag may become soiled. When this happens, you will need to "double bag" the items. Two staff members are needed for double bagging. In Figure 9-23 Joe is inside the room and Juanita is helping him to double bag by standing outside the room with a clean bag.

1. Joe places the soiled item(s) into a bag and seals the bag.
2. Juanita holds open a clean bag. The top of the clean bag is folded back over Juanita's hands to form a cuff.
3. Joe places the soiled bag into the clean bag.
4. Juanita seals the clean bag and disposes of it according to facility policy.

Remember, **YOU** are important in breaking the chain of infection. When you use the correct precautions for each patient and task, you will help to prevent the spread of infections in your facility.

HOW & WHY

Juanita folded the top of the clean bag over her gloved hands to help protect herself from having contact with the soiled bag.

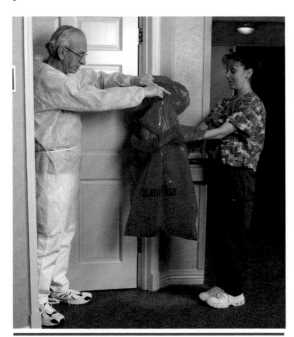

Figure 9-23 Two staff members are needed for double bagging.

CHAPTER REVIEW

1. What causes infections?

2. List 4 signs or symptoms of an infection.

3. What is the chain of infection?

4. What are Standard Precautions?

Circle the one BEST response.

5. What is the goal of an infection control program?
   a. To keep the institution in compliance with state regulations
   b. To prevent the spread of infections to other facilities
   c. To keep the facility as germ-free as possible
   d. To treat patient with infections as quickly as possible

6. When should hands be washed?
   a. Before and after patient contact
   b. Before handling food trays
   c. After using the bathroom
   d. All of the above

7. Ms. Leong has tuberculosis. What type of Transmission-Based Precautions would you expect to use when caring for her?
   a. Airborne
   b. Contact
   c. Droplet
   d. Protective

Answers are on page 705.

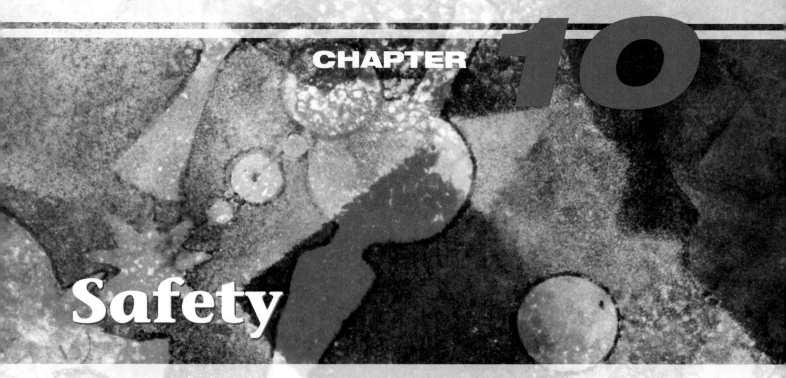

CHAPTER 10

Safety

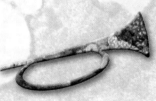

What you will learn

- Accident risk factors and how to prevent them
- How to handle an emergency
- Personal safety measures
- Do's and don'ts of restraint use

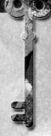

KEY TERMS

Hemorrhage A large amount of sudden uncontrolled bleeding

Incident Any unexpected situation that can cause harm to a person

Restraint Any manual or chemical item or device that restricts a person's freedom of movement or body access

Seizure (convulsion) Sudden uncontrolled muscle contraction resulting from abnormal brain activity

Accident Risk Factors and How to Prevent Them

Keeping your patients safe is the job of each employee of the hospital or nursing home. You must help keep your patients safe each day. It is also important to keep co-workers, visitors, and volunteers safe.

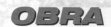

OBRA requires that all long-term care (LTC) centers follow safety policies and procedures. It is important to provide the nursing home resident with a safe environment while still encouraging independence.

An accident may also be called an incident. An **incident** is any unexpected situation that can cause harm to a person. You can prevent incidents by:

- Knowing the safety policies and procedures at your facility
- Thinking about safety each day
- Using only equipment you have been properly trained to use
- Doing only those jobs for which you have been trained
- Telling your supervisor about equipment that is broken or missing parts
- Using equipment only for its intended use

Safety

The most important thing you can do to prevent accidents is to be aware of what is going on around you.

People in hospitals and nursing homes are often at higher risk of injury due to accidents. Some of these people have disabilities, vision or hearing problems, or are weak. Some may be taking medicines that make them drowsy. Others may be confused or have dementia and are unable to think clearly.

As a nursing assistant, you will care for many different patients each time you work. Each of your patients has different needs and receives different types of diets and treatments.

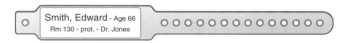

Figure **10-1**　Patient identification bracelet.

It is important that you give the right care to the right person. Giving the wrong care to your patient can cause injury or even death.

When people are admitted to a health care facility, they usually receive a patient identification (ID) bracelet that lists the person's name (Figure 10-1). Other information such as the room number, doctor's name, and the name of the facility may also be listed on the ID bracelet. An allergy bracelet that lists all of the person's allergies may also be applied on admission. An allergy bracelet is usually red. To provide a more homelike environment, many LTC settings use a photo of the patient taken on admission to identify the person.

It is important for you to know what method your facility uses to identify patients and to use it correctly.

How to Handle an Emergency

Falls are a common type of accident, especially in older people. Most falls happen during busy times in the facility such as mealtimes, bedtimes, and change of shift. Patients may become confused because of vision or hearing problems or because of medications they are taking.

Most health care agencies install hand rails in halls, stairways, and bathrooms to help prevent falls. Properly installed and maintained hand rails give support to people who are weak or unsteady when they are walking or using the bathroom (Figure 10-2). Equipment such as wheelchairs, stretchers, beds, and shower chairs rely on wheels to make them movable. Because these items are movable, when a person sits in a wheelchair or on a bed with wheels, the wheelchair or bed may move, resulting in a fall. Always lock the wheels on movable equipment before assisting a patient into or out of the equipment (Figure 10-3). These measures help to keep both patients and visitors safe.

HOW&*WHY*

Dangers such as a wet floor, dim lighting, or broken equipment can also lead to falls.

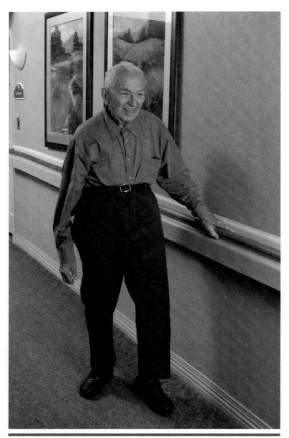

Figure 10-2 Most health care agencies install hand rails in halls, stairways, and bathrooms to help prevent falls.

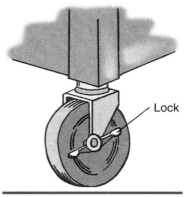

Figure 10-3 Lock on a bed wheel.

NOTES ON
❄ *Older Adults*

Falls are the most common accident in nursing homes. As people get older, their risk of falling increases. If a person has fallen in the past, the person's risk of falling again also increases. Patients over the age of 65 have a higher risk of falling than patients who are younger.

Even with the best safety measures in place, accidents sometimes occur. You need to know what to do if you see a resident or patient fall in your facility or if you find a person who has fallen. If you are caring for a person who starts to fall:

- Do not try to stop the fall. You might hurt yourself, or both of you could fall and make the situation worse.
- Ease the person to the floor as gently as you can, and call for help.
- Always stay with the patient until the charge nurse arrives.
- Do not try to lift a patient who has fallen until the nurse has checked for injuries. You could make the injury worse by trying to get the patient up (Figure 10-4).

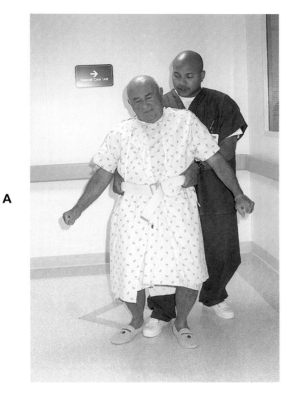
A

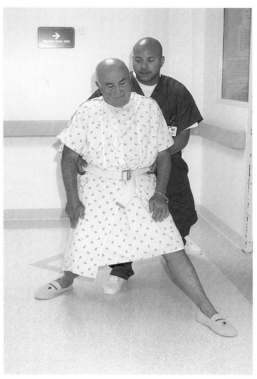
B

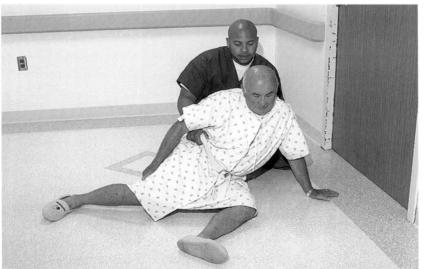
C

Figure 10-4   Supporting a falling person. **A,** With your feet about shoulder width apart, place one foot between the patient's feet. **B,** Pull the patient back against your leg, and let the patient slide against it to the floor. **C,** Bend your knees, and slowly help the patient to sit on the floor.

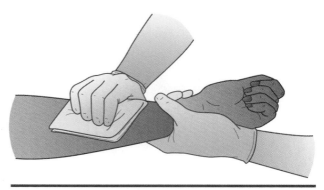

Figure 10-5   Apply firm pressure with a gloved hand to the bleeding area.

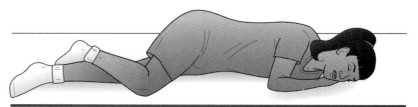

Figure 10-6   Position the patient on her side if she is on the floor or in bed.

Patients who fall may cut themselves and bleed. A large amount of bleeding is called a hemorrhage. If you find a patient who is bleeding:

- Immediately call for help.
- Apply firm pressure with a gloved hand to the bleeding area (Figure 10-5).
- If the injury is to an arm or a leg, raise the limb above the level of the heart to slow the bleeding.
- Always stay with the patient until help arrives.
- If the patient is standing, help her back to bed or into a chair so that she does not faint from loss of blood and fall.
- Follow the directions given to you by the charge nurse.

Some patients may experience a seizure. A seizure is a sudden attack of the muscles contracting and relaxing. If patients are having a **seizure:**

- Call for help.
- Position patients on their side if they are on the floor or in bed (Figure 10-6).
- If patients are standing, ease them to the floor gently so they are not injured.
- Clear the area around patients, and put a pillow or blanket under their head.

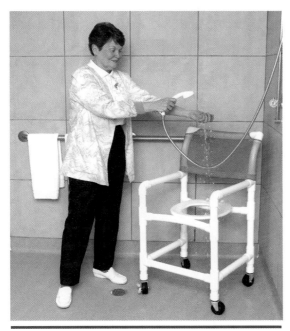

***Figure* 10-7**   Before beginning a bath or
shower, check the temperature of the water.

- Do NOT try to hold patients down or control their movements.
- Never put your fingers or any object into patients' mouth.
- Stay with patients until the seizure has ended or until the charge nurse arrives.
- Make a mental note of the time the seizure started and report the length of the seizure to the charge nurse.

Burns are the second most common injury to patients in health care agencies. Burns can occur if the temperature of the water in the shower or tub is too hot. Hot food or liquids served at mealtime may burn patients. By checking the water temperature before beginning a bath or shower, the chance of burns can be reduced (Figure 10-7).

Smoking causes a fire hazard. Most health care facilities do not allow smoking within the building or limit smoking to restricted areas. The best way to prevent a fire is to keep it from starting in the first place. Be alert to any hazards that could cause a fire. Broken electrical equipment, frayed cords (Figure 10-8), and equipment that overheats can all cause fires. Using extension cords or plugging too many things into an outlet is also danger-ous (Figure 10-9). Three-pronged plugs are used on all electrical equipment (Figure 10-10). The third prong is called the ground. It helps to prevent shocks when using electrical equipment

NOTES ON
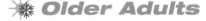 *Older Adults*

Older patients may have a de-creased feeling of pain or tempera-ture and not realize that water or liquids are too hot.

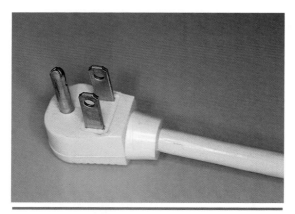

Figure **10-8** A frayed electrical cord.

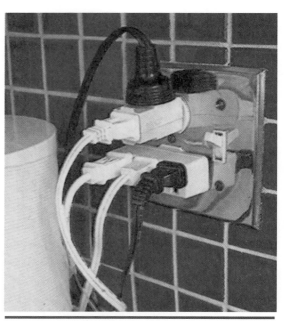

Figure **10-9** This electrical outlet is over-loaded and could cause a fire.

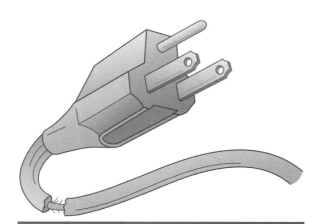

Figure **10-10** A three-pronged plug.

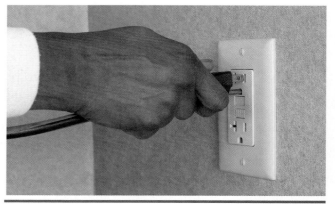

Figure **10-11** When plugging in or unplugging equipment, always hold the plug by its base.

HOW & WHY

When plugging in or unplugging equipment, always hold the plug by its base (see Figure 10-11). Never unplug a piece of equipment by pulling on the cord, which can cause sparking.

(Figure 10-11). If you notice a fire hazard or piece of equipment that is damaged, report it to your supervisor immediately.

Every employee should know where the fire alarms, fire extinguishers, and exit doors are in the building. Never block an alarm, extinguisher, or exit door with carts or other equipment. Fire drills are held on a regular basis to practice the fire emergency procedures.

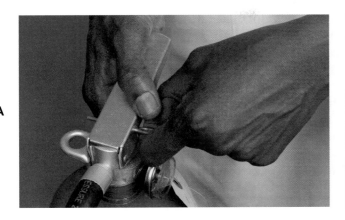
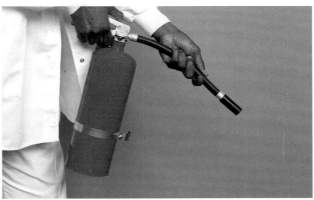
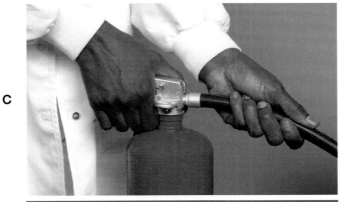

Figure 10-12   Using a fire extinguisher. **A,** Pull
the safety pin out of the handle of the extinguisher.
B, Aim the hose at the base of the fire—this helps
keep the fire from spreading. **C,** Squeeze the handle
of the extinguisher.

In case of a fire, remember to RACE:
R—Rescue any patients in danger by moving them away
from the fire.
A—Activate the alarm system.
C—Contain the fire by closing doors and windows.
E—Extinguish the fire if it is small.

Many agencies require that all employees know how to use a
fire extinguisher. There are different types of fire extinguishers for
different types of fires. Fire extinguishers are marked according to
their use: oil/grease fires, electrical fires, and paper/wood fires.
Some agencies use an all-purpose fire extinguisher in patient
care areas. A fire extinguisher is very easy to use; just remember
PASS (Figure 10-12).

P—Pull the safety pin out of the handle of the extinguisher.

A—Aim the hose at the *base* of the fire—this helps keep the fire from spreading.

S—Squeeze the handle of the extinguisher.

S—Sweep the nozzle back and forth across the base of the fire to extinguish it.

Each facility has policies and procedures to follow if it is necessary to evacuate (remove) the patients from the facility. The charge nurse will decide if it is necessary to evacuate and will tell you what to do. Unless instructed otherwise, you first remove the patients who are closest to the fire. Those who can walk should be helped to go to a safe place. Patients in wheelchairs are the second group to be evacuated, and bed-bound patients are evacuated last. Figures 10-13 and 10-14 show how to evacuate people who cannot walk.

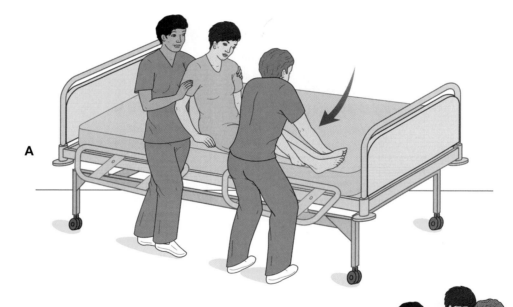

A

B

Figure **10-13**   Evacuating a person who cannot walk—2-person carry. **A,** Assist the person to a sitting position on the side of the bed. **B,** Place the person's arms over your shoulder. With one caregiver on each side, reach behind the person's back and grasp the shoulder of your co-worker. Reach under the person's legs, and grasp your co-worker's arm. Carry the person to a safe area.

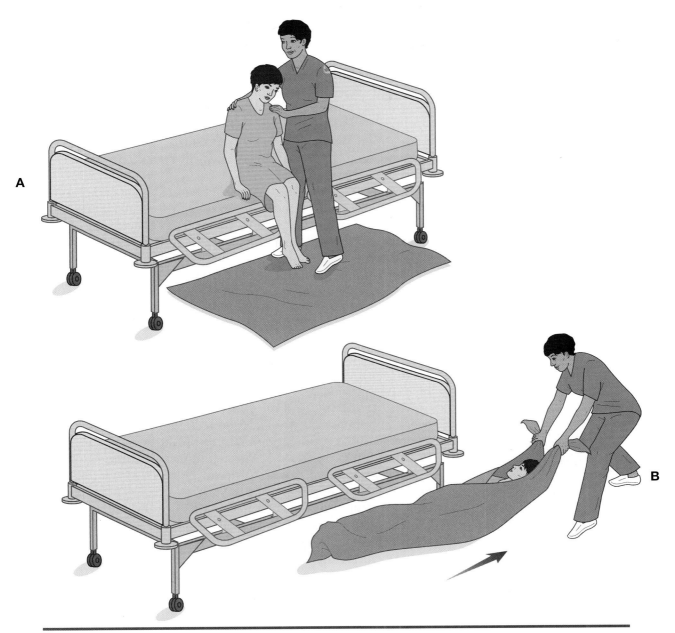

Figure 10-14   Evacuating a person who cannot walk—1-person carry. **A,** Spread a large blanket on the floor, making sure that it is large enough to extend from the person's feet to beyond his head. Assist the person in sitting on the side of the bed. Grasp the person from behind by reaching under her arms and crossing your hands over her chest. Lower her to the floor by sliding her gently down one of your legs. **B,** Wrap the blanket around the person. Grasp the blanket over the head, and pull the person to a safe area.

Once the fire department arrives, they will direct the evacuation and assist in moving the patients to safety.

Using oxygen is also a safety concern. It is important that patients receive the oxygen that they need to treat their condition. It is also important that the patient remain safe. When a patient is receiving oxygen therapy, a fire can ignite more easily and burn more quickly than it could without the extra oxygen. Remember, oxygen does not cause the fire; it makes the fire burn faster and hotter. Even a small spark can start a fire if there is an oxygen tank on.

An "OXYGEN IN USE" sign must be posted on the door of any patient who is receiving oxygen. Keep all electrical equipment, such as radios or televisions, away from the oxygen tank. Do not use anything flammable, such as nail polish remover, on a patient who is receiving oxygen. Even though a facility does not permit smoking, some visitors and patients may not follow the rules. Notify your supervisor immediately if a patient or visitor is smoking or has matches in a patient care area.

There are many hazardous substances in the workplace. The federal government has designed a program called the "Written Hazardous Communication Program" that requires all employers to teach their employees about the possible dangers they will be exposed to.

A material safety data sheet (MSDS) must be provided for every chemical you are exposed to (Figure 10-15). Even things as common as soaps and cleaning products have the potential to cause harm. Keep these items in a locked cabinet so that patients do not have access to them. Hazardous chemicals must have warning labels (Figure 10-16). Words, pictures, and symbols tell you what type of safety measures are needed.

Each year your employer will ask you to attend a special training program to help you to remember where to find information about the chemicals in your facility and what to do if there is an accident involving those chemicals.

HOW & WHY

The "Written Hazardous Communication Program" is also called the "Right to Know" program.

NOTES ON
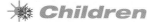
Children

Accidental poisonings are a concern when caring for children. The phone number for your local poison control center should be posted by each telephone for emergency use.

NOTES ON
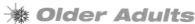
Older Adults

Accidental poisonings are a concern when caring for confused elderly patients. The phone number for your local poison control center should be posted by each telephone for emergency use.

MATERIAL SAFETY DATA SHEET
(MSDS)

Date of Issue: 4/28/02		Date of Revision: 8/8/03

SECTION 1 IDENTIFICATION

CHEMICAL NAME: Glutaraldehyde	INFORMATION TELEPHONE NUMBER: 1 (800) 733-8690
TRADE NAME: Aldecide	EMERGENCY TELEPHONE NUMBER:
MANUFACTURER'S NAME: Brennan Corporation	1 (800) 331-0766
MFG. ADDRESS: P.O. Box 93	
CITY: Camden STATE: NJ ZIP: 08106	

SECTION 2 COMPOSITION OF INGREDIENTS

CAS NUMBER	CHEMICAL NAME OF INGREDIENTS	PERCENT	PEL	TLV
111-30-8	Glutaraldehyde	2.5	0.2 ppm	0.2 ppm
7732-18-5	Water	97.4	None	None
7632-00-0	Sodium Nitrite	<1	None	None

SECTION 3 PHYSICAL AND CHEMICAL PROPERTIES

BOILING POINT: 212° F	SPECIFIC GRAVITY (H_2O = 1): 1.004
VAPOR PRESSURE (mm Hg): 0.20 at 20° C	VAPOR DENSITY (AIR = 1): 1.1
ODOR: Sharp odor	pH: 7.5-8.5
SOLUBILITY IN WATER: Complete (100%)	MELTING POINT: n/a
APPEARANCE: Bluish-green liquid	FREEZING POINT: 32° F
EVAPORATION RATE: 0.98 (Water = 1)	ODOR THRESHOLD: 0.04 ppm

SECTION 4 FIRE AND EXPLOSION HAZARD DATA

FLASH POINT: Not flammable (aqueous solution)

FLAMMABILITY LIMITS: LEL: n/a   UEL: n/a

EXTINGUISHING MEDIA: n/a (aqueous solution)

SPECIAL FIRE FIGHTING PROCEDURES: n/a

UNUSUAL FIRE/EXPL HAZARDS: None

SECTION 5 REACTIVITY DATA

STABILITY: Stable

CONDITIONS TO AVOID: Avoid temperatures above 200° F.

INCOMPATIBILITY (MATERIAL TO AVOID): Acids and alkalines will neutralize active ingredient.

HAZARDOUS DECOMPOSITION BYPRODUCTS: None

HAZARDOUS POLYMERIZATION: Will not occur

***Figure* 10-15** A material safety data sheet (MSDS) must be available for every chemical in the workplace.

Continued

MATERIAL SAFETY DATA SHEET

PAGE 2

SECTION 6 HEALTH HAZARD DATA

ROUTE OF ENTRY: SKIN: yes   **EYES:** yes   **INHALATION:** yes   **INGESTION:** yes

SIGNS AND SYMPTOMS OF OVEREXPOSURE:

SKIN: Moderate irritation. May aggravate existing dermatitis.

EYES: Serious eye irritant. May cause irreversible damage.

INHALATION: Vapors may be irritating and cause stinging sensations in the eyes, nose, and throat.

INGESTION: May cause irritation or chemical burns of the mouth, throat, esophagus, and stomach. May cause vomiting, diarrhea, dizziness, faintness, and general systemic illness.

CARCINOGENICITY DATA: **NTP:** No   **AIRC:** No   **OSHA:** No

SECTION 7 EMERGENCY FIRST AID PROCEDURES

SKIN: Wash skin with soap and water for 15 minutes. If irritation persists, seek medical attention.

EYES: Immediately flush with water for 15 minutes. Seek medical attention.

INHALATION: Remove to fresh air. If irritation persists, seek medical attention.

INGESTION: Do not induce vomiting. Give large amounts of water. Seek medical attention.

SECTION 8 PRECAUTIONS FOR SAFE HANDLING AND USE

SPILL PROCEDURES: Ventilate area, wear protective gloves and eye gear. Wipe with sponge, mop, or towel. Flush with large quantities of water. Collect liquid and discard it.

WASTE DISPOSAL METHOD: Container must be triple rinsed and disposed of in accordance with federal, state, and/or local regulations. Used solution should be flushed thoroughly with water into sewage disposal system in accordance with federal, state, and/or local regulations.

PRECAUTIONS IN HANDLING AND STORAGE: Store in a cool, dry place (59-86° F) away from direct sunlight or sources of intense heat. Keep container tightly closed when not in use.

SECTION 9 CONTROL MEASURES

VENTILATION: Adequate ventilation to maintain recommended exposed limit.

RESPIRATORY PROTECTION: None normally required for routine use.

SKIN PROTECTION: Wear protective gloves. Butyl rubber, nitrile rubber, polyethylene, or double-gloved latex.

EYE PROTECTION: Safety goggles or safety glasses

WORK/HYGIENE PRACTICES: Prompt rinsing of hands after contact. Handle in accordance with good personal hygiene and safety practices. These practices include avoiding unnecessary exposure.

Figure 10-15, *cont'd* A material safety data sheet (MSDS) must be available for every chemical in the workplace.

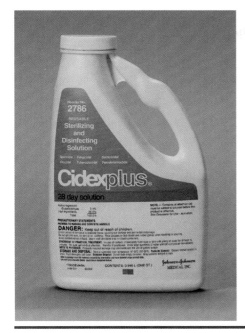

PRECAUTIONARY STATEMENTS
HAZARDS TO HUMANS AND DOMESTIC ANIMALS
DANGER: Keep out of reach of children.
Direct contact is corrosive to exposed tissue, causing eye damage and skin irritation/damage. Do not get into eyes, on skin or on clothing. Wear goggles or face shield and rubber gloves when handling or pouring. Avoid contamination of food. Use in well ventilated area in closed containers.
STATEMENT OF PRACTICAL TREATMENT: In case of contact, immediately flush eyes or skin with plenty of water for at least 15 minutes. For eyes, get medical attention. Harmful if swallowed. Drink large quantities of water and call a physician immediately.
NOTE TO PHYSICIAN: Probable mucosal damage may contraindicate the use of gastric lavage.
STORAGE AND DISPOSAL: Store at controlled room temperature 15°-30°C (59°-86°F).
Pesticide disposal: Discard residual solution in drain. Flush thoroughly with water.
Container disposal: Do not reuse empty container. Wrap container and put in trash.
Refer to package insert for material compatibility information and more detailed usage/product data.
Use with polycarbonate plastic could cause equipment failure.

*TRADEMARK   CONTENTS: 0.946 L (ONE QT.)
2786 C2-1   830006

Figure **10-16**   All hazardous chemicals must have warning labels.

The events of September 11, 2001, made us realize how important it is for every health care worker to know how to deal with an emergency. Your facility has a disaster plan, and your employer will review it with you each year. Tornadoes, earthquakes, or bomb threats, in addition to fires, may affect you.

In the event of a tornado:
- Move all patients away from windows.
- Remove any heavy objects, such as plants, from windowsills.
- Close the drapes or blinds.
- Pull the privacy curtains around any patients who remain in their beds.

The National Weather Service may be able to provide you with a warning if a tornado is sighted in your area. If you are involved in a tornado, stay calm and follow the directions of your supervisor.

During an earthquake the layers of earth move back and forth over each other. If an earthquake occurs, try to stay calm. During the actual earthquake you will not be able to help your patients.
- If you are inside the building, stay there and take cover under a heavy table or in a doorway.
- After the earthquake is over, do not use matches or candles. During the movement of the ground, gas pipes can break and an open flame can cause an explosion.
- Follow your supervisor's directions for providing care after the earthquake is over.

If your job includes answering the telephone, you could be involved in a bomb threat. If you receive this type of call:
- Make note of the exact time of the call.
- Be calm and courteous; do not interrupt the caller.
- Pay special attention to any noises in the background such as music, machinery, or other voices.
- Write down exactly what the caller says, and notify your supervisor as soon as the caller hangs up.
- Always take a bomb threat seriously.

Personal Safety Measures

Personal safety is an issue for all employees. The Occupational Safety and Health Administration (OSHA) reports that more assaults occur in health care and social service industries than any other. Hospital emergency departments frequently deal with patients and visitors who are under the influence of drugs or alcohol. Poorly lit parking areas are a risk to staff who enter or leave the building when it is dark. There are many things you can do to stay safe, including:
- Try to park in a well-lit area.
- If you have to walk to your car in the dark, use the buddy system.
- Keep the building safe by reporting any unauthorized visitors or suspicious activity.
- Promptly report any violent or threatening incidents to your supervisor.
- Be sensitive to racial and cultural differences.
- Treat others with respect.

Most employers offer a workplace safety program to help you to stay safe.

HOW & WHY

The safety program may include information about security cameras or monitors if installed in your facility.

Do's and Don'ts of Restraint Use

The use of restraints in health care agencies has been a topic of debate for almost 20 years. A **restraint** is defined as any manual or chemical item or device that is attached to or next to the person's body that limits the person's freedom of movement or body access that the person cannot easily remove. Examples of restraints include:

- Wrist restraints (Figure 10-17)
- Mitten restraints (Figure 10-18)
- Vest restraints (Figure 10-19)
- Jacket restraints (Figure 10-20)
- Belt restraints (Figure 10-21)
- Full side rails/bed rails

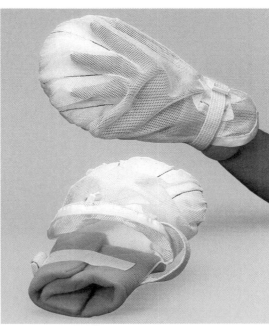

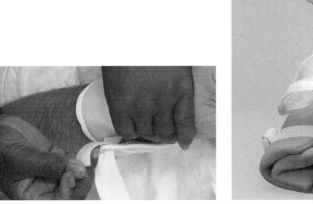

Figure **10-17**   Wrist restraints.

Figure **10-18**   Mitten restraints.

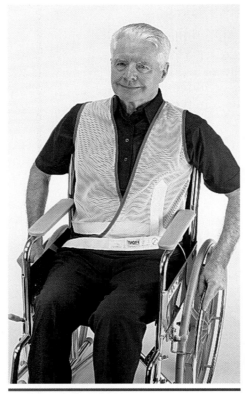

***Figure* 10-19**   Vest restraint.

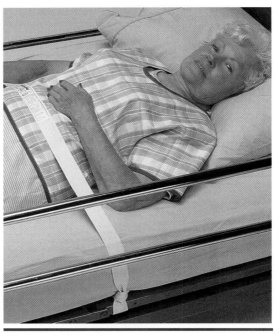

***Figure* 10-20**   Jacket restraint. Always ensure the side rails are covered to prevent patients from attempting to exit through or between rails.

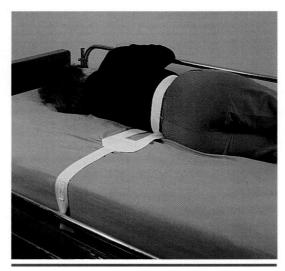

***Figure* 10-21**   Belt restraint.

In years past, physical restraints were commonly used in an attempt to prevent patient injuries and falls. Current studies show that the use of restraints does not decrease falls and actually increases the number of injuries in health care settings. Even full side rails, which were routinely used with most patients in the past, are considered a restraint and can cause injury (Figure 10-22). Restraint use has been mentioned in some strangulation deaths in the United States. In these cases, the patients died because of the way the restraint was used (Figures 10-23 and 10-24).

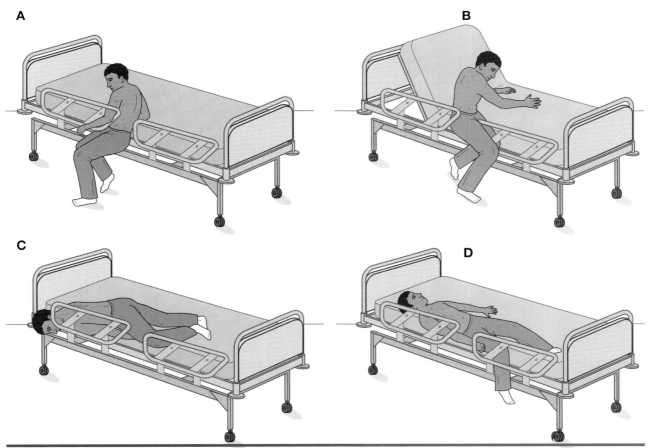

Figure 10-22 Full side rails are considered a restraint and may pose a safety risk. **A,** Person is trapped between the bars of the side rail. **B,** Person is trapped between the upper and lower side rails. **C,** Person is trapped between the headboard and the side rail. **D,** Person is trapped between the mattress and the side rail.

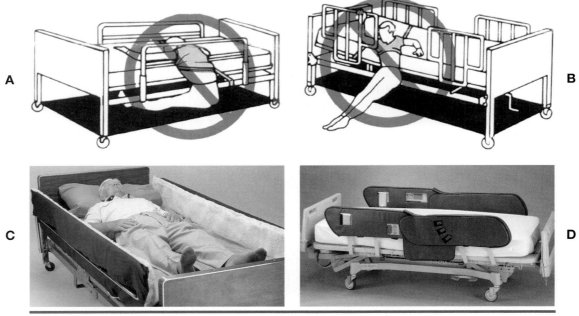

***Figure* 10-23**   With a waist restraint in place, a person may become trapped between the upper and lower side rails, resulting in injury or death. **A,** A padded side rail prevents the person from being caught between the rails. **B,** Unprotected half-length bed rails are dangerous for restrained persons. **C,** Full-length bed rails. **D,** Full-length bed rails.

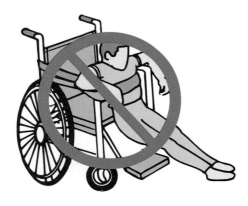

Straps to prevent sliding should always be over the thighs—NOT around the waist or chest. Straps should be at a 45-degree angle and secured to the chair under the seat, not behind the back. They should be snug but comfortable and not restrict breathing. If a belt or vest is too loose or applied around the waist, the person may slide partially off the seat—resulting in possible suffocation and death.

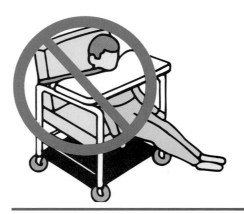

Tray tables (with or without a belt or vest) pose potential danger if the person should slide partly under the table and become caught. This could result in suffocation and death. Make sure the person's hips are positioned at the back of the chair—this may necessitate the use of an anti-slide material (Posey Grip), a pommel cushion, or a restrictive device if the person shows any tendency to slide forward.

***Figure* 10-24**   When the person slides down or forward with a restraint on, injury or strangulation can occur.

Freedom from restraints is a resident right under OBRA guidelines. There may be some situations in which the use of restraints is permitted. OBRA permits a person to be restrained if:

- The restraint is necessary to treat the person's physical, emotional, or behavioral problems and is part of the plan of care.
- The restraint is necessary to protect other patients or persons from harm.
- The doctor has ordered the restraint for medical reasons and includes in the order the body part to be restrained, the device to be used, and the amount of time the restraint is to be used.
- The least restrictive method is used.
- The person agrees to the use of the restraint.
- The person's dignity and quality of life are protected.

Each facility has policies and procedures in place for using restraints. Basic guidelines for restraint use include:

- NEVER apply a restraint without fully understanding how the device should be used.
- If a person is restrained, the restraint and skin under the restraint must be checked at least every 15 minutes and released and the person repositioned at least every 2 hours.
- NEVER apply a restraint without a doctor's order.
- NEVER apply a restraint if the person refuses it.

Most agencies have a "restraint alternative" program that help to keep patients safe and still upholds their right to be restraint free. Alternative to restraints include:

- Bed alarms to alert staff if a patient gets up without help (Figure 10-25)
- Floor cushions or pads next to the bed to decrease injuries if a person does fall when getting out of bed (Figure 10-26)
- Barriers such as stop signs posted on doors to discourage confused patients from wandering into the area (Figure 10-27)

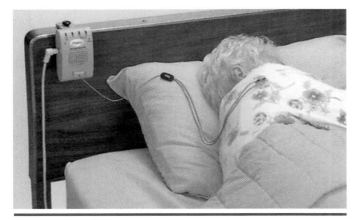

Figure **10-25** Bed alarm.

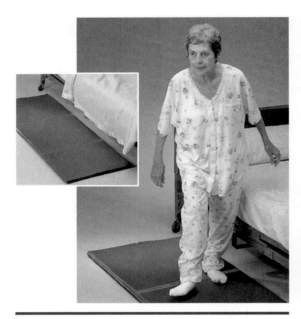

***Figure* 10-26** Floor cushion next to the bed.

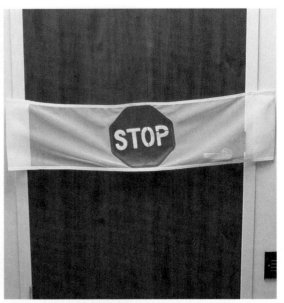

***Figure* 10-27** Barrier with a stop sign to discourage wandering.

- Partial bed rails to prevent patients from rolling out of the bed while allowing them freedom to get up if they wish to (Figure 10-28)
- Wedge cushions applied to wheelchairs to prevent forward sliding (Figure 10-29)
- Wheelchair/chair alarms to alert staff if the person slides forward or tries to get up without help (Figure 10-30)
- Activities and diversions such as games, movies, and music
- Pillows, wedges, and other positioning devices
- Furniture that meets the person's needs such as low beds, rocking chairs, or recliners
- Easy-release belts that the person can remove if desired

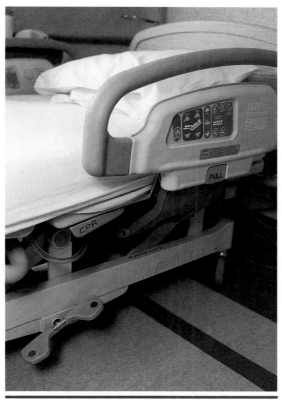

Figure **10-28**   A partial bed rail provides
safety without restraining the patient.

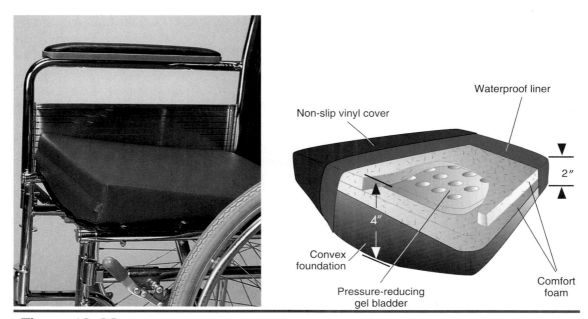

Figure **10-29**   A wedge cushion helps to prevent the person from sliding out of the wheelchair.

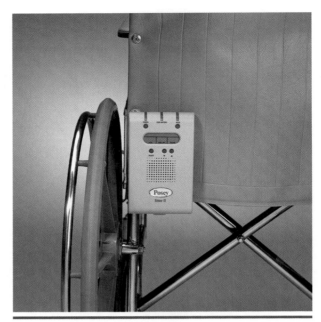

***Figure* 10-30** Wheelchair alarms are triggered by a change in weight.

It is important to remember the definition of a restraint when deciding if something you are using is a restraint. For example:

It is 4:00 AM, and the certified nursing assistant (CNA), Loretta, has assisted Mr. Henderson back to bed 6 times in the last hour. Mr. Henderson is slightly confused and keeps returning to the nurses' station asking if it is time to make breakfast. Mr. Henderson has fallen several times in the last month, and Loretta is worried that he will fall and hurt himself. Loretta thinks about helping Mr. Henderson back to bed and putting his side rails up to remind him not to get up without help. When she reviews his care plan, she sees that Mr. Henderson was a cook and always started work at 3:00 in the morning. The care plan tells Loretta that the best way to deal with this situation is to assist Mr. Henderson to a comfortable chair near the nurses' station and provide him with a snack as allowed on his diet. Loretta also encourages Mr. Henderson to tell her about his job as a cook. Mr. Henderson is calm and remains safe sitting in the chair at the nurses' station, where he can be more closely observed.

Loretta knew that using side rails on this patient would be considered a restraint. By reviewing the care plan, she not only provided Mr. Henderson with a safe environment, but she also treated him with dignity and respect, which makes his quality of life better.

Certainly not all situations are handled this easily. With creative problem solving, most persons can be safe and restraint free. When restraints are not readily available and staff are encouraged to use other methods to treat problems, patients are much happier and safer.

CHAPTER REVIEW

1. List 4 ways that you can prevent accidents or incidents in your facility.

2. What should you do if a patient you are caring for falls?

3. What should you do if a patient or resident you are caring for has a seizure?

4. What are the 4 things you should do if there is a fire in your facility? (Remember to RACE.)

5. What should you do in case of a tornado?

6. How should you handle a bomb threat?

7. What are some things you can do to stay safe at work?

8. What is a restraint?

Circle the one BEST response.

9. Whose job is it to keep the patients in your hospital or nursing home safe?
   a. The administrator
   b. The director of nursing
   c. The security department
   d. All employees

10. A large amount of bleeding is called a(n)
   a. Seizure
   b. Hemorrhage
   c. Burn
   d. Incident

11. Ms. Lester is mildly confused and sometimes forgets that she needs help when getting up from her wheelchair to walk to the bathroom. Which of the following methods could be used to help her stay safe while keeping her free from restraints as required by OBRA?
   a. An easy-release belt that she can remove if she wishes to
   b. A chair alarm that alerts staff that she is attempting to stand
   c. Encouraging her to participate in activities such as games or movies so that she can be more closely observed
   d. All of the above

Answers are on pages 705 to 706.

CHAPTER 11

Body Mechanics

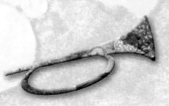

What you will learn

- The principles of body mechanics
- How to move and position a patient in bed
- How to transfer patients safely
- How to use a mechanical lift

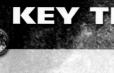

KEY TERMS

Body alignment The correct positioning of the head, back, neck, and limbs

Dangling Allowing the patient to sit on the side of the bed for 1 to 2 minutes to adjust to the change from a lying to a sitting position

Fowler's position/semi-Fowler's position The head of the bed is raised 60 to 90 degrees for Fowler's position and 30 to 60 degrees for semi-Fowler's position. The patient's knees are elevated just a little to avoid pressure on the back of the legs

Orthostatic hypotension A rapid drop in blood pressure that occurs with a change in position

Prone position The patient is on the abdomen

Sims' position The patient begins in a side-lying position and is turned toward the abdomen

Supine position The patient rests on the back with arms and legs straight down at sides

Trapeze A bar hung above the patient's bed to assist the person with moving in the bed

The Principles of Body Mechanics

As a nursing assistant, one of your duties is to help patients move. You need to know how to do this so that you do not injure the patient or yourself. Using good body mechanics means that you use your body to lift and move patients without putting too much strain on your body. Using good body mechanics help you by:

- Protecting you from injury when moving patients or objects
- Reducing fatigue and strain on your back
- Making your muscles work with you to maximize strength
- Making lifting, transferring, and moving objects and patients easier
- Giving you balance and stability when lifting

Correct posture is essential to good body mechanics because it puts the body parts in proper alignment (Figure 11-1). When standing, your feet should be flat on the floor about 12 inches apart. Your back and neck should be straight. Your arms should be relaxed at your sides and abdominal muscles tucked in. With your head up and your eyes straight ahead, an imaginary line could be drawn straight from your head through the center of your body to your feet. This correct positioning of your head, back, body, and limbs is called **body alignment**. Body alignment is important for your patients too. When your patient is sitting in the chair or lying in bed, the body should be in proper alignment (Figure 11-2).

HOW & WHY

Back injuries from moving patients are the most common cause of on-the-job injuries for nursing assistants. Using good body mechanics can help prevent injuries.

NOTES ON
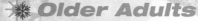
Older Adults

When moving an older person, move slowly and carefully to avoid causing pain. The skin of the older person is more fragile, and joints may be stiff.

NOTES ON
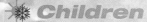
Children

Body alignment is important when positioning children, as well as adults.

HOW & WHY

Good body mechanics are important at home and at work. If you think about what you are doing before you do it, you are less likely to get hurt.

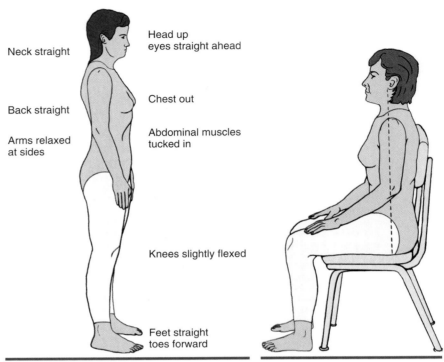

Neck straight

Back straight

Arms relaxed at sides

Head up eyes straight ahead

Chest out

Abdominal muscles tucked in

Knees slightly flexed

Feet straight toes forward

***Figure* 11-1**   Correct standing body alignment.

***Figure* 11-2**   Correct sitting body alignment.

Safety

When getting ready to lift a patient or move an object, always start in good body alignment. Here are some guidelines to help you to stay safe when lifting:

1. Ask for help whenever possible. Never try to lift something that you feel is too heavy for you to lift safely.
2. Ask the patients to help move parts of their bodies if they are able to.
3. Keep your feet about shoulder width apart for a broad base of support.
4. Bend at the hips and knees instead of at the waist (Figure 11-3).
5. Use the large muscles of the arms, legs, and thighs instead of the back muscles when lifting.
6. Keep whatever you are moving close to your body.
7. Whenever possible, push, pull, or roll an object rather than lifting it.
8. Avoid jerking or tugging motions. Use a smooth motion to lift an object.
9. When working with others, **count to three** so that everyone is working together.
10. Avoid twisting your body. Turn your whole body to face the object you are lifting.

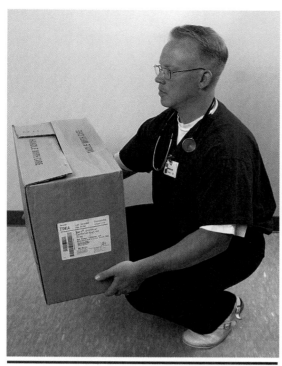

***Figure* 11-3**   Bending at the hips and knees lets the strong muscles of the legs do the lifting and prevents back strain.

Moving a Patient in Bed

When moving patients in bed, you should encourage them to help as much as possible so the sheet will not rub against the patient's skin. Using a lift sheet will decrease the friction of sliding a patient's skin over the sheets. A **trapeze** (bar hung above the patient's bed) will help the patient to raise the buttocks off the bed and move easier (Figure 11-4). Before moving a patient in the bed, you will need to decide how much help you will need. If the patient is heavy or unable to assist, you will need to ask another nursing assistant for help.

Moving a person who is unable to help or is very weak requires at least 2 people. This helps to protect you and the patient from injury.

NOTES ON
⑨ *Culture*

If the people you are moving are unable to understand what you are telling them because of a language barrier, you can use gestures to show them what you want them to do.

Safety

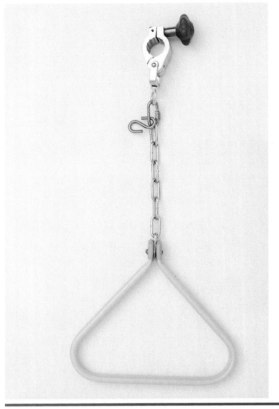
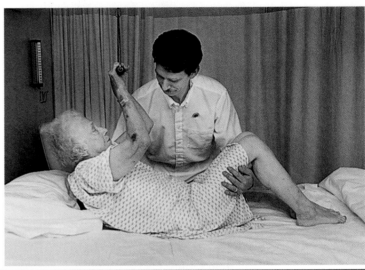

Figure **11-4**   **A,** Trapeze. **B,** Moving a patient with a trapeze.

Procedure
MOVING THE PATIENT UP IN BED

EQUIPMENT
- **A lift sheet for the dependent patient**
  Get help if needed

◆ **COMPLETE STANDARD BEGINNING STEPS (see inside front cover)**

1 Raise the bed to a comfortable working height.
Raise the side rail on the far side of the bed.

2 Remove any positioning devices or pillows used for the current position.

3 Lower the head of the bed so that the bed is flat.

MOVING THE PATIENT UP IN BED—cont'd

4 Turn the patient onto her back, and place the pillow against the headboard to protect the patient's head (Figure 11-5).

5 If the patient **can** assist:

   a. Ask the patient to bend both knees and place her feet flat on the bed.

   b. Ask the patient to hold on to the side rail or the trapeze.

   c. Place one of your arms under the patient's shoulders and the other arm under her upper thighs. Ask the patient to put her chin on her chest.

   d. With a rocking motion of the hips and legs, and on the count of three, push toward the head of the bed with your arms while the patient lifts her hips off the bed and pushes toward the head of the bed with both feet.

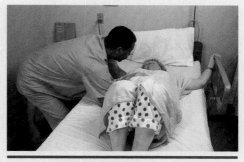

Figure **11-5**   Step 4.

6 If the patient **cannot** assist (requires 2 people):

   a. With the patient on her side, place a lift sheet under the patient by rolling up the edge of the sheet close to her and placing it firmly against her back from the shoulders to the hips.

   b. Roll the patient onto her other side, and pull the sheet through.

   c. Turn the patient onto her back.

   d. Roll or fanfold the sheet close to the patient's side.

   e. Place one foot slightly in front of the other about shoulder width apart (Figure 11-6).

   f. Grasp the sheet close to the patient with one hand near her shoulder and the other at her hip.

   g. With your hips and knees bent a little, count to three and together lift the patient toward the head of the bed.

   h. Smooth out the lift sheet.

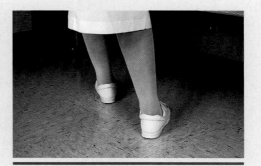

Figure **11-6**   Step 6e.

Procedure
MOVING THE PATIENT UP IN BED—cont'd

7 Assist the patient to a comfortable position using the turning schedule or as the charge nurse instructs.

8 Replace the pillow under the patient's head.

9 Place the signal light and personal care items where the patient can reach them.

◆ **COMPLETE STANDARD ENDING STEPS (see inside front cover)**

Positioning a Patient in Bed

Positioning a patient does four things: (1) it makes the patient more comfortable, (2) it improves blood flow, (3) it prevents contractures and respiratory problems (Chapter 12), and (4) it relieves pressure over bony areas such as the hips and heels. In general, patients who are unable to move on their own should be turned and repositioned at least every 1½ to 2 hours if they are in bed and every 20 to 30 minutes if they are sitting in a chair. Frequent position changes help to prevent pressure ulcers.

It is important that the patient's body be kept in proper alignment. There are several positions that are commonly used for patients while in bed.

Supine Position

In the **supine position** patients rest on their back with their arms and legs straight down at their sides (Figure 11-7). The bed is flat, and patients may be supported with pillows to help make them comfortable and to help them stay in the correct position.

Fowler's and Semi-Fowler's Position

The **Fowler's position** is a variation of the supine position. The patient begins in the supine position. The head of the bed is raised **60 to 90 degrees**, and the patient's knees are elevated a little to avoid pressure on the back of the legs. This position may be used when the patient is eating, reading, or watching television. In the **semi-Fowler's position** the head of the bed is raised **30 to 60 degrees**, and the patient's knees are elevated a little to avoid pressure on the back of the legs (Figure 11-8). The patient can use this position when watching television or talking to visitors.

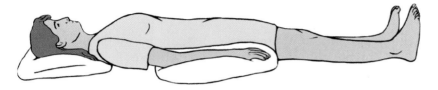

***Figure* 11-7** Supine position and upper arms parallel to the body and supported.

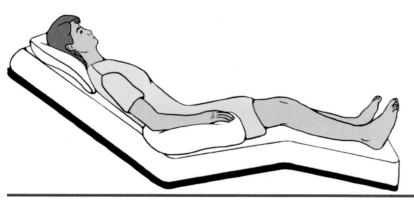

***Figure* 11-8** Semi-Fowler's position.

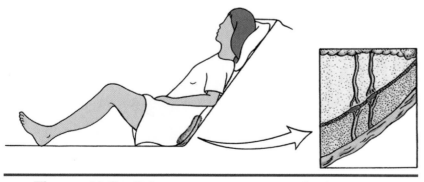

***Figure* 11-9** Sliding movement can cause skin breakdown.

HOW&WHY

Both the Fowler's and semi-Fowler's position cause pressure on the patient's coccyx (tailbone). If the head of the bed is higher than 30 degrees, the patient may slide down in the bed. This sliding movement can cause skin breakdown (Figure 11-9).

Side-Lying and Side-Lying Oblique Position

These positions move the pressure from the bony areas of the back. In both positions the patient starts in the supine position with the head of the bed no higher than **30 degrees.** After injury or surgery the patient may be logrolled, keeping the head, back, and legs in a straight line, into a side-lying position. This keeps the neck and spine aligned.

Prone Position

The **prone position** places patients on their abdomen (Figure 11-10). The position may be used to eliminate pressure over the back and hips.

Sims' Position

The **Sims' position** is a variation of the prone position. In the Sims' position the patient begins in a side-lying position and is turned toward the abdomen. This position also decreases pressure on the back (Figure 11-11).

Pillows and foam wedges may be used to help keep the patient in proper alignment.

NOTES ON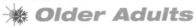

The prone position is not commonly used and may be uncomfortable for elderly patients.

NOTES ON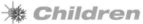

The prone or stomach-lying position is not recommended for infants as it may increase the risk of sudden infant death syndrome (SIDS).

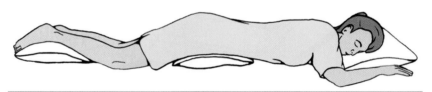

***Figure* 11-10**   Prone position.

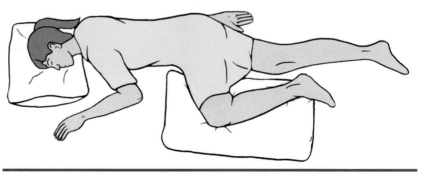

***Figure* 11-11**   Sims' position.

Procedure
POSITIONING THE PATIENT IN BED

EQUIPMENT

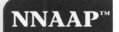

- Pillows
- Foam wedge or positioning devices as ordered
  Get help if needed

◆ **COMPLETE STANDARD BEGINNING STEPS (see inside front cover)**

1 Raise the bed to a comfortable working height.

2 Remove any positioning devices or pillows used for the current position.

3 Lower the head of the bed so that the bed is flat.

4 Position the patient according to the turning schedule or direction from your charge nurse.

   a. Supine position
     1) Lower the head of the bed so that the bed is flat. Use heel pads or a small pillow or towel rolled up under the ankles to prevent pressure on the heels.
     2) Maintain the upper arms parallel with the body, and support the forearms with a small pillow or folded blanket (see Figure 11-7).

   b. Fowler's or semi-Fowler's position
     1) Begin with the patient in the supine position.
     2) Elevate the head of the bed **60 to 90 degrees** for the Fowler's position or **30 to 60 degrees** for the semi-Fowler's position.
     3) Elevate the knee section of the bed slightly to prevent sliding (Figure 11-12).

   c. Side-lying or oblique side-lying position
     1) Begin with the patient in the supine position.
     2) Stand on the side of the bed to which you will turn the patient.
     3) Place one of your hands on the patient's far shoulder and the other on her far hip.

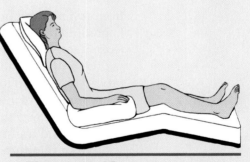

***Figure* 11-12**   Fowler's position.

Continued

Procedure
POSITIONING THE PATIENT IN BED—cont'd

4) Roll the patient smoothly toward you onto her hip. A lift sheet may also be used to turn the patient toward you (Figure 11-13).

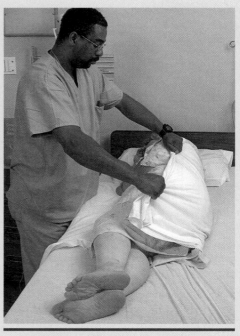

***Figure* 11-13** Step 4 c(4).

5) Place a pillow lengthwise along the patient's back, and tuck in smoothly to prevent the patient from rolling onto her back. Logrolling a patient requires at least 3 caregivers and can be done with or without a lift sheet. The procedure used to logroll a patient is the same as turning a patient onto her side except that the body is turned as a unit and remains straight at all times. This procedure is used for patients who have had spine surgery or an injury that requires that the spine be kept straight (Figure 11-14).

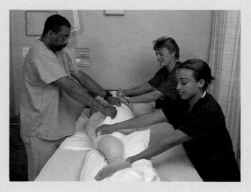

A

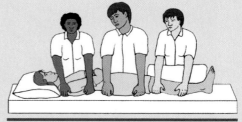

B

***Figure* 11-14** **A,** Logrolling a patient using a lift sheet. **B,** Logrolling a patient without a lift sheet.

Procedure
POSITIONING THE PATIENT IN BED—cont'd

6) Bend both of the patient's knees after the turn, and place a pillow or folded blanket between the legs from the knees to the feet to prevent pressure.

7) Position the lower arm so that the patient is not lying on the arm (Figure 11-15, *A*).

8) Position the upper arm on a pillow (Figure 11-15, *B*).

9) For the oblique side-lying position, move the shoulder blade next to the bed forward toward you.

10) Make sure the pillow under the head is smooth and that the ear is flat.

11) Flex the arm next to the mattress, and raise the hand.

12) Support the upper arm with a pillow so that it is level with the shoulder.

13) Pull the lower hip slightly forward.

d. Prone position

1) Begin with the patient in the supine position.

2) Stand on the side of the bed to which you will turn the patient.

3) Place a small pillow against the patient's abdomen below the ribs.

4) Place the patient's arms straight at her sides.

5) Place one of your hands on the patient's far shoulder and the other on her far hip.

6) Roll the patient smoothly toward you onto her abdomen. A lift sheet may also be used to turn the patient toward you.

7) The patient should be centered in the bed.

8) Place a small pillow under the patient's head, and turn the head to one side (Figure 11-16).

9) Make sure the pillow under the head is smooth and that the ear is flat.

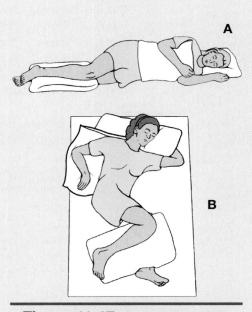

Figure **11-15**   Step 4c(7) and (8).

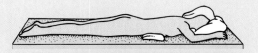

Figure **11-16**   Step 4d(8).

Continued

Procedure
POSITIONING THE PATIENT IN BED—cont'd

10) Position the arms at shoulder level with the elbows bent and the palms flat on the bed.

11) Place a pillow under the lower legs from the knees to the feet.

e. Sims' position

1) Begin with the patient in a side-lying position

2) Place one of your hands on the patient's far shoulder and the other on her far hip.

3) Roll the patient smoothly toward you partly onto her abdomen. A lift sheet may also be used to turn the patient toward you.

4) Straighten the leg on the far side, and bend the knee of the leg closest to you.

5) Place the bent knee on a small pillow or folded blanket.

6) Straighten the arm on the far side, and bend the elbow of the arm closest to you. Position the arm closest to you palm side down (Figure 11-17).

5 Place the signal light and personal care items where the patient can reach them.

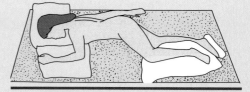

***Figure* 11-17** Step 4e(6).

◆ **COMPLETE STANDARD ENDING STEPS (see inside front cover)**

How to Transfer Patients Safely

Lifting and transferring patients also requires the use of proper body mechanics. The patient may be independent or need minimal assistance with transfers. Other patients may be totally dependent on their caregivers to be transferred to a chair, wheelchair, or stretcher. Patients who have been in bed for a long period of time, may become dizzy when they attempt to sit up or stand. This dizziness occurs when the blood pressure drops suddenly and is called **orthostatic hypotension**. Gradually changing the patient's position gives the patient's body a chance to adjust to the new position.

Two common transfers that you will perform are moving the patient from the bed to a chair or a wheelchair and moving the patient from a bed to a stretcher. Wheelchairs and stretchers are commonly used to transport patients to another area of the facility.

To use a transfer or gait belt safely, always follow the manufacturer's instructions. A transfer or gait belt is always applied over clothing to avoid injuring the skin.

NOTES ON
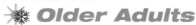
Older Adults
Always move patients toward their stronger side if they have one-sided weakness, such as after a stroke.

HOW&*WHY*
To perform a 2-person transfer, position one nursing assistant on either side of the patient.

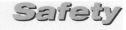

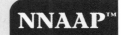

Procedure
TRANSFERRING THE PATIENT FROM THE BED TO A CHAIR OR WHEELCHAIR

EQUIPMENT

- Wheelchair or chair
- Transfer or gait belt
  Get help if needed.
- Slippers or shoes and socks
- Robe

NNAAP™

◆ **COMPLETE STANDARD BEGINNING STEPS (see inside front cover)**

1 Place the wheelchair or chair parallel to the patient's bed with the seat facing the head of the bed. Lock the wheels on the wheelchair, and swing the footrests out of the way if possible.

2 With the bed in its lowest position and the wheels locked, raise the head of the bed so that the patient is sitting up in the bed.

3 Place the slippers or socks and shoes on the patient.

Continued

Procedure

TRANSFERRING THE PATIENT FROM THE BED TO A CHAIR OR WHEELCHAIR—cont'd

4 Assist the patient to a sitting position by lifting the upper body as the legs swing over the edge of the bed (Figure 11-18). Encourage the patient to assist as much as possible.

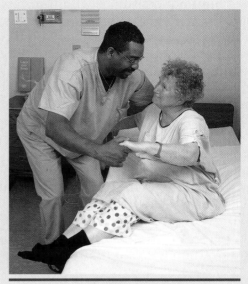

Figure **11-18** Step 4.

5 Allow the patient to sit on the side of the bed for 1 to 2 minutes to adjust to the change in position. This is called **dangling** (Figure 11-19).

6 Help the patient to put on her robe.

7 Place the transfer or gait belt around the patient's waist and secure (per facility policy). Make sure the belt is *under* the breasts when using with a female patient.

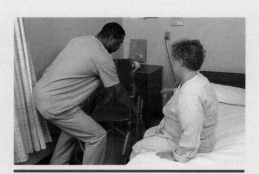

Figure **11-19** Step 5.

8 Assist the patient to stand by positioning yourself in front the patient with your feet shoulder width apart.

9 If you are using a gait belt, grasp both sides of the belt firmly. If the patient is able to help, ask her to place her hands flat on the bed and push up to assist with standing.

Procedure

TRANSFERRING THE PATIENT
FROM THE BED TO A CHAIR OR WHEELCHAIR—cont'd

10 If you are not using a gait belt, place your hands under the patient's arms. If the patient is able to help, ask her to place her hands flat on the bed and push up to assist with standing.

11 Keeping your back straight, bend at the knees and on the count of three bring the patient to a standing position. To keep the patient's feet from sliding forward, place your feet in front of the patient's feet. Putting non-skid slippers or shoes and socks on the patient before assisting her with transfer also prevents the feet from sliding forward (Figure 11-20).

12 Turn and move the patient towards her stronger side so that her back is toward the chair or wheelchair.

13 Have the patient reach back for the arm of the chair.

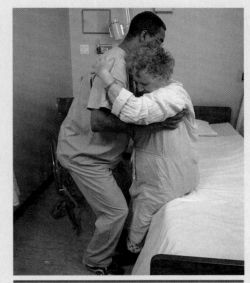

Figure **11-20**   Step 11.

14 With the back of the patient's legs against the seat of the chair, lower the patient into a sitting position in the chair, bending your knees and keeping your back straight (Figure 11-21).

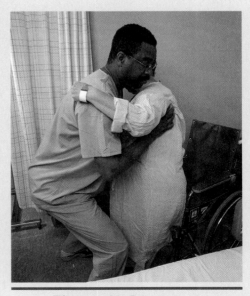

Figure **11-21**   Step 14.

Continued

Procedure

TRANSFERRING THE PATIENT FROM THE BED TO A CHAIR OR WHEELCHAIR—cont'd

15 Position the patient in proper alignment in the chair so that the spine is straight.

16 Assist the patient with placing her feet on the footrests of the wheelchair if using footrests.

◆ **COMPLETE STANDARD ENDING STEPS (see inside front cover)**

Safety

If the patient is unable to assist with the transfer, ask another nursing assistant for help.

NEVER allow patients to place their hands or arms around your neck when helping them to stand to transfer. This can cause a serious neck or back injury to the nursing assistant.

Patients are usually transferred onto a stretcher to be moved from place to place within the facility for tests or x-ray films. The patient may also be moved onto a stretcher to be transported to another facility by ambulance. A patient who is independent will be able to move over onto the stretcher with minimal assistance. The dependent patient may require the help of 3 or more staff members to be transferred onto a stretcher. Some facilities may use a roller board, which helps to move the patient onto the stretcher. The basics of performing a transfer from the bed to a stretcher are the same whether a roller board is used or not.

Procedure

TRANSFERRING THE PATIENT FROM A BED TO A STRETCHER

EQUIPMENT

- Bed
- Stretcher
  Additional staff members
- 1 bath blanket or flat sheet

◆ **COMPLETE STANDARD BEGINNING STEPS (see inside front cover)**

1 Lock the wheels of the bed, and raise it to the same height as the stretcher.

2 Begin with the patient in the supine position with the head of the bed flat.

3 Fold the top covers to the foot of the bed, making sure the feet are uncovered.

4 Remove any positioning devices or wedges from the bed, and cover the patient with a bath blanket or sheet.

5 Place a lift sheet under the patient as described in the procedure *Moving the Patient Up in Bed,* p. 226.

6 With at least one nursing assistant on each side of the bed, grasp the lift sheet and move the patient to the side of the bed nearest to the stretcher.

7 Place the stretcher on the side of the bed, and lock the wheels.

8 With 2 nursing assistants on the far side of the stretcher, grasp the lift sheet and pull the patient onto the stretcher on the count of three (Figure 11-22).

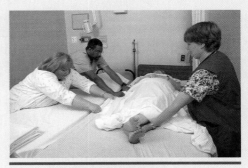

***Figure* 11-22**   Step 8.

Continued

Procedure

TRANSFERRING THE PATIENT FROM A BED
TO A STRETCHER—cont'd

9 Have the third nursing assistant stand on the opposite side of the bed and assist with lifting and guiding the patient onto the stretcher (Figure 11-23).

10 Place a pillow under the patient's head, and fasten the safety belt over the patient. Raise the side rails on the stretcher.

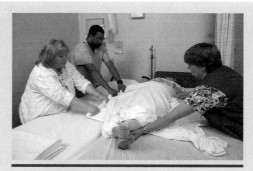

Figure 11-23 Step 9.

◆ **COMPLETE STANDARD ENDING STEPS (see inside front cover)**

HOW & WHY
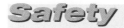
Being transferred with a mechanical lift can be a frightening experience for the patient.

HOW & WHY
The patient will remain on the sling to allow for ease in transferring the patient back to the bed.

Safety
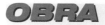

OBRA

Using a Mechanical Lift

Mechanical lifts are used for patients who are unable to assist with the transfer process. They can be used to transfer a patient from the bed to a wheelchair. Some facilities require the use of a mechanical lift for any patient who is unable to stand with assistance. There are many different brands of mechanical lifts available. Some lifts are manual, and others work off a rechargeable battery.

It is important that you be trained to use the lift provided by your employer. Never use a piece of equipment that you are not familiar with or have not been taught to use. If you are not familiar with the type of lift provided, ask your charge nurse for assistance.

Most mechanical lifts require 2 staff members to safely operate them. Check your facility policy regarding the use of mechanical lifts before using it.

OBRA requires that nursing homes provide care that enhances each person's quality of life, safety, and health. Using good body mechanics and safe transfer techniques helps to protect residents from harm. Remember to provide privacy when positioning the resident by closing the door and privacy curtain.

Procedure
TRANSFERRING THE PATIENT FROM THE BED TO A CHAIR USING A MECHANICAL LIFT

EQUIPMENT
- Chair or wheelchair
- Mechanical lift with sling

Additional staff member

◆ COMPLETE STANDARD BEGINNING STEPS (see inside front cover)

1 Place the wheelchair or chair at the patient's bedside.

2 Lock the wheels if transferring into a wheelchair and lock the wheels

3 Raise the bed to a comfortable working height and lock the wheels.

4 Begin with the patient in the supine position.

5 Using the procedure for turning a patient, turn the patient onto her side and place the sling behind her back

6 The sling should extend from the patient's knees to her head. (Follow the manufacturer's directions regarding proper placement of the sling.)

7 Turn the patient onto her back, and ask her to cross her arms over her chest.

8 Position the lift at the side of the bed, and spread the base of the lift.

9 Lower the boom, and attach the shorter chains at the shoulder area of the sling to the hooks on the boom.

10 Raise the boom slightly, and attach the longer chains at the hip area of the sling to the hooks on the boom.

11 Adjust the sling so that the patient's weight is evenly supported.

12 Raise the boom to lift the patient off the bed. Depending on the model being used, the boom may be controlled with a hand-operated pump or an electric controller (Figure 11-24).

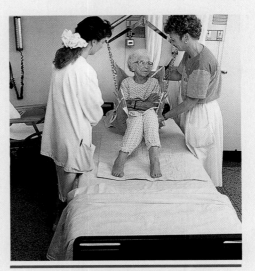

***Figure* 11-24**   Step 12.

Continued

Procedure

TRANSFERRING THE PATIENT FROM THE BED TO A CHAIR USING A MECHANICAL LIFT—cont'd

13 Raise the patient just high enough so that her hips are not resting on the bed and her legs can be guided over the side of the bed.

14 While supporting the patient, guide the lift toward the chair or wheelchair so that when the patient is lowered she will be properly positioned in the seat (Figure 11-25).

15 Slowly lower the patient into the seat so that she is in proper alignment.

16 Pay close attention to the patient's head so that she does not hit her head on the boom while she is being lowered into the chair.

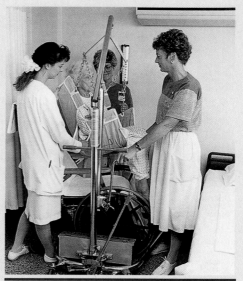

Figure 11-25 Step 14.

17 When the patient is securely seated, lower the boom enough to remove the chains from the boom (Figure 11-26).

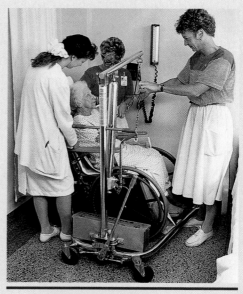

Figure 11-26 Step 17.

◆ **COMPLETE STANDARD ENDING STEPS (see inside front cover)**

CHAPTER REVIEW

1. List 5 reasons good body mechanics are important.

2. List 4 things positioning patients accomplishes.

Circle the one BEST response.

3. Why is a lift sheet used when moving a patient up in bed?
   a. To protect the bed from soiling
   b. To allow the patient to help with the move
   c. To decrease rubbing against the patient's skin
   d. To make the transfer easier on the nursing assistant

4. In general, how often should patients who are unable to move on their own be turned and repositioned?
   a. At least every 1½ to 2 hours if they are in bed and every 20 to 30 minutes if they are sitting in a chair
   b. At least every 2 to 3 hours if they are in bed and every 30 to 60 minutes if they are sitting in a chair
   c. At least every 1 to 2 hours if they are in bed and every 30 to 60 minutes if they are sitting in a chair
   d. At least every 3 to 4 hours if they are in bed and every 20 to 30 minutes if they are sitting in a chair

5. The charge nurse has instructed you to place Ms. Henderson in the supine position. This means that you will position her on her
   a. Side
   b. Back
   c. Abdomen
   d. Hip

6. Mr. Lee is a patient who has left-sided weakness from a stroke. When transferring him from his bed to the chair, you should
   a. Position the chair directly in front of him
   b. Position the chair on his left side
   c. Position the chair on his right side
   d. Position the chair directly behind him

Mark T for true or F for false.

7. _____ All mechanical lifts work exactly the same way.

Answers are on page 706.

CHAPTER 12

Rest, Exercise, and Ambulation

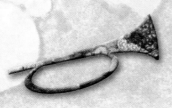

What you will learn

- The importance of comfort, rest, and sleep
- How to care for the patient on bedrest
- The purpose of range-of-motion exercises
- How to perform range-of-motion exercises
- How to assist a patient with ambulation
- How to assist a falling patient

KEY TERMS
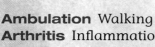

Ambulation Walking

Arthritis Inflammation of the joints

Atrophy Decrease in muscle size

Contractures Joints that do not have a normal shape, which is caused by shortening of the muscle

Fracture Broken bone

Orthostatic hypotension A rapid drop in blood pressure that occurs with a change in position

Pneumonia Inflammation/infection of the lungs

Pressure ulcers An inflammation or sore that develops over areas where the skin and tissue underneath are injured due to lack of blood flow and oxygen supply as a result of constant pressure

The Importance of Comfort, Rest, and Sleep

Proper rest and sleep are important to good health. They are even more important to a person who is recovering from an injury or illness. A person who is well rested can deal with pain better and has a better response to pain medications.

The amount of sleep a person needs changes over the course of his lifetime (Table 12-1). Newborns normally sleep about 16 hours each day. By children's first birthday, they are sleeping between 12 and 14 hours a day. By the time they are teenagers, they will spend about 8 hours sleeping. A healthy adult needs anywhere from 5 to 10 hours of sleep per day. As we get older, the amount of time we sleep at night begins to decrease.

There are many things that affect our sleep patterns. Environmental factors such as a room that is too hot or too cold can interfere with our ability to sleep well. Drinking liquids that contain caffeine, such as coffee, tea, or soda, can interfere with sleep. A person who is ill or in pain may have trouble sleeping. Some people worry at night and are unable to sleep. Students who stay up late studying and people who work evening and night shifts may also have a hard time getting enough rest. In a hospital or a nursing home, noise, lights, and an unfamiliar environment make it more difficult to sleep soundly.

Residents of nursing homes have the right to make decisions about how they want to live their lives. This includes deciding what time to go to bed and what time to get up. Encouraging the residents to make as many decisions as possible and respecting their requests promotes quality of life and dignity.

NOTES ON
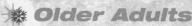
Older Adults

Many older adults awaken more at night, but they may also nap more often during the day.

NOTES ON
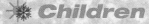
Children

Many children continue to take a nap in the afternoon even after beginning school.

NOTES ON
Culture

In some cultures it is the custom to close all businesses and have a short rest period between lunch and dinner.

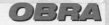

Table 12-1

HOURS OF SLEEP REQUIRED	
Age	Per day requirements (in hours)
Newborns (to 1 month)	14-18
Infants (to 1 year)	12-14
Toddlers (to 3 years)	11-12
Preschoolers (to 6 years)	11-12
Mid to late childhood (to 12 years)	10-11
Adolescents (to 18 years)	8-9
Young adults (to 40 years)	7-8
Middle-age adults (to 65 years)	7
Older adults (older than 65)	5-7

Many of the patients that you take care of as a nursing assistant will experience pain or discomfort. A patient who has had surgery will have pain. Many medical conditions such as cancer and **arthritis** (inflammation of the joints) can also cause pain. Pain is very personal. There is no way to measure other people's pain or discomfort. You must rely on their description to know if their pain is getting better or worse.

A scale is often used to help patients to rate their level of pain. The most common scale is a number scale (Figure 12-1). Patients are asked to rate their pain from 0 (no pain) to 10 (the worst pain possible). This type of scale will help you to know if the patient's pain is better or worse and if the comfort measures you provide are helpful. When you ask people about their pain, ask them to point to the area that hurts (Figure 12-3). Ask the person to describe the pain (Box 12-1).

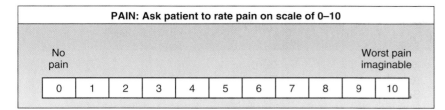

Figure 12-1   Pain number rating scale.

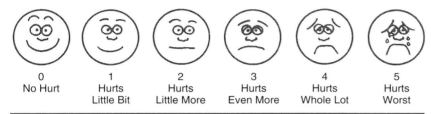

Figure 12-2   FACES pain rating scale.

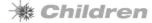
Children may find a picture scale that uses faces more helpful than a number scale (see Figure 12-2).

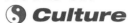
When caring for a person who has difficulty speaking English, you may prefer the picture scale that uses faces.

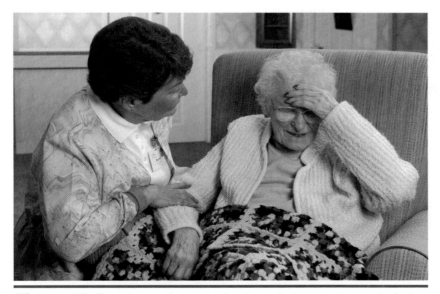

Figure 12-3   When asking people about their pain, it may be helpful to have them point to the area that hurts.

Box 12-1

PAIN DESCRIPTION WORDS

Dull	Stabbing	Numbing
Aching	Squeezing	Pressure
Sore	Sharp	Tender
Burning	Crushing	Unbearable
Throbbing	Tiring	Viselike
Cramping	Miserable	

NOTES ON
⑨ *Culture*

In some cultures, expressing pain is seen as a sign of weakness. You may need to offer the person pain relief measures more than one time.

HOW & WHY

Some patients may be afraid if the room is totally dark. Leaving the bathroom light or a night-light on may make them feel more secure in unfamiliar surroundings.

For example, patients who have arthritis in their knees may rate their pain as a 7 when they get up in the morning. After a warm whirlpool bath, a person rates the pain as a 3. This helps the health care team to know that the heat of the whirlpool has decreased the patient's pain.

More information about care of the patient after surgery is in Chapter 28.

There are many things that you can do to make the patient who is in pain more comfortable. Some of the options involve the administration of pain medications that are given by mouth or by injection. This is usually done by the charge nurse. A patient-controlled analgesia pump allows the people to administer their own pain medication through an intravenous (IV) line. The pump is set to deliver the amount of medication ordered by the doctor. Use of heat and cold can lessen discomfort and may be ordered by the doctor. (Additional information on the use of heat and cold is in Chapter 24.) Some patients may use a small electrical stimulator attached to electrodes to block pain. This type of a device is called a transcutaneous electrical nerve stimulation (TENS) unit.

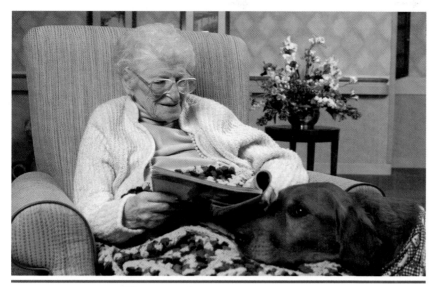

***Figure* 12-4** Patient reading.

As a nursing assistant, there are several things that you can do to make your patients more comfortable. These comfort measures do not include the use of medications. Some patients have a hard time relaxing. When people are tense, their muscles are tight and pain can be worse. You can help a patient to relax by making sure the bed is clean and comfortable. Also, bright lights can make it difficult to relax. Ask patients if they are more comfortable with the lights on or off.

If their diet permits, a light snack at bedtime may make it easier to relax. Some patients enjoy reading or listening to soothing music or tapes of the ocean or wind (Figure 12-4).

NOTES ON
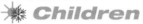 *Children*

When caring for a child, ask the parent(s) how the child normally sleeps at home. A night-light or special toy may help the child to sleep and feel more secure.

HOW & WHY

Your facility's activities department may be able to provide books or music.

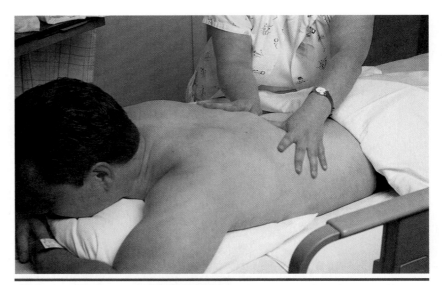

Figure **12-5** A back rub can help to relax muscles and relieve tension.

HOW&WHY

Cold hands and cold lotions can cause the patient to tense and pull away.

A back rub can help to relax muscles and relieve tension (Figure 12-5). A back rub also stimulates circulation and provides an opportunity for you to look at the condition of the patient's skin. Steps for the procedure for giving a back rub can be found in Chapter 23. If a patient is on bedrest, a back rub should be given each morning and evening to decrease the chance of **pressure ulcers** (skin breakdown due to constant pressure on the skin). (Additional information regarding pressure ulcers is included in Chapter 23.)

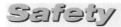

Safety

Do not massage any areas that are red. Reddened skin can be a sign of skin breakdown. Massaging the red areas can increase the damage to the skin.

Caring for the Patient on Bedrest

The patient on bedrest has been confined to the bed by the doctor's orders. It is important for you to know why the patient must remain in the bed. Some patients are placed on bedrest for the first 12 to 24 hours after a diagnostic procedure or surgery. Some patients may be on bedrest to allow an injury to heal, such as a **fracture** (broken bone). There are several levels of bedrest.

Strict bedrest means that people are not allowed to do anything for themselves.

Bedrest usually means that people can do their bathing and grooming as long as they remain in the bed.

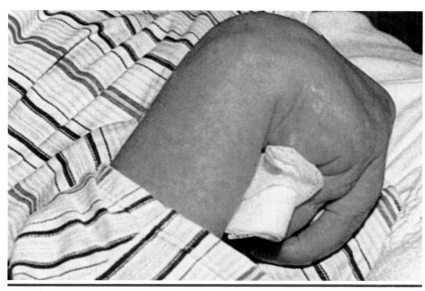

***Figure* 12-6**   A contracture.

Bedrest with commode or bathroom privileges means that people can get out of bed to use the bedside commode or to walk
to the bathroom.

It is important to check with the charge nurse to find out
what type of restriction your patient has and for how long.

Bedrest and lack of exercise can cause serious health problems. Pressure ulcers can form because of pressure on a bony
area. Lack of exercise can cause constipation and blood clots
too. **Pneumonia/inflammation** (infection of the lungs) is also
a complication of bedrest. When patients are not moving, they
become weak. Muscles begin to shrink in size, a condition called
atrophy. Muscles also shorten, causing deformities of the joints
called **contractures** (Figure 12-6). **Orthostatic hypotension**, a
drop in the blood pressure when the person moves from a lying
or sitting to a standing position, can cause the patient to faint.

There are several things you can do to prevent the problems
that occur when a patient is on bedrest.

1. Turn patients, and put them in a different position at least
   every 1½ to 2 hours. This increases circulation, and pressure is not applied to the same areas for a long time.
2. Encourage deep breathing and coughing to help prevent
   pneumonia.
3. Perform range-of-motion (ROM) exercises as permitted by
   the patient's condition. The exercise increases circulation
   and exercises the muscles and joints. ROM exercises can
   help prevent atrophy, contractures, and blood clots. ROM
   can also help prevent constipation.

HOW&*WHY*

Taking deep breaths helps to expand the lungs and loosen secretions. When the person coughs,
the secretions are removed and
pneumonia is prevented.

HOW&*WHY*

Performing ROM exercises to the
legs causes the abdominal muscle
to move. This movement stimulates
the intestines and helps to prevent
constipation.

NOTES ON
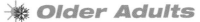
Older Adults

Some older patients find head exercises very uncomfortable because of arthritis in the neck. Do not continue with an exercise that causes pain.

Performing Range-of-Motion Exercises

Range-of-motion (ROM) exercises can be done actively or passively. Active range of motion (AROM) means that patients participate in the exercises or are able to do them on their own or with your help. Passive range of motion (PROM) means that they need you to do the exercises for them. It is important for you to know which joint(s) to exercise and if there are any exercises that you should not do. Each ROM exercise should be repeated 3 to 5 times. Your charge nurse will instruct you on how many times a day the exercises should be done.

Safety

Always stop the exercises and notify your charge nurse if the patient complains of pain. Support the limb above and below the joint to avoid causing harm to the joint.

Procedure
RANGE-OF-MOTION EXERCISES

EQUIPMENT
* **Bath blanket or top sheet**

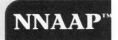

◆ **COMPLETE STANDARD BEGINNING STEPS (see inside front cover)**

1 If permitted, encourage the patient to do as many of the exercises as she can. Instructions are given for performing passive range-of-motion (ROM) exercises. Begin with the patient comfortably seated in a chair or lying in the bed.

   a. Head
      1) Support the head with your hands, and bring the head forward until the chin touches the chest.
      2) Extend the neck by lifting the chin so that the patient looks upward.
      3) Turn the head so that the patient looks over the right shoulder and then the left shoulder (Figure 12-7).

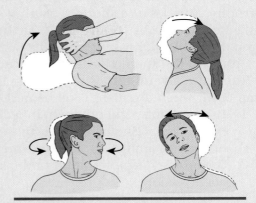

***Figure* 12-7** Step 1a.

Procedure

RANGE-OF-MOTION EXERCISES—cont'd

b. Shoulder/Elbow

1) Support the arm at the wrist and elbow, and lift the arm forward and toward the ceiling. Lower the arm to the patient's side (Figure 12-8).

2) Support the arm at the wrist and elbow, and lift the arm out to the side and toward the ceiling. Lower the arm to the patient's side.

3) Support the arm at the elbow and wrist. Bend the arm at the elbow to touch the shoulder, and then straighten the arm.

4) Hold the arm in a handshake position, supporting it at the elbow. Turn the palm of the hand toward the ceiling and then toward the floor (Figure 12-9).

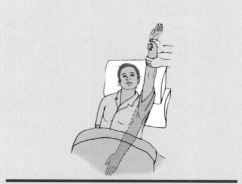

Figure **12-8**   Step 1b(1).

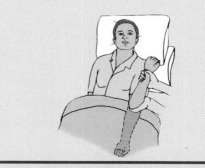

Figure **12-9**   Step 1b(4).

c. Wrist

1) Support the hand and the arm above the wrist. Bend the wrist forward and then straighten. Bend the wrist backwards and then straighten (Figure 12-10).

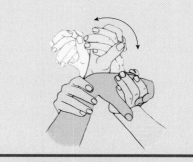

Figure **12-10**   Step 1c(1).

2) Support the hand and the arm above the wrist. Move the hand from side to side at the wrist (Figure 12-11).

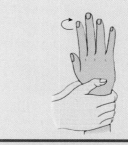

Figure **12-11**   Step 1c(2).

Continued

Procedure
RANGE-OF-MOTION EXERCISES—cont'd

    d.   Fingers

       1)   Support the hand at the wrist. Assist the patient with making a fist with the thumb on the outside of the fingers, then open the hand fully (Figure 12-12, *A*).

       2)   Move each finger toward and then away from the finger next to it (Figure 12-12, *B*).

       3)   Touch the tip of the thumb to the tip of each finger.

       4)   Move the thumb in a circular motion in one direction and then in the other direction (Figure 12-12, *C*).

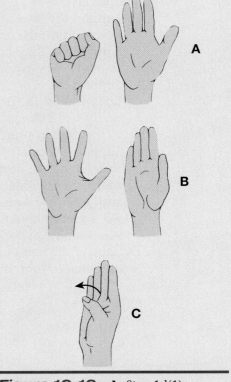

Figure **12-12**   **A,** Step 1d(1). **B,** Step 1d(2). **C,** Step 1d(4).

    e.   Hip and knee

       1)   Support the leg at the knee and ankle joints. Keeping the leg straight, raise and lower the leg.

       2)   Bend the knee, and move the leg toward the chest, then straighten the leg (Figure 12-13).

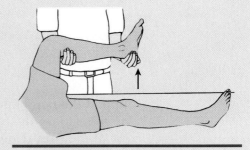

Figure **12-13**   Step 1e(2).

Procedure

RANGE-OF-MOTION EXERCISES—cont'd

3) Move the leg out toward the side of the body and then back toward the center of the body (Figure 12-14).

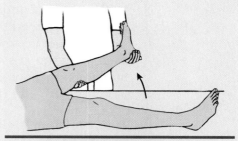

Figure 12-14   Step 1e(3).

f. Ankle
   1) With the leg straight, support the knee and ankle joints, and move the foot so that the toes point toward the center of the body and then toward the side of the body (Figure 12-15).

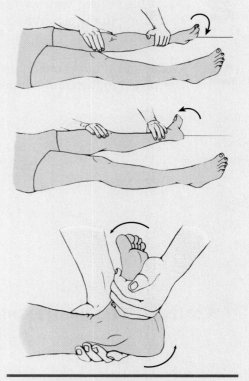

Figure 12-15   Step 1f(1).

Continued

Procedure
RANGE-OF-MOTION EXERCISES—cont'd

2) With one hand under the ankle and the other hand on the ball of the foot, bend the foot up toward the chin and then point the toes downward to straighten the foot.

g. Toes
1) Bend and then straighten the toes (Figure 12-16).
2) Move each toe toward and then away from the toe next to it.

2 Assist the patient back to a comfortable position, and put the signal light where the patient can reach it.

3 Wash your hands, and report the procedure completed to the charge nurse.

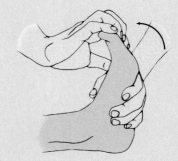
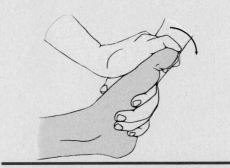

***Figure* 12-16** Step 1g(1).

◆ COMPLETE STANDARD ENDING STEPS **(see inside front cover)**

Assisting With Ambulation

The term **ambulation** means walking. Patients who have been ill or are recovering from an injury may be weak or unsteady when they walk. You will assist the patient with ambulating so that he can get his strength back safely. Some patients will walk with the assistance of a cane or walker. It is also important for you to know what to do if a patient begins to fall so that neither you nor the patient is injured.

OBRA requires that all residents receive care that enhances their quality of life. This includes care that prevents the complications of immobility such as pneumonia, pressure ulcers, and contractures. Keep in mind that residents of long-term care centers also have the right to *refuse* care. If a resident refuses care, let your charge nurse know.

OBRA

If the patient begins to fall, step behind the patient with your feet slightly apart and your hands on the gait belt under the person's arms. Pull the patient's body close to your body, and slowly lower the person to the floor using the muscles in your legs. Keep your back as straight as possible, bending at the knees and hips as you support the patient (Figure 12-17). Call for help at once.

Safety

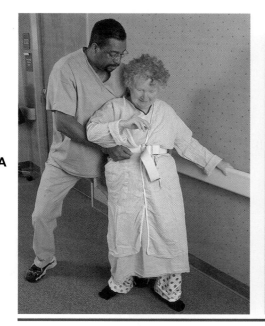
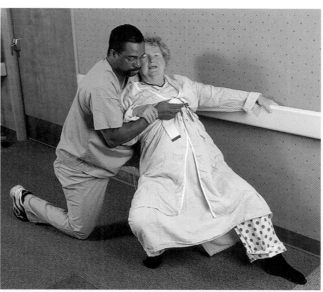

Figure **12-17 A,** Step behind patient. **B,** Lower the patient.

Procedure
ASSISTING WITH AMBULATION

EQUIPMENT

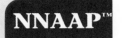

- Robe
- Slippers or shoes with non-skid soles
- Socks
- Gait belt (per facility policy)
- Walker or cane if needed

◆ **COMPLETE STANDARD BEGINNING STEPS (see inside front cover)**

1 Assist the patient with putting on her robe, socks, and shoes or slippers.

2 Place the gait belt around the patient's waist according to the procedure for using a gait belt (Chapter 11).

3 Assist the patient to a standing position, allowing her to regain her balance after standing.

4 Standing on the patient's weaker side, place one hand on the gait belt in front of her waist and the other hand in back under the gait belt (Figure 12-18).

5 Walk in the same pattern as the patient, both taking a step with the left foot and then the right foot at the same time.

6 When ambulating in a hallway with a hand rail, encourage the patient to hold on to the handrail with the stronger arm while you walk on the opposite side.

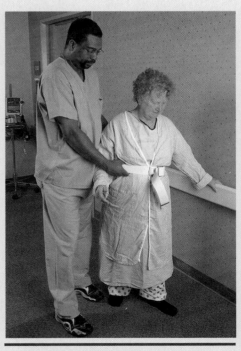

Figure 12-18   Step 4.

Continued

Procedure
ASSISTING WITH AMBULATION—cont'd

When Ambulating a Patient With a Cane (steps 7 to 12)

7 Follow steps 1 to 5 above.

8 Place the cane in the patient's stronger hand (Figure 12-19).

9 Instruct the patient to move the cane forward 6 to 8 inches and to the outside of the stronger leg.

10 Assist the patient with stepping forward with the weaker leg. The toe of the weaker foot should be even with the tip of the cane.

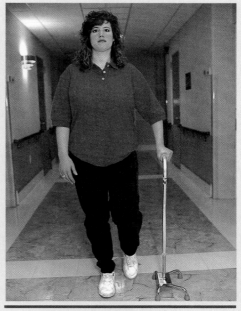

Figure **12-19** Step 8.

11 Instruct the patient to put her weight on the cane and the weaker leg while stepping forward with the stronger leg so that the stronger foot is now next to the weaker foot (Figure 12-20).

12 Walk in the same pattern as the patient, both stepping forward with the left foot and then the right foot.

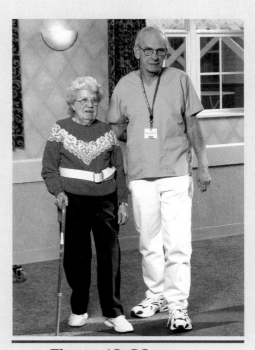

Figure **12-20** Step 11.

Continued

Procedure
ASSISTING WITH AMBULATION—cont'd

When Ambulating a Patient With a Walker (steps 13 to 18)

13 Follow steps 1 to 5 above.

14 Assist the patient with positioning herself within the frame of the walker (Figure 12-21).

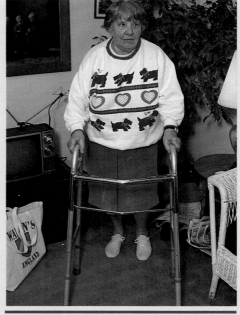

Figure **12-21**   Step 14.

15 Instruct the patient to move the walker forward by lifting it and setting it down if it is a non-wheeled walker or rolling the walker forward if it has wheels (Figure 12-22).

16 Assist the patient with taking a step forward into the walker with the weaker leg.

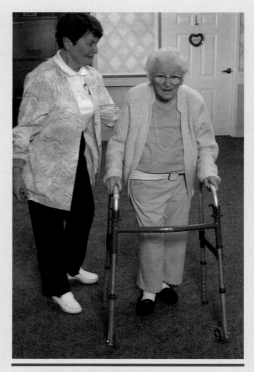

Figure **12-22**   Step 15.

Procedure

ASSISTING WITH AMBULATION—cont'd

17 Instruct the patient to move the strong leg forward (Figure 12-23).

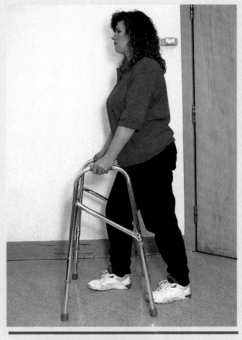

Figure **12-23**   Step 17.

18 Walk in the same pattern as the patient, both stepping forward with the left foot and then the right foot (Figure 12-24).

19 Encourage the patient to keep her chin up and eyes looking forward as she walks.

20 Ambulate the patient the distance instructed by the charge nurse.

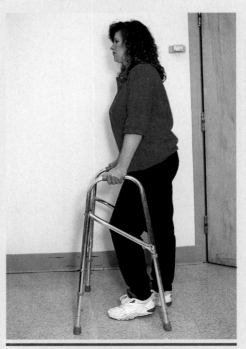

Figure **12-24**   Step 18.

Continued

Procedure

ASSISTING WITH AMBULATION—cont'd

21 Return the patient to her bed or chair, and remove the gait belt if used. Make sure the patient is comfortable, with the signal light within reach.

22 Return the walker or cane to storage if used per facility policy.

23 Report the procedure completed to the charge nurse.

◆ COMPLETE STANDARD ENDING STEPS **(see inside front cover)**

CHAPTER REVIEW

1. Why is proper rest and sleep important?

2. List 4 complications of bedrest.

3. What is the difference between active and passive range-of-motion exercises?

Circle the one BEST response.

4. How many hours of sleep does a healthy adult need per day?
   a. 5 to 10 hours
   b. 8 to 10 hours
   c. 12 to 24 hours
   d. 16 to 18 hours

5. Why are range-of-motion exercises done?
   a. To decrease circulation
   b. To increase atrophy
   c. To prevent contractures
   d. To encourage blood clots

6. When ambulating a patient with a cane
   a. Stand on the patient's stronger side.
   b. Have the patient place the cane in the weaker hand.
   c. Instruct the patient to step forward with the weaker foot first.
   d. Place the tip of the cane in front of the weaker foot.

7. What should you do if the patient you are walking with begins to fall?
   a. Step in front of the patient, put your arms around the patient waist, and slowly lower the patient to the floor.
   b. Stand behind the patient, and hold the patient close to your body until help arrives.
   c. Step behind the patient, pulling the patient close to your body, and slowly lower the patient to the floor.
   d. Stand to the side of the patient, grasp the patient by the arms, and assist the patient into a chair.

Fill in the blank with the correct term.

8. A _____ can relax muscles, relieve tension, and stimulate circulation.

Answers are on page 706.

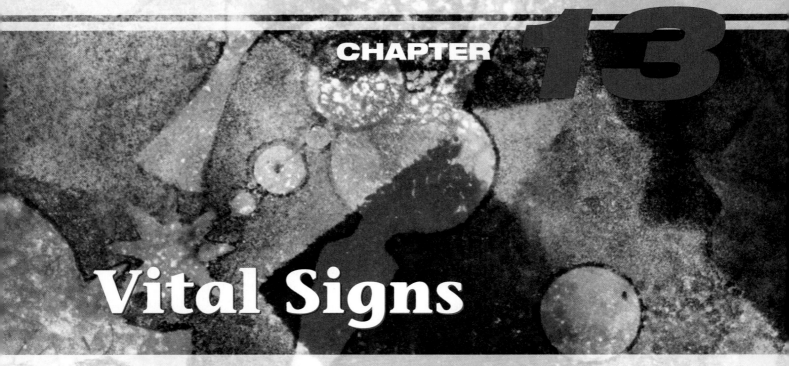

CHAPTER *13*

Vital Signs

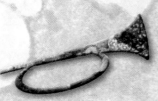

What you will learn

- What vital signs are
- Factors that affect vital signs
- How to report and record vital signs measurements
- Normal ranges of oral, rectal, axillary, and aural/tympanic membrane temperatures
- How to take oral, rectal, axillary, and aural/tympanic membrane temperatures
- Normal ranges of pulse, respiration, and blood pressure measurements
- How to take a radial and apical pulse
- How to count respirations
- How to take a blood pressure
- How to measure height and weight

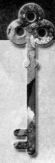

KEY TERMS

Aural temperature Temperature taken in the ear, same as tympanic membrane temperature

Axilla/axillary temperature Temperature taken under the arm or in the armpit

Blood pressure The pressure of blood in an artery

Body temperature A measurement of the amount of heat in the body

Bradycardia A heart rate below 60 beats per minute

Centigrade or Celsius (C) A scale used for measuring temperature

Diastolic pressure The lower (or bottom) number of a blood pressure reading obtained while the heart muscle is relaxed and the pressure in the artery is lower

Fahrenheit (F) A scale used for measuring temperature

Force Strength of the pulse

Graphic forms Forms in the medical record used for recording vital signs

Heart rate The number of pulse beats, or heartbeats, that are counted in 1 minute

Hypertension (high blood pressure) Blood pressure reading above 140/90 mm Hg

Hypotension (low blood pressure) Blood pressure reading below 100/60 mm Hg

Irregular pulse The heart is beating in an uneven way, with different amounts of time between heartbeats

Oral temperature Temperature taken in the mouth

Pulse The throbbing felt over the artery as the heart beats

Rectal temperature Temperature taken in the rectum

Regular pulse The heart is beating in an even, steady way

Respiration The cycle of breathing in and out

Rhythm Pattern of the pulse, described as regular or irregular

Sphygmomanometer An instrument used to measure blood pressure

Stethoscope An instrument that has two earpieces attached by flexible tubing to a diaphragm that is placed against the patient's skin to hear heart and lung sounds

Systolic pressure The higher (or top) number of a blood pressure reading obtained while the heart muscle is contracting and the pressure in the artery rises

Tachycardia A heart rate above 100 beats per minute

Tympanic membrane temperature Temperature taken in the ear, same as aural temperature

Vital signs Temperature, pulse, respiration, and blood pressure

What Are Vital Signs?

The word *vital* means life. The four **vital signs** are temperature, pulse, respiration, and blood pressure. Measurements of vital signs provide a picture of what is happening to the basic life functions of the body. These functions include regulation of body temperature, breathing, and heartbeat.

Height and weight are not considered vital signs but are two additional measurements that are used when looking at a person's level of wellness or illness. Height and weight are usually measured on admission and are recorded on the same form in the chart. Height and weight are also covered in this chapter.

Factors That Affect Vital Signs

Many factors affect vital signs. A person's vital signs are not always the same throughout a 24-hour period.

Activity, stress, eating, emotions, weather, illness, and medications can affect vital signs. Vital signs tell how a person is responding to medical treatment. They can also signal a life-threatening emergency.

When Are Vital Signs Measured?

Vital signs are usually measured at these times:
- When a person is admitted to a health care facility
- During a physical examination
- On a schedule as ordered by the doctor
- Before and after surgery, certain medical procedures, or diagnostic tests
- Before and after certain nursing procedures
- When medications are taken that affect heartbeat, circulation, or breathing
- When a person complains of pain, illness, shortness of breath, changes in heartbeat, and fever or chills

Reporting and Recording Vital Signs

Small changes in vital signs may be due to important changes in a patient's medical condition.

Safety

Measuring, recording, and reporting vital signs accurately is a very important skill. If you are unsure about any measurement or reading, ask a nurse to repeat the measurement.

Vital signs are usually taken when a person is sitting quietly or lying down. Report vital signs immediately to a nurse when any measurement is:
- Changed from a previous measurement
- Above the normal range
- Below the normal range

Vital signs are recorded on **graphic forms** or on log sheets (Figure 13-1). Graphic forms and log sheets allow the nurse or doctor to examine and compare changes in a patient's vital signs over time. Types of forms and procedures for recording these measurements will vary from facility to facility.

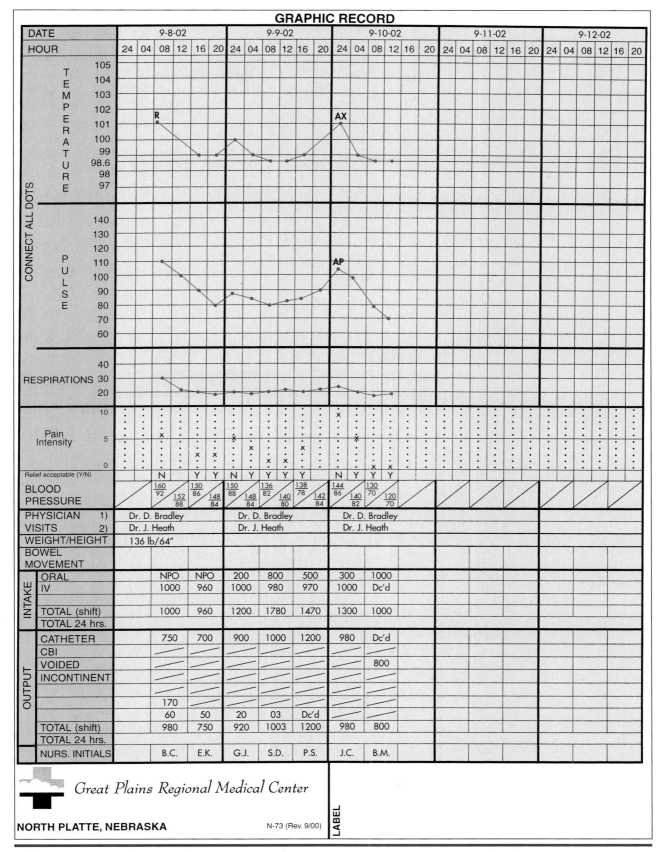

Figure 13-1 Vital signs are recorded on graphic forms or on log sheets.

Body Temperature

Body temperature is a measurement of the amount of heat in the body. The body produces heat when cells use food for energy. Heat is lost through breathing, the skin, urine, and stool. The temperature regulation center in the brain works to keep a balance between heat produced and heat lost. Body temperature is lower in the morning and higher in the late afternoon and evening. In addition to the factors listed at the beginning of the chapter, body temperature is also affected by pregnancy and the menstrual cycle.

Temperature is measured using the **Fahrenheit (F)** and **centigrade** or **Celsius (C)** scales (Figure 13-2). A small ° before either capital letter is used to indicate degrees (Table 13-1). Body temperature is usually measured in one of four body areas:

Table 13-1

FAHRENHEIT TO CELSIUS SCALES	
Fahrenheit	Celsius (centigrade)
95.0°	35.0°
95.9°	35.5°
96.8°	36.0°
97.7°	36.5°
98.6°	37.0°
99.5°	37.5°
100.4°	38.0°
101.3°	38.5°
102.2°	39.0°
103.1°	39.5°
104.0°	40.0°
104.9°	40.5°

To change Celsius to Fahrenheit, multiply by 9/5 and add 32.
To change Fahrenheit to Celsius, subtract 32 and multiply by 5/9.

- The mouth **(oral)** is the most common and easiest place.
- The ear **(tympanic membrane or aural)** takes the least amount of time.
- The underarm **(axilla/axillary)** is the least accurate and takes the longest. The axillary temperature is normally 1° F lower than an oral temperature taken on the same person.
- The rectum **(rectal)** is the most accurate. A rectal temperature is normally 1° F higher than an oral temperature taken on the same person.

Remember to follow Standard Precautions when taking an oral or rectal temperature. Both of these procedures place you at risk of having contact with mucous membranes and body fluids.

Each site has a normal baseline value and range. Body temperature higher than the normal range for the patient may be called a fever. Tables 13-2 and 13-3 shows the normal ranges in body temperatures in adults and children.

Thermometers are used to measure temperature. The most common types are digital (Figure 13-3), electronic (Figure 13-4), and tympanic thermometers (Figure 13-5). Glass thermometers (Figure 13-6) are used less often. Schools and clinics may use a disposable single-use thermometer strip (Figure 13-7). Measuring body temperature is a common nursing assistant task.

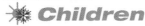

NOTES ON

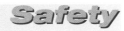
Children

Body temperature is less stable in children. Children are more likely to have a high temperature when they are ill than an adult is.

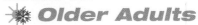

NOTES ON

Older Adults

Body temperature in an older person is usually lower because of a slower metabolism. The average body temperature in older adults is 96.8° F. The normal range in an older adult is 96° to 98° F.

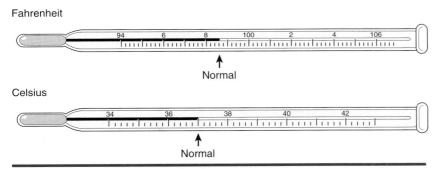

Figure 13-2 Temperature is measured using a Fahrenheit (F) *(top)* or centigrade/Celsius (C) *(bottom)* scale.

Table 13-2

ADULT TEMPERATURE VARIATIONS	Oral	Axillary	Rectal	Tympanic
Average temperature	98.6° F	97.6° F	99.6° F	98.6° F
Normal temperature range	97.6°-99.6° F	96.6°-98.6° F	98.6°-100.6° F	97.6°-99.6° F

Table 13-3

AVERAGE ORAL/TYMPANIC TEMPERATURES IN INFANTS AND CHILDREN	
Age	Temperature
3 months	99.4° F
6 months	99.5° F
1 year	99.7° F
3 years	99.0° F
5 years	98.6° F
9 years	98.0° F

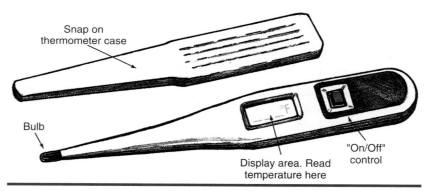

Figure 13-3 Digital thermometer.

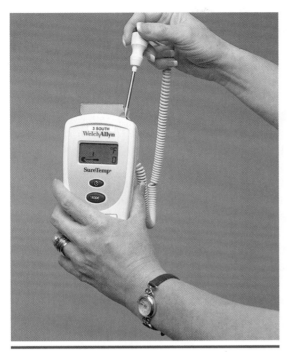

Figure 13-4 Electronic thermometer.

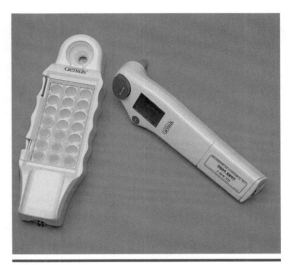

Figure 13-5 Tympanic thermometer.

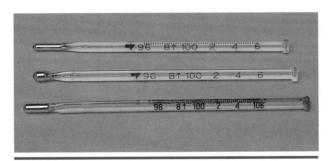

Figure 13-6 Glass thermometers.

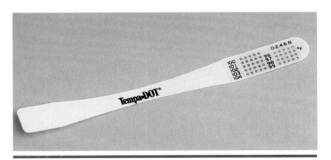

Figure 13-7 Disposable thermometer.

Glass Thermometers

Glass thermometers are most often used in the home setting or for patients in isolation. Many health care facilities no longer use glass thermometers because of the risk or danger of mercury poisoning. This can occur if a person comes into contact with mercury spilled from a broken or shattered glass thermometer.

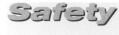

Mercury can be very toxic even in small amounts. If you accidentally break a thermometer or other piece of medical equipment containing mercury, follow your facility's policies and procedures for cleaning up the spill.

A glass thermometer is a hollow tube containing an inner column filled with mercury. The two main parts of the thermometer are the bulb and the stem. Figure 13-8 shows the different parts of a glass thermometer.

Body heat makes mercury expand and move along the stem of the thermometer. Lines marked on the stem show temperature readings in degrees. Markings on a Fahrenheit thermometer usually range from 92° to 94° to 106° or 108° F. Each long line represents an even degree. Each short line represents 0.2 (two tenths) of a degree. Figure 13-2 shows a Fahrenheit thermometer with a temperature reading of 98.6° F.

Markings on a centigrade thermometer usually range from 34° to 43° C. Each long line represents an even degree. Each short line represents 0.1 (one tenth) of a degree. Figure 13-2 shows a centigrade thermometer with a temperature reading of 37° C.

To read a glass thermometer, follow these steps:
- Hold the thermometer near the end of its stem and at eye level.
- Rotate the stem until you can see the number and line markings.
- Turn the stem back and forth slowly until you can see the column of mercury.
- The point where the mercury stops is the patient's temperature.
- Read the temperature to the nearest degree (long line) and tenth of a degree (short line) (see Figure 13-8).

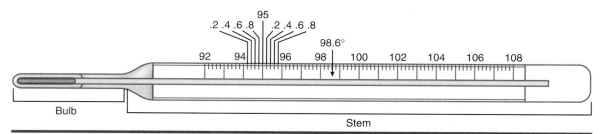

Figure 13-8 Markings on a glass thermometer.

Caring for Glass Thermometers

Follow these guidelines when using glass thermometers to prevent spread of infection and injury to the patient:

- Use only the patient's own thermometer.
- Do not use a thermometer that has been used to take a rectal temperature to take an oral or axillary temperature.
- Inspect the thermometer for cracks or chips before every use.
- Before use, rinse the thermometer in cold running water if it has been soaked in a disinfectant solution. Wipe the tip and stem dry with tissues.
- Shake down the mercury column below the number and line markings by holding the thermometer stem and briskly snapping the wrist in a downward motion. Stand away from objects that you could strike with the thermometer while shaking it down.
- Use plastic covers or sheaths according to facility policy. Each cover is used only once, then thrown away.
- After use, clean the thermometer according to facility policy. Wipe off visible secretions using dry tissues before rinsing the thermometer with cold running water.
- Between uses, store the thermometer in a closed case or a container filled with disinfectant solution.

Procedure
TAKING A TEMPERATURE USING A GLASS THERMOMETER

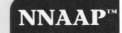

EQUIPMENT
- **Glass oral thermometer and storage container**
- **Dry tissues**
- **Notepad and pen**
- **Plastic cover or sheath, if used**
- **Gloves (per facility policy)**

The patient should not eat, drink, smoke, or chew gum for at least 20 minutes before taking an oral temperature.

SPECIAL CONSIDERATIONS
- Do not take an oral temperature if a person is:
  - An infant or child younger than age 5
  - Unconscious, confused, disoriented, or restless
  - Recovering from surgery to the face, mouth, nose, neck, or throat
  - Using oxygen or has a nasogastric tube in place
  - Breathing through the mouth or has a sore mouth
  - Paralyzed on one side of the body

Continued

Procedure

TAKING A TEMPERATURE USING A GLASS THERMOMETER—cont'd

PRECAUTIONS

- Ask the patient not to talk or bite down on thermometer while it is in place.
- Oral temperatures are usually taken on adults and older children who are awake, alert, and able to follow directions.

1 Remove thermometer from storage container and prepare it for use:

   a. Inspect the thermometer for chips or cracks.
   b. Rinse and dry the thermometer.
   c. Shake down mercury column (Figure 13-9).

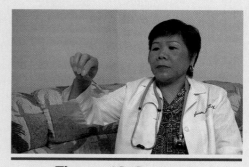

***Figure* 13-9** Step 1c.

2 Place plastic cover or sheath over thermometer, if used.

3 For oral temperature:

   a. Ask patient to moisten his lips and open his mouth, then place tip of thermometer under the patient's tongue (Figure 13-10).
   b. Ask the patient to close his lips around the thermometer to hold it in place. Leave thermometer in place for 3 minutes.

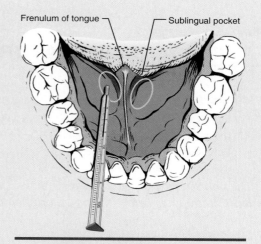

Frenulum of tongue — Sublingual pocket

***Figure* 13-10** Step 3a.

Continued

Procedure

TAKING A TEMPERATURE USING A GLASS THERMOMETER—cont'd

    c. Remove thermometer from patient's mouth. Discard the plastic cover, if used. Wipe excess secretions from the thermometer with dry tissues.

    d. Read the temperature (Figure 13-11).

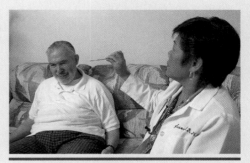

Figure **13-11** Step 3d.

4 For axillary temperature:

    a. Follow steps 1 to 3.

    b. Help patient to remove an arm from the gown.

    c. Dry axilla with a towel.

    d. Place thermometer in axilla, then place patient's arm next to or across his chest to help hold thermometer in place (Figure 13-12).

    e. Leave thermometer in place for 5 to 10 minutes.

    f. Remove thermometer and read temperature.

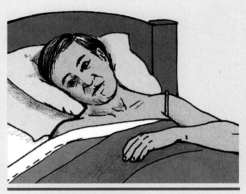

Figure **13-12** Step 4d.

5 For rectal temperature:

    a. Put on gloves and follow steps 1 to 3.

    b. Assist the patient with turning onto his side while lying in bed.

    c. Lubricate the tip of the thermometer with water-soluble lubricant placed on a tissue.

    d. Fold top bed linens to expose anal area.

    e. Raise upper buttock to expose anus (Figure 13-13).

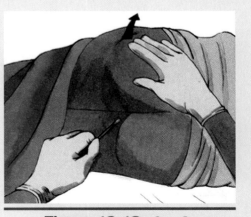

Figure **13-13** Step 5e.

Continued

Procedure
TAKING A TEMPERATURE USING A GLASS THERMOMETER—cont'd

f. Insert the thermometer 1 inch into the rectum (Figure 13-14).

g. Hold the thermometer in position for 2 to 3 minutes.

h. Remove thermometer, and wipe excess secretions and lubricant off with dry tissue. Read temperature.

i. Wipe anal area with dry tissue to remove excess lubricant. Discard used tissue.

j. Remove your gloves, and wash your hands.

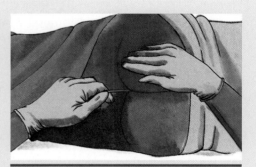

***Figure* 13-14**   Step 5f.

6 Record the reading, and report any abnormalities to the nurse.

COMPLETE STANDARD ENDING STEPS (see inside front cover)

Electronic Thermometers

Electronic thermometers are hand-held, battery-operated devices that measure temperature rapidly. The temperature is digitally shown on a panel at the top or the front of the thermometer. Most units have separate color-coded oral and rectal probes, blue for oral or axillary and red for axillary or rectal. A disposable plastic cover (sheath) is placed over the probe before taking a patient's temperature. This plastic cover is thrown away after use to help prevent spread of infection. The thermometer is attached to a battery-charging unit when not in use (Figure 13-15).

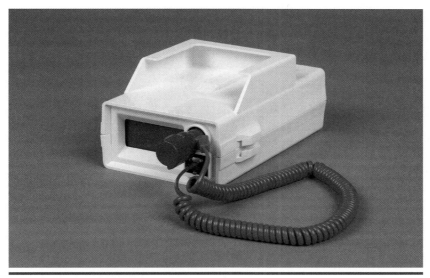

Figure 13-15   Electronic thermometer.

Procedure
TAKING A TEMPERATURE USING AN ELECTRONIC THERMOMETER

EQUIPMENT

- Electronic thermometer with probe (blue probe for oral or axillary temperature, red probe for rectal temperature) (Figure 13-16)
- Disposable plastic cover (sheath)
- Tissue (for rectal temperature)
- Water-soluble lubricant (for rectal temperature)
- Towel (for axillary temperature)
- Notepad and pen
- Gloves (per facility policy)

The patient should not eat, drink, smoke, or chew gum for at least 20 minutes before taking an oral temperature.

PRECAUTION

- Do not take an axillary temperature immediately after a patient takes a bath.
- Do not take a rectal temperature if a person:
  - Has diarrhea
  - Has a rectal disorder or injury
  - Has had rectal surgery
  - Has serious heart disease

NNAAP™

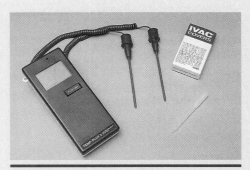

Figure 13-16   Electronic thermometer with blue and red probes.

Continued

Procedure

TAKING A TEMPERATURE USING AN ELECTRONIC THERMOMETER—cont'd

◆ **COMPLETE STANDARD BEGINNING STEPS (see inside front cover)**

1 Plug proper probe into thermometer unit.

2 Provide for patient privacy, then move the patient to the correct position for taking oral, axillary, or rectal temperature.

3 Place plastic cover over probe (Figure 13-17).

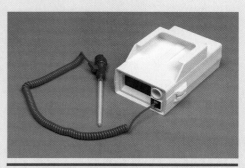

Figure **13-17**   Step 3.

4 For oral temperature:

a. Ask patient to moisten her lips and open mouth, then place probe under patient's tongue (Figure 13-18).
b. Ask patient to close lips around the probe to hold it in place.
c. Leave probe in place until you hear a tone or see a flashing or steady light on the readout panel. Read the temperature on the display.

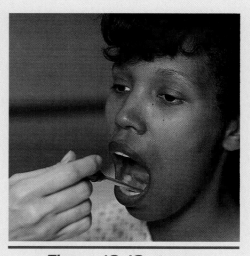

Figure **13-18**   Step 4a.

Procedure

TAKING A TEMPERATURE USING AN ELECTRONIC THERMOMETER—cont'd

d. Remove the probe. Press the eject button on the blunt end of the probe to loosen the plastic cover. Discard the probe cover (Figure 13-19).

e. Replace probe in holder.

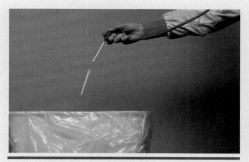

***Figure* 13-19**   Step 4d.

 5 For axillary temperature:

a. Help patient to remove an arm from the gown.

b. Dry axilla with a towel.

c. Place probe in axilla (Figure 13-20, *A*).

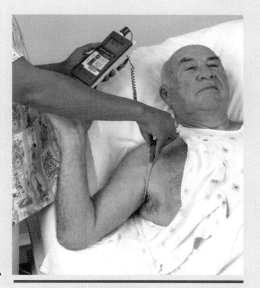

A

***Figure* 13-20**   **A**, Step 5c.

Continued

Procedure

TAKING A TEMPERATURE USING AN ELECTRONIC THERMOMETER—cont'd

d. Then place patient's arm next to or across his chest to help hold probe in place (Figure 13-20, *B*).

e. Follow steps 5c to 5e above.

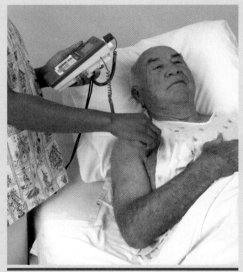

B

***Figure* 13-20, cont'd, *B*,** Step 5d.

6   *For rectal temperature:*

a. 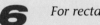 Put on gloves.

b. Assist the patient with turning onto his side while lying in bed.

c. Lubricate the tip of the probe cover with water-soluble lubricant placed on a tissue.

d Fold top bed linens to expose anal area.

e. Raise upper buttock to expose anus.

f. Insert the probe $\frac{1}{2}$ inch into the rectum (Figure 13-21).

g. Follow steps 5c to 5e above.

h. Wipe anal area with dry tissue to remove extra lubricant. Discard used tissue.

i. Remove your gloves and wash your hands.

7   Record the reading, and report any abnormalities to the nurse.

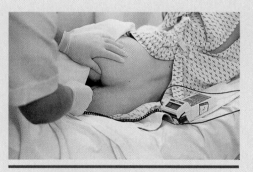

***Figure* 13-21**   Step 6f.

◆ **COMPLETE STANDARD ENDING STEPS (see inside front cover)**

Tympanic Membrane (Aural) Thermometers

Tympanic membrane (aural) thermometers are hand-held, battery-operated units that measure temperature at the tympanic membrane (eardrum) of the ear. A covered probe tip is placed in the ear canal, and the temperature result is ready in 1 to 3 seconds. These units are especially useful for measuring temperature in children. The unit is placed in a battery-charging device when not in use.

Procedure
TAKING A TYMPANIC MEMBRANE (AURAL) TEMPERATURE

EQUIPMENT
- **Tympanic membrane (aural) thermometer**
- **Plastic disposable probe cover**

◆ **COMPLETE STANDARD BEGINNING STEPS (see inside front cover)**

1 Place plastic cover over probe (Figure 13-22).

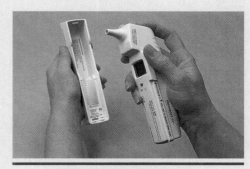

***Figure* 13-22** Step 1.

Continued

Procedure

TAKING A TYMPANIC MEMBRANE (AURAL) TEMPERATURE—cont'd

2 Ask patient to turn her head so her ear is facing you (Figure 13-23).

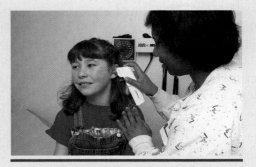

Figure **13-23**   Step 2.

3 Insert the probe gently into the ear canal, and then gently pull back on the edge of the ear to straighten out the ear canal (Figure 13-24). In children under the age of 2, pull the earlobe down and back to straighten the ear canal.

4 Press the "Start" button on the thermometer.

5 Leave the thermometer in place until you hear a tone or see a flashing light on the readout display. Read the temperature reading on the display.

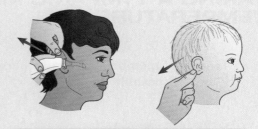

Figure **13-24**   Step 3.

6 Remove the probe from the ear, and let go of the ear.

7 Press the eject button to loosen the probe cover. Throw away the probe cover. Replace the probe in its resting place in the base unit.

8 Record the reading, and report any abnormalities to the nurse.

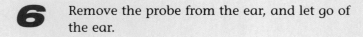

COMPLETE STANDARD ENDING STEPS (see inside front cover)

Digital Thermometers

Digital thermometers are small, battery-powered, hand-held devices most frequently used in a home setting or for a patient in isolation. The devices have an on/off button and signal that a patient's temperature measurement is reached by making an electronic beeping noise. Plastic sheath covers cover the probe tip and should be thrown away after use. The probe tip is cleansed with an alcohol swab and a dry tissue after each use. These devices may be used for oral and axillary temperatures. It may take 30 to 90 seconds for a temperature to be measured with this device (see Figure 13-3).

Pulse

When the heart beats, it pumps blood through the blood vessels of the body. A **pulse** is the throbbing that you can feel over the artery as the heart beats. You feel a pulse as you hold your fingertips over an artery close to the surface of the skin. Common locations for taking a pulse include the radial (wrist), carotid (neck), and brachial (elbow) arteries (Figure 13-25). The radial pulse is most frequently used when taking routine vital signs. You can also hear a pulse by using a stethoscope to listen over the apical area of the chest (Figure 13-26).

You take a pulse to determine a person's **heart rate**. The heart rate is the number of pulse beats, or heartbeats, that you count in 1 minute.

Other information you gather while you are taking a pulse are the **rhythm** (pattern) and **force** (strength) of the pulse. The rhythm of a pulse is described as **regular** or **irregular**. A regular pulse means the heart is beating in an even, steady pattern. An irregular pulse means the heart is beating in an uneven pattern, with different amounts of time between heartbeats.

Terms used to describe a pulse that is easy to feel include strong, bounding, or forceful. A pulse that is difficult to feel may be described as weak, thready, or faint.

Never use your thumb to feel a pulse. There is a pulse in your thumb that you may mistake for the patient's pulse.

The normal range of heart rate for an adult is 60 to 100 beats per minute. This normal range varies by age-group, as shown in Table 13-4. Heart rate is affected by many factors (Table 13-5). Two terms frequently used to describe abnormal heart rates are **tachycardia** and **bradycardia**. In an adult, tachycardia is defined as a heart rate above 100 beats per minute. Bradycardia is a heart rate below 60 beats per minute.

Text continued on p. 288

HOW & WHY

Heart rate = number of pulse beats counted in 1 minute.

NOTES ON
❋ *Older Adults*

As a person ages, his heart rate slows. Older people can have a heart rate as low as 50 beats per minute.

NOTES ON
❋ *Children*

It is normal for the heart rate of a child to be faster than an adult.

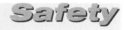

HOW & WHY

Tachy = rapid or fast; brady = slow.

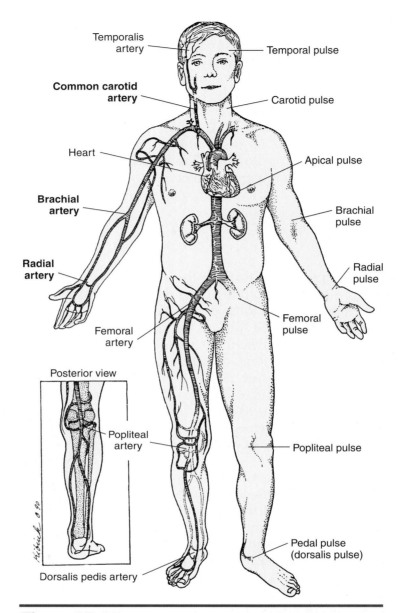

Temporalis
artery

Temporal pulse

**Common carotid
artery**

Carotid pulse

Heart

Apical pulse

**Brachial
artery**

Brachial
pulse

Radial
pulse

**Radial
artery**

Femoral
pulse

Femoral
artery

Posterior view

Popliteal
artery

Popliteal pulse

Pedal pulse
(dorsalis pulse)

Dorsalis pedis artery

***Figure* 13-25** Common locations for taking a pulse in-
clude the radial (wrist), carotid (neck), and brachial (elbow)
arteries.

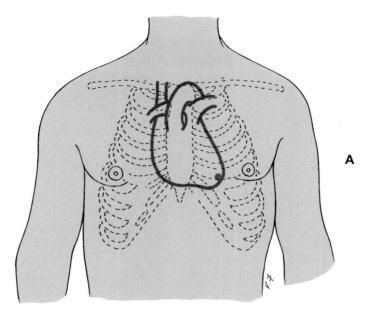

A

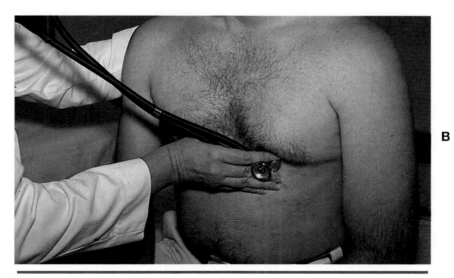

B

***Figure* 13-26** **A,** Location of the heart in the chest. **B,** Using a stethoscope to take an apical pulse.

Table 13-4

PULSE RATES	
Age	Average pulse rate at rest (beats per minute)
Normal range	60-100
Newborn	120-160
1 year	110
5 years	95
Adult woman	76-80
Adult man	72

Table 13-5

PULSE RATE FACTORS	
Factor	Results
Age	Rate decreases with age.
Body form	Rate is slower for tall, thin people.
Body temperature	Rate increases with higher temperatures.
Blood pressure	Rate decreases when pressure is higher.
Drugs	Rate increases with stimulants; rate decreases with depressants.
Emotional state	Rate increases with anxiety.
Blood loss	Rate increases with large blood loss.
Exercise	Rate increases with more exercise.
Pain	Rate increases with pain.

Procedure
TAKING A RADIAL PULSE

EQUIPMENT

* Watch or clock with second hand
* Notepad and pen

The patient should be sitting or lying down.

◆ **COMPLETE STANDARD BEGINNING STEPS (see inside front cover)**

1 Press your index and middle finger of your hand lightly over the radial artery, which is located on the thumb side (and inner aspect) of the wrist (Figure 13-27).

2 Pay attention to the rhythm—regular or irregular—and force (strength) of the pulse.

3 Count the number of pulse beats you feel for 1 full minute.

4 Write down the pulse rate, rhythm, and quality on a notepad.

5 Record the reading, and report any abnormalities to the nurse.

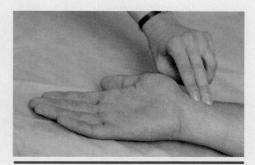

Figure 13-27   Step 1.

◆ **COMPLETE STANDARD ENDING STEPS (see inside front cover)**

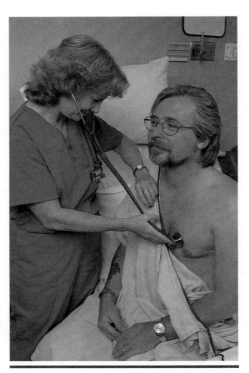

***Figure* 13-28** An apical pulse measurement may be taken on adults who have heart problems or are taking medications that affect the heart.

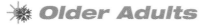
Apical Pulse

An apical pulse measurement is taken in infants and preschool-age children. The nurse may also ask you to take an apical pulse measurement in adults who have heart problems or are taking medications that affect the heart (Figure 13-28). When taking an apical pulse measurement, a **stethoscope** is used to listen to the heart rate. A stethoscope is an instrument that is placed against the patient's body to hear heart or lung sounds.

When you listen to an apical pulse, you will notice that each heartbeat makes two sounds very close together, *a lub* and a *dub.* You hear them when the two sets of valves in the heart close. The *lub-dub* sound counts as one beat.

Procedure
TAKING AN APICAL PULSE

EQUIPMENT
- Watch or clock with second hand
- Notepad and pen
- Stethoscope
- Alcohol wipes

The patient should be sitting or lying down.
Cleanse earpieces and diaphragm of stethoscope with alcohol wipe. Throw away wipe.

◆ **COMPLETE STANDARD BEGINNING STEPS (see inside front cover)**

1 Expose left side of patient's chest.

2 Place earpieces of stethoscope in your ears.

3 Place diaphragm (chest piece) of the stethoscope over the apical area of heart, which is located 2 to 3 inches to the left of the sternum below the nipple (Figure 13-29).

4 Pay attention to the rhythm—regular or irregular—and force (strength) of the pulse.

5 Count the number of pulse beats you hear in 1 full minute (see Figure 13-28).

6 Remove the stethoscope from patient's chest and the earpieces from your ears.

7 Rearrange the patient's clothing to cover the chest.

8 Write down the pulse rate, rhythm, and quality on notepad.

9 Clean the earpieces and diaphragm (chest piece) of the stethoscope with alcohol wipes. Throw away the wipe.

10 Record the reading, and report any abnormalities to the nurse.

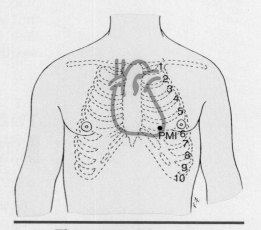

Figure **13-29**   Step 3.

◆ **COMPLETE STANDARD ENDING STEPS (see inside front cover)**

Respiration

Respiration, also known as breathing, has two parts—inhalation and exhalation. When a person inhales or breathes in, the chest expands, and air is taken into the lungs. When a person exhales or breathes out, the chest returns to its resting position, and "used" air moves out of the lungs. One inhalation plus one exhalation make up one respiration.

A normal respiratory rate in an adult is 12 to 20 respirations (or breaths) per minute. Normal respiratory rates vary by age-group and are noted in Table 13-6. Normal respirations are quiet and have an even pattern. Factors that affect the pulse rate can also affect respiration.

Respirations are counted when a person is resting quietly and positioned so you can observe the rise and fall of the chest. Respirations are counted right after taking a pulse, while your hand is still on a patient's wrist or while your stethoscope is still placed on a patient's chest. This way the patient will not see that you are counting respirations. When patients know that their respirations are being counted, they often change their breathing pattern.

HOW & WHY

1 inhalation + 1 exhalation = 1 respiration.

NOTES ON
✳ *Children*

Respirations in a child are usually faster than in an adult.

Table 13-6

AVERAGE RESPIRATION RANGES	
Age	Respirations (per Minute)
Newborn	30-80
Infant	20-40
Child	20-30
Adolescent	16-20
Adult	12-20
Elderly	16-20

Procedure
COUNTING RESPIRATIONS

EQUIPMENT

- Watch or clock with second hand
- Notepad and pen
- Stethoscope
- Alcohol wipes

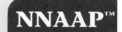

The patient should be sitting or lying down.
Cleanse earpieces and diaphragm of stethoscope with alcohol wipe. Throw away wipe.

◆ **COMPLETE STANDARD BEGINNING STEPS (see inside front cover)**

1 With fingers still placed on patient's wrist or with stethoscope placed on patient's chest after taking the pulse, count the patient's respirations (Figure 13-30).

2 Count the number of respirations you observe in 1 full minute.

3 Remove your fingers from the patient's wrist, or remove stethoscope from the patient's chest.

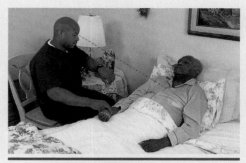

Figure **13-30**   Step 1.

4 Write down respiratory rate and pattern on notepad.

5 Record the reading, and report any abnormalities to the nurse.

◆ **COMPLETE STANDARD ENDING STEPS (see inside front cover)**

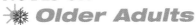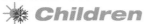
Blood Pressure

Blood pressure measures the pressure of blood in an artery. When the heart muscle contracts, blood pushes against the walls of an artery and pressure in the artery rises. This time period is known as systole, and the blood pressure number obtained is known as the **systolic pressure.** This is the higher (or top) number of a blood pressure reading. The time period in between heartbeats is called diastole. During this time, the heart muscle is relaxed and pressure in the artery is lower. The blood pressure number obtained during this time is called the **diastolic pressure** and is the lower (or bottom) number of a blood pressure reading. Blood pressure is measured in millimeters of mercury (mm Hg) and recorded as follows:

$$\frac{124}{74} \quad \begin{array}{l}\text{systolic pressure} \\ \text{diastolic pressure}\end{array}$$

Many factors affect blood pressure. Some of these factors include stress, medications, and activity. Blood pressure also varies with age (Table 13-7). The normal systolic blood pressure for an adult ranges from 100 to 140 mm Hg, while the normal diastolic pressure range is 60 to 90 mm Hg.

Table 13-7

AVERAGE BLOOD PRESSURE LEVELS	
Age	Blood pressure (mm Hg)
Newborn	35/40
4 years	85/60
6 years	95/62
10 years	100/65
12 years	108/67
16 years	118/75
Adult	100-140/60-90
Elderly	100-160/60-100

Blood pressure readings higher than 140/90 mm Hg are known as **hypertension** (high blood pressure). A blood pressure reading lower than 100/60 mm Hg is known as **hypotension** (low blood pressure).

Readings higher or lower than the normal ranges need to be reported to a nurse.

Safety

Using Blood Pressure Equipment

A stethoscope and a **sphygmomanometer** are used to take a blood pressure. The sphygmomanometer is a device used to measure blood pressure. It has two connected parts—a cuff device that is wrapped around the upper arm and a unit for measuring the pressure in millimeters of mercury (mm Hg). You will most likely use one of three types of sphygmomanometer—aneroid, mercury, or electronic. Figure 13-31 shows examples of each type.

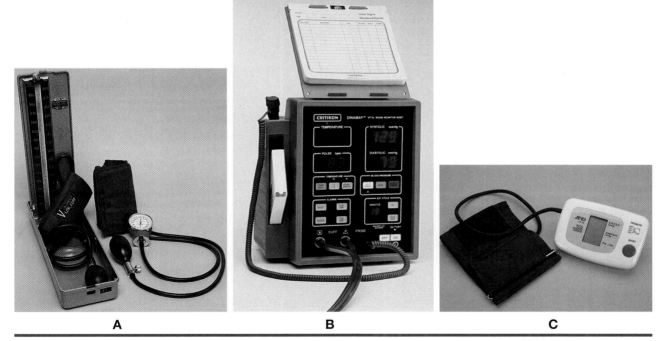

A   **B**   **C**

Figure **13-31**   **A**, Mercury *(left)* and aneroid *(right)* sphygmomanometers. **B**, Automatic blood pressure monitor. **C**, Electronic sphygmomanometer.

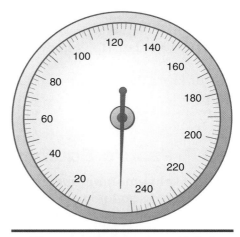

Figure 13-32 Aneroid dial.

The aneroid device has a round dial and a needle indicator that moves as the cuff is inflated or deflated (Figure 13-32). Markings on the dial are given in 2 mm Hg increments. The longer markings indicate 10, 20, 30, 40 mm Hg, and so on. This device is compact and portable.

A mercury device has a cuff connected to a unit containing a vertical column of mercury. As the cuff is inflated or deflated, the mercury moves up or down the column. Markings along the column indicate 2 mm Hg increments. The longer markings again indicate 10, 20, 30, 40 mm Hg, and so on (Figure 13-33). Results for both these units are recorded in even numbers. Most people believe the mercury device is more accurate than the aneroid device.

An electronic device has a cuff attached to a measurement unit with a display panel that gives a digital readout of the blood pressure. Many of these units also display a pulse measurement. Battery-operated units are useful for home settings. A variety of electronic units are available, so you will need to read operating instructions to use the different devices.

This is an overview of what happens when you take a blood pressure. After you wrap the cuff around the upper arm, you place the diaphragm of the stethoscope over the brachial artery. You will be able to listen to sounds produced by blood flow through the artery. As the cuff is inflated, the increased air pressure in the cuff blocks off blood flow to the lower arm. As the cuff is slowly deflated, air pressure in the cuff decreases. The first sound, or pulsation, you hear as blood begins to flow through the brachial artery is the systolic pressure. You will

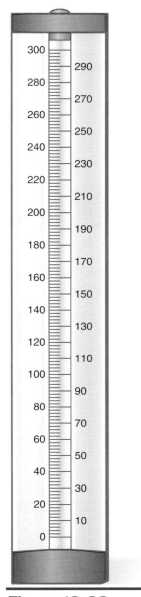

Figure 13-33
Mercury column.

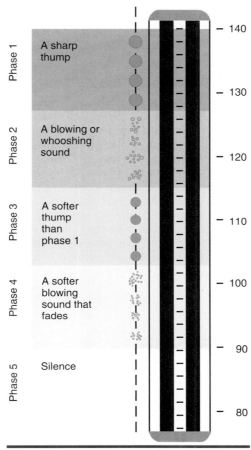

Figure 13-34   Sounds heard during
blood pressure measurement.

continue to hear pulsations as the cuff continues to deflate. The
point where the pulsation sounds stop, or become very quiet
and less clear, is the diastolic pressure. You then deflate the cuff
completely, remove the diaphragm of the stethoscope from the
brachial artery, and write down the blood pressure reading
(Figure 13-34).

NOTES ON
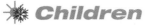
✳ *Children*

Many children require the use of a smaller cuff to obtain an accurate reading.

NOTES ON
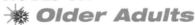
✳ *Older Adults*

Many thin elderly patients require the use of a smaller cuff to obtain an accurate reading.

Taking Accurate Blood Pressure Measurements

Taking an accurate blood pressure measurement is an important skill. Follow the guidelines in Box 13-1 to help you take an accurate measurement. If you are still unsure about your results, ask a nurse to retake the patient's blood pressure.

Box 13-1

GUIDELINES FOR TAKING AN ACCURATE BLOOD PRESSURE

- Do not take blood pressure on an arm with an intravenous (IV) line, a cast, or a dialysis access site.
- Do not take blood pressure on an arm that has an injury or surgery.
- Do not take a blood pressure on the same side as a mastectomy (removal of the breast).
- Allow a patient to rest quietly for 10 to 20 minutes before taking blood pressure, if possible.
- Choose the correct size of cuff. A cuff that is too small or too large for the patient's arm will not give an accurate measurement. Follow the size guidelines on the cuff.
- Put the cuff over bare skin; do not put the cuff over clothing.
- Make sure the patient room is as quiet as possible.

Procedure
TAKING A BLOOD PRESSURE

EQUIPMENT
- **Stethoscope**
- **Sphygmomanometer**
- **Alcohol wipes**
- **Notepad and pen**

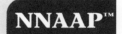

Find out a patient's normal blood pressure from the medical record, if available.
Position patient in a relaxed sitting or lying position.

◆ **COMPLETE STANDARD BEGINNING STEPS (see inside front cover)**

1 Cleanse the earpieces and diaphragm of the stethoscope with an alcohol wipe. Throw away wipe.

2 Loosen or remove clothing on patient's upper arm.

Continued

Procedure
TAKING A BLOOD PRESSURE—cont'd

3 Place patient's arm at the level of his heart, with palm up and upper arm exposed (Figure 13-35).

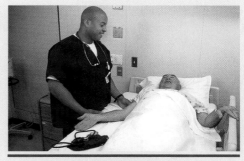

Figure **13-35**   Step 3.

4 Open the valve on the bulb by turning it in a counterclockwise direction. Squeeze cuff to expel any remaining air in the cuff, then close valve on the bulb by turning it in a clockwise direction until valve no longer moves (Figure 13-36).

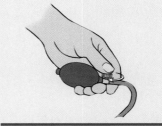

Figure **13-36**   Step 4.

5 Locate and feel for the pulsation of the brachial artery (Figure 13-37).

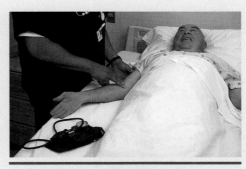

Figure **13-37**   Step 5.

Continued

Procedure
TAKING A BLOOD PRESSURE—cont'd

6 Wrap the cuff around the patient's upper arm, placing the arrow marking on the cuff over the brachial artery (Figure 13-38). The bottom of the cuff should be 1 inch above the elbow.

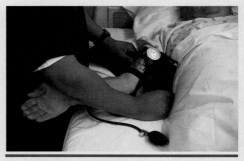

Figure **13-38**   Step 6.

7 The cuff should fit closely and not slide down the arm (Figure 13-39).

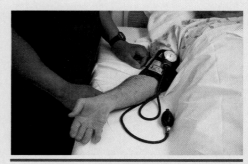

Figure **13-39**   Step 7.

8 Position the diaphragm of the stethoscope over the brachial artery (Figure 13-40). Make sure the entire surface of the diaphragm touches the patient's skin.

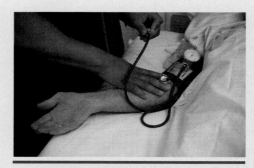

Figure **13-40**   Step 8.

Procedure
TAKING A BLOOD PRESSURE—cont'd

9   Quickly inflate the cuff to 30 mm Hg above the patient's usual systolic reading (Figure 13-41).

10   Gently open the valve on the bulb, and allow the cuff to deflate at a rate of 2 to 3 mm Hg per second.

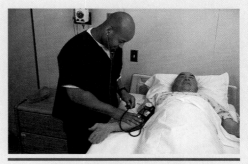

Figure **13-41**   Step 9.

11   Note the point where you hear the first pulsation, or sound. This is the systolic pressure (Figure 13-42).

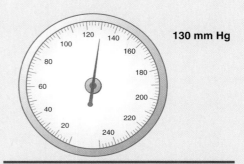

Figure **13-42**   Step 11.

12   Continue to let the cuff deflate. Listen for the point when you hear the pulsation sound disappear or become very quiet. This is the diastolic pressure (Figure 13-43).

13   Allow the cuff to deflate completely. You may have to open the valve more to allow all the air in the cuff to escape.

14   Remove the diaphragm of the stethoscope from the patient' arm, and take the earpieces out of your ears.

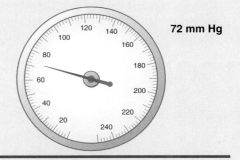

Figure **13-43**   Step 12.

Continued

Procedure
TAKING A BLOOD PRESSURE—cont'd

15 If you wish to recheck your results or are unsure of your readings, wait 30 seconds before taking the blood pressure again (Figure 13-44).

16 Unwrap and remove the cuff from the patient's arm.

17 Write down the blood pressure on a notepad.

18 Record the reading, and report any abnormalities to the nurse.

◆ **COMPLETE STANDARD ENDING STEPS (see inside front cover)**

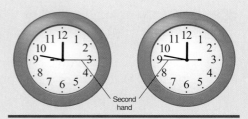

Second hand

Figure 13-44   Step 15.

NOTES ON
❄ *Children*

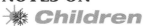

Height and weight for infants and children are regularly measured as part of their well-child examinations.

OBRA

NOTES ON
❄ *Older Adults*

Residents of long-term care centers are usually weighed each month. A weight gain or loss of 5 pounds or more should be reported to the nurse.

Measuring Height and Weight

Height and weight are measured when a patient is admitted to a health care facility and when a patient visits a doctor's office (Figure 13-45).

A variety of types of weight scales are used in health care facilities—including chair scales and lift scales. Figure 13-46 shows a caregiver using a lift type of scale to weigh a bedridden patient. You will most often use a standing scale for measuring height and weight.

Remember to respect the resident's right to dignity and privacy by keeping him covered and exposing only the body parts needed to perform the procedures. Explain what you are going to do before performing the procedure to make the resident more relaxed. The resident's vital signs and weight are considered private information and should not be shared with visitors or people not directly involved in the resident's care.

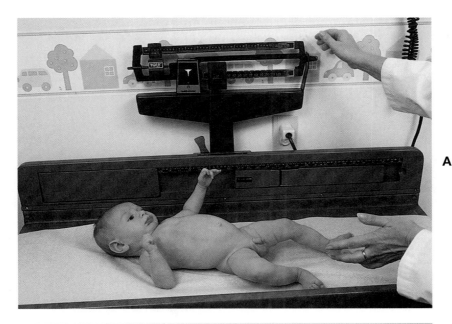

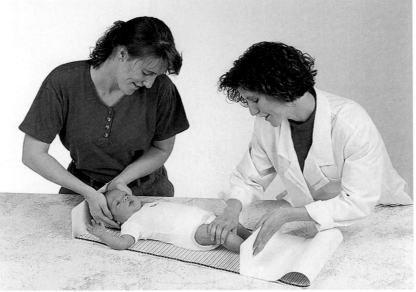

Figure 13-45   **A,** Weighing an infant. **B,** Measuring the length of the infant.

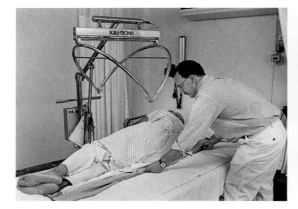
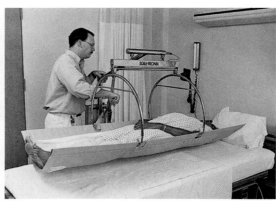

A   B

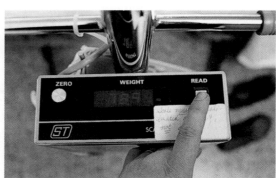

C

Figure 13-46   Lift scale. **A,** The sling is placed under the patient. **B,** The patient is lifted. **C,** A digital reading of the patient's weight is displayed.

Procedure
MEASURING HEIGHT AND WEIGHT USING A STANDING SCALE

EQUIPMENT

- **Standing scale**
- **Notepad and pen**

NNAAP™

Ask the patient to urinate to empty her bladder.
Ask if the patient needs help to remove extra clothing and shoes,
and then help the patient if she wants help.

◆ COMPLETE STANDARD BEGINNING STEPS **(see inside front cover)**

1   Raise the height rod on the scale to a level above the patient's height.

Procedure

MEASURING HEIGHT AND WEIGHT USING A STANDING SCALE—cont'd

2   Assist the patient with stepping on the scale. Ask patient to hold her arms straight at her sides (Figure 13-47).

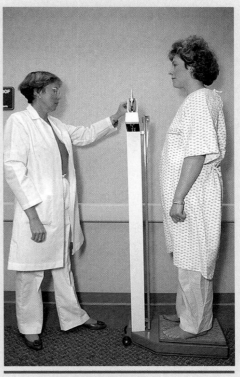

Figure 13-47   Step 2.

3   Slide and adjust the scale weights until the pointer balances in the middle position (Figure 13-48).

4   Note and record weight on notepad.

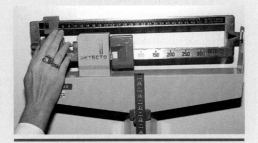

Figure 13-48   Step 3.

Continued

Procedure

MEASURING HEIGHT AND WEIGHT USING A STANDING SCALE—cont'd

5   Ask patient to stand straight and still.

6   Fold movable part of height rod so it is at a 90-degree angle to the remaining part of the rod, then slide entire rod slowly and gently down until it touches the top of the patient's head (Figure 13-49).

7   Assist patient with stepping off the scale.

8   Note and record height on notepad.

9   Record the reading, and report any abnormalities to the nurse.

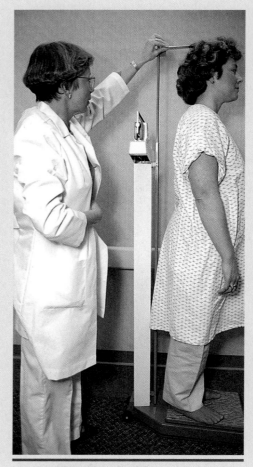

Figure 13-49   Step 6.

◆ **COMPLETE STANDARD ENDING STEPS (see inside front cover)**

CHAPTER REVIEW

1. What are the 4 things measured when taking vital signs?

2. When should vital signs readings be reported to the nurse?

3. Which sites are most commonly used for temperature measurement?

4. What is the normal range of heart rate for an adult who is resting quietly?

5. It is time to take Mr. Thompson's blood pressure. You obtain a reading of 82/52 mm Hg. What do you know about this reading?

6. Mr. Longwood has a blood pressure of 138/82 mm Hg. Which number is the systolic, and which number is the diastolic in this reading?

7. What do the "systolic" and "diastolic" numbers measure?

8. When are height and weight measured?

Circle the one BEST response.

9. Which of these factors can affect a person's vital signs?
   a. Emotions and activity
   b. Medications and illness
   c. Time of day and eating
   d. All of the above

10. You take Ms. James's oral temperature and get a reading of 97.7° F. What do you know about this result?
    a. It is within the normal range.
    b. Ms. James has a fever.
    c. Ms. James has been drinking hot coffee.
    d. The result should be reported immediately to a nurse.

11. Mr. Thompson is a patient on the surgical floor. He just had rectal surgery. He is wearing an oxygen mask. He also wears hearing aids in both ears. The RN asks you to take his temperature. Which site is the best choice for taking Mr. Thompson's temperature?
    a. Oral (mouth)
    b. Axillary
    c. Rectal
    d. Ear (tympanic membrane)

CHAPTER REVIEW

12. You take Mr. Thompson's radial pulse. It is 134 beats per minute. What do you know about this result?
   a. This rate is within the normal range for an adult.
   b. Mr. Thompson has bradycardia.
   c. Mr. Thompson has tachycardia.
   d. Mr. Thompson has hypertension.

13. When you observe Mr. Thompson's respirations, his breathing is labored and you count a rate of 36 breaths per minute. What should you do?
   a. Report these findings to the nurse.
   b. Record the results on the graphic record; the nurse can read the results later in the shift.
   c. Do nothing; these are normal findings.
   d. Ask Mr. Thompson to calm down and breathe more slowly.

14. Ms. James shows you a record of the blood pressure readings she has obtained at home using her electronic sphygmomanometer. The most recent three readings are 164/92, 176/94, and 182/92 mm Hg. When you take her blood pressure, you obtain a reading of 188/94. What do you know about these readings?
   a. These readings are in the normal range for an adult.
   b. These readings indicate hypertension.
   c. These readings indicate hypotension.
   d. These readings are critically high, and Ms. James needs to be hospitalized immediately.

Answers are on page 707.

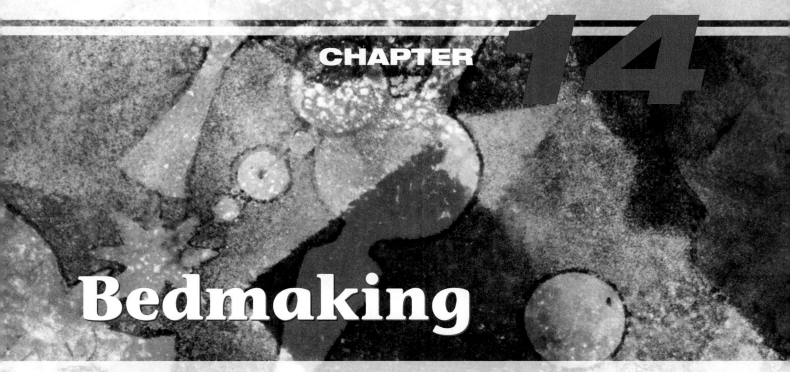

CHAPTER 14

Bedmaking

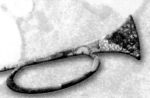

What you will learn

- Why a clean and neatly made bed is important
- Linens needed to make a bed
- How to handle clean and dirty linens
- How often to change linens on a bed
- The difference between an occupied and an unoccupied bed
- How to make a closed bed, an open bed, an occupied bed, and a surgical bed
- How to put linens onto special mattresses
- How to make a bed with cradle or foot board in place

KEY TERMS

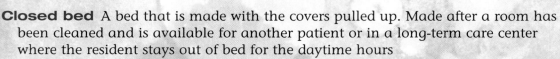

Closed bed A bed that is made with the covers pulled up. Made after a room has been cleaned and is available for another patient or in a long-term care center where the resident stays out of bed for the daytime hours

Cradle (overbed cradle) A frame placed at the foot of the bed to prevent bed linens from resting on the feet and lower legs

Drawsheet A small sheet placed sideways across the bed to cover the area of the bed between the patient's shoulders and thighs. Can be changed if it becomes dirty or may be used to reposition the patient in the bed. Sometimes called a lift sheet

Foot board A frame placed at the foot of the bed to prevent bedclothes from resting on the feet and lower legs

Lift sheet A small sheet placed sideways across the bed to cover the area of the bed between the patient's shoulders and thighs. Can be changed if it becomes dirty or may be used to reposition the patient in the bed. Sometimes called a draw sheet

Mattress pad A pad placed between the mattress and the bottom sheet that absorbs moisture and keeps the patient from perspiring if the mattress is covered with plastic

Mitered corner A method of folding the sheets at the corners at a right angle that has a neat appearance

Occupied bed A bed that is made while the patient is in it

Open bed A bed that is made with the covers fanfolded to the foot of the bed in preparation for a new admission or a patient who will return to the bed after the linens are changed

Pressure ulcer An inflammation or sore that develops over areas where the skin and tissue underneath are injured due to the lack of blood flow and oxygen supply as a result of constant pressure

Protective pad An absorbent pad that is placed over the bottom sheet or the drawsheet to give additional protection. Pads are cloth or disposable. Frequently used with patients who are incontinent, vomiting, or bleeding. Sometimes called an underpad

Surgical bed A bed that is made with the covers fanfolded to the side so that the transfer from a stretcher to the bed is easier

Toe pleat A 3- to 4-inch fold in the top covers across the foot of the bed that allows patients to freely move their feet under the top covers

Underpad An absorbent pad that is placed over the bottom sheet or the drawsheet to provide additional protection. Pads are cloth or disposable. Frequently used with patients who are incontinent, vomiting, or bleeding. Sometimes called a protective pad

Unoccupied bed A bed that is made while the patient is out of the bed

Why Is a Clean and Neatly Made Bed Important?

The bed is one of the most important parts of patients' environment while they are in a health care setting. Many patients in hospitals and nursing homes spend most of their day in bed. A clean, wrinkle-free bed is especially important for the patient who is on bedrest. The comfort and appearance of the bed are important to the patient.

Wrinkles are uncomfortable and can lead to the development of skin breakdown or **pressure ulcers** (Chapter 23).

Safety

Linens Needed to Make a Bed

Beds in most health care facilities are made with the following linens:

- **Mattress pad**—A mattress pad absorbs moisture and keeps the patient from perspiring if the mattress is covered in plastic.
- **Bottom sheet**—A bottom sheet is either flat or fitted. A fitted sheet is either contoured or has elastic edges to fit tightly over the edges of the mattress.
- **Drawsheet or lift sheet**—The drawsheet or lift sheet is a small sheet placed sideways across the bed to cover the area of the bed between the patient's shoulders and thighs. This sheet can be changed if it becomes dirty or may be used to lift or move the patient in the bed.
- **Underpad/protective pad**—This is placed over the bottom sheet or the drawsheet to provide additional protection. Pads are cloth or disposable.
- **Top sheet**
- **Pillowcase**
- **Blanket and/or bedspread**

How to Handle Clean and Dirty Linens

For the health and safety of the patient and the employee, good infection control practices should be followed when handling dirty linens. Gloves and other personal protective equipment may be required (Chapter 9). Hands should always be washed before handling clean linens.

Safety

Clean linens are stored in a closet or on the clean linen cart in the hallway. The door to the linen closet must be kept closed when it is not in use. The clean linen cart is always kept covered, and the cover is replaced after removing the required linens. Take only the linens you need into the patient's room.

Linens should be stacked on a clean surface in the order they will be used.

As dirty linens are removed from the bed, roll them toward the center of the bed with the dirty areas on the inside. Dirty linens are covered with germs and should never be shaken. Place the dirty linens in a covered linen hamper. Some facilities do not permit linen hampers to be taken into patient rooms. Dirty linens may be placed in a pillowcase or in a plastic bag before transporting them to the hamper. Dirty linens are never placed on other surfaces such as the chair, nightstand, or floor. Dirty linen hampers should be returned to the appropriate storage area according to facility policy. Dirty linen hampers should be kept covered to control odors and decrease the spread of germs. The dirty linen hamper is never placed next to the clean linen cart.

When handling both clean and dirty linens, avoid contact with your uniform. Linens that touch the floor or have been taken into a patient room but not used are considered dirty and should be placed in a dirty linen hamper.

How Often to Change Linens on a Bed

Change linens as often as necessary to keep the bed clean, dry, and free from wrinkles. The frequency of linen changes depends on facility policy and on the needs of the patient. Most hospitals change bed linens at least once a day. In a nursing home, the linens may be changed 2 to 3 times per week on the days the resident gets a shower or bath. If a patient's bed is wet or dirty from perspiration, stool, urine, vomiting, or bleeding, it will need to be changed more often. Regardless of the setting, if the linens are wet or dirty, they should be changed to keep the patient comfortable.

The Difference Between an Occupied and an Unoccupied Bed

An **occupied bed** is a bed that is made while the patient is in it. Changing the linens on an occupied bed may be done after giving a bed bath or as part of giving incontinent care (Chapter 15). When the bed is made with the patient out of the bed, it is called an **unoccupied** bed. A **closed bed** is a bed that is not currently being used by the patient. A closed bed is made after the room has been cleaned and is available for another patient. A closed bed is also made in long-term care centers where the residents remain out of bed for the daytime hours.

Open beds and **surgical beds** are also considered unoccupied beds because there is no patient in the bed when the linens are changed. An open bed means that the covers are turned back in preparation for the patient. An open bed is made when a new patient is being admitted or if the patient will be returning to the bed after the linens have been changed. A surgical bed is made in preparation for a patient being moved from a stretcher into the bed. This may be a patient returning to the room from surgery or a procedure or a patient arriving by ambulance. The bed is made in a way that allows an easy transfer from the stretcher to the bed.

Safety　To prevent injury to your back, adjust the bed to a comfortable working height, lower the back and knee rest, and lock the wheels.

Safety　Bed linens may be contaminated with blood or body fluids. Follow Standard Precautions and the Bloodborne Pathogen Standard when handling dirty linens.

Procedure
MAKING AN UNOCCUPIED BED (CLOSED)

EQUIPMENT
- Clean linens
- Dirty linen hamper
- Gloves and other personal protective equipment needed

◆ **COMPLETE STANDARD BEGINNING STEPS (see inside front cover)**

1 Arrange the linens in the order they will be used. The items needed first should be on the top, and the items needed last should be on the bottom (Figure 14-1).

2 Place the linens on a clean chair close to the bed.

3 Adjust the bed to a comfortable working height, lower the back and knee rest, and lock the wheels.

4 Put on gloves if linens are soiled with blood or body fluids.

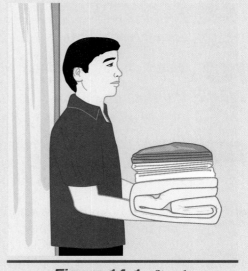

Figure 14-1 Step 1.

Continued

Procedure
MAKING AN UNOCCUPIED BED (CLOSED)—cont'd

5 Loosen the linens on one side of the bed by lifting the mattress with one hand and drawing the linens out with the other hand.

6 Fold the spread or blanket to the foot of the bed, and remove it if it is to be used again (Figure 14-2).

7 Remove the pillow from the bed. Grab the pillow with one hand; using the other hand, gather the pillowcase and pull it back over the pillow so it is inside out. Place the pillow on a chair, and put the dirty pillowcase in the dirty linen hamper.

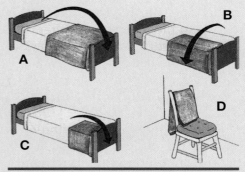

***Figure* 14-2**   Step 6. **A,** Fold top edge of blanket down to the bottom edge. **B,** Fold blanket over from far side of bed to near side. **C,** Fold top edge of blanket down to bottom edge. **D,** Place folded blanket on a chair.

8 Gather all dirty linens by folding the edges inward so that the dirtiest side is on the inside (Figure 14-3).

9 Move to the other side of the bed, and repeat steps 5 and 8. Place the dirty linens in the dirty linen hamper.

10 Remove gloves if used and wash hands.

11 If the mattress pad is to be reused, straighten it and allow it to remain on the mattress.

12 If the mattress pad has been removed, place the clean mattress pad on the bed lengthwise with the fold in the center of the bed.

13 Place the bottom sheet lengthwise on the bed with the fold in the center of the bed. Place the sheet with the rough edges of the hem facing down, away from the patient.

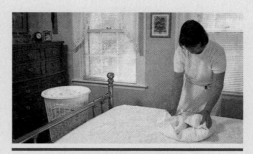

***Figure* 14-3**   Step 8.

Continued

Procedure

MAKING AN UNOCCUPIED BED (CLOSED)—cont'd

14 If using a flat bottom sheet, the lower edge of the sheet should be even with the foot of the mattress.

15 Tuck the bottom sheet under the head of the mattress.

16 Miter the corner by facing the head of the bed and with the hand closest to the bed, pick up the edge of the sheet about 12 to 14 inches from the edge of the bed, making a triangle. Lay the triangle on top of the mattress. Tuck the hanging portion of the sheet under the mattress. Holding the fold at the top of the mattress, bring the triangle down and tuck it in (Figure 14-4).

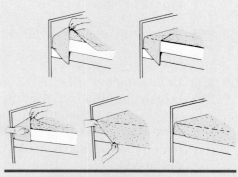

17 Tuck the bottom sheet under the side of the mattress.

Figure 14-4   Step 16.

18 If using a drawsheet/lift sheet, place the folded drawsheet/lift sheet across the bed so that it will extend from the patient's shoulders to the patient's hips. Tuck in the drawsheet/lift sheet per facility policy.

19 Unfold the clean top sheet and place wrong side up, top hem even with the top edge of the mattress and centerfold line on the center of the bed.

20 Unfold the blanket with the centerfold line on the center of the bed, and place over the top sheet. Allow enough of the top sheet to extend beyond the top edge of the blanket to allow for 2 inches of sheet to fold over the top edge of the blanket. Fold the top sheet over the upper edge of the blanket/spread so that the sewn edge of the hem faces down toward the blanket/spread to make a cuff on one side of the bed (Figure 14-5).

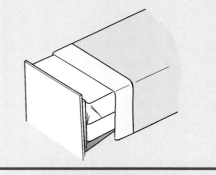

Figure 14-5   Step 20.

21 Lift the bottom of the mattress with one hand, and tuck the top sheet and blanket under the mattress on that side with the other hand.

22 Miter the corner.

Continued

Procedure

MAKING AN UNOCCUPIED BED (CLOSED)—cont'd

23 Move to the other side of the bed.

24 Beginning at the head of the bed, tuck in the bottom sheet, pulling tightly as you move toward the foot of the bed (Figure 14-6). Miter the top corner (see step 16).

25 Tuck in the drawsheet/lift sheet per facility policy.

26 Unfold the top sheet and blanket, keeping both centered on the bed. Fold the top sheet over the upper edge of the blanket/spread so that the sewn edge of the hem faces downward toward the blanket/spread to make a cuff on this side of the bed.

27 Lift the bottom of the mattress with one hand and tuck the top sheet and blanket under the mattress with the other hand.

28 Miter the corner (Figure 14-7).

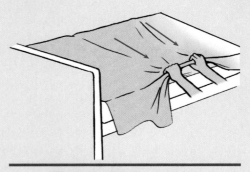

Figure 14-6   Step 24.

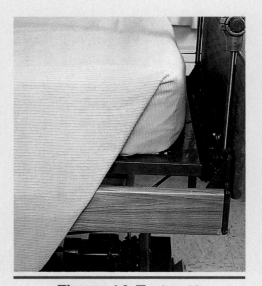

Figure 14-7   Step 28.

Continued

Procedure

MAKING AN UNOCCUPIED BED (CLOSED)—cont'd

29 Make a **toe pleat** by grasping both sides of the top covers at the mitered corner and gently pulling the top covers toward the foot of the bed to make a 3- to 4-inch fold across the foot of the bed (Figure 14-8).

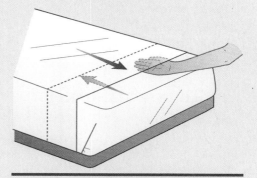

Figure 14-8   Step 29.

30 Put the clean pillowcase on the pillow. Hold the end seam of the pillowcase at the center, and turn the pillowcase back over your hand. Grasp the pillow through the pillowcase at the center of one end of the pillow. Bring the pillowcase over the pillow, and fit the corners of the pillow into the corners of the pillowcase (Figure 14-9).

31 Place the pillow on the bed with the open side of the pillowcase away from the door.

32 Place the signal light near the head of the bed.

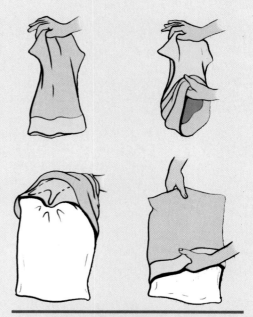

Figure 14-9   Step 30.

◆ **COMPLETE STANDARD ENDING STEPS (see inside front cover)**

Procedure
MAKING AN UNOCCUPIED BED (OPEN)

EQUIPMENT
- Clean linens
- Dirty linen hamper

- Gloves and other personal protective equipment needed

◆ **COMPLETE STANDARD BEGINNING STEPS (see inside front cover)**

Follow steps 1 to 29 as listed for making a closed bed.

30 Grasp the top cuff of the top sheet and blanket with both hands.

31 Fanfold the top linens to the foot of the bed and smooth (Figure 14-10).

32 Place the signal light near the head of the bed.

33 Put the clean pillowcase on the pillow. Hold the end seam of the pillowcase at the center, and turn the pillowcase back over your hand. Grasp the pillow through the pillowcase at the center of one end of the pillow. Bring the pillowcase over the pillow, and fit the corners of the pillow into the corners of the pillowcase (see Figure 14-9).

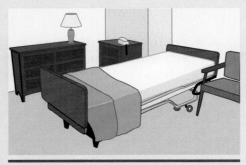

***Figure* 14-10**   Step 31.

34 Place the pillow on the bed with the open side of the pillowcase away from the door.

◆ **COMPLETE STANDARD ENDING STEPS (see inside front cover)**

Procedure
MAKING A SURGICAL BED

EQUIPMENT

- Clean linens
- Dirty linen

- Gloves and other personal hamperprotective equipment needed

◆ **COMPLETE STANDARD BEGINNING STEPS (see inside front cover)**

Follow steps 1 to 22 as listed for making a closed bed.

23 Tuck in the drawsheet/lift sheet per facility policy.

24 Unfold the top sheet and blanket, keeping both centered on the bed.

25 Fold top linen to form a triangle (Figure 14-11).

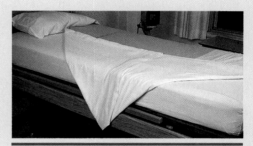

Figure **14-11**   Step 25.

26 Fanfold the blanket and top sheet to the far side of the bed (Figure 14-12).

27 Put the clean pillowcase on the pillow. Hold the end seam of the pillowcase at the center, and turn the pillowcase back over your hand. Grasp the pillow through the pillowcase at the center of one end of the pillow. Bring the pillowcase over the pillow, and fit the corners of the pillow into the corners of the pillowcase (see Figure 14-9).

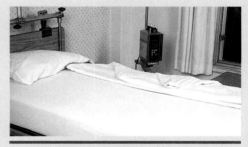

Figure **14-12**   Step 26.

28 Place the pillow against the headboard with the open side of the pillowcase away from the door.

29 Place the signal light near the head of the bed.

◆ **COMPLETE STANDARD ENDING STEPS (see inside front cover)**

Procedure
MAKING AN OCCUPIED BED

EQUIPMENT
- Clean linens
- Dirty linen hamper
- Gloves and other personal protective equipment needed

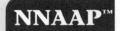

◆ **COMPLETE STANDARD BEGINNING STEPS** (see inside front cover)

1 Arrange the linens in the order they will be used. The items needed first should be on the top, and the items needed last should be on the bottom.

2 Place the linens on a clean chair close to the bed.

3 Identify the patient, and inform her of what you are going to do.

4 Provide privacy by closing the door and pulling the privacy curtain around the bed.

5 Adjust the bed to a comfortable working height; lower the back and knee rest if allowed for that patient. Lock the wheels (Figure 14-13).

6 Raise the side rail on the opposite side from where you are working.

7 Put on gloves if linens are soiled with blood or body fluids.

8 Loosen the linens at the foot of the bed.

9 Fold the spread or blanket to the foot of the bed, and remove it if it is to be used again (see Figure 14-2).

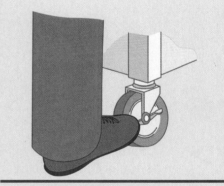

***Figure* 14-13**   Step 5.

10 Place a bath blanket over the top sheet. Ask the patient to hold the bath blanket or tuck it under the patient's shoulders while you remove the top sheet (Figure 14-14).

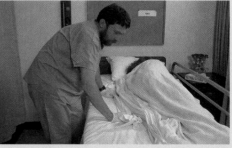

***Figure* 14-14**   Step 10.

Continued

Procedure
MAKING AN OCCUPIED BED—cont'd

11 Remove the top sheet, and place it in the dirty linen hamper.

12 Turn the patient toward the raised side rail with a pillow under her head. Loosen the bottom linens, and roll them toward the patient's back (Figure 14-15). If the mattress pad is to be reused, straighten it and allow it to remain on the mattress.

13 If the mattress pad has been removed, place the clean mattress pad on the bed lengthwise with the fold in the center of the bed.

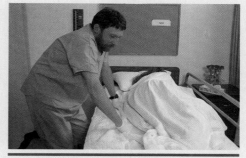

Figure 14-15 Step 12.

14 Place the bottom sheet lengthwise on the bed with the fold in the center of the bed. Place the sheet with the rough edges of the hem facing down, away from the patient. Push the folded bottom sheet under the rolled dirty linens that will be removed (Figure 14-16).

15 If using a flat bottom sheet, the lower edge of the sheet should be even with the foot of the mattress.

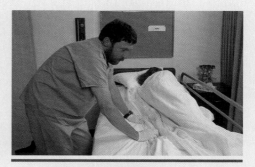

Figure 14-16 Step 14.

16 Tuck the bottom sheet under the head of the mattress.

17 Miter the corner by facing the head of the bed and with the hand closest to the bed, pick up the edge of the sheet about 12 to 14 inches from the edge of the bed, making a triangle. Lay the triangle on top of the mattress. Tuck the hanging portion of the sheet under the mattress. Holding the fold at the top of the mattress, bring the triangle down and tuck it in (Figure 14-17).

18 Tuck the bottom sheet under the side of the mattress.

19 Fanfold the bottom sheet close to the patient's back.

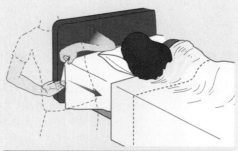

Figure 14-17 Step 17.

Continued

Procedure
MAKING AN OCCUPIED BED—cont'd

20 If using a drawsheet/lift sheet, place the folded drawsheet/lift sheet across the bed so that it extends from the patient's shoulders to her hips. Fanfold the sheet close to the patient's back on top of the bottom sheet (Figure 14-18). Tuck in the drawsheet/lift sheet per facility policy.

21 Raise the side rail on the side on which you have been working.

22 Move to the other side of the bed, and lower the side rail.

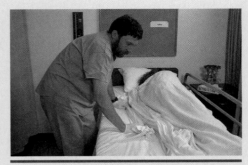

Figure 14-18   Step 20.

23 Roll the patient away from you, over the linens and onto the clean side (Figure 14-19). Explain to the patient that she will feel a large "lump" as she rolls over the linens. Keep the patient covered with the bath blanket while she is being turned.

24 Move the pillow so that it remains under the patient's head.

25 Remove the dirty linens, and place them in the dirty linen hamper.

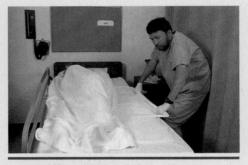

Figure 14-19   Step 23.

26 Remove gloves if used and wash hands.

27 Pull the clean linens toward you. Tuck in the bottom sheet, and miter the corner at the head of the bed. Tuck in the lift sheet/drawsheet per facility policy.

28 Assist patient to the center of the bed.

29 Place the clean top sheet over the patient with the sewn edges of the hem facing up and away from the patient's face. Ask the patient to hold the top sheet or tuck it under her shoulders (Figure 14-20).

30 Remove the bath blanket from the patient, keeping her covered with the sheet (see Figure 14-20). Place the bath blanket in the dirty linen hamper.

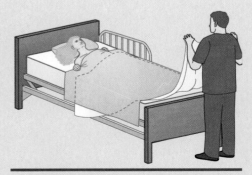

Figure 14-20   Steps 29 and 30.

Continued

Procedure
MAKING AN OCCUPIED BED—cont'd

31 Apply the blanket or spread to the bed 2 inches below the upper edge of the top sheet. Fold the top sheet over the upper edge of the blanket/spread so that the sewn edge of the hem faces down toward the blanket/spread to make a cuff.

32 At the foot of the bed lift the mattress with one hand, and tuck the top bed linens under the mattress on that side (Figure 14-21). Make a **mitered corner.**

33 Raise the side rail, and move to the opposite side of the bed.

34 Lower the side rail. At the foot of the bed lift the mattress with one hand, and tuck the top bed linens under the mattress on that side. Make a mitered corner.

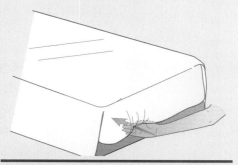

***Figure* 14-21**   Step 32.

35 Make a toe pleat by grasping both sides of the top covers at the mitered corner and gently pulling the top covers toward the foot of the bed to make a 3- to 4-inch fold across the foot of the bed (Figure 14-22).

36 Remove the pillow from under the patient's head, and remove the pillowcase.

37 Place the dirty pillowcase in the dirty linen hamper.

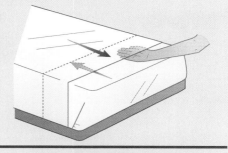

***Figure* 14-22**   Step 35.

38 Put the clean pillowcase on the pillow. Hold the end seam of the pillowcase at the center, and turn the pillowcase back over your hand. Grasp the pillow through the pillowcase at the center of one end of the pillow. Bring the pillowcase over the pillow, and fit the corners of the pillow into the corners of the pillowcase (see Figure 14-9).

39 Place the pillow under the patient's head with the open side of the pillowcase away from the door.

Continued

Procedure
MAKING AN OCCUPIED BED—cont'd

40 Place the signal light near the head of the bed.

41 Lower side rail per care plan and facility policy.

◆ **COMPLETE STANDARD ENDING STEPS (see inside front cover)**

How to Put Linens Onto Special Mattresses

Patients who spend most of their time in bed often have problems with pressure ulcers. Many manufacturers have designed special beds and mattresses to meet the needs of patients on prolonged bedrest. Figure 14-23, shows pictures of several types of specialty beds. Each manufacturer provides specific instructions regarding the procedure for placing linens on their mattresses.

Safety   It is important to follow the manufacturer's guidelines when making a bed with a special mattress. The charge nurse can provide you with instructions.

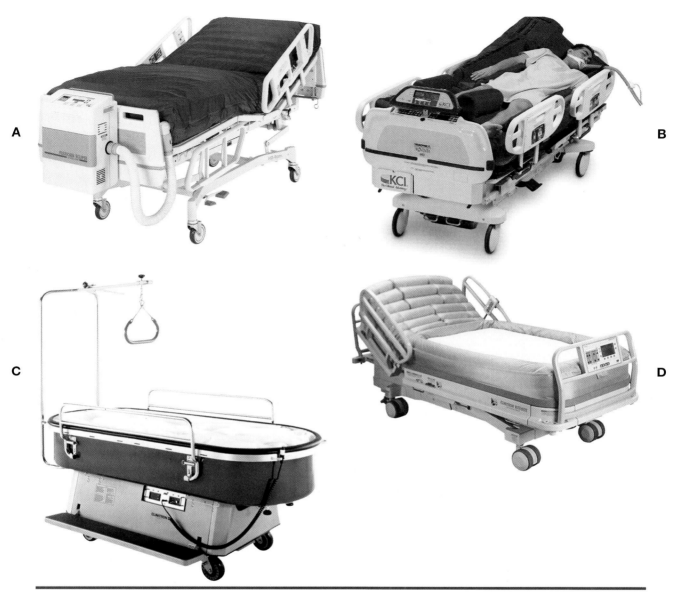

Figure 14-23   Specialty beds. **A,** Low-air-loss bed. **B,** Lateral rotation bed. **C,** Air-fluidized therapy bed. **D,** Combination air-fluidized therapy and low-air-loss bed.

How to Make a Bed With a Cradle or Foot Board in Place

A **cradle** or a **foot board** is applied to the foot of the bed to keep the linens from resting on the patient's feet and/or lower legs (Figure 14-24). A cradle or foot board may be used for a patient who has had foot or lower leg surgery, suffers from foot pain due to poor circulation, or has a pressure ulcer on the foot. When placing the top sheet and blanket on the bed, they are placed over the cradle or foot board and then tucked in at the bottom of the mattress. If the linens are large enough, the corners can be mitered. A patient with a cradle or foot board does not require a toe pleat in the top linens.

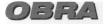

Many nursing home residents bring bedspreads, blankets, quilts, or afghans from home. This helps the person to feel more comfortable. The resident should be encouraged to make as many decisions about his environment as possible. All resident belongings should be marked with the person's name so that they can be promptly returned after being washed.

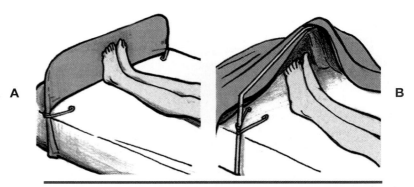

Figure **14-24**   **A**, Foot board. **B**, Bed cradle.

CHAPTER REVIEW

1. Why is a clean and neatly made bed important?

2. While you are making Mr. Henderson's bed, the clean pillowcase falls onto the floor. What action should you take?

3. What linens are usually needed to make a bed?

Circle the one BEST response.

4. Which of the following pieces of linen absorbs moisture and keeps the patient from perspiring if the mattress is enclosed in a plastic cover?
   a. Top sheet
   b. Pillowcase
   c. Mattress pad
   d. Lift sheet

5. How should clean linens be stored?
   a. On an uncovered linen cart outside of the patient's room
   b. In a linen closet with the door kept closed
   c. In the patient's nightstand or closet
   d. In a dirty linen hamper

6. Where should dirty linens be placed after they are removed from the bed?
   a. On the floor next to the bed
   b. On the patient's overbed table
   c. In the linen closet
   d. In the dirty linen hamper

7. Ms. Harmon, a nursing home resident, is incontinent of stool and urine. How often should her linens be changed?
   a. Every day according to facility policy
   b. 2 to 3 times a week on the days she is bathed
   c. Whenever her family asks that they be changed
   d. As often as needed to keep the bed clean and dry

8. What is an occupied bed?
   a. A bed that is made while the patient is in it
   b. A bed that is made with the patient out of the bed
   c. A bed that is made in preparation for a new patient
   d. A bed that is made in preparation for a patient returning from surgery

9. How are linens changed on a special mattress?
   a. Linens on special mattresses are changed in the same manner as a regular mattress.
   b. Linens are not used on special mattresses because of their special design.
   c. Linens on special mattresses are changed according to the manufacturer's instructions.
   d. Linens on special mattresses are changed according to the patient's request.

CHAPTER REVIEW

10. When is a cradle or foot board used on the patient's bed?
  a. For patients who are likely to fall out of the bed
  b. For patients who have had foot surgery
  c. For patients who complain of cold feet
  d. For patients who have good circulation

Mark T for true or F for false.

11. _____ Residents in a nursing home are allowed to use their own blanket or bedspread from home if they desire.

Answers are on page 707.

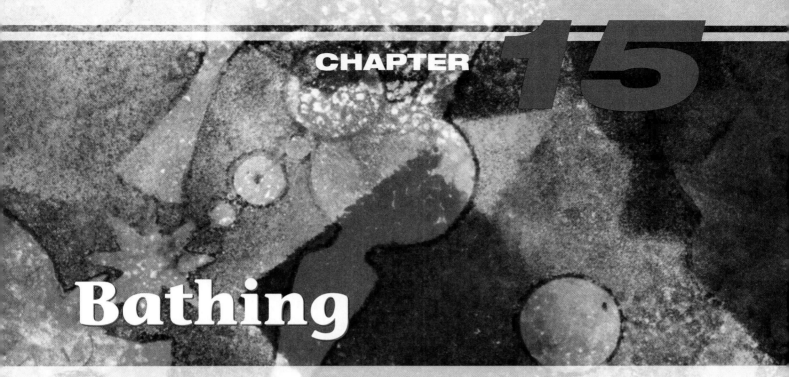

CHAPTER 15

Bathing

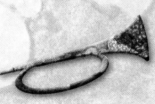

What you will learn

- General guidelines for bathing
- How to give a partial and complete bed bath
- How to give a tub bath
- How to give a shower
- How to perform perineal care

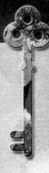

KEY TERMS

Continent In control of bowel and/or bladder functioning
Incontinent Not in control of bowel and/or bladder functioning

General Guidelines for Bathing a Patient

Bathing is an important part of personal hygiene. Some patients are able to bathe themselves without help. Other patients need partial or total assistance with their bath. People who are patients in a hospital setting are usually helped to bathe every day. People who are residents in a nursing home are usually bathed 2 to 3 times a week or as often as needed to keep the skin clean and prevent odors.

Bathing accomplishes 4 things. Bathing cleanses the skin of dirt and waste products, makes the patient more comfortable, stimulates circulation to the skin, and gives the nursing assistant an opportunity to look at the condition of the patient's skin.

Important things to consider when bathing a patient include:

- Floors, tubs, and showers become slippery when wet.
- Water used for the bath should be warm, 105° F for a tub bath or shower and 115° F for a bed bath. Allow the patient to feel the water before applying it to his skin.
- Water over 120° F can burn the skin.
- The room temperature should be 75° to 80° F and free from drafts to keep the patient from becoming chilled during the bath.
- Because warm water can stimulate the urge to urinate, always offer the bedpan or take the patient to the bathroom *before* beginning the bathing process.
- Providing privacy for the patient during the bath is important.
- All patients should be encouraged to be as independent as possible with their hygiene, including bathing.
- Rinse all soap from the skin. Soap left on the skin is drying and can cause itching.
- A washcloth mitt/mitten should be used when bathing a patient (Figure 15-1). This prevents dripping water onto the patient from the corners of the washcloth.

NOTES ON
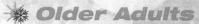
Older Adults

The skin of the elderly person tends to be dry. Nursing home residents are usually bathed 2 to 3 times a week. Bathing more often causes the skin to become dry. Elderly people also have less body fat and become chilled more easily.

Safety

Safety

NOTES ON
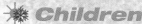
Children

In some families it is important to the parents to participate in the care of their child. Assisting with the bath is a good chance for parents to care for their child; this also helps the child to feel safe during the bath.

NOTES ON
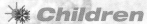
Children

Small children and infants may chill easily. Keep them covered as much as possible while bathing.

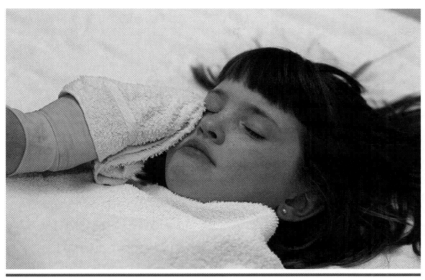

Figure 15-1   Washcloth mitt/mitten.

- Many facilities use a liquid soap. If using bar soap, do not leave the soap in the tub or bath basin. The soap will melt and make the water soapy.
- When giving a bed bath, change the water in the basin when it becomes cold, soapy, or dirty.

Residents in long-term care centers should be encouraged to do as much of their personal care as possible. This promotes independence and allows the person to be in control of his activities of daily living.

Giving a Partial or Complete Bed Bath

A complete bed bath involves washing the entire body. A partial bed bath involves washing the face, hands, underarms, and the genital/perineal area. A complete bed bath is given to a patient who is unable to get out of bed, such as a patient who has just had surgery. A partial bed bath is given to a patient who does not need a complete bath, such as on the days between complete baths or in the morning or at bedtime.

When giving a bath, protect yourself from contact with blood, body fluids, or open skin by following Standard Precautions and the Bloodborne Pathogen Standard.

Text continued on p. 337

NOTES ON

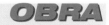 **Culture**

People from some cultures may not be comfortable with a caregiver of the opposite sex helping them to bathe. Your charge nurse will give you direction on how to care for people with cultural beliefs different from your own.

OBRA

HOW & WHY

Linens are usually changed after completion of a bed bath. Bedmaking is covered in Chapter 14.

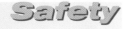

Procedure
COMPLETE BED BATH

EQUIPMENT

- Bath basin
- Soap and soap dish
- 3 or 4 bath towels
- 2 or 4 washcloths
- Bath blanket
- Linen bag
- Clean gown or clothes
- Personal care items such as lotion, powder, or deodorant
- Gloves

COMPLETE STANDARD BEGINNING STEPS (see inside front cover)

1 Fill bath basin ⅔ full of warm water (115° F) (Figure 15-2). Place on the overbed table next to the bed.

2 Raise the side rail on the opposite side of the bed, and raise the bed to a comfortable working height.

3 Place patient in the supine (lying on his back) position on the side of the bed nearest to you.

4 Put on gloves.

5 Offer the patient the bedpan or urinal.

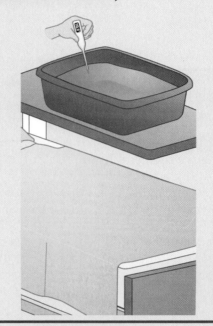

Figure 15-2   Step 1.

6 Cover the top sheet with a bath blanket. Ask the patient to hold the bath blanket in place, and remove the top sheet/blanket without disturbing the bath blanket (Figure 15-3).

7 Remove the patient's gown or pajamas.

8 Place a towel across the patient's chest.

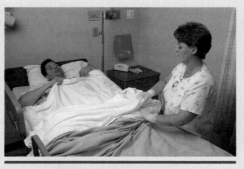

Figure 15-3   Step 6.

Procedure
COMPLETE BED BATH—cont'd

9   Wet the washcloth, wring it out, and fold it into a mitt/mitten (Figure 15-4).

    a.   Place your right hand under the lower right hand corner of the washcloth.

    b.   Secure the washcloth with your thumb, and wrap the washcloth around the back of your hand.

    c.   Fold the washcloth over the palm of your hand, and secure with your thumb. There will now be 2 layers of washcloth over the palm of your hand and under your thumb.

    d.   Fold the washcloth down over the tips of your covered fingers, and tuck the top edge under the lower edge of the washcloth.

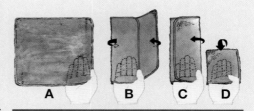

***Figure* 15-4**   Step 9.

10   Using one corner of the mitt/mitten, wash the eyes starting at the inner corner of the eyes and wiping out (Figure 15-5). USE A DIFFERENT CORNER OF THE MITT/MITTEN FOR EACH EYE. This prevents spreading germs from one eye to the other if the patient has an eye infection.

11   Wash, rinse, and dry the face and ears. Use soap on the face only if the patient requests it.

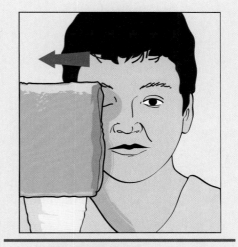

***Figure* 15-5**   Step 10.

12   Wash, rinse, and dry the neck (Figure 15-6).

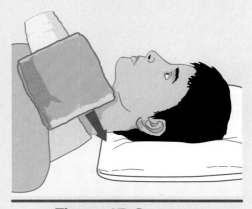

***Figure* 15-6**   Step 12.

Continued

Procedure
COMPLETE BED BATH—cont'd

13 Expose the arm on the far side of the bed, and place a bath towel under the arm up to the shoulder.

14 If the patient is able to, place the basin of water on the bed and place the patient's hand in the basin.

15 Wash and rinse the hand, arm, underarm, and shoulder on the far side of the bed (Figure 15-7).

16 Remove the basin of water, and dry the hand, arm, underarm, and shoulder on the far side of the bed.

17 Repeat steps 13 to 16 with the arm nearest to you.

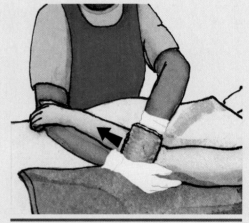

Figure 15-7 Step 15.

18 Place a towel across the chest and fold the bath blanket down to the abdomen (Figure 15-8).

19 Wash, rinse, and dry the chest and under the breasts, keeping the patient covered for privacy and warmth.

20 Keep the towel over the chest, and fold the bath blanket down to the pubic area.

21 Wash, rinse, and dry the abdomen.

22 Remove towel, and cover the patient with the bath blanket.

23 Raise the side rail on the side of the bed nearest to you for safety.

24 Change the water in the bath basin, put the dirty washcloth and towel in the linen bag, and obtain a clean washcloth.

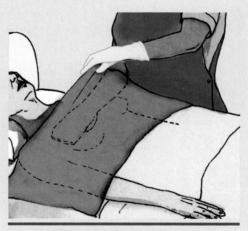

Figure 15-8 Step 18.

Procedure
COMPLETE BED BATH—cont'd

25 Lower the side rail on the side of the bed closest to you.

26 Expose the leg on the far side of the bed, bend the knee, and place a towel under the leg from the foot to the hip. If possible, place the foot in the basin of water (Figure 15-9).

27 Wash, rinse, and dry the foot and leg.

28 Repeat steps 26 and 27 with the leg on the near side of the bed.

29 Raise the side rail on the side of the bed nearest to you for safety.

30 Change the water in the bath basin. Put the dirty washcloth and towel in the linen bag, and obtain a clean washcloth.

31 Lower the side rail on the side of the bed closest to you.

32 Assist the patient to turn onto his side with his back toward you.

33 Fold the bath blanket over the patient's side to expose his back and buttocks.

34 Place a clean towel parallel to the patient's back from his shoulders to his hips (Figure 15-10).

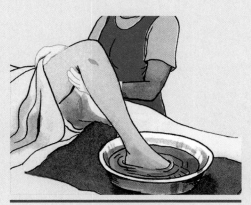

Figure 15-9   Step 26.

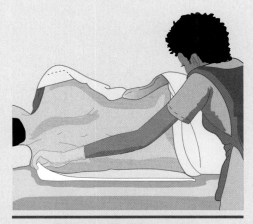

Figure 15-10   Step 34.

Continued

Procedure
COMPLETE BED BATH—cont'd

35 Wash, rinse, and dry the back and buttocks (Figure 15-11).

36 Turn the patient onto his back, and place a towel under his buttocks.

37 If the patient is able, give him a clean washcloth, soap, and towel to wash the perineal area. If the patient is unable to assist, provide perineal care as outlined in this chapter.

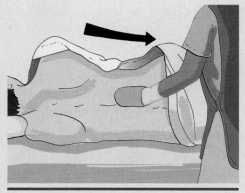

Figure **15-11** Step 35.

38 Apply lotion, deodorant, or powder as desired by the patient. When applying powder, sprinkle a small amount of the powder into the palm of your hand away from the patient. Apply a thin layer of powder to the patient's skin (Figure 15-12). NEVER shake the powder directly onto the patient's skin. Breathing in the powder can cause lung irritation.

39 Put a clean gown or clothing on the patient without exposing him (Chapter 18).

40 Return the bed to the lowest position, and put the side rails down as ordered. Make sure the patient's signal light is where the patient can reach it.

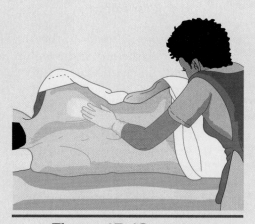

Figure **15-12** Step 38.

41 Remove, clean, and store equipment according to facility policy.

42 Remove your gloves and wash your hands.

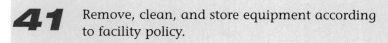

◆ **COMPLETE STANDARD ENDING STEPS (see inside front cover)**

Procedure
PARTIAL BED BATH

EQUIPMENT

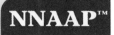

- Bath basin
- Soap and soap dish
- 3 or 4 bath towels
- 3 or 4 washcloths
- Bath blanket
- Linen bag
- Clean gown or clothes
- Personal care items such as lotion, powder, or deodorant
- Gloves

◆ **COMPLETE STANDARD BEGINNING STEPS (see inside front cover)**

1 Fill bath basin ⅔ full of warm water (115° F).

2 Raise the bed to a comfortable working height, and raise the side rail on the opposite side of the bed (Figure 15-13).

3 Place patient in the supine position on the side of the bed nearest to you.

4 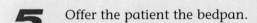 Put on gloves.

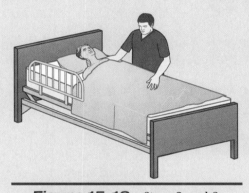

***Figure* 15-13**　Steps 2 and 3.

5 Offer the patient the bedpan.

6 Cover the top sheet with a bath blanket. Ask the patient to hold the bath blanket in place, and remove the top sheet/blanket without disturbing the bath blanket.

7 Remove the patient's gown or pajamas.

8 Place a towel across the patient's chest (Figure 15-14).

9 Wet washcloth, wring out, and fold into a mitt/mitten.

10 Using one corner of the mitt/mitten, wash the eyes starting at the inner corner of the eyes and wiping out. USE A DIFFERENT CORNER OF THE MITT/MITTEN FOR EACH EYE.

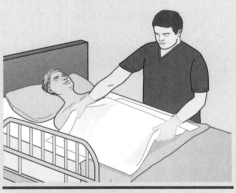

***Figure* 15-14**　Step 8.

11 Wash, rinse, and dry the face and ears. Use soap on the face only if the patient requests it.

Continued

Procedure
PARTIAL BED BATH—cont'd

12 Expose the arm on the far side of the bed, and place a bath towel under the arm up to the shoulder.

13 If the patient is able to, place the basin of water on the bed and place the patient's hand in the basin (Figure 15-15).

14 Wash and rinse the hand and underarm (axilla) on the far side of the bed.

15 Remove the basin of water, and dry hand and underarm (axilla) on the far side of the bed.

16 Repeat steps 12 to 15 with the hand and underarm (axilla) nearest to you.

17 Raise the side rail on the side of the bed nearest to you for safety.

18 Change the water in the bath basin, put the dirty washcloth and towel in the linen bag, and obtain a clean washcloth (Figure 15-16).

19 Lower the side rail on the side of the bed closest to you.

20 Place a towel under the patient's buttocks.

21 If the patient is able, provide him with a clean washcloth, soap, and towel to wash the perineal area. If the patient is unable to assist, provide perineal care as outlined in this chapter.

22 Apply lotion, deodorant, or powder as desired by the patient.

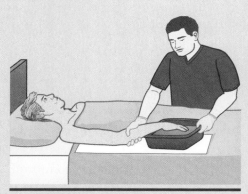

Figure 15-15 Step 13.

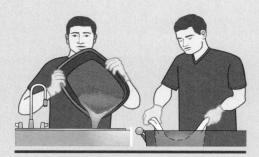

Figure 15-16 Step 18.

Procedure
PARTIAL BED BATH—cont'd

23 Put a clean gown or clothing on the patient without exposing him (Figure 15-17).

24 Return the bed to the lowest position, and put the side rails down as ordered. Make sure the patient's signal light is where the patient can reach it.

25 Remove, clean, and store equipment according to facility policy.

26 Remove your gloves and wash your hands.

◆ **COMPLETE STANDARD ENDING STEPS (see inside front cover)**

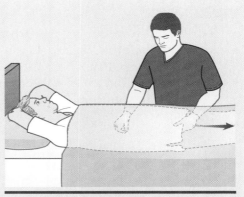

***Figure* 15-17** Step 23.

Giving a Tub Bath

A tub bath is more commonly given in a long-term care center. A tub bath may provide a greater sense of relaxation than a shower and may be preferred by some patients.

Fill the tub with enough water to cleanse the patient, usually mid-chest level. You will need to know how to operate the tub in your facility. Most tubs are equipped with whirlpool jets. Many tubs have a built-in thermometer so that you can check the temperature of the water. A water temperature of 105° F is safe and comfortable for most patients. Let patients feel the temperature of the water and adjust it according to their preference.

Most patients stay in the tub for 10 to 15 minutes. A longer period of time allows the water to cool, and the patient may become chilled.

Never leave a patient unattended in the tub!

NOTES ON
❄ *Older Adults*

The elderly may have a decreased sensation of hot or cold and are more prone to burns. Check the temperature of the water carefully to make sure it is not too hot.

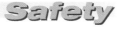

Procedure
GIVING A TUB BATH

EQUIPMENT

- 3 or 4 bath towels
- 3 or 4 washcloths
- Soap and soap dish
- Tub chair if used
- Disinfecting solution and cloth

- Bathmat or additional bath towel
- Linen bag
- Clean gown or clothes
- Personal care items such as lotion, powder, or deodorant
- Gloves

◆ **COMPLETE STANDARD BEGINNING STEPS (see inside front cover)**

1 Clean the bathtub and tub chair according to facility policy using disinfectant. Rinse well (Figure 15-18).

2 Place a bathmat or towel on the floor next to the tub.

3 Assist the patient to the tub room.

4 Put on gloves.

5 Assist the patient with using the bathroom if needed.

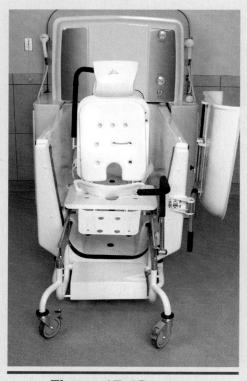

Figure **15-18**   Step 1.

Procedure
GIVING A TUB BATH—cont'd

6 Fill the tub at least ½ full with warm water (105° F), and check the temperature of the water with the thermometer or on the inside of your arm (Figure 15-19).

7 Assist the patient with undressing.

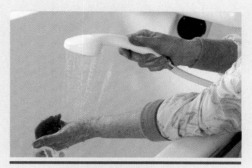
***Figure* 15-19** Step 6.

8 Assist the patient into the tub according to facility policy and procedures. Allow the patient to test the temperature of the water for comfort before placing him in the tub. Adjust the water temperature according to his preference (Figure 15-20).

9 Assist the patient with bathing as needed. If the patient is unable to assist, wet the washcloth, wring it out, and fold it into a mitt/mitten.

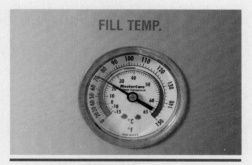
***Figure* 15-20** Step 8.

10 Using one corner of the mitt/mitten, wash the eyes, starting at the inner corner of the eyes and wiping out. USE A DIFFERENT CORNER OF THE MITT/MITTEN FOR EACH EYE.

11 Wash and rinse the face, neck, chest, arms, hands, abdomen, and back. Use soap on the face only if the patient requests it.

12 Wash and rinse legs and feet. Discard the dirty washcloth into a linen bag.

13 If desired, a shampoo may be given at this time. Cover the head with a clean dry towel (Chapter 17) (Figure 15-21).

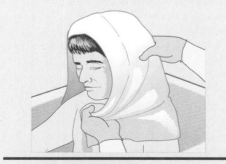
***Figure* 15-21** Step 13.

Continued

Procedure

GIVING A TUB BATH—cont'd

14 Assist the patient with turning slightly to one side. Wash and rinse perineal area, and put the washcloth into the linen bag.

15 Assist the patient out of the tub, and cover with a bath blanket.

16 Drain the tub.

17 Uncover the patient one area at a time, and dry the skin thoroughly.

18 Apply lotion, powder, or deodorant as desired.

19 Assist the patient with dressing in a clean gown or clothing (Figure 15-22).

20 Remove your gloves and wash your hands.

21 Assist the patient back to his room

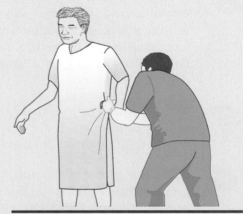

Figure 15-22 Step 19.

22 Return to the tub room, remove soiled articles and linens, and clean the tub with a disinfecting solution; rinse well (Figure 15-23).

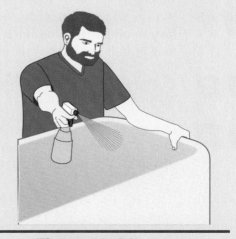

Figure 15-23 Step 22.

Giving a Shower

A shower may be preferred by some patients because of personal preference or difficulty in getting in and out of the tub. Most facility showers will be equipped with a shower chair and a long hose on the shower nozzle (Figure 15-24).

When placing patients in the shower stall, make sure that they are facing the side wall or the door of the shower. This allows you to help patients if they lean forward.   *Safety*

When using a shower chair with wheels, always lock the wheels when the chair is in the shower stall. Many showers have a built-in thermometer so that you can check the temperature of the water. A water temperature of 105° F is safe and comfortable for most patients. Let patients feel the temperature of the water and adjust it according to their preference.

The elderly may have a decreased sensation of hot or cold and can get burned. Check the temperature of the water carefully to make sure it is not too hot.   *Safety*

Unless patients are independent in their care, never leave them unattended in the shower!   *Safety*

When giving a tub or shower bath, remember to clean the tub and/or chair with the disinfectant provided by your facility. This will prevent spreading germs from one patient to another. It is important to follow the manufacturer's direction when using disinfectants. Most chemicals will damage the skin, and equipment should rinsed well before using.   *Safety*

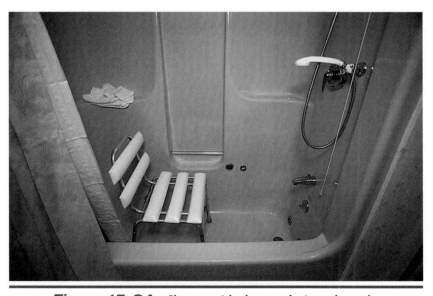

***Figure* 15-24**   Shower with shower chair and nozzle.

Procedure
GIVING A SHOWER

EQUIPMENT

- 3 or 4 bath towels
- 3 or 4 washcloths
- Soap and soap dish
- Shower chair if used
- Disinfecting solution and cloth
- Bathmat or additional bath towel

- Bath blanket
- Linen bag
- Clean gown or clothes
- Personal care items such as lotion, powder, or deodorant
- Gloves

◆ **COMPLETE STANDARD BEGINNING STEPS (see inside front cover)**

1 Clean the shower chair according to facility policy using disinfectant; rinse well.

2 Place a bathmat or towel on the floor next to the shower.

3 Assist the patient to the shower room.

4 Put on gloves.

5 Assist him with using the bathroom if needed.

6 Assist the patient with undressing.

7 Assist the patient into the shower chair according to facility policy and procedures (Figure 15-25). Allow the patient to test the temperature of the water for comfort before placing him in the shower. Adjust the water temperature according to his preference.

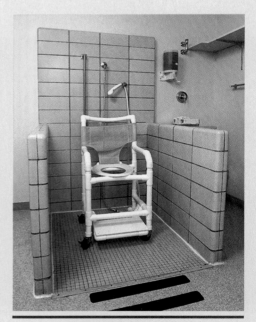

***Figure* 15-25**   Step 7.

Procedure
GIVING A SHOWER—cont'd

8 Assist the patient with bathing as needed. Keeping the spray of the water on the patient will help him to stay warm (Figure 15-26).

9 If the patient is unable to assist, wet washcloth, wring out, and fold into a mitt/mitten.

10 Using one corner of the mitt/mitten, wash the eyes, starting at the inner corner of the eyes and wiping out. USE A DIFFERENT CORNER OF THE MITT/MITTEN FOR EACH EYE.

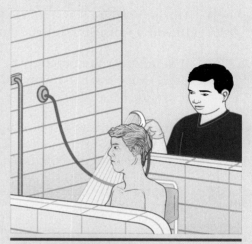

Figure 15-26 Step 8.

11 Wash and rinse the face, neck, chest, arms, hands, abdomen, and back (Figure 15-27). Use soap on the face only if the patient requests it.

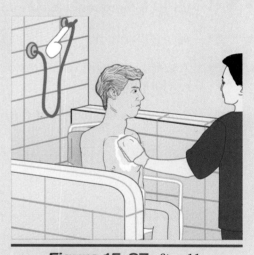

Figure 15-27 Step 11.

Continued

Procedure

GIVING A SHOWER—cont'd

12 Wash and rinse legs and feet (Figure 15-28). Put the dirty washcloth into a linen bag.

13 If desired, a shampoo may be given at this time. Cover the head with a clean dry towel (Chapter 17).

14 Assist the patient with turning slightly to one side. Wash and rinse perineal area, and put the dirty washcloth into the linen bag.

15 Assist the patient out of the shower, and cover with a bath blanket.

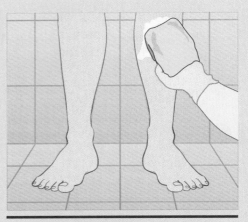

Figure 15-28   Step 12.

16 Uncover the patient one area at a time, and dry the skin thoroughly (Figure 15-29).

17 Apply lotion, powder, or deodorant as desired.

18 Assist the patient with dressing in a clean gown or clothing.

19 Remove your gloves and wash your hands.

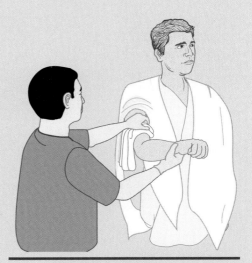

Figure 15-29   Step 16.

Procedure

GIVING A SHOWER—cont'd

19 Assist the patient back to his room (Figure 15-30).

20 Return to the shower room, remove soiled articles and linens, and clean the shower chair with a disinfecting solution; rinse well.

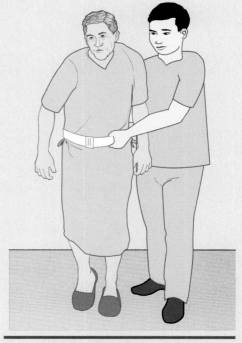

***Figure* 15-30**   Step 19.

◆ **COMPLETE STANDARD ENDING STEPS (see inside front cover)**

How to Perform Perineal Care

Perineal care, also called "pericare," may be a part of the bathing procedure or a separate procedure. Pericare involves cleaning the genitals and the anal area.

The purposes of pericare include:
- Preventing skin breakdown in the perineal area
- Preventing itching, burning, and odor
- Preventing infections
- Cleaning the area for a patient who is unable to do so for himself

Patients who are **continent**, or in control of the bladder and bowel functions, should have pericare daily with their morning grooming. If a patient is **incontinent** or not in control of bowel or bladder functions, pericare should be performed after each voiding or stool. If a patient has an indwelling catheter, pericare should be performed each morning with grooming and after each bowel movement.

When assisting with or performing pericare, you should observe your patient for discharge, odors, or signs of skin breakdown such as redness, irritation, or rashes.

Some facilities use special products when performing pericare. Other facilities instruct you to use soap and warm water. If you use a special product for pericare, make sure to read the manufacturer's instructions before using it.

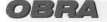

Residents of long-term care centers have the right to make decisions regarding their care and treatment. Allow residents to decide if they prefer a tub bath or a shower and if they want to bathe in the morning or before bedtime. This information should be included in the residents' care plan. Remember to provide privacy when giving personal care by closing doors and privacy curtains.

Procedure
PERINEAL CARE

EQUIPMENT

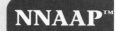

- Basin of warm water
- Washcloths (2)
- Bed protector
- Bedpan

- Towel
- Bath blanket
- Soap and soap dish or pericare product
- Gloves

◆ **COMPLETE STANDARD BEGINNING STEPS (see inside front cover)**

1 Put on gloves.

2 Assist the patient with using the bedpan or urinal if needed.

3 Assist the patient to the supine or side-lying position.

4 Place the bed protector under the patient's hips.

5 Cover the patient with the bath blanket (Figure 15-31).

   a. Position the bath blanket like a diamond with a corner at the patient's head and a corner at the feet.

   b. Wrap the blanket around the patient's legs by bringing one corner under each leg and over the top. Tuck one corner under each hip.

6 Expose the perineal area.

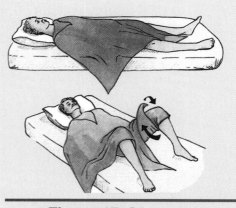

Figure 15-31 Step 5.

Continued

Procedure
PERINEAL CARE—cont'd

7 Male pericare

    a. Using a circular motion, gently wash the penis by lifting it and cleaning from the tip downward (Figure 15-32).

    b. Rinse and dry the penis.

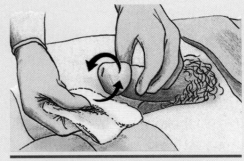

***Figure* 15-32** Step 7a.

    c. If the patient is uncircumcised, pull back the foreskin, wash, rinse, and dry the penis. Then pull the skin over the end of the penis (Figure 15-33).

    d. Wash, rinse, and dry the scrotum.

    e. Wash, rinse, and dry the skin area between the legs.

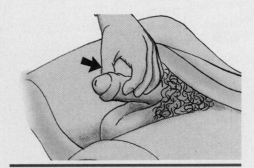

***Figure* 15-33** Step 7c.

    f. Turn the patient onto his side. Wash, rinse, and dry the anal area, washing from front to back (Figure 15-34).

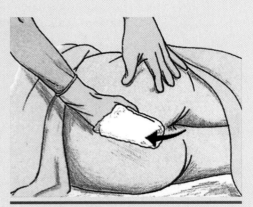

***Figure* 15-34** Step 7f.

Procedure
PERINEAL CARE—cont'd

8   Female pericare

     a.   Using a clean area of the washcloth for each wipe of the peri area, gently open all skin folds and wash the inner area from front to back (Figure 15-35).

     b.   Wash and rinse the inner labia from front to back.

     c.   Wash and rinse the outer skin folds from front to back.

     d.   Wash the inner legs and outer perineal area along the outside of the labia.

     e.   Turn the patient onto her side; wash and rinse the anal area, washing from front to back.

     f.   Dry the perineal area.

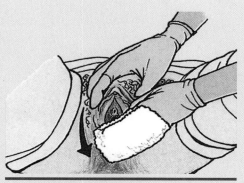

***Figure* 15-35**   Step 8a.

9   Remove the bed protector and the bath blanket.

10   Remove, clean, and store equipment according to facility policy.

11   Remove your gloves and wash your hands.

12   Make the patient comfortable, with the signal light within reach.

◆ **COMPLETE STANDARD ENDING STEPS (see inside front cover)**

CHAPTER REVIEW

1. List the 4 things accomplished by bathing.

2. What body parts are washed in a partial bed bath?

3. What is the difference between a patient who is continent and one who is incontinent?

Circle the one BEST response.

4. What water temperature should be used for a tub bath or shower?
   a. 105° F
   b. 110° F
   c. 115° F
   d. 120° F

5. If a patient has an indwelling catheter, when should pericare be performed?
   a. Once a day with morning grooming
   b. After each voiding or stool
   c. Each morning with grooming and after each bowel movement (BM)
   d. Each morning and at bedtime

Fill in the blanks with the correct term related to the health care system.

6. Soap left on the skin is _____ and can cause _____.

Answers are on page 707.

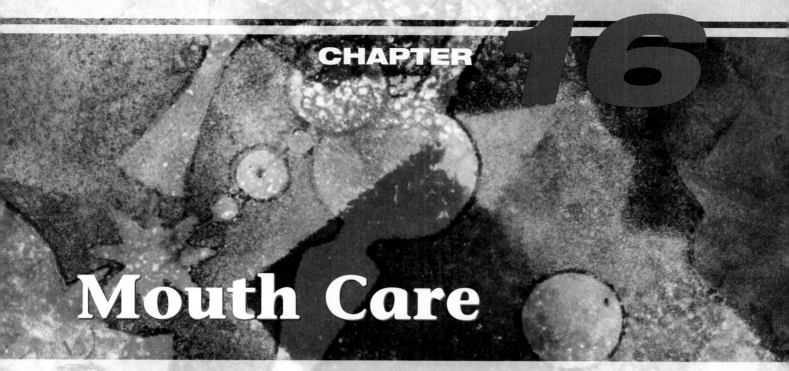

CHAPTER 16

Mouth Care

What you will learn

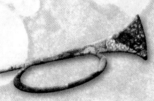

- General guidelines for mouth care
- Assisting with mouth care
- Denture care
- Mouth care for the unconscious patient

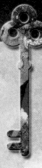

KEY TERMS

Halitosis Bad breath

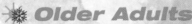

NOTES ON
✳ *Older Adults*

The older person makes less saliva and may have a very dry mouth. The older person may need oral care more often than 2 times a day.

NOTES ON
✳ *Children*

Young children will need assistance with oral care. This is a good chance for the parents to help in caring for their child. You may need to show the parents how to do oral care the correct way.

NOTES ON
☯ *Culture*

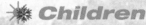

Although good oral care is important to the physical health of all people, not all cultures feel that fresh breath is important. It is important to respect the beliefs and values of all patients.

OBRA

Safety

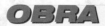

General Guidelines for Mouth Care

A clean mouth is very important to the physical and mental well-being of the patient. Mouth care is also called oral care or oral hygiene. Mouth care removes food particles, stimulates circulation to the gums, and prevents **halitosis** (bad breath). Mouth care also helps to prevent cavities in the teeth and mouth infections. People with poor oral hygiene may have a bad taste in the mouth that can affect their appetite. Some medications can also cause an unpleasant taste in the mouth. A patient who is unconscious or unable to take food or fluids by mouth may have a very dry mouth.

Mouth care for the conscious patient should be provided on a regular basis, at least 2 times a day. Mouth care is usually given in the early morning before breakfast and before bedtime. Most dentists recommend brushing the teeth after each meal. Some patients may need mouth care more often. Your charge nurse will instruct you if your patient has special needs.

When helping the patient with his mouth care, you should look for signs of problems such as:

- Loose or broken teeth
- Red or swollen gums
- Dry, cracked, or coated tongue
- Sores or white patches in the mouth or on the tongue
- Black or brown areas on the teeth, which could be signs of tooth decay
- Poorly fitting dentures
- Changes in eating habits, which could mean mouth pain

Report any problems to the charge nurse.

Residents of long-term care centers should continue to receive regular dental care to enhance their quality of life.

When assisting with mouth care, you can protect yourself by following Standards Precautions and the Bloodborne Pathogen Standard. While performing this procedure, you may have contact with blood, body fluids, or mucous membranes.

Procedure
ASSISTING WITH MOUTH CARE

EQUIPMENT

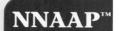

- Drinking glass
- Emesis basin or sink
- Water

- Toothbrush
- Hand towel
- Toothpaste

- Mouthwash
- Dental floss
- Gloves

◆ COMPLETE STANDARD BEGINNING STEPS (see inside front cover)

1 Assist the patient to the bathroom, or raise the head of the bed 45 to 90 degrees so that the patient is sitting upright.

2 Wet the toothbrush and apply toothpaste.

3 Put on gloves.

4 Instruct or help the patient to brush the gum line and then to brush the teeth up and down on both sides (Figure 16-1, *A*).

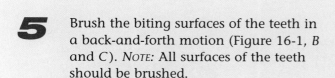

5 Brush the biting surfaces of the teeth in a back-and-forth motion (Figure 16-1, *B* and *C*). *NOTE:* All surfaces of the teeth should be brushed.

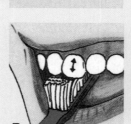
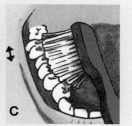

6 Gently brush the tongue (Figure 16-1, *D*).

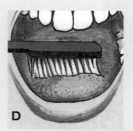

Figure 16-1 Steps 4, 5, and 6.

Continued

Procedure
ASSISTING WITH MOUTH CARE

7 Instruct or help the patient to rinse his mouth and spit the water into the emesis basin or the sink (Figure 16-2).

8 Obtain 12 to 16 inches of dental floss.

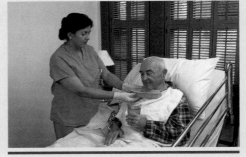

Figure 16-2   Step 7.

9 Loosely wrap the floss around the middle finger on each hand (Figure 16-3).

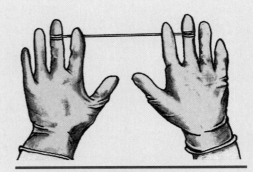

Figure 16-3   Step 9.

10 Using index fingers and thumbs, gently work the floss between each tooth, moving up to the gum line and back down to the tooth edge (Figure 16-4).

11 Dilute the mouthwash, ½ water and ½ mouthwash. Full-strength mouthwash has a strong taste and may sting the inside of the mouth.

12 Instruct or assist the patient to rinse his mouth with the mouthwash and spit it into the emesis basin or the sink. *NOTE:* Use of mouthwash does not replace brushing the teeth.

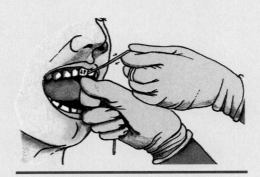

Figure 16-4   Step 10.

13 Assist the patient with wiping his face with the towel.

Procedure
ASSISTING WITH MOUTH CARE—cont'd

14 Assist the patient to a comfortable position with the signal light where he can reach it.

15 Remove your gloves and wash your hands.

◆ **COMPLETE STANDARD ENDING STEPS (see inside front cover)**

Denture Care

Patients who have dentures (false teeth) and who are weak or ill may need assistance with cleaning their dentures.

It is important to be very careful when handling your patient's dentures. Dentures are expensive, and if they are broken, the patient may be unable to eat a regular diet.

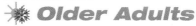

Using a paper towel or washcloth to grip the dentures will keep them from slipping out of your gloved hand. When dentures are not in the mouth, store them in cool water in a container marked with the patient's name. Some people prefer to soak their dentures in a cleaning solution. Using a cleaning solution does not replace the need to brush the dentures.

Cleaning or storing dentures in hot water can cause them to change shape or become warped.

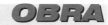

Dentures are cleaned so that they do not irritate the gums or cause the patient to have bad breath or an unpleasant taste in the mouth. Clean the dentures in the morning before breakfast and at bedtime. Some patients keep their dentures in their mouth while they sleep; others remove their dentures and soak them overnight.

NOTES ON
❋ *Older Adults*

Some people in long-term care leave their dentures out of their mouth during their hours of sleep.

Residents of long-term care centers have the right to receive courteous and dignified care. Residents' personal care items should be labeled with their name. Residents should be encouraged to be as independent as possible in their care. This promotes self-esteem and a sense of dignity for the person.

OBRA

Procedure
DENTURE CARE

EQUIPMENT

- Drinking glass
- Emesis basin or sink
- Water
- Toothbrush
- Hand towel
- Toothpaste
- Mouthwash
- Denture cup
- Gloves

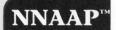

◆ **COMPLETE STANDARD BEGINNING STEPS (see inside front cover)**

1 Assist the patient to the bathroom, or raise the head of the bed 45 to 90 degrees so that the patient is sitting upright.

2 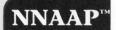 Put on gloves.

3 Ask the patient to remove his dentures.

4 If the patient is unable to remove his dentures, run your gloved finger along the upper gum as you gently push the upper edge of the denture forward and down. Remove lower denture by pushing forward and up.

5 Place dentures in a clean denture cup marked with the patient's name (Figure 16-5).

6 Dilute the mouthwash, ½ water and ½ mouthwash.

7 Instruct or assist the patient to rinse his mouth with the mouthwash and spit it into the emesis basin or the sink. If desired, the patient can gently brush his gums with toothpaste and a soft toothbrush or toothette (a small sponge attached to the end of a stick).

8 Wipe the mouth with a towel.

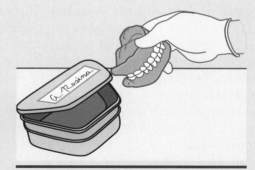

Figure 16-5 Step 5.

Procedure
DENTURE CARE—cont'd

9 Fill a clean sink with 3 to 4 inches of cool water, and place a clean washcloth on the bottom of the sink (Figure 16-6). (This will prevent the dentures from breaking if they are dropped.)

10 Wet the toothbrush and apply toothpaste.

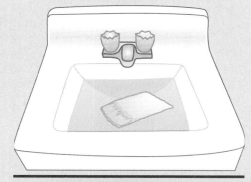

Figure 16-6 Step 9.

11 Thoroughly brush the dentures on all sides (Figure 16-7).

12 Rinse the dentures in cool running water, and place them in a clean denture cup. Rinsing or soaking the dentures in hot water can cause them to warp or to bend.

13 If the resident is going to wear the dentures, replace them in the mouth, upper dentures first.

14 If the resident is not going to wear the dentures, store the dentures in a clean denture cup filled with cool water and marked with the resident's name.

15 Remove, clean, and store equipment.

16 Assist the patient to a comfortable position with the signal light where the patient can reach it.

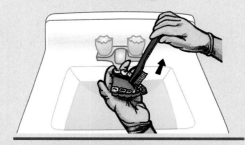

Figure 16-7 Step 11.

17 Remove your gloves and wash your hands.

◆ COMPLETE STANDARD ENDING STEPS **(see inside front cover)**

Mouth Care for the Unconscious Patient

A patient who is unconscious needs mouth care more frequently. The unconscious person frequently breathes only through the mouth, causing the mouth to become dry and crusty. These dry secretions can cause halitosis. The patient who is unable to take food or fluids by mouth is also at risk of developing a dry mouth. Mouth care should be given to the unconscious resident every 2 hours to keep the lining of the mouth moist.

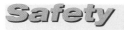

Unconscious residents should be turned onto their side so that they do not choke on the solution used to perform mouth care.

Procedure
MOUTH CARE FOR THE UNCONSCIOUS PATIENT

EQUIPMENT

- Drinking glass
- Emesis basin or sink
- Water
- Toothbrush
- Hand towel
- Mouthwash
- Lip balm
- Gloves

◆ **COMPLETE STANDARD BEGINNING STEPS (see inside front cover)**

1 Raise the bed to a comfortable working height.

2 Turn the patient onto her side facing you.

3 Lower the side rail.

4 Put on gloves.

5 Place a towel under the patient's head.

6 Place the emesis basin under the patient's mouth and chin (Figure 16-8).

7 Dilute the mouthwash, ½ water and ½ mouthwash.

8 Wet the toothbrush with the mouthwash-water solution.

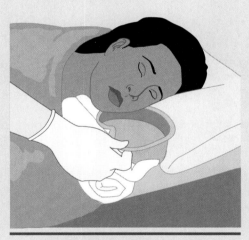

Figure 16-8 Step 6.

Continued

Procedure
MOUTH CARE FOR THE UNCONSCIOUS PATIENT—cont'd

9 Brush the gum line, and then brush the teeth up and down on both sides (Figure 16-9).

10 Brush the biting surfaces of the teeth in a back-and forth-motion. *NOTE:* All surfaces of the teeth should be brushed.

11 Gently brush the tongue.

12 Wipe the mouth and lips with the towel.

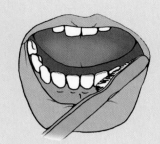
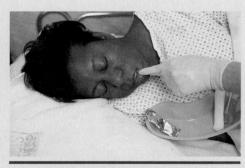

Figure **16-9**   Step 9.

13 Apply lip balm to the lips (Figure 16-10).

14 Remove, clean, and store equipment.

15 Assist the patient to a comfortable position with the signal light where the patient can reach it.

16 Remove your gloves and wash your hands.

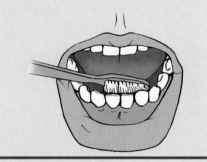

Figure **16-10**   Step 13.

◆ **COMPLETE STANDARD ENDING STEPS (see inside front cover)**

CHAPTER REVIEW

1. Why is mouth care done?

2. When should the conscious resident be provided with mouth care?

3. List 3 things the certified nursing assistant (CNA) should look for when providing mouth care.

Circle the one BEST response.

4. How should dentures be stored when they are not in the mouth?
   a. In a glass on the resident's sink
   b. In a box in the nightstand
   c. Wrapped in a washcloth in the overbed table
   d. In cool water in a denture cup

5. How often does the unconscious resident need mouth care?
   a. Every 1 hour
   b. Every 2 hours
   c. Every 3 hours
   d. Every 4 hours

Mark T for true or F for false.

6. _____ Soaking the dentures in a cleaning solution replaces the need to brush the dentures.

Answers are on pages 707 to 708.

CHAPTER 17

Personal Care and Comfort Measures

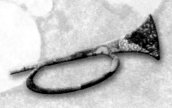

What you will learn

- The basics of hair care
- How to give a shampoo
- How to shave a person
- Nail and foot care
- Care of eyeglasses and hearing aids

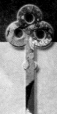

KEY TERMS

Lice Tiny white insects that attach to the hair strands
Podiatrist Foot doctor

Hair Care

We all like to look our best. Brushing and combing the hair not only helps the patient to look better, but it also cleans the hair of dirt particles, prevents tangling of the hair, and stimulates circulation of the scalp. Illness, malnutrition, and stress can affect the condition of the hair. Some medications, such as those used to treat cancer, can cause hair loss.

Hair should be combed or brushed each morning and throughout the day as needed to maintain a neat appearance. Hair should be washed at least weekly. Younger patients may need to have their hair washed every day because their hair is oilier.

Some patients are able to comb or brush their own hair. This provides good exercise to the patients' arms and encourages them to be more independent. Other patients may need total assistance with their hair care.

When providing hair care, use only the patient's own supplies. Never borrow a comb or a brush from another patient; this can spread germs and infections!

When providing hair care, you should look for bumps, cuts, sores, or swollen areas. Small white spots on the hair that do not brush or comb off may be head **lice**. Report your observations to the charge nurse.

NOTES ON
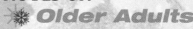
Older Adults

In long-term care centers, female residents may go to the beauty shop each week to have their hair shampooed and styled. You should not wash the hair of the resident who goes to the beauty shop unless instructed to by the charge nurse.

NOTES ON
☯ Culture

When caring for people from a different culture, ask them about their method of hair care or any cultural restrictions.

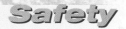

HOW & WHY
Nursing staff are not permitted to cut the hair of their patients.

Procedure
COMBING AND BRUSHING THE HAIR

EQUIPMENT

- Patient's comb or brush
- Towel
- Mirror, if available
- Gloves, if needed

◆ **COMPLETE STANDARD BEGINNING STEPS (see inside front cover)**

1 Assist the patient to a sitting position by raising the head of the bed 45 to 90 degrees, or assist the patient with sitting in a chair at the bedside.

2 Place the towel under the patient's head if she is in bed or around her shoulders if she is sitting in the chair (Figure 17-1).

3 Remove any eyeglass or hearing aids.

4 If the patient has sores or open areas on the scalp, put on gloves.

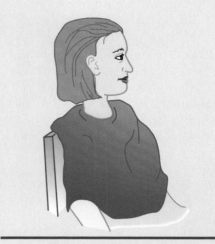

***Figure* 17-1** Step 2.

5 Brush or comb the hair in downward strokes (Figure 17-2).

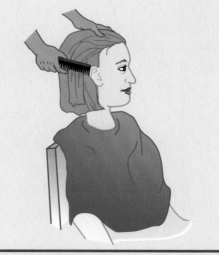

***Figure* 17-2** Step 5.

Procedure
COMBING AND BRUSHING THE HAIR—cont'd

6   To remove tangles, start at the bottom of the hair and work toward the scalp.

7   Style the hair according to the patient's request (Figure 17-3).

8   Replace any eyeglasses or hearing aids.

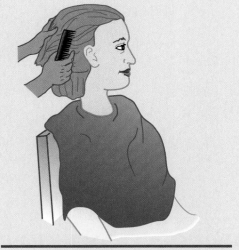

Figure 17-3   Step 7.

9   Allow the resident to view herself in the mirror if one is available (Figure 17-4).

10   Assist the resident to a comfortable position with the signal light where the patient can reach it.

11   Remove gloves if used, and wash your hands.

12   Remove, clean, and store equipment according to facility policy.

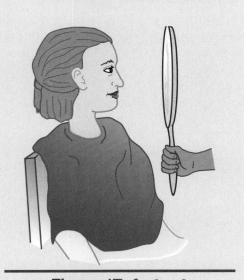

Figure 17-4   Step 9.

◆ **COMPLETE STANDARD ENDING STEPS (see inside front cover)**

Giving a Shampoo

If a patient is in the hospital for a short stay, it may not be necessary to shampoo the hair. Patients who are admitted for a longer stay or those who are in nursing homes need to have their hair shampooed on a regular basis. Older patients usually need their hair washed 1 to 2 times a week when they are bathed. Younger patients may need both bathing and shampooing of the hair every day because the hair is oilier.

It is easiest to shampoo the hair while bathing the patient in the tub or shower.

Safety
Do not use the *fingernails* when washing the hair. This can scratch the scalp. Be careful not to allow the shampoo to run into the patient's eyes.

Safety
Be careful when using a hairdryer in a shower or tub room. Never stand in water when using an electric appliance or use an electric hair dryer on a person who is in water.

Procedure
GIVING A SHAMPOO IN THE TUB OR SHOWER

EQUIPMENT

- **Bath towels (2)**
- **Washcloth**
- **Shampoo**
- **Conditioner (optional)**
- **Patient's comb or brush**
- **Gloves, if needed**

◆ **COMPLETE STANDARD BEGINNING STEPS (see inside front cover)**

1 Assist the patient to the tub or shower room.

2 Adjust the water temperature to 105° F (Figure 17-5).

3 Allow the patient to check the temperature of the water.

4 If giving a shampoo during a bath, the certified nursing assistant (CNA) would have gloves on. For a shampoo not given with a bath, put on gloves if the patient has sores or open areas on the scalp.

5 Assist the patient with undressing and help her into the tub or shower according to the procedure in Chapter 15.

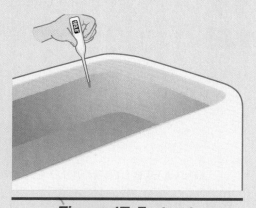
Figure 17-5 Step 2.

Procedure

GIVING A SHAMPOO IN THE TUB OR SHOWER—cont'd

6 Ask the patient to hold a clean folded wash-cloth over her eyes (Figure 17-6).

7 Ask the patient to tilt her head back slightly if she is able to.

8 Using the nozzle, thoroughly wet the patient's hair.

9 Apply a small amount of shampoo, and wash the hair thoroughly with the tips of the fingers.

10 Rinse the hair thoroughly from front to back using the nozzle.

11 Apply conditioner if desired by the patient, and rinse thoroughly from front to back.

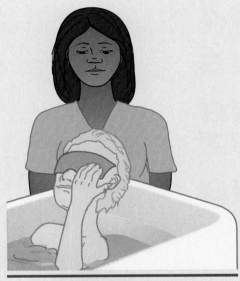

Figure 17-6   Step 6.

12 Towel dry the hair, and place a clean dry towel over the patient's head to keep her warm (Figure 17-7).

13 When finished with bathing, assist the patient from the tub or shower as indicated in Chapter 15.

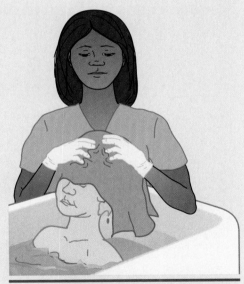

Figure 17-7   Step 12.

Continued

Procedure

GIVING A SHAMPOO IN THE TUB OR SHOWER—cont'd

14 Finish towel drying the hair. If desired, the hair can be dried using a hair dryer (Figure 17-8).

15 Comb or brush the hair as desired by the patient.

16 Remove gloves if used, and wash your hands.

17 Remove, clean, and store equipment according to facility policy.

18 Assist the patient back to her room.

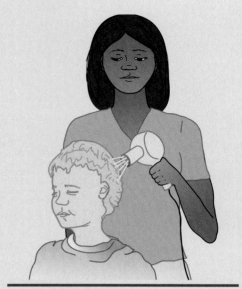

Figure 17-8   Step 14.

◆ COMPLETE STANDARD ENDING STEPS **(see inside front cover)**

Bed or Stretcher Shampoo

If a patient is on bedrest and cannot move into the tub or shower, the hair can be washed while the patient is in bed or on a stretcher.

To shampoo the hair while the person is on a stretcher, place the stretcher in front of the sink. Place a towel under the patient's neck over the edge of the sink. Assist the patient with moving toward the head of the stretcher until the head is tilted over the sink.

Use a small pitcher, cup, or hand-held nozzle to wet and rinse the hair (Figure 17-9).

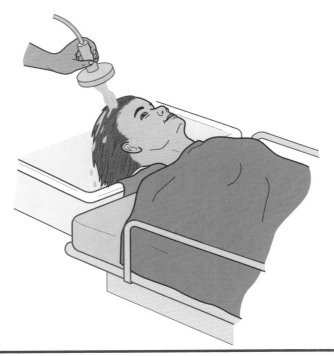

Figure 17-9   Shampooing the hair while the person is on a stretcher.

To shampoo the hair while a person is in bed, a special bed shampoo tray is used. There are many different styles and models of shampoo trays. Place the shampoo tray under the patient's head. The tray is attached to a drainage tube that drains the water from the tray into a bucket that is next to the bed. Use a small pitcher or cup to wet and rinse the hair. It is hard to keep the water from running out along the patient's neck and getting the bed wet during this procedure. If necessary, change the linens on the bed after giving a bed shampoo. A bed shampoo is usually given at the same time as a complete bed bath (Figure 17-10).

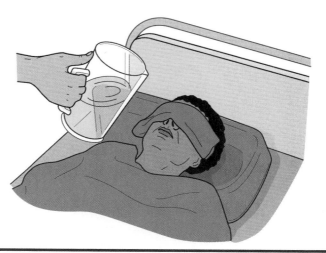

Figure 17-10 Shampooing the hair while the person is in bed with a bed shampoo tray.

Shaving

Shaving should be done according to your facility's policy. For male patients, shaving is a part of their normal daily hygiene and may be done before or after the bath. Many patients shave on days that they are not bathing. If a patient is able to shave himself, he should be encouraged to do so. Shaving provides good exercise for the arms. If the patients have their own electric razors, they can use them. Many electric razors are now cordless and are only plugged into an electrical outlet to recharge them.

Some female patients shave parts of their body as well. Women shave the legs, underarms, and facial hairs. Legs and underarms are usually shaved during or after bathing or showering.

NOTES ON Culture

Shaving practices vary among different cultures. It is important to respect your patient's wishes regarding shaving or not shaving. Never shave a beard or mustache without the person's permission.

Some facilities do not permit the use of safety or disposable razors and require that all patients be shaved with an electric razor. Always use an electric razor when shaving a confused person.

Safety

Never use an electric razor on a patient who is receiving oxygen as this could present a fire hazard.

Safety

Dispose of the disposable razors in a sharps container. Protect yourself from exposure to blood by following Standard Precautions and the Bloodborne Pathogen Standard.

Safety

To prevent the spread of germs or infections, the head of an electric razor should be cleaned between patients. Follow your facility's policy for cleaning the electric razor. Many facilities clean the heads of the electric razor with an alcohol wipe. Make sure that the razor is unplugged before cleaning it.

Safety

Procedure

SHAVING WITH A SAFETY OR DISPOSABLE RAZOR

EQUIPMENT

- Basin or sink with warm water
- Razor
- Shaving cream
- Washcloth

- Towel
- Mirror
- After-shave lotion, if desired
- Gloves

◆ **COMPLETE STANDARD BEGINNING STEPS (see inside front cover)**

1 Assist the patient to a sitting position by raising the head of the bed 45 to 90 degrees or assist the patient with sitting in a chair at the bedside or at the sink.

2 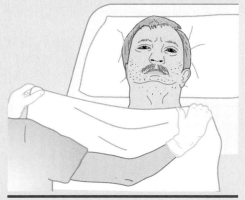 Put on gloves.

3 If the patient has dentures, make sure they are in his mouth.

4 Spread a towel across the patient's chest under his chin (Figure 17-11).

5 If the patient is able to shave himself, allow him to complete the procedure. If the patient requires your assistance, proceed with steps 5 to 17.

Figure 17-11 Step 4.

6 Using the washcloth, thoroughly wet the face with warm water (Figure 17-12).

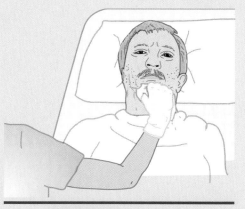

Figure 17-12 Step 6.

Procedure
SHAVING WITH A SAFETY OR DISPOSABLE RAZOR—cont'd

7 Apply shaving cream ⅛-inch thick to the face.

8 Leave the lather in place 15 to 30 seconds to help soften the beard.

9 Pull the skin tight with the fingers of one hand. With the other hand, hold the razor at a 45-degree angle to the patient's face and shave in the direction that the hair grows. Shave down on the face and up on the neck (Figure 17-13).

10 Continue shaving over the chin and neck using short, firm strokes.

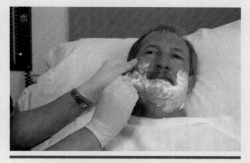

Figure 17-13 Step 9.

11 Rinse the razor often in the water (Figure 17-14).

12 When finished, rinse the face with clean warm water.

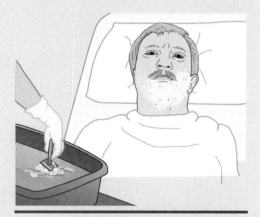

Figure 17-14 Step 11.

Continued

Procedure

SHAVING WITH A SAFETY OR DISPOSABLE RAZOR—cont'd

13 Pat the face dry with a towel (Figure 17-15).

14 Apply after-shave lotion if the patient requests it.

15 Make the patient comfortable with the signal light where the patient can reach it.

16 Remove your gloves and wash your hands.

17 Remove, clean, and store equipment according to facility policy. Dispose of razors in a sharps container.

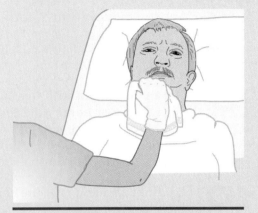

Figure 17-15   Step 13.

 COMPLETE STANDARD ENDING STEPS (see inside front cover)

Procedure
SHAVING WITH AN ELECTRIC RAZOR

EQUIPMENT

- Electric Razor (Figure 17-16)
- Towel
- Mirror
- Pre-shave and after-shave lotion, if desired

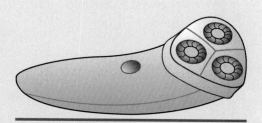

Figure 17-16   Electric razor.

◆ **COMPLETE STANDARD BEGINNING STEPS (see inside front cover)**

1 Assist the patient to a sitting position by raising the head of the bed 45 to 90 degrees, or assist the patient with sitting in a chair at the bedside or at the sink.

2 If the patient has dentures, make sure they are in his mouth (Figure 17-17).

3 Spread a towel across the patient's chest under his chin.

4 Apply pre-shave lotion if the patient requests it.

5 If the patient is able to shave himself, allow him to complete the procedure. If the patient requires your assistance, proceed with steps 6 to 11.

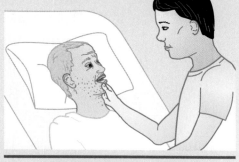

Figure 17-17   Step 2.

6 Start shaving from the sideburns, holding the skin tight and using a circular motion (Figure 17-18).

7 Shave the neck and around the mouth.

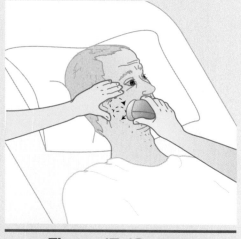

Figure 17-18   Step 6.

Continued

Procedure

SHAVING WITH AN ELECTRIC RAZOR—cont'd

8   Apply after-shave lotion if the patient requests it (Figure 17-19).

9   Sanitize the razor head according to your facility policy.

10   Make the patient comfortable with the signal light where the patient can reach it.

11   Remove, clean, and store equipment according to facility policy.

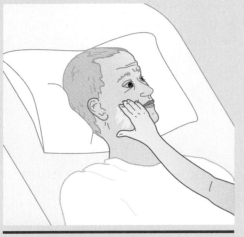

Figure 17-19   Step 8.

◆ **COMPLETE STANDARD ENDING STEPS (see inside front cover)**

Nail and Foot Care

Nail and foot care should be included in the patient's daily hygiene. The best time to perform nail and foot care is right after the patient's bath. Nail care can also be given after soaking the patient's hands or feet in warm water for 5 to 10 minutes to soften the nails. Fingernails should be cleaned daily. Confused patients should have their nails trimmed short to avoid scratches.

Never cut the toenails of a patient who has diabetes. Notify the charge nurse if the toenails of a patient with diabetes need to be cut. The podiatrist also provides this service.

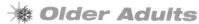
NOTES ON Older Adults

Older patients often have thickened nails or conditions that require the services of a **podiatrist,** or foot doctor.

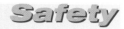
Safety

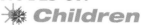
NOTES ON Children

It is best to cut the fingernails of small children or infants with manicure scissors while they are asleep.

Procedure
FINGERNAIL CARE

EQUIPMENT

- Nail clippers
- Emery board
- Orange stick
- Basin of warm soapy water
- Lotion
- Goggles
- Towels (3)
- Gloves

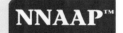
NNAAP™

◆ **COMPLETE STANDARD BEGINNING STEPS (see inside front cover)**

1 Assist the patient to a sitting position by raising the head of the bed 45 to 90 degrees, or assist the patient with sitting in a chair at the bedside.

2 Put on gloves.

3 Place the basin of warm soapy water on a towel on the overbed table (Figure 17-20).

4 Assist the patient with placing her hands in the water, and allow them to soak for 5 to 10 minutes to soften the nails. *NOTE:* If the patient has just been bathed, steps 2 and 3 may be omitted.

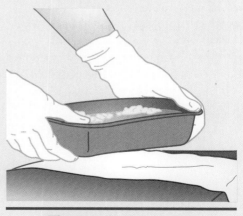
Figure 17-20 Step 3.

Continued

Procedure
FINGERNAIL CARE—cont'd

5 Gently remove dirt from under and around each fingernail using the orange stick (Figure 17-21). Use a paper towel to clean the orange stick after you clean each fingernail and as needed.

6 Rinse the hands with clean warm water, and dry the hands with a towel.

7 Place a clean towel under the patient's dry hands.

8 Put on goggles, and trim the fingernails if needed. Trim the nails in a gentle curve to avoid sharp corners (Figure 17-22).

9 Remove goggles.

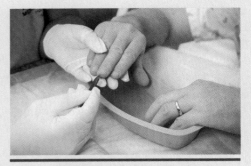

Figure 17-21   Step 5.

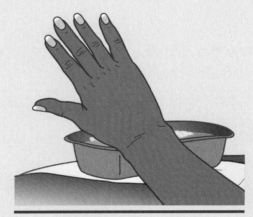

Figure 17-22   Step 8.

10 Shape and smooth the nails with an emery board (Figure 17-23).

11 Rub lotion onto the hands.

12 Remove your gloves and wash your hands.

13 Make the patient comfortable, with the signal light where the patient can reach it.

14 Remove, clean, and store equipment according to facility policy.

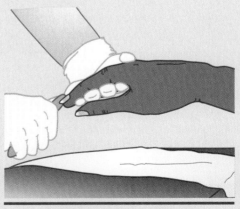

Figure 17-23   Step 10.

◆ **COMPLETE STANDARD ENDING STEPS (see inside front cover)**

Procedure
FOOT CARE

EQUIPMENT

- Nail clippers
- Emery board
- Orange stick
- Basin of warm soapy water
- Lotion
- Goggles
- Towels (3)
- Gloves

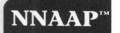

◆ **COMPLETE STANDARD BEGINNING STEPS (see inside front cover)**

1 Assist the patient to a sitting position on the side of the bed, or assist the patient with sitting in a chair at the bedside.

2 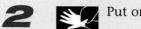 Put on gloves.

3 Place the basin of warm soapy water on a towel on the floor (Figure 17-24).

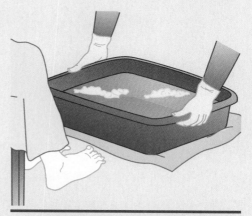

Figure 17-24 Step 3.

4 Assist the patient with placing the feet in the water, and allow them to soak for 5 to 10 minutes to soften the nails (Figure 17-25). *NOTE:* If the patient has just been bathed, steps 2 and 3 may be omitted.

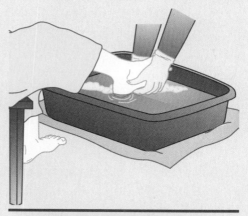

Figure 17-25 Step 4.

Continued

Procedure
FOOT CARE—cont'd

5 Gently remove dirt from under and around each toenail using the orange stick. Use a paper towel to clean the orange stick as needed.

6 Rinse the feet with clean warm water, and dry the feet with a towel (Figure 17-26).

7 Place a clean towel under the patient's dry feet.

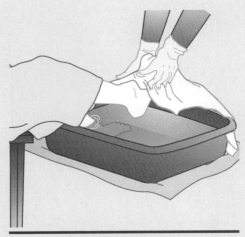

Figure 17-26 Step 6.

8 Put on goggles, and trim the toenails if needed. Trim the nails straight across (Figure 17-27).

9 Remove goggles.

10 Shape and smooth the nails with an emery board.

11 Rub lotion onto the feet.

12 Remove your gloves and wash hands.

13 Make the patient comfortable, with the signal light within reach.

14 Remove, clean, and store equipment according to facility policy.

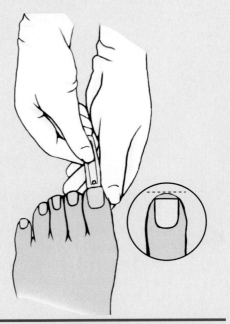

Figure 17-27 Step 8.

◆ **COMPLETE STANDARD ENDING STEPS (see inside front cover)**

Care of Eyeglasses and Hearing Aids

Most eyeglasses today have plastic lenses that scratch more easily than glass lenses. To clean eyeglasses use clean warm water and a soft, lint-free cloth to wipe dry.

Do not use a paper towel or tissue to clean eyeglass. Paper products contain wood fibers that can scratch the lenses.

Eyeglasses should be stored in an eyeglass case in the nightstand when not in use. Never place eyeglasses on a table with the lenses facing down. This also scratches the lenses.

OBRA requires that residents who need eyeglasses or hearing aids be provided with these items each day. This allows residents to be as independent as possible and enhances their quality of life.

Hearing aids increase sounds and are used by people who have hearing loss. There are several types of hearing aids. The most common types of hearing aids are those that are attached to a patient's eyeglasses, those that are placed in the ear canal (Figure 17-28), and those with an over-the-ear style (Figure 17-29). The level of sound on a hearing aid can be adjusted to meet the patient's needs. Hearing aids are powered by a small battery (Figure 17-30). Hearing aids should be cleaned daily according to the manufacturer's instructions and stored in the "OFF" mode in their protective case when not in use. Be careful not to drop the hearing aid or get it wet. Always remove the patient's hearing aid during bathing.

If your patients use eyeglasses and/or a hearing aid, they will need to have these items so that they are as independent as possible.

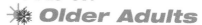

Safety

OBRA

NOTES ON
❄ *Older Adults*

Residents of long-term care centers should have their names marked on their eyeglasses in case they are misplaced. The eye doctor usually has a special tool that can be used to mark the glasses with the resident's name.

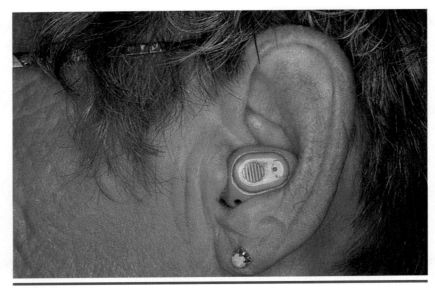

***Figure* 17-28**   Hearing aid.

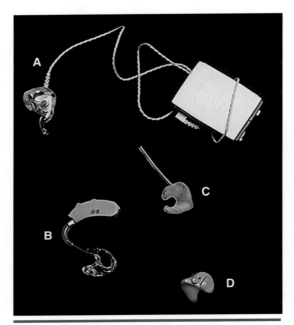

***Figure* 17-29**   Types of hearing aids. *A,* Older aid with a battery pack worn on the body and a wire connected to the ear mold. *B,* Behind-the-ear (BTE) battery with ear mold. *C,* In-the-ear (ITE) mold with battery. *D,* Small in-the-canal (ITC) mold.

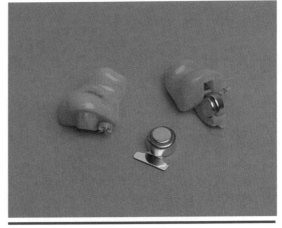

***Figure* 17-30**   Hearing aids are powered by a small battery.

CHAPTER REVIEW

1. How often should hair be combed or brushed?

2. Where should you dispose of a disposable razor after you are finished using it?

3. Where should eyeglasses be stored when not in use?

4. How should hearing aids be cleaned and stored?

Circle the one BEST response.

5. If you are working in a long-term care center and your female resident has a weekly beauty shop appointment, you should
   a. Wash her hair before she goes to the beauty shop
   b. Wash her hair after she returns from the beauty shop
   c. Allow the beauty shop to wash her hair

6. What water temperature should be used when shampooing the hair?
   a. 95° F
   b. 100° F
   c. 105° F
   d. 110° F

7. What should you do if you notice cuts or sores on your patient's head while performing hair care?
   a. Notify the charge nurse.
   b. Notify the doctor.
   c. Notify the patient's family.
   d. Notify the beautician.

8. What kind of a doctor is the podiatrist?
   a. Eye doctor
   b. Ear doctor
   c. Heart doctor
   d. Foot doctor

Fill in the blank with the correct term.

9. Borrowing a comb or brush from another patient can spread _____.

Answers are on page 708.

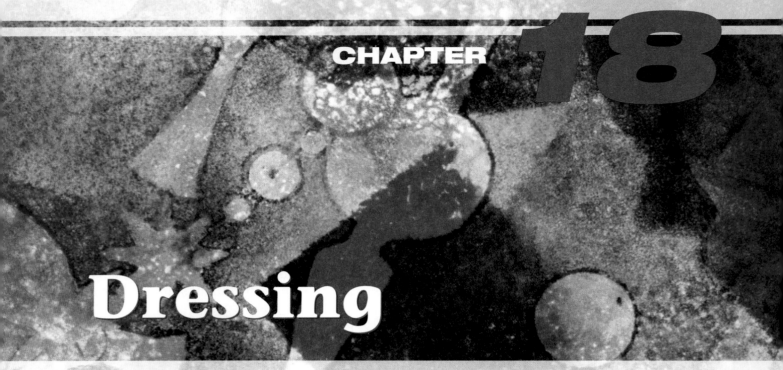

CHAPTER 18

Dressing

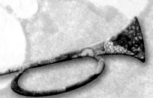

What you will learn

- The key points of dressing and undressing
- How to change a hospital gown
- How to change the gown of a patient with an IV
- How to assist with undressing and dressing

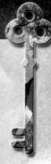

KEY TERMS

Hospital gown A thin cotton garment provided to patients that ties behind the neck and waist to secure an open back seam

IV (intravenous) A needle inserted into a vein to allow medications or fluids to be given to a patient

The Key Points of Dressing and Undressing

While in a health care facility, many patients wear **hospital gowns** that are provided by the facility. The patient's gown is changed when it is dirty or after bathing. For patients with an **IV (intravenous)**, it is usually more convenient for the patient to wear a hospital gown. In many facilities, hospitals gowns have snaps on the shoulders to make it easier to dress a person with an IV. Some patients prefer to wear their own nightclothes or pajamas.

When caring for a patient with an IV on an IV pump, ask the nurse to assist you by disconnecting the tubing from the pump while you change the hospital gown. Never disconnect the IV from a pump!

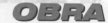

In a nursing home or long-term care (LTC) center, the resident usually dresses in street clothes each day. Appropriate daytime dress depends upon the time of year and the resident's plans for the day. For example, a resident who is going out to the doctor on a cold day should have a coat or jacket.

Residents of LTC centers should be dressed in clothes that are clean and in good condition. Most long-term care centers mark residents' clothing with their name. It is not appropriate to "borrow" clothing from one resident for another.

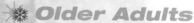

The nursing assistant helps the resident with dressing and undressing. Clothing that opens down the front or back makes it easier to dress residents who have limited movement.

There are special aids that can be used to help the residents to dress themselves. Long-handled shoehorns and clothing with Velcro fasteners allow the resident to be more independent when dressing (Figure 18-1).

NOTES ON
❄ *Older Adults*

Because they have less body fat, many elderly patients feel cold when the nursing assistant does not. Assisting patients with dressing in layers such as a blouse and a sweater or a shirt and a jacket allows the patients to remove the outer layer of clothing if they become too warm.

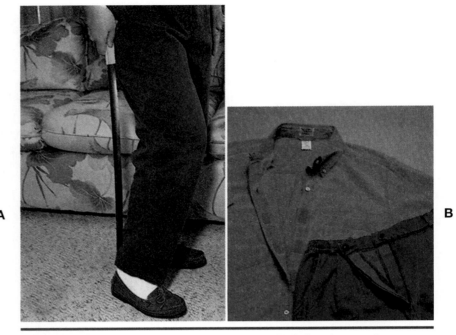

***Figure* 18-1** Dressing aids. **A,** Long-handled shoe horn reduces bending. **B,** Clothing with Velcro makes it easy to dress and undress.

OBRA Residents should be encouraged to make choices about what they are going to wear whenever possible.

Procedure
CHANGING A HOSPITAL GOWN

EQUIPMENT
- Clean hospital gown
- Dirty linen hamper
- Gloves and other personal protective equipment needed

◆ **COMPLETE STANDARD BEGINNING STEPS (see inside front cover)**

1 Provide privacy for the patient.

2 If there is a risk of contact with blood or body fluids, put on gloves.

3 Assist the patient with turning onto his side so that you can untie the gown at the neck and waist (Figure 18-2). Assist the patient to return to the supine position.

4 If the patient is unable to turn, reach behind the neck and waist to untie the gown.

5 Loosen the gown around the body.

6 Unfold the clean gown, and lay it over the patient's chest.

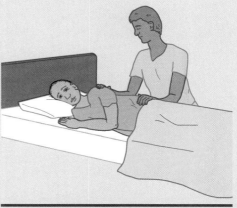

***Figure* 18-2**   Step 3.

7 Remove one arm at a time from the sleeve, leaving the dirty gown over the patient's body (Figure 18-3). If the patient has weakness on one side, begin by removing the stronger arm first.

8 Slide each arm through a sleeve of the clean gown. If the patient has weakness on one side, begin with the weaker arm first, making sure to support the arm as you slide it through the sleeve.

9 Remove the dirty gown from under the clean gown.

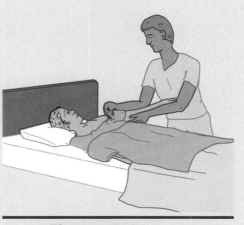

***Figure* 18-3**   Step 7.

Continued

Procedure
CHANGING A HOSPITAL GOWN—cont'd

10 Adjust the clean gown, and fasten the ties behind the neck and waist (Figure 18-4).

11 Remove gloves if worn and wash your hands.

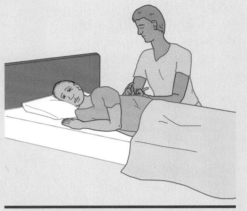

Figure 18-4   Step 10.

◆ COMPLETE STANDARD ENDING STEPS **(see inside front cover)**

Procedure

CHANGING A HOSPITAL GOWN WHEN THE PATIENT HAS AN IV

EQUIPMENT
- Clean hospital gown
- Dirty linen hamper
- Gloves and other personal protective equipment needed

◆ **COMPLETE STANDARD BEGINNING STEPS** (see inside front cover)

1 Provide privacy for the patient (Figure 18-5).

2 🖐 If there is a risk of contact with blood or body fluids, put on gloves.

3 Assist the patient with turning onto her side so that you can untie the gown at the neck and waist. Assist patient to return to the supine position.

4 If the patient is unable to turn, reach behind the neck and waist to untie the gown.

5 Loosen the gown around the body.

6 Unfold the clean gown, and lay it over the patient's chest.

7 Remove the gown from the arm without the IV first.

8 Move the gown down the arm that has the IV. Slowly remove the arm and hand from the sleeve (Figure 18-6).

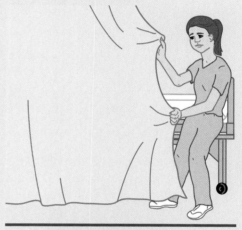

Figure 18-5   Step 1.

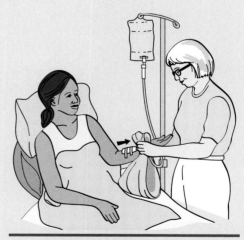

Figure 18-6   Step 8.

Continued

Procedure

CHANGING A HOSPITAL GOWN WHEN THE PATIENT HAS AN IV—cont'd

9 Keep the sleeve gathered, and slide your hand along the tubing to the IV bag or bottle (Figure 18-7).

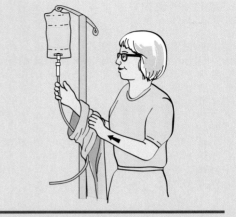

Figure 18-7   Step 9.

10 Remove the IV bag or bottle from the pole. Slide the dirty gown up and over the top of the IV bag or bottle, being careful not to pull on the IV tubing (Figure 18-8). It is important to keep the IV bag or bottle higher than the patient at all times.

11 Replace the IV bag or bottle on the pole. *NOTE:* If the gown has snaps on the shoulder, unsnap the gown and remove the gown from the patient's body without taking the IV bag from the IV pole.

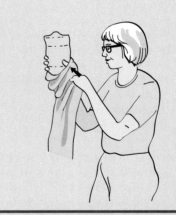

Figure 18-8   Step 10.

Procedure

CHANGING A HOSPITAL GOWN WHEN THE PATIENT HAS AN IV—cont'd

12   Gather the sleeve of the clean gown that will go on the arm with the IV. Remove the IV bag or bottle from the pole, and slip the sleeve over the bag or bottle (Figure 18-9).

13   Replace the IV bag or bottle on the pole.

14   Gently slide the sleeve over the tubing, hand, and arm up onto the patient's shoulder.
NOTE: If the gown has snaps on the shoulder, unsnap the gown and put the gown on the patient without taking the IV bag from the IV pole. Fasten the snaps after the gown is in place.

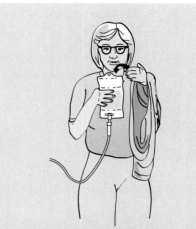

***Figure* 18-9**   Step 12.

15   Slide the other arm through a sleeve of the clean gown.

16   Remove the dirty gown from under the clean gown.

17   Adjust the clean gown, and fasten the ties behind the neck and waist.

18   If gloves were worn, remove and wash hands.

◆ COMPLETE STANDARD ENDING STEPS **(see inside front cover)**

Procedure
ASSISTING THE PATIENT WITH UNDRESSING AND DRESSING

EQUIPMENT

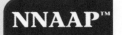

- Dirty linen hamper
- Clothing appropriate for the environment, selected by the patient
- Gloves and other personal protective equipment needed

◆ **COMPLETE STANDARD BEGINNING STEPS (see inside front cover)**

Undressing

1 Provide privacy for the patient.

2 If there is a risk of contact with blood or body fluids, put on gloves.

3 Assist the patient to a comfortable position. Open all of the clothing by unbuttoning buttons and unzipping zippers.

4 Remove a dress or pullover shirt by moving the garment up the body. Guide each arm out of the garment, and gently slip the garment over the patient's head (Figure 18-10).

5 Remove a button-down shirt or blouse by removing one arm at a time from the sleeve. If the patient has a weak side, remove the stronger arm first.

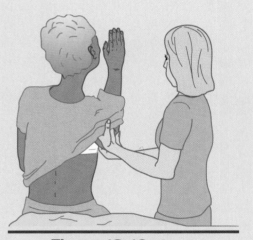

Figure 18-10 Step 4.

Procedure

ASSISTING THE PATIENT WITH UNDRESSING AND DRESSING—cont'd

6 If the patient is wearing a bra, open the hooks and slip off the bra (Figure 18-11).

7 For a patient wearing an undershirt or full slip, follow step 4.

8 If dressing the patient in pajamas or a hospital gown, put the top garments on at this time so that the patient is not left uncovered.

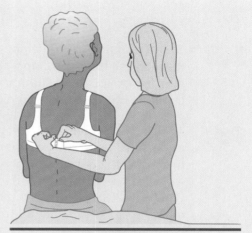

Figure 18-11 Step 6.

9 Help the patient to lie down, and remove shoes and socks (Figure 18-12).

10 Pull pants or pantyhose gently down the legs from the waist and remove.

11 Remove underpants, and replace with clean underpants if the patient desires.

12 If dressing the patient in pajamas, put the pajama bottoms on by putting both legs in the pajama legs and sliding the bottoms up over the legs and hips.

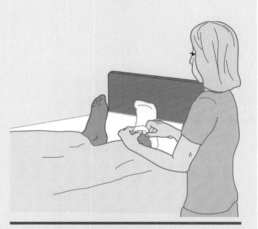

Figure 18-12 Step 9.

Continued

Procedure

ASSISTING THE PATIENT WITH UNDRESSING AND DRESSING—cont'd

Dressing

13 To put a bra on a female patient, slide her arms through the bra straps, and adjust the cups to fit over her breasts. Adjust the shoulder straps and close the hooks in the front or back as required.

14 To put on a patient's pullover shirt, full slip, or undershirt, assist the patient with putting both arms into the garment. If the patient has a weak side, begin with the weaker arm first (Figure 18-13). Gently pull the garment up and over the patient's head, adjusting the neck opening.

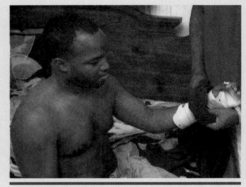

***Figure* 18-13**   Step 14.

15 To put on a button-down shirt or blouse, place one arm at a time through each sleeve. If the patient has a weaker side, start by dressing the weak arm first. Slide the shirt up the arms, and adjust the garment over the patient's shoulder (Figure 18-14). Button the buttons.

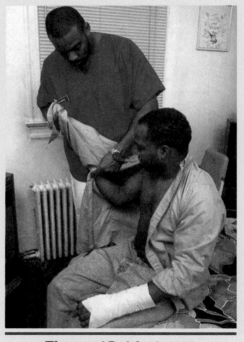

***Figure* 18-14**   Step 15.

Procedure
ASSISTING THE PATIENT WITH UNDRESSING AND DRESSING—cont'd

16 To put on pants or slacks, put both legs in pants and slide garment up to hips (Figure 18-15). Have the patient lift his hips, and pull pants up. Adjust garment, zip the zipper, and fasten if needed.

17 Roll socks or stockings from the opening to just below the heel. Support the patient's ankle, and slip the rolled sock or stocking over the toes. Adjust the sock over the heel, and pull it smoothly up the leg.

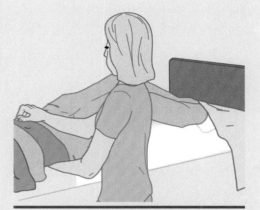

Figure 18-15   Step 16.

18 Assist the patient to a sitting position. Loosen the shoelaces, and pull the tongue of the shoe up and forward. Support the patient's ankle, and gently slide the toes, foot, and heel into the shoe. Use a shoehorn if necessary (Figure 18-16). Tie the shoelaces.

19 If gloves were worn, remove and wash hands.

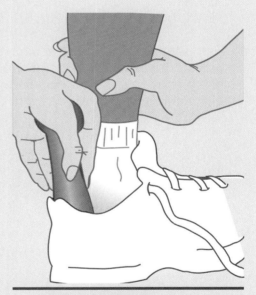

Figure 18-16   Step 18.

◆ **COMPLETE STANDARD ENDING STEPS (see inside front cover)**

CHAPTER REVIEW

1. How should a nursing home resident be dressed?

2. Why does the elderly patient feel cold even when the nursing assistant is not?

Circle the one BEST response.

3. When is the patient's hospital gown changed?
   a. Every morning before breakfast
   b. In the evening or after dinner
   c. When it is dirty or after bathing
   d. At bedtime or before bathing

4. When changing a patient's hospital gown, the nursing assistant should
   a. Remove the dirty gown completely before putting on the clean gown
   b. Provide privacy for the patient
   c. Place the dirty gown on the chair when he is finished
   d. Remove the weaker arm from the gown first

5. When changing the hospital gown of a patient who has an IV, the correct procedure is
   a. Remove the gown from the arm without the IV first
   b. Keep the IV bag or bottle lower than the patient at all times
   c. Remove both arms from the gown at the same time
   d. Place the clean gown on the arm without the IV first

6. How does the nursing assistant remove a dress or pullover style shirt when assisting a patient with undressing?
   a. Pull the garment up and over the patient's head and arms at the same time.
   b. Always begin by removing the right arm from the garment first.
   c. Guide the garment over the patient's head, then remove both arms.
   d. Guide each arm out of the garment, then slip it over the patient's head.

Answers are on page 708.

CHAPTER 19

Nutrition and Fluids

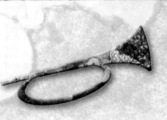

What you will learn

- The basics of good nutrition and hydration
- Different types of diets
- Enteral and parenteral nutrition/intravenous (IV) therapy
- How to measure intake and output (I&O)
- How to assist a person with eating

KEY TERMS

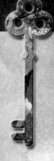

Aspiration Taking in, such as aspirating fluids into the lungs

Dehydration Excessive loss of fluids from the body tissues

Edema Swelling, build up of fluid in the tissues

Enteral nutrition Giving nutrients through the digestive tract using a tube

Nutrients Substances in food that support life

Parenteral nutrition Giving nutrients through a tube that does not enter the digestive system such as intravenous (IV) fluids

The Basics of Good Nutrition and Hydration

Food and water are needed to keep our bodies working properly. The amount and types of food and fluids in our diet affect our physical and mental health. A well-balanced diet provides energy and helps you fight off illnesses. A good diet is also important to help your body grow and to repair injured tissues.

Food provides the **nutrients** necessary to keep your body working. Nutrients are divided into 5 categories.

1. *Carbohydrates*—Carbohydrates provide energy to the cells. They are the fuel of the body much like gasoline is fuel for your car. Carbohydrates are found in cereals, breads, pastas, rice, potatoes, fruits, vegetables, and sugars. If more carbohydrates are taken in than are needed, your body stores them as fat.

2. *Proteins*—Proteins make and repair body tissue, help build blood, and provide energy. Proteins are in meats, eggs, fish, poultry, dairy products, nuts, and beans. If you eat more protein than your body needs, your body stores it as fat.

3. *Fats*—Fats are needed to carry vitamins, provide energy and heat, and help with growth. Fats include butter, oils, salad dressings, whole milk, meats, fish, and nuts.

4. *Vitamins*—Vitamins are important for the proper breakdown and use of nutrients by the body. A well-balanced diet contains enough of the vitamins. The vitamins your body needs are identified by letters such as A, B, C, D, E, and K. Vitamins in food can be destroyed by overcooking or exposure to air. Different foods contain different vitamins. For example, oranges are a good source of Vitamin C, and milk is a good source of Vitamin D.

5. *Minerals*—The body needs many different types of minerals to keep it working properly. A well-balanced diet will contain enough of the minerals your body needs. Minerals keep bones and teeth strong, keep muscles and nerves working properly, and help you to have a stable balance of water in the body. Calcium, potassium, sodium, and iron are just a few of the minerals found in foods.

In addition to nutrients, your body needs fluid and fiber to keep it going. About 60% to 70% of your body weight is water. Water is essential to life. It carries nutrients to the cells through the bloodstream and carries waste away from the cells. Water regulates body temperature, lubricates joints, and aids in digestion. A person can live only a few days without water. For good health the body needs about 8 glasses (2000 to 3000 ml) of fluid a day. At least 1000 ml of the fluids you drink each day should be water. Juices, coffee, tea, milk, and soft drinks are also fluids (Figure 19-1). *Making sure that your patients receive enough fluids each day is an important part of your job!* Unless a patient is on a special diet or is unable to take in anything by mouth, fresh drinking water should be at the bedside at all times.

Some conditions can upset the fluid balance in the body. If a patient has a fever, is vomiting, or has diarrhea, the patient will lose body fluids rapidly. This excessive loss of fluids from the body tissues is called **dehydration** (Figure 19-2).

Fiber or roughage is another important part of the diet. Fiber is in all plant foods such as fruits, vegetables, whole grains, and nuts. Fiber is the part of the plant that absorbs water. Dietary fiber helps prevent constipation and is needed for healthy elimination of stool.

The United States Department of Agriculture (USDA) provides recommendations for a well-balanced diet using a Food Guide Pyramid (Figure 19-3). The Food Guide Pyramid divides food into 6 separate groups. The groups in the Food Guide Pyramid, beginning at the bottom, are:

Breads, cereals, rice, and pasta—These are all foods made from grains such as wheat, oats, and rice. This group contains carbohydrates and fiber. Examples of items from this food group include bread, bagels, noodles, and pasta. You need 6 to 11 servings from this group each day.

Vegetables—We need 3 to 5 servings of food from this group each day. Vegetables provide vitamins, carbohydrates, and fiber. Examples of vegetables include carrots, spinach, and corn.

Fruit—Fruits provide carbohydrates, fiber, and vitamins. Apples, pears, grapes, and bananas are examples of fruits. You need 2 to 4 servings from this group daily.

Milk, yogurt, and cheese—This group provides minerals and fats. We need 2 to 3 servings from this group each day.

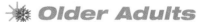

NOTES ON
Older Adults

Elderly people may not feel thirsty even though they are dehydrated. Elderly people also tend to become dizzy and confused when they are dehydrated. It is especially important to encourage your older patients to drink enough fluids each day.

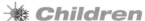

NOTES ON
Children

During periods of rapid growth, children need more protein, vitamins, and minerals.

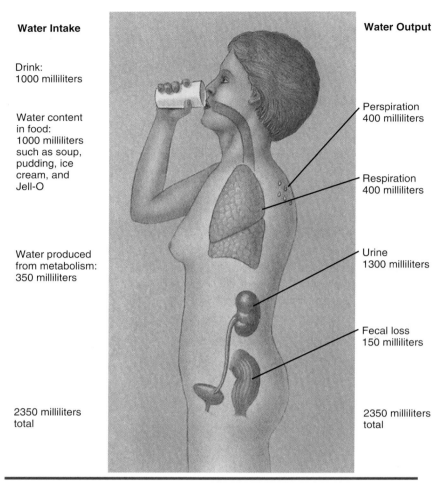

Water Intake

Drink:
1000 milliliters

Water content
in food:
1000 milliliters
such as soup,
pudding, ice
cream, and
Jell-O

Water produced
from metabolism:
350 milliliters

2350 milliliters
total

Water Output

Perspiration
400 milliliters

Respiration
400 milliliters

Urine
1300 milliliters

Fecal loss
150 milliliters

2350 milliliters
total

Figure **19-1**   Water balance.

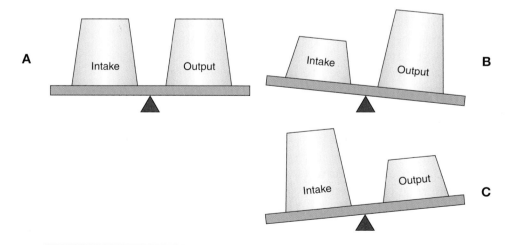

Figure **19-2**   Alterations in fluid balance. **A,** Fluid balance. **B,** Output
greater than intake = dehydration. **C,** Intake greater than output =
fluid accumulation in the body.

DIETARY GUIDELINES
for
AMERICANS

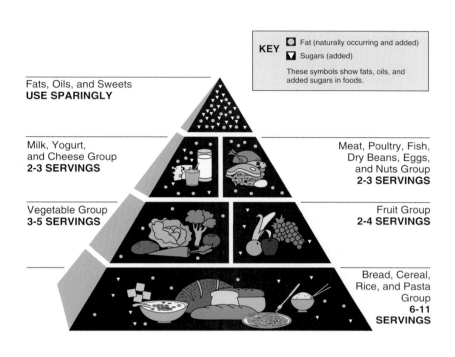

KEY ☐ Fat (naturally occurring and added)
     ▼ Sugars (added)

These symbols show fats, oils, and added sugars in foods.

Fats, Oils, and Sweets
USE SPARINGLY

Milk, Yogurt,
and Cheese Group
2-3 SERVINGS

Meat, Poultry, Fish,
Dry Beans, Eggs,
and Nuts Group
2-3 SERVINGS

Vegetable Group
3-5 SERVINGS

Fruit Group
2-4 SERVINGS

Bread, Cereal,
Rice, and Pasta
Group
**6-11
SERVINGS**

DIETARY GUIDELINES
for
AMERICANS

EAT A VARIETY OF FOODS to get the energy, proteins, minerals, and fiber you need for good health.

BALANCE THE FOODS YOU EAT WITH PHYSICAL ACTIVITY–MAINTAIN OR IMPROVE YOUR WEIGHT to reduce your chances of having high blood pressure, heart disease, a stroke, certain cancers, and the most common kind of diabetes.

CHOOSE A DIET WITH PLENTY OF GRAIN PRODUCTS, VEGETABLES, AND FRUITS which provide needed vitamins, minerals, fiber, and complex carbohydrates and can help you lower your intake of fat.

CHOOSE A DIET LOW IN FAT, SATURATED FAT, AND CHOLESTEROL to reduce your risk of heart attack and certain types of cancer and to help you maintain a healthy weight. CHOOSE A DIET MODERATE IN SUGARS. A diet with lots of sugars has too many calories and too few nutrients for most people and can contribute to tooth decay.

CHOOSE A DIET MODERATE IN SALT AND SODIUM to help reduce your risk of high blood pressure.

IF YOU DRINK ALCOHOLIC BEVERAGES, DO SO IN MODERATION. Alcoholic bever-ages supply calories, but little or no nutrients. Drinking alcohol is also the cause of many health problems and accidents and can lead to addiction.

Figure 19-3   The Food Guide Pyramid.

Meat, poultry, fish, dried beans, eggs, and nuts—These foods also provide minerals and fats and include beef, pork, chicken, turkey, and peanut butter. You need to eat 2 to 3 servings of this group each day.

Fats, oils, and sweets—This group is at the top of the pyramid, and we should use only a little of these. Cakes, pies, cookies, butter, and salad dressings belong to this group.

Eating a well-balanced diet is the first step to good health (Box 19-1). The USDA suggests that you eat a variety of foods from each food group and keep a healthy body weight. At different times in your life, your dietary needs are different. For example, women who are pregnant or breast-feeding need more milk than men or older women (Table 19-1).

NOTES ON
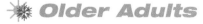
Older Adults

As the body ages, it needs the same amount of nutrients but fewer calories. Many older people suffer from chronic diseases that decrease their appetite. You can assist the older person by offering a variety of foods from the Food Guide Pyramid.

Box 19-1

WHAT IS ONE SERVING?

Bread, Cereal, Rice, and Pasta
1 slice of bread
3 or 4 crackers
½ cup cooked cereal
1 cup dry cereal
½ cup cooked rice or pasta

Fruit
1 melon wedge
1 medium-size whole fruit (size of tennis ball)
¾ cup fruit juice
½ cup cooked or canned fruit
¼ cup dried fruit (for example, raisins, prunes, figs)

Vegetable
¾ cup of vegetable juice
1 cup raw leafy vegetables
½ cup chopped or cut raw vegetables
½ cup cooked vegetables
1 small potato

Meat, Poultry, Fish, Dry Beans, Eggs, and Nuts
2½ to 3 ounces cooked lean meat, poultry, or fish (size of a deck of cards)
½ cup cooked dry beans
1 egg
2 tablespoons peanut butter
½ cup nuts

Milk, Yogurt, and Cheese
1 cup milk
1½ ounces natural cheese
2 ounces processed cheese (2 slices)
2 cups cottage cheese
1 cup yogurt

Fats and Sweets
Use sparingly

Table 19-1

AMOUNT OF SERVINGS NEEDED DAILY

	Women and some older adults	Most children, teenage girls, active women, and most men	Teenage boys, active men, and some very active women
Calorie level*	About 1600	About 2200	About 2800
Bread group	6	9	11
Vegetable group	3	4	5
Fruit group	2	3	4
Milk group	2-3†	2-3†	2-3†
Meat group	2 (for a total of 5 ounces)	2 (for a total of 6 ounces)	3 (for a total of 7 ounces)

Data from United States Department of Agriculture, 2000.

*These are the calorie levels if you choose low-fat, lean foods from the five major food groups and use foods from the fats and sweets group sparingly.

†Women who are pregnant or breast-feeding, teenagers, and young adults to age 24 may need three servings.

Types of Diets

Doctors may order a special diet to treat a person's disease or condition. Some special diets are ordered to decrease certain items in the diet or for weight control.

In the long-term care setting, federal guidelines require that each person's dietary needs be met. Meals must be well balanced, attractive, and tasty. Each resident of a nursing home must receive 3 meals a day and be offered a snack at bedtime.

Table 19-2 lists the most commonly seen diets and why they are used.

In addition to the diets listed in Table 19-2, some facilities provide other specialty diets such as renal diets that are low in sodium, protein, and fluids. Some facilities also provide diets that are high in one specific nutrient such as protein.

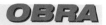

HOW & WHY

Some nursing home residents receive thickened liquids to aid in swallowing. Liquids are thickened to nectar, honey, or pudding consistency by adding a powdered thickening substance. Follow the manufacturer's directions about the amount of thickener to add to achieve the desired thickness.

Table 19-2

COMMON DIETS		
Diet	**Use**	**Foods allowed**
Regular diet	Patients who have no special dietary needs	Any food the patient desires
Clear liquid	After surgery or if nauseated or vomiting	Water, ice chips, tea, coffee (without cream), broth, plain gelatin, Popsicles, clear juices (apple, grape, and cranberry), lemon-lime soda
Full liquid	If clear liquids are tolerated After surgery, if nauseated or vomiting	All items on clear liquid plus milk, all juices, plain ice cream or sherbet, pudding, custard, strained soups, creamed cereals
Soft/pureed	If full liquids are tolerated for difficulty chewing or swallowing	All liquids, eggs, chopped or shredded meats, cooked or canned fruit or vegetables, plain cakes
Sodium restricted/ no added salt	Patients with heart disease, fluid retention, or kidney disease	No salt added to cooking or at the table. No salty or processed foods (canned soups, chips, luncheon meats)
Diabetic/no concentrated sweets (NCS)	Patients with diabetes	No sugar or sweets (cookies, cakes, pies, jelly)

Enteral and Parenteral Nutrition/ Intravenous (IV) Therapy

Patients who are unable to chew or swallow often receive enteral or parenteral nutrition. **Enteral nutrition** is giving nutrients through the digestive tract using a tube. Enteral nutrition can be given through a nasogastric (NG) tube, which enters the nose and delivers liquid feedings into the stomach (Figure 19-4, *A*). For long-term use a tube is placed directly into the abdomen, called a gastrostomy or G-tube (Figure 19-4, *B*). Enteral feedings are frequently called "tube feedings" because the liquid nutrients come through a tube. There are many different brands of enteral feedings. Doctors order the type of feeding they feel is best for their patient based on each individual's needs (Figure 19-5). A patient can be maintained for a long time on tube feedings that provide all of the necessary nutrients. Abdominal cramping and diarrhea are frequent side effects of tube feedings. If your patient has diarrhea, you should notify your charge nurse. Patients who receive tube feedings are at risk of **aspiration**. This means that the tube feeding enters the lungs during the feeding. The tube feeding irritates the lining of the lungs and can lead to pneumonia. To help avoid this problem, the head of the patient's bed is elevated at least 30 degrees during the feeding and for at least $\frac{1}{2}$ hour after the feeding is finished (Figure 19-6). This helps to prevent aspiration.

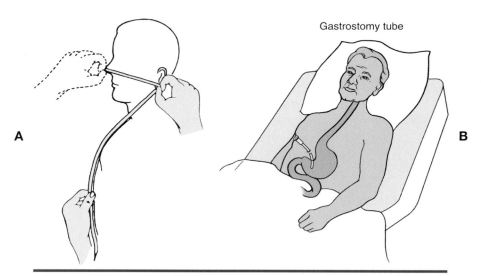

Gastrostomy tube

A

B

***Figure* 19-4**   **A,** Enteral nutrition can be given through a nasogastric (NG) tube, which enters the nose and delivers liquid feedings into the stomach. **B,** Patient receiving tube feeding.

Parenteral nutrition provides the daily nutritional requirements through an IV route. Parenteral nutrition is used when the digestive tract cannot be used or does not absorb enough nutrients to provide good nutrition. The intravenous method of administration can be used to provide fluids with or without nutrients or medications added. If your patient is receiving parenteral nutrition or IV therapy, it is your job to make sure the tubing is not twisted and that the patient does not lie on the IV tubing. An electronic pump monitors many IV and parenteral fluids. When dressing and undressing the patient, you may need to ask the charge nurse to help with the pump. Never unplug the pump or change the settings on the device. It is also important to report any redness or drainage from the site where the tubing enters the body. The most common site for an IV is in the arm or hand. Some types of IVs are placed in the neck or directly into the chest wall. If you have questions about caring for the patient with an IV, always ask your charge nurse for help.

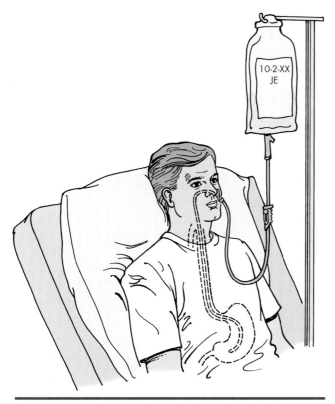

Figure 19-5   Patient receiving tube feeding.

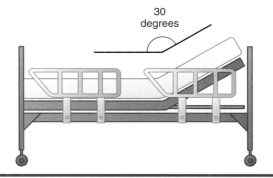

Figure 19-6   Head of bed elevated 30 degrees.

Measuring Intake and Output

It is your job as a nursing assistant to make sure that your patients have an adequate fluid intake each day. *The average person needs 2000 to 3000 ml (70 to 100 ounces) of fluid each day. At least 1000 ml of a person's fluid intake should be water. If people take in more fluid than they put out through urine, perspiration, feces, or emesis,* **edema** *or swelling occurs. The signs of edema are:*

- Weight gain
- Swelling of fingers, hands, feet, ankles, and face
- Decreased urination
- Fluid collection in the abdomen

If people lose more fluids than they take in, dehydration occurs. The signs of dehydration are:

- Thirst
- Constipation
- Decreased urination
- Low blood pressure
- Weak, rapid pulse
- Confusion or disorientation
- Dry lips and mucous membranes
- Rapid weight loss

A healthy person's intake and output should be about equal each day. If doctors suspect that there is a fluid imbalance, they will request that the patient's intake and output (I&O) be measured. Some patients are placed on a fluid restriction to prevent edema or swelling. The charge nurse tells you which patients need their intake and output measured. This information is also part of the care plan and the nursing assistant assignment sheet if used by your facility.

To measure fluid intake it is necessary to accurately measure and record ALL OF THE FLUIDS a resident takes in. Foods such as gelatin and ice cream that become liquid at room temperature are considered fluids and must be measured and recorded. The nursing assistant checks and records the fluids taken at mealtimes and between meals. Fluids given through tube feedings and IV fluids are measured and recorded by the nurse. Most facilities use containers that hold standard amounts of fluids (Table 19-3). The measurements may be listed at the bottom of the I&O sheet that is kept at the patient's bedside. For example, the average coffee cup holds 8 ounces or 240 ml. A juice glass or container of ice cream holds 4 ounces or 120 ml. Some containers, such as milk cartons and soft drink cans, list the volume

NOTES ON
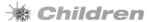 **Children**

Infants and young children are more likely to become dehydrated in a short period of time due to diarrhea or vomiting.

Table 19-3

COMMON VOLUMES OF FOOD CONTAINERS*	
Container	**Volume**
Coffee cup	240 ml
Iced tea glass	300 ml
Juice glass	120 ml
Wax drinking cup	180 ml
Styrofoam cup	180 ml
Large glass	240 ml
Cream package	15 ml
Sherbet	120 ml
Soup, clear	120 ml
Soup, thick	180 ml
Gelatin (Jell-O)	90 ml
Milk carton	240 ml

*May vary from one facility to another.

of liquid they contain. If a container is marked in ounces, you will need to convert the ounces into ml (milliliters) so that the intake can be recorded.

$$1 \text{ ounce} = 30 \text{ ml}$$

If the resident drinks an 8-ounce glass of water, you would record 240 ml ($8 \times 30 = 240$).

If the resident has a 6-ounce bowl of thick soup, you would record 180 ml ($6 \times 30 = 180$).

Intake is totaled and recorded at the end of each shift and at the end of the 24-hour period.

Procedure
MEASURING ORAL INTAKE

EQUIPMENT
* I&O form
* Pen or pencil
* List of volume of commonly used containers used in your facility

◆ **COMPLETE STANDARD BEGINNING STEPS (see inside front cover)**

1 Measure and record all fluids consumed by the patient on your shift.

   a.   Record intake after each meal before the tray is removed (Figure 19-7).
   b.   Record other intake as it is consumed.
   c.   Check the water pitcher for water consumed during your shift.

2 Total the amount of fluids consumed by the patient on your shift.

DATE	11/17/04			11/18/04					
HOUR	0600	1400	2200	0600	1400	2200	0600	1400	2200
INTAKE Oral	180	560	380	120	620	380			
Intravenous	475	550	550	350	350	350			
IVPB Piggyback									
Transfusion									
8 hr. Total									
24 hr. Total			2695			2170			
OUTPUT Urine	650	980	850	500	850	820			
Emesis									
Gastric-Duo									
8 hr. Total									
24 hr. Total			2480			2170			
Stool									
Weight									

Figure 19-7   Step 1.

3 If the patient's intake has been less than 1000 to 1500 ml on the day and evening shift, tell your charge nurse (Figure 19-8).

4 If the patient is on a fluid restriction and has consumed more than the amount of liquid permitted, tell your charge nurse.

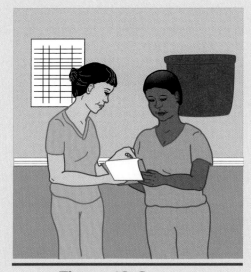

Figure 19-8   Step 3.

◆ **COMPLETE STANDARD ENDING STEPS (see inside front cover)**

It is also important to measure patients' output to determine their fluid balance. In most facilities, all patients with an indwelling catheter are required to have their urinary output measured. If the patient uses a bedpan, bedside commode, or urinal, the urine can be easily collected and measured. If the patient uses the toilet, a special collection container, sometimes called a "hat" because of its shape, is used (Figure 19-9). The specimen collection container fits over the toilet between the top edge of the stool and the seat. Liquid stools are also measured. The specimen collection container can be used to measure liquid stool, and a graduated measuring device, similar to a measuring cup, is usually used to measure emesis. The urine is usually discarded in the toilet after it is measured (Figure 19-10).

Always hold the measuring device at eye level to make sure it is accurate. Output is totaled and recorded at the end of each shift and at the end of the 24-hour period.

Maintaining accurate I&O records is an important function of the nursing assistant.

When measuring urine output, remember to follow Standard Precautions and the Bloodborne Pathogens Standard.

Safety

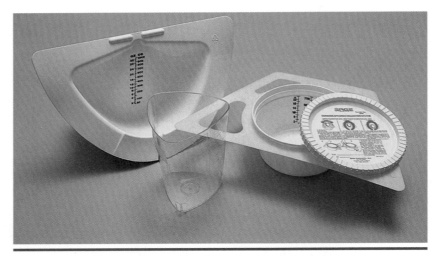

***Figure* 19-9** Specimen "hat," Specipan, and graduated measuring container used for measuring urine.

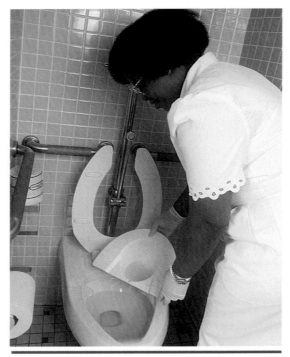

***Figure* 19-10** Unless instructed otherwise, the urine can be discarded in the toilet after it is measured.

Procedure
MEASURING OUTPUT

EQUIPMENT

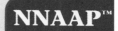

- Measuring device
- I&O form
- Pen or pencil
- Gloves

◆ **COMPLETE STANDARD BEGINNING STEPS (see inside front cover)**

1 Measure and record all fluid output including urine, stool, and emesis on your shift.

2 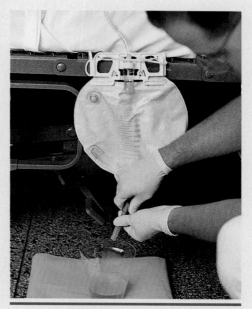 Put on gloves.

3 If the patient has a urinary catheter:

a. Place the measuring device below the level of the catheter bag.

b. Carefully open the drain outlet from the catheter bag, making sure the drain outlet does not touch the floor or the inside of the measuring device (Figure 9-11).

c. Allow the bag to drain completely.

d. Reattach the drain outlet to the collection container.

4 Remove your gloves and wash your hands.

5 Total the amount of output the patient has had on your shift.

Figure **19-11**   Step 3b.

◆ **COMPLETE STANDARD ENDING STEPS (see inside front cover)**

NOTES ON
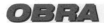 *Culture*

It is important for you to respect the cultural and personal preferences your patients have about their meals. For example, some religions prohibit eating certain foods on religious holidays.

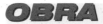

OBRA requires that long-term care centers provide residents with assistive devices such as adaptive utensils and plate guards to help them to be more independent at mealtime.

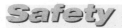

OBRA requires food to be at the correct temperature when it is served to the resident. Hot foods such as meat and potatoes must be hot, and cold foods such as Jell-O and salad must be cold.

Safety

Check the temperature of the food by feeling the container. *Never blow on the food to cool it.*

Assisting the Person With Eating

Meals are an important part of maintaining and restoring health. Food means many things to people (Box 19-2). We celebrate holidays and special events with food.

Many patients look forward to their mealtimes as the most enjoyable part of the day. Patients may be served a tray in their room or may eat together in a common dining room. Many patients are independent with their meals, but others need assistance or require feeding.

Regardless of the type of diet patients are receiving, where they eat their meals, or the amount of help they need, you can make each meal a pleasant experience.

Box 19-2

EXAMPLES OF CULTURAL OR RELIGIOUS BELIEFS RELATED TO FOOD

The theory of hot and cold foods predominates in many cultures. Filipinos, Caribbean Islanders, Mexicans, and Latinos may plan their meals based on these beliefs. Food classification as hot or cold is slightly different from culture to culture.

Mexicans believe hot is warmth, strength, and reassurance, whereas cold is menacing and weak. Classification has nothing to do with spiciness. Hot foods include rice, grains, alcohol, beef, lamb, chili peppers, chocolate, and cheese. Cold foods include beans, citrus fruits, dairy products, most vegetables, honey, raisins, chicken, fish, and goat. Foods can be made hot or cold depending on how they are prepared.

Orthodox Judaism requires kosher food preparation and does not allow eating pork, some fowl, shellfish, blood, and mixing of milk or dairy products with meat dishes. No cooking is done on the Sabbath (Saturday). For all Jewish people, no leavened bread is eaten during Passover.

The Church of Jesus Christ of Latter-Day Saints (Mormons) does not allow the use of alcohol, tobacco, and caffeine.

Seventh-Day Adventists encourage a vegetarian diet and do not allow the eating of pork, shellfish, or alcohol.

Procedure
ASSISTING THE PERSON WITH EATING

EQUIPMENT
- Food tray
- Napkin, towel, or clothing protector
- Overbed table if patient is eating in his room
- Chair

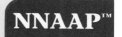

◆ **COMPLETE STANDARD BEGINNING STEPS (see inside front cover)**

1 Provide before-meal care for the patient by assisting him with using the bathroom and washing his hands and face.

2 Assist the patient to an upright position in the bed or in a chair (Figure 19-12).

3 Wash your hands.

4 Protect the patient's clothing with a napkin, towel, or clothing protector.

5 Obtain the patient's tray, and check that he has received the correct diet.

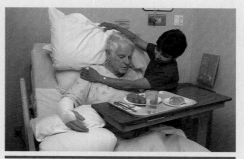

Figure **19-12** Step 2.

6 Check the tray for any assistive devices the patient needs (Figure 19-13).

7 Place the tray on the overbed table or the table in front of the patient.

8 Face the patient, and explain that you will be assisting him with his meal.

9 Remove the plate covers, and arrange the dishes so they are convenient for the patient to reach.

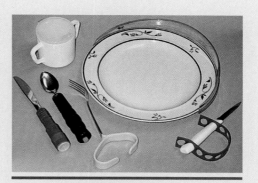

Figure **19-13** Step 6.

10 Describe the food on the tray so the patient knows what has been sent.

Continued

Procedure
ASSISTING THE PERSON WITH EATING—cont'd

11 Prepare the food by cutting the meat, buttering the bread, pouring milk, and so on as needed (Figure 19-14).

12 Season the food as the patient wishes according to his dietary guidelines. *NOTE:* Assist the patient only as much as needed, and encourage the patient to be as independent as possible.

13 If the patient is visually impaired, describe the location of the food using the face of a clock to describe where each item is located on the tray (Figure 19-15).

14 If patients can feed themselves, make sure they have started eating before leaving the room.

15 If the patient must be fed, ask the patient the desired order for eating the different foods.

16 Using a spoon, fill the spoon ½ full and give small bites. Feed the patient slowly, giving the patient time to chew and swallow (Figure 19-16).

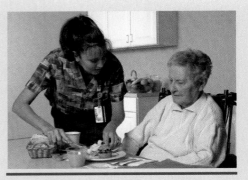

***Figure* 19-14**   Step 11.

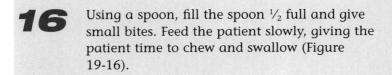

***Figure* 19-15**   Step 13.

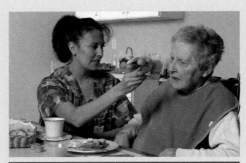

***Figure* 19-16**   Step 16.

Procedure
ASSISTING THE PERSON WITH EATING—cont'd

17 Alternate liquids and solids. If the patient has difficulty drinking, use a bendable straw if permitted (Figure 9-17).

18 Wipe the patient's mouth as needed.

19 When the patient is finished, note the amount of food and fluids consumed and remove the tray or dishes.

20 If required, record the intake.

21 Provide after-meal care: wash the patient's hands and face, and remove the napkin, towel, or clothing protector.

22 Make sure the patient is comfortable, and if in the patient's room, make sure the signal light is where the patient can reach it.

23 Wash your hands.

◆ COMPLETE STANDARD ENDING STEPS **(see inside front cover)**

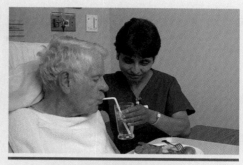

Figure **19-17** Step 17.

CHAPTER REVIEW

1. Why is a well-balanced diet important?

2. List the 5 categories of nutrients, and give an example of each.

3. In addition to nutrients, what else does your body need to keep it going?

4. List the 6 food groups listed in the USDA Food Guide Pyramid.

5. What is enteral nutrition?

6. List 3 signs of dehydration.

7. Mr. Long is on I&O. Listed below are the items on his breakfast tray. Calculate his total fluid intake in ml (milliliters).
   4 ounces scrambled eggs
   2 slices of toast with butter and jelly
   6 ounces coffee
   4 ounces corn flakes
   3 ounces milk
   4 ounces orange juice
   1 banana
   Total _____

Circle the one BEST response.

8. Excessive loss of fluids from the body tissues is called
   a. Aspiration
   b. Dehydration
   c. Edema
   d. Hydration

9. What type of diet would you expect a patient with diabetes to receive?
   a. Soft
   b. Full liquid
   c. Sodium restricted
   d. No concentrated sweets

10. Ms. Hughes has an order to receive a clear liquid diet after her recent abdominal surgery. Which item should NOT be on her tray?
    a. Ice cream
    b. Grape juice
    c. Plain gelatin
    d. Coffee

11. How much fluid does the average person need each day?
    a. 500 to 750 ml
    b. 800 to 1200 ml
    c. 1000 to 2000 ml
    d. 2000 to 3000 ml

12. Which of the following statements **best** describes the nursing assistant's role when assisting a person with eating?
    a. All residents should be fed by the nursing assistant.
    b. The nursing assistant should stand to feed a person who needs assistance.
    c. Hot foods should be cooled by gently blowing on them.
    d. Patients should be fed using a spoon.

Answers are on page 708.

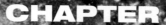

Urinary Elimination

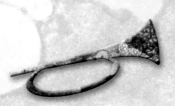

What you will learn

- Normal and abnormal urinary functions
- Measures to promote normal urination patterns
- How to assist a person with toileting
- How to care for urinary catheters

KEY TERMS

Bedpan A container made of metal or plastic used by a bedridden person to collect stool and/or urine

Bedside commode A chair with an opening for a bedpan or a container

Bladder A muscular sac that stores urine

Condom catheter An external device applied to a male patient's penis and attached to a drainage bag

Dysuria Painful or difficult urination

Frequency Urinating at frequent intervals

Hematuria Blood in the urine

Incontinence Inability to control the release of urine from the bladder or stool through the rectum

Indwelling catheter A tube inserted into the bladder and attached to a drainage bag

Kidneys Bean-shaped urinary organs that filter the blood

Nephrons Filter unit of the kidney

Nocturia Frequent urination at night

Oliguria Less than 500 ml of urine in a 24-hour period

Polyuria Abnormally large amounts of urine

Ureters Small tubes that connect the kidneys to the urinary bladder

Urethra A small tube that drains urine from the bladder

Urgency The need to urinate right away

Urinal A plastic container used by men to urinate

Void To urinate

Normal and Abnormal Urinary Functions

The urinary system is made up of your **kidneys**, **ureters**, urinary **bladder**, and **urethra** (see Figure 7-21). People are born with two kidneys. The kidneys are located on either side of your spine in the small of your back at the lower edge of the rib cage. Blood enters the kidneys and travels through the **nephrons**, where it is cleaned. The substances that the body does not need are filtered out and create urine. The ureters are tiny tubes that connect the kidneys to the urinary bladder. The urinary bladder stores urine. When the bladder becomes full, receptors in the bladder send a message to the brain and you experience a strong need to urinate or **void**. This need is usually felt when the bladder contains about 200 ml of urine. The tube that carries the urine from the bladder to the outside of the body is called the urethra. In a female this tube is about $1\frac{1}{2}$ inches long. In a male it is about 8 inches long. Since this tube opens outside of the body, it is possible for an infection to enter the body here.

A healthy adult makes 1000 to 2000 ml of urine a day. There are several factors that can affect urine production, including:

- *Age*—The elderly need to urinate more frequently as the kidneys do not work as well as in younger patients.
- *Diseases*—Such as diabetes.
- *Amount and kinds of liquids taken in*—For example, caffeine increases urinary output.
- *Body temperature*—A fever can decrease the amount of urine produced.
- *Drugs*—Medications for high blood pressure can increase urinary output.
- *Amount of salt in the diet*—A diet high in salt causes the body to retain fluid and decreases urinary output.

Measures to Promote Normal Urination Patterns

Normal urine is clear and light yellow in color. Some drugs and foods such as beets, carrots, and red food coloring change the color of urine. Most people urinate when they get up in the morning, before meals, and at bedtime. Some people need to urinate every 2 to 3 hours and may need to get up at night to use the bathroom. Some people who are ill may need help getting to the bathroom, and others may use a bedpan or urinal. To help the patient to maintain normal urinary elimination you should:

- Follow the person's normal voiding routine and habits
- Provide for privacy
- Allow enough time for the person to urinate; do not rush the person
- Provide 2000 to 3000 ml of fluid per day unless instructed otherwise by the charge nurse
- Answer signal lights quickly

Let your charge nurse know if you notice anything abnormal about the patient's urine or if the patient complains of difficulty when urinating. A urinary tract infection is the most common cause of difficult or painful urination. Other common urinary problems include:

- **Dysuria**—painful or difficult urination
- **Frequency**—urinating at frequent intervals
- **Hematuria**—blood in the urine
- **Incontinence**—inability to control the release of urine from the bladder
- **Nocturia**—frequent urination at night
- **Oliguria**—less than 500 ml of urine in a 24-hour period
- **Polyuria**—abnormally large amounts of urine
- **Urgency**—the need to urinate right away

NOTES ON
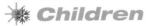
Children

Between the age of 2½ and 4 most children are able to control their bladder functioning. If children are ill or hospitalized, they may return to a less developed way of behavior and lose control over their bladder.

OBRA

NOTES ON
⑨ Culture

Some people may have a difficult time allowing the nursing assistant to help them with toileting. They may be embarrassed or feel that these bodily functions are private. It is important to respect your patient's culture and to provide care in a respectful manner.

Bladder training programs help some people with urinary incontinence regain control of their urinary function. Some people need bladder training after the removal of an indwelling catheter. Your charge nurse will instruct you about a patient's bladder retraining program. If the patient has a catheter, the catheter may be clamped to prevent urine from draining out of the bladder. Your charge nurse will tell you how long to leave the catheter clamped. At the end of that amount of time, the catheter is unclamped for 15 minutes to allow the urine to drain into the bag and then the clamp is re-applied. Later, the catheter is removed and the patient is encouraged to void at regular intervals.

Regaining control of bladder function makes people feel better about themselves and increases their quality of life.

Another type of bladder retraining is used with people who are incontinent but do not have a catheter in place. The person is helped to use the bathroom, commode, bedpan, or urinal at regular intervals according to the care plan. The nursing assistant documents whether the person was wet or dry before being helped to the toilet and if the person was able to urinate. Not all patients are able to regain control of their bladder function. It is important to treat patients with respect whether they are successful with bladder retraining or not.

Patients who are incontinent may use some type of a protective pad or undergarment. These products are either washable or disposable (Figure 20-1). Your charge nurse will tell you which type of product best suits the needs of your patient. It is important to keep your patients clean and dry. Incontinence is embarrassing and uncomfortable for the patient, and patients who are incontinent are likely to develop skin breakdown in the perineal area (Chapter 23).

Safety

When assisting with urinary elimination, remember to follow Standard Precautions and the Bloodborne Pathogen Standard.

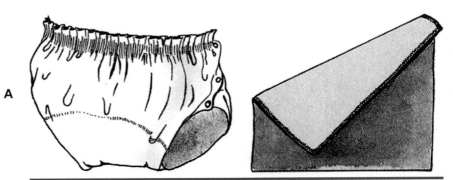

Figure 20-1 Incontinence products. **A,** Reusable undergarment. **B,** Reusable bed pad.

How to Assist a Person With Toileting

Some patients need help with urinary elimination. Some patients may not be able to go to the bathroom and may use a bedside commode, a bedpan, or a urinal (Figures 20-2 and 20-3). A **bedside commode** is a chair with an opening for a bedpan or a container. The commode allows a normal position for elimination.

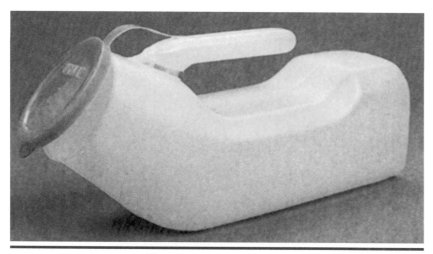

***Figure* 20-2**   Urinal.

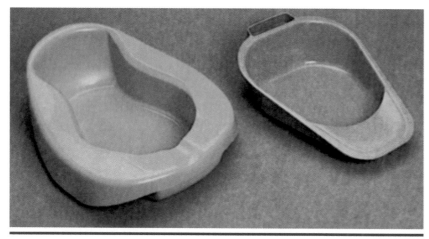

***Figure* 20-3**   Bedpans. **A,** Regular bedpan. **B,** Fracture pan.

Procedure
ASSISTING THE PATIENT TO THE COMMODE

EQUIPMENT
- Commode
- Toilet tissue
- Bath blanket
- Towel(s)
- Washcloth(s)
- Basin of warm water
- Soap
- Gloves

◆ **COMPLETE STANDARD BEGINNING STEPS (see inside front cover)**

1 Put on gloves.

2 Place the commode next to the bed, and re-move the cover or lid (Figure 20-4).

3 Help the patient to sit on the side of the bed, and put on a robe and slippers.

4 Help the patient to the commode using a trans-fer belt (Chapter 11).

5 Cover the patient with a bath blanket, and place the toilet tissue and signal light where the patient can reach them.

6 Ask the patient to signal when he is finished, and provide as much privacy as possible. (If necessary for safety, stay with the patient.)

7 Remove your gloves and wash your hands (Figure 20-5).

8 When the patient signals he is finished, wash your hands and put on gloves.

9 Help the patient with perineal hygiene if neces-sary (Chapter 15).

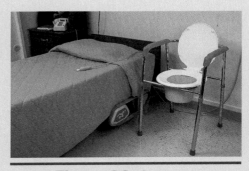
Figure 20-4   Step 2.

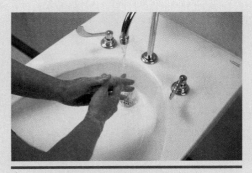
Figure 20-5   Step 7.

Procedure
ASSISTING THE PATIENT TO THE COMMODE—cont'd

10 Help the patient to return to bed, and remove his robe and slippers (Figure 20-6).

11 Remove the commode container, and cover with a towel.

12 Take the container to the bathroom to be emptied. Look for any abnormalities (such as blood or an unusual odor), and notify the charge nurse before emptying the container.

13 Measure urine if the patient is on intake and output (I&O) (Chapter 19).

14 Empty, clean, and disinfect the container according to your facility's policies.

15 Clean the commode according to your facility's policies.

16 Return the container to the commode (Figure 20-7).

17 Return the commode and other supplies to their proper place.

18 Assist the patient with washing his hands.

19 Remove your gloves and wash your hands.

20 Record urinary output on chart if needed.

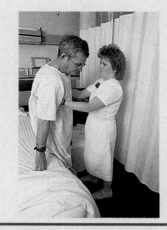

Figure 20-6   Step 10.

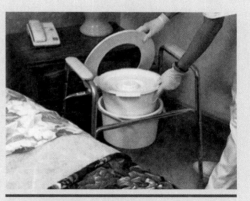

Figure 20-7   Step 16.

◆ **COMPLETE STANDARD ENDING STEPS (see inside front cover)**

A **bedpan** is used when a person cannot get out of bed. There are two types of bedpans, standard bedpans and fracture pans (see Figure 20-3). Bedpans are made of metal or plastic. A metal bedpan should be warmed by placing it under warm running water and drying it before use. A fracture pan has a thinner edge that is placed under the buttocks of a person with a leg, hip, or back injury.

Procedure
ASSISTING THE PATIENT WITH USING THE BEDPAN

EQUIPMENT

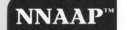

- Bedpan
- Bedpan cover
- Toilet tissue
- Bath blanket
- Towel(s)

- Washcloth(s)
- Basin of warm water
- Soap
- Gloves

 COMPLETE STANDARD BEGINNING STEPS (see inside front cover)

1 Put on gloves.

2 Warm and dry the bedpan if necessary.

3 Lower the head of the bed and the side rail nearest to you.

4 Assist the patient into the supine position (Chapter 11).

5 Fanfold the top linens down, keeping the legs covered.

Procedure

ASSISTING THE PATIENT WITH USING THE BEDPAN—cont'd

6   Ask the patient to raise her hips off of the bed, and slide the bedpan under the patient (Figure 20-8).

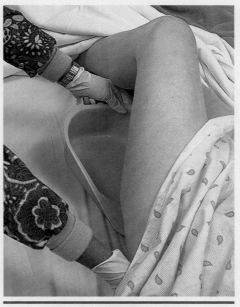

Figure 20-8   Step 6.

7   If the patient is unable to raise her hips off of the bed, turn the patient onto her side facing away from you. Place the bedpan firmly against the buttocks, and turn the patient onto her back (Figure 20-9).

8   Cover the patient with a bath blanket.

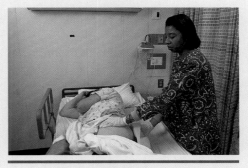

Figure 20-9   Step 7.

9   Raise the head of the bed so that the patient is in a sitting position, and make sure that she is properly positioned on the bedpan (Figure 20-10).

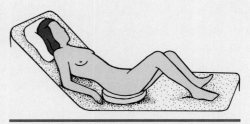

Figure 20-10   Step 9.

Continued

Procedure

ASSISTING THE PATIENT WITH USING THE BEDPAN—cont'd

10 Raise the side rail if needed for safety, and place the toilet tissue and signal light within reach. Ask the patient to signal when she is finished using the bedpan.

11 Remove your gloves and wash your hands.

12 Provide privacy.

13 When the patient signals she is finished, wash your hands and put on gloves (Figure 20-11).

14 Lower the side rail nearest to you and the head of the bed.

15 Help the patient with perineal hygiene if necessary (Chapter 15).

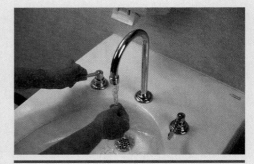

Figure 20-11 Step 13.

16 Remove the bedpan, and cover with a bedpan cover (Figure 20-12).

17 Take the bedpan to the bathroom to empty it. Look for any abnormalities, and notify the charge nurse before you empty the bedpan.

18 Measure urine if the patient is on I&O (Chapter 19).

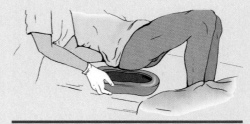

Figure 20-12 Step 16.

19 Empty, clean, and disinfect the bedpan according to your facility's policies.

20 Return the bedpan and other supplies to their proper place.

21 Assist the patient with washing her hands.

Procedure

ASSISTING THE PATIENT WITH USING THE BEDPAN—cont'd

22 Remove your gloves and wash your hands (Figure 20-13).

23 Record urinary output on chart if needed.

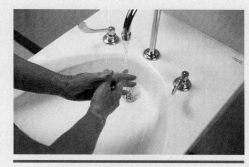

Figure 20-13   Step 22.

◆ **COMPLETE STANDARD ENDING STEPS (see inside front cover)**

A **urinal** is a plastic container used by men to urinate (see Figure 20-2). A urinal has a cap and handle that allows it to be hung on the side rail within the patient's reach if facility policy permits. After the urinal is used, the cap is closed to prevent spills.

OBRA requires that all residents in long-term care centers receive care that makes the quality of life better. This includes providing proper hygiene and answering signal lights promptly to avoid problems with incontinence.

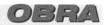

Procedure

ASSISTING THE PATIENT WITH USING A URINAL

EQUIPMENT

- Urinal
- Towel(s)
- Washclolth(s)
- Basin of warm water
- Soap
- Gloves

 COMPLETE STANDARD BEGINNING STEPS (see inside front cover)

1 Put on gloves.

2 Find out if the patient will use the urinal while he is in bed, sitting on the side of the bed, or standing, according to instructions from the charge nurse.

   a.   If the patient uses the urinal while in bed, raise the head of the bed (Figure 20-14) and assist him with placing his penis in the urinal if needed.

   b.   If the patient uses the urinal while sitting, assist him to a sitting position on the side of the bed and assist him with placing his penis in the urinal if needed.

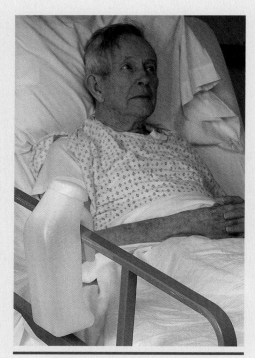

Figure 20-14   Step 2a.

Procedure
ASSISTING THE PATIENT WITH USING A URINAL

   c. If the patient uses the urinal while standing, assist him with putting on slippers and standing at the side of the bed (Figure 20-15). Assist the patient with placing his penis in the urinal if needed.

3 Place the signal light within reach, and provide privacy as safety permits.

4 Remove your gloves and wash your hands if you leave the room.

5 When the patient signals he is finished using the urinal, wash your hands and put on gloves.

6 Close the cap on the urinal.

7 Help the patient with perineal hygiene if necessary (Chapter 15).

8 Take the urinal to the bathroom to be emptied. Look for any abnormalities, and notify the charge nurse before you empty the urinal.

9 Measure urine if the patient is on I&O (Chapter 19).

10 Empty, clean, and disinfect the urinal according to your facility's policies.

11 Return the urinal and other supplies to their proper place.

12 Assist the patient with washing his hands.

13 Remove your gloves and wash your hands.

14 Record urinary output on chart if needed (Figure 20-16).

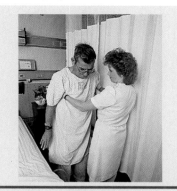

Figure 20-15   Step 2c.

	DATE	11/17/04			11/18/04					
	HOUR	0600	1400	2200	0600	1400	2200	0600	1400	2200
INTAKE	Oral	180	560	380	120	620	380			
	Intravenous	475	550	550	350	350	350			
	IVPB Piggyback									
	Transfusion									
	8 hr. Total									
	24 hr. Total			2695			2170			
OUTPUT	Urine	650	980	850	500	850	820			
	Emesis									
	Gastric-Duo									
	8 hr. Total									
	24 hr. Total			2480			2170			
	Stool									
	Weight									

Figure 20-16   Step 14.

◆ **COMPLETE STANDARD ENDING STEPS (see inside front cover)**

How to Care for Urinary Catheters

A urinary catheter is a tube used to drain urine. A straight catheter is put into the bladder and removed after the bladder is emptied. An **indwelling catheter** is put into the bladder and attached to a drainage bag. An indwelling catheter has a balloon near the tip that is inflated with sterile water to prevent the catheter from slipping out of the bladder (Figure 20-17). A nurse or doctor usually inserts the catheter using a sterile procedure. Catheters are usually used for patients who have surgery or are too weak or ill to use a bedpan, urinal, or commode. If a patient has a wound or a pressure ulcer, a catheter can prevent urine contact with the open area. Indwelling catheters are not routinely used for patients who are incontinent since they increase the chance of a urinary tract infection. Indwelling catheter care is normally provided with morning and bedtime care and after each bowel movement (BM) if the patient is incontinent of stool.

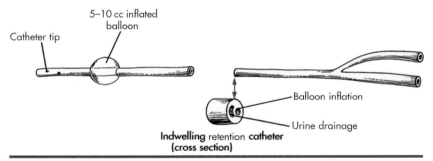

Figure 20-17 An indwelling catheter.

NOTES ON
❄ *Older Adults*

The elderly female patient may find it difficult to lie on her back for catheter care because of arthritis or stiffness. You can assist the patient onto her side with her top leg bent at the knee and supported by pillows to provide catheter care (Figure 20-18).

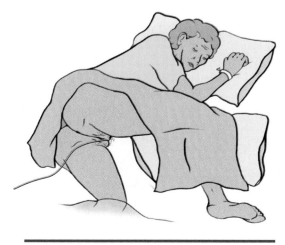

Figure 20-18 Positioning of an elderly female patient for catheter care.

Procedure
PROVIDING INDWELLING CATHETER CARE

EQUIPMENT

- Bed protector
- Bath blanket
- Towel(s)
- Washcloth(s)
- Basin of warm water
- Soap and soap dish or pericare product
- Gloves

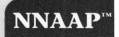

◆ **COMPLETE STANDARD BEGINNING STEPS** (see inside front cover)

1 Put on gloves.

2 Assist the patient to a supine or side-lying position.

3 Place the bed protector under the patient's hips.

4 Cover the patient with the bath blanket.

5 Expose the perineal area.

6 Male catheter and pericare

  a. Using a circular motion, gently wash the penis by lifting it and cleaning from the tip downward toward the scrotum with warm water and soap (Figure 20-19).
  b. Rinse and dry the penis.
  c. If the patient is uncircumcised, pull back the foreskin, wash, rinse, and dry, and pull the skin over the end of the penis.
  d. Using a clean washcloth, hold the catheter near the tip of the penis and clean the first 4 inches of the catheter, washing from the penis toward the drainage bag using warm water and soap. Rinse the catheter, using a clean area of the washcloth. *Do not pull on the catheter during cleaning.*
  e. Wash, rinse, and dry the scrotum.

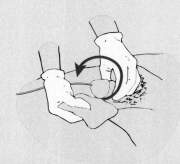

Figure 20-19 Step 6a.

Continued

Procedure
PROVIDING INDWELLING CATHETER CARE—cont'd

f.   Wash, rinse, and dry the skin area between the legs.

g.   Wash, rinse, and dry the anal area, washing from front to back (Figure 20-20).

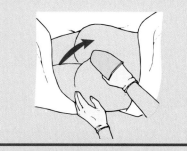

Figure 20-20   Step 6g.

7   Female catheter and pericare

a.   Using a clean area of the washcloth for each wipe of the perineal area, gently open all skin folds and wash the inner area from front to back (Figure 20-21).

b.   Wash and rinse the inner labia from front to back.

c.   Wash and rinse the outer skin folds from front to back.

d.   Wash the inner legs and outer perineal area along the outside of the labia with warm water and soap.

e.   Using a clean washcloth, hold the catheter near the opening of the urethra and clean the first 4 inches of the catheter, washing from the body toward the drainage bag with warm water and soap.

f.   Rinse the catheter, using a clean area of the washcloth. *Do not pull on the catheter during cleaning.*

g.   Wash and rinse the anal area, washing from front to back (Figure 20-22).

h.   Dry the perineal area.

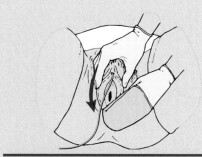

Figure 20-21   Step 7a.

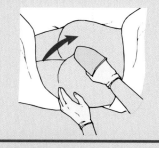

Figure 20-22   Step 7g.

Procedure
PROVIDING INDWELLING CATHETER CARE—cont'd

8 Secure the catheter according to facility policy (Figure 20-23).

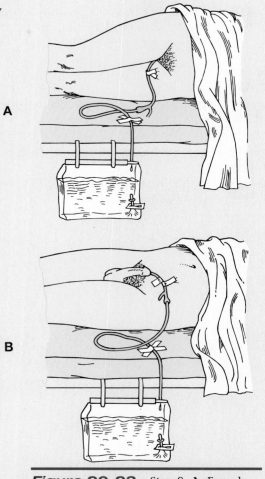

Figure 20-23   Step 8. **A**, Female. **B**, Male.

Continued

Procedure

PROVIDING INDWELLING CATHETER CARE—cont'd

9 Make sure that the drainage bag is below the level of the bladder and does not touch the floor (Figure 20-24).

10 Remove the bed protector and the bath blanket.

11 Remove, clean, and store equipment according to facility policy.

12 Remove your gloves and wash your hands.

13 Make the patient comfortable, with the signal light within reach.

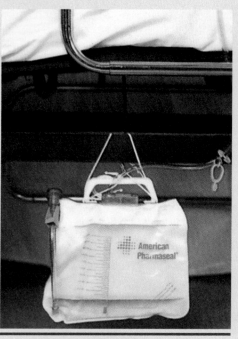

Figure 20-24   Step 9.

A closed drainage system is used for indwelling catheters. Nothing is allowed to enter the system, and the system remains sterile. If germs enter the system, they can travel into the bladder and kidneys, causing a life-threatening infection. The drainage system contains tubing and a drainage bag. The tubing is attached to the catheter at one end and the drainage bag at the other end. The drainage bag hangs from the bed frame, chair, or wheelchair. The bag must be lower than the bladder but must not touch the floor.

Never hang a drainage bag from the bed side rail. When the rail is raised, the bag can be raised higher than the patient's bladder and the urine will not drain into the bag properly. It is also possible to injure the patient by pulling the catheter out when raising or lowering a side rail.

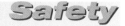

Some patients wear a leg bag when they are up during the day. The leg bag is attached to the thigh or calf and is covered by clothing (Figure 20-25). Both drainage bags and leg bags are emptied, and the urine is measured. Bags should be emptied at the end of each shift, when they become full, and anytime the bag is changed.

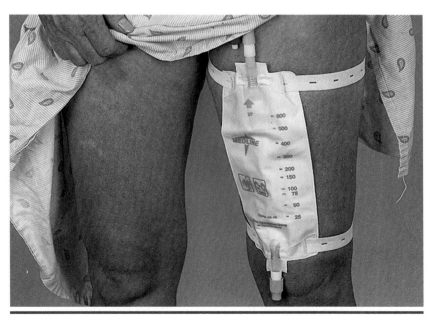

Figure 20-25　The leg bag is attached to the thigh or calf and is covered by clothing.

Procedure
EMPTYING A URINARY DRAINAGE BAG

EQUIPMENT
- Measuring container or graduate
- Paper towels
- Gloves

◆ **COMPLETE STANDARD BEGINNING STEPS** (see inside front cover)

1 Put on gloves.

2 Place the paper towels on the floor.

3 Place the graduate (or measuring container) on top of the paper towels under the drain on the bag.

4 Open the clamp on the drain.

5 Let all of the urine drain into the graduate, being careful not to allow the end of the drain to touch the inside of the graduate (Figure 20-26).

6 Close the drain.

7 Measure the urine. Look for any abnormalities, and notify the charge nurse before you empty the container.

8 Remove and throw away the paper towels.

9 Dispose of the urine.

10 Empty, clean, and disinfect the graduate according to your facility's policies.

11 Return the graduate to the proper place.

12 Remove your gloves and wash your hands.

13 Record urinary output on chart.

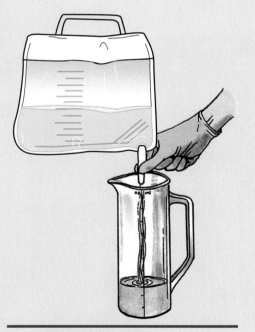

Figure 20-26 Step 5.

◆ **COMPLETE STANDARD ENDING STEPS** (see inside front cover)

Drainage bags may be changed from a leg bag or a drainage bag in the morning and again at bedtime. It may also be necessary to change a drainage bag if it begins to leak or according to facility policy to reduce the chance of infection.

Procedure
CHANGING A DRAINAGE BAG

EQUIPMENT

- Measuring container or graduate
- Paper towels
- Antiseptic wipes
- Sterile cap and plug (if changing from a drainage bag to a leg bag)

- Catheter clamp
- Bath blanket
- Gloves

◆ **COMPLETE STANDARD BEGINNING STEPS (see inside front cover)**

1 Put on gloves.

2 Fanfold the covers back, and cover the patient with a bath blanket.

3 Empty the leg bag or drainage bag according to the procedure.

4 Expose the connection between the catheter and the drainage bag or leg bag tubing.

5 Clamp the catheter (Figure 20-27).

6 Raise the bed to a comfortable working height for good body mechanics.

7 Place the bed protector under the connection between the catheter and the drainage or leg bag tubing.

8 Place a clean paper towel on the overbed table next to the bed.

9 Open the antiseptic wipes, and place them on the clean paper towels.

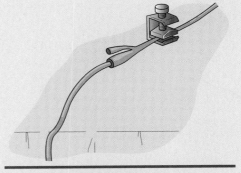

Figure 20-27   Step 5.

Continued

Procedure
CHANGING A DRAINAGE BAG—cont'd

10 Open the package with the sterile cap and plug, and set the opened package on the paper towels (Figure 20-28). *Do not allow the cap or plug to touch anything other than the inside of the package.*

11 Open the package with the new drainage or leg bag and tubing.

12 Disconnect the catheter from the current tubing. Do not allow the catheter to touch anything.

13 Insert the sterile plug into the end of the catheter. Only touch the end of the plug. Do not touch the portion of the plug that goes into the catheter.

14 If it will be re-used, place the sterile cap on the end of the tubing attached to the bag (Figure 20-29).

15 Remove the cap from the new drainage or leg bag tubing and the plug from the end of the catheter.

16 If the end of the catheter or the tubing is touched, clean the end thoroughly with the antiseptic wipes before proceeding.

17 Place the new drainage or leg bag tubing end into the end of the catheter.

18 Remove the clamp from the catheter.

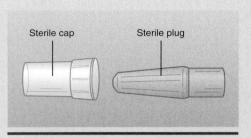

Sterile cap   Sterile plug

Figure **20-28**   Step 10.

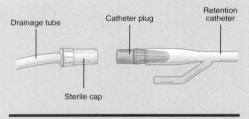

Drainage tube   Catheter plug   Retention catheter

Sterile cap

Figure **20-29**   Step 14.

Procedure
CHANGING A DRAINAGE BAG—cont'd

19 Position the bag on the side of the bed or chair or on the patient's leg if using a leg bag (Figure 20-30).

20 Cover the patient, and remove the bath blanket.

21 Return the bed to its lowest position.

22 Follow facility policy regarding storage or disposal of the previously used bag.

23 Remove your gloves and wash your hands.

24 Record urinary output on chart.

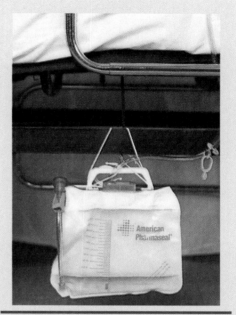

Figure 20-30 Step 19.

◆ **COMPLETE STANDARD ENDING STEPS (see inside front cover)**

A **condom catheter** may be used for incontinent male patients. They are sometimes called external catheters, Texas catheters, or urinary sheaths. A condom catheter slides over the penis and is secured to the skin with an elastic type of tape that comes with the catheter (Figure 20-31). Some condom catheters have a flap of adhesive on the catheter itself (Figure 20-32). A condom catheter can be attached to either a leg bag or a drainage bag.

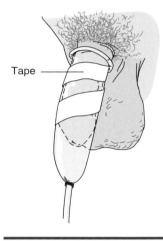

Tape

***Figure* 20-31** A condom catheter.

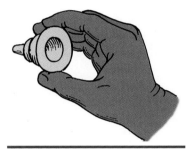

***Figure* 20-32** Some condom catheters have a flap of adhesive on the catheter itself.

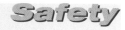

It is important to use the elastic tape that comes with the catheter. Using adhesive or surgical tape can cut off the flow of blood to the penis, causing injury. Follow the manufacturer's directions when you apply a condom catheter. If you are not sure how to apply the catheter after reading the directions, ask your charge nurse for help.

There is little risk of urinary tract infection from a condom catheter because it is applied on the outside of the penis. You will need to remove the condom catheter each day (or more frequently according to your facility policy) to check for skin redness or irritation and to cleanse the penis.

NOTES ON
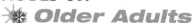
Older Adults

The skin on the penis of an older patient may be fragile and likely to tear. Be careful when you apply and remove the tape on a condom catheter.

Procedure
APPLYING A CONDOM CATHETER

EQUIPMENT

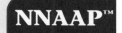

- **Bath blanket**
- **Condom catheter and drainage or leg bag**
- **Basin of warm water**
- **Soap and soap dish**
- **Washcloth(s)**
- **Towel(s)**
- **Bed protector**
- **Gloves**

 COMPLETE STANDARD BEGINNING STEPS (see inside front cover)

1 Put on gloves.

2 Fanfold the covers back, and cover the patient with a bath blanket.

3 Secure the drainage bag to the bed frame, or have a leg bag ready.

4 Raise the bed to a comfortable working height for good body mechanics.

5 Place a bed protector under the patient's buttocks.

Continued

Procedure
APPLYING A CONDOM CATHETER—cont'd

6 Expose the genital area.

7 Provide perineal care (Chapter 15).

8 Apply catheter by rolling it smoothly onto the penis, leaving 1 to 2 inches between the end of the penis and the tip of the catheter (Figure 20-33).

9 Using the elastic tape provided by the manufacturer, wrap the strip of tape over the catheter in a spiral to secure it.

10 If using a self-adhesive catheter, follow the manufacturer's directions.

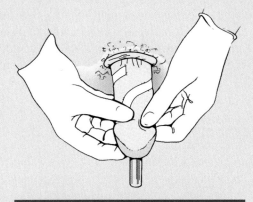

Figure 20-33 Step 8.

11 Attach the catheter tubing to the drainage or leg bag (Figure 20-34).

12 Remove and dispose of the bed protector.

13 Cover the patient, and return the bed to its lowest position.

14 Remove your gloves and wash your hands.

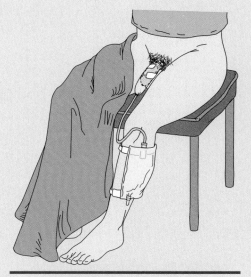

Figure 20-34 Step 11.

◆ **COMPLETE STANDARD ENDING STEPS (see inside front cover)**

CHAPTER REVIEW

1. List the 4 main parts of the urinary system.

2. Where is urine stored?

3. List 3 factors that can affect urine production.

4. How can you help your patients to maintain normal urinary elimination?

5. How does helping your patients regain control of their bladder functioning through bladder retraining benefit the patients?

6. What types of equipment can a person who cannot walk to the bathroom use?

7. What is a condom catheter?

Circle the one BEST response.

8. How much urine does a healthy adult make each day?
   a. 500 to 1000 ml
   b. 1000 to 2000 ml
   c. 2000 to 2500 ml
   d. 2500 to 3500 ml

9. Blood in the urine is called
   a. Dysuria
   b. Frequency
   c. Hematuria
   d. Nocturia

10. Ms. Lester gets up to urinate frequently at night. This condition is known as
    a. Nocturia
    b. Oliguria
    c. Polyuria
    d. Urgency

11. What should the nursing assistant do if he notices anything abnormal in the urine of a patient who is using a bedside commode or bedpan for urinary elimination?
    a. Notify the charge nurse before emptying the container
    b. Notify the charge nurse after emptying the container
    c. Notify another nursing assistant before emptying the container
    d. Notify another nursing assistant after emptying the container

12. What is the correct way to clean a catheter when providing indwelling catheter care?
    a. Pull the tubing tight, and wash back and forth.
    b. Use soap and water, and wash the first 12 inches of the catheter.
    c. Clean the catheter using antiseptic wipes.
    d. Clean the catheter washing from the body towards the bag.

Answers are on pages 708 to 709.

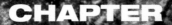

CHAPTER 21

Bowel Elimination

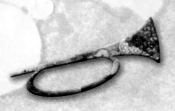

What you will learn

- Normal and abnormal bowel functions
- Measures to promote normal bowel function
- How to give an enema
- Use of a rectal tube
- How to care for a person with an ostomy

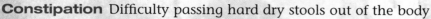

KEY TERMS

Constipation Difficulty passing hard dry stools out of the body

Defecation A bowel movement (BM)

Diarrhea Frequent passage of liquid stools

Enema Putting a liquid solution into the rectum

Feces Semisolid mass of waste products from the intestine

Flatulence Excessive amounts of air or gas in the stomach and intestines

Impaction A buildup of feces in the rectum

Incontinence Inability to control the release of urine from the bladder or stool through the rectum

Ostomy A surgical procedure in which an opening is made to allow the passage of urine from the bladder or intestinal contents from the bowel to exit the body through an opening in the abdomen called a stoma

Peristalsis Wavelike movement

Rectal tube A tube inserted about 4 inches into the patient's rectum to relieve flatulence and abdominal bloating or distention

Stoma Opening

Suppository A medication put into the rectum

Normal and Abnormal Bowel Functions

The digestive system is a 30-foot-long tube that begins at the mouth and goes to the anus. It is also called the gastrointestinal (GI) tract. This system takes in and digests food for the body and eliminates body waste. Partially digested food and fluids move from the stomach into the small intestine and then the large intestine, where fluid is absorbed. The semisolid mass of waste products is called **feces**. Feces is moved through the large intestine to the rectum by a wavelike movement called **peristalsis**. The feces remains in the rectum until it is excreted from the body through the anus during **defecation** or a bowel movement (BM).

Some people have several bowel movements a day. For other people, it may be normal to have a bowel movement every 2 or 3 days. There are several factors that can affect bowel elimination, including:

- *Age*—the elderly are more likely to have **constipation**, difficulty passing hard dry stools
- *Diseases*
- *Food and fluid intake*—a diet with enough fiber and fluids is necessary for healthy bowel functioning
- *Drugs*—some medications can cause constipation or **diarrhea**, the frequent passage of liquid stools

Measures to Promote Normal Bowel Function

Normal stools are soft formed and brown. Bleeding in the stomach or small intestine can cause stools to be black. Bleeding in the lower colon and rectum causes stools to be red. Some foods also affect the color of stool. Diseases can cause the stool to be clay colored or green. People who are ill may need help with elimination. Some need help getting to the bathroom, and others use a bedpan. To help the patient to maintain normal bowel elimination you should:

- Follow the person's normal bowel routine and habits
- Provide for privacy
- Allow enough time for the person to defecate; do not rush the person
- Provide 2000 to 3000 ml of fluid per day unless the charge nurse tells you otherwise
- Encourage a diet with adequate fiber such as fresh fruits and vegetables
- Encourage activity such as walking to increase peristalsis
- Answer the signal light promptly

Tell the charge nurse if you notice anything abnormal about the patient's stool or if the patient complains of difficulty with bowel elimination. Common bowel problems include:

- Constipation—difficulty passing hard dry stools. This may be caused by a diet lacking in fiber or fluids, drugs, aging, inactivity, and some diseases.
- Diarrhea—frequent passage of liquid stools. This may be caused by infections, drugs, some foods, and germs in food or water.
- **Flatulence**—excessive amounts of air or gas in the stomach and intestines.
- **Impaction**—a buildup of feces in the rectum (Figure 21-1). A fecal impaction can occur from untreated constipation. The person may have liquid stools that pass around the impaction.
- **Incontinence**—inability to control the release of stool through the anus.

Bowel training programs can help people with fecal incontinence get control of their bowel function again. Some people need bowel training after an illness or injury.

OBRA requires that facilities provide care in a way that maintains each person's highest level of well-being and independence. Regaining control of bowel function makes the people feel better about themselves and increases their quality of life.

Bowel retraining also helps the person to develop a regular bowel elimination routine and helps to avoid constipation and

NOTES ON
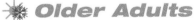 **_Older Adults_**

Older people who are ill, have a fever, and are spending most of their time in bed may become dehydrated and develop a fecal impaction.

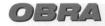

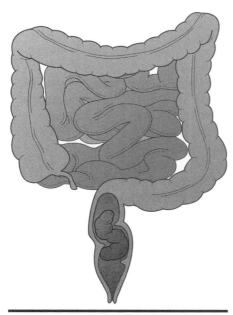

***Figure* 21-1**   Fecal impaction.

impaction. Your charge nurse will instruct you regarding the patient's normal bowel pattern. You will have to assist the person with using the bathroom, commode, or bedpan at those times. Many people also are on diets high in fiber and fluids. The doctor may order a medication to help stimulate the patient to defecate.

The nursing assistant documents whether the person was able to have a bowel movement. Not all patients are able to get control of their bowel function again. It is important to treat patients with respect whether they are successful with bowel retraining or not.

OBRA

It is important to provide privacy to the resident when assisting with bowel elimination. It is important to respect residents' rights to make decisions that affect their life and to be encouraged to participate in their care as much as possible. For example, the resident who has had an ostomy for a long time may be able to care for it with minimal assistance.

As you learned in Chapter 20, patients who are incontinent may use some type of a protective pad or undergarment. It is important to keep your patients clean and dry at all times. Incontinence is embarrassing and uncomfortable for the patient, and patients who are incontinent are more likely to develop skin breakdown in the perineal area (Chapter 23).

Safety

When assisting with bowel elimination, remember to follow Standard Precautions and the Bloodborne Pathogen Standard.

How to Administer an Enema

An **enema** is the introduction of a liquid solution into the rectum. Enemas remove feces from the colon, relieve constipation or flatulence, and help remove an impaction. Enemas are also given to clean the bowel before surgery or diagnostic tests. The most common types of enemas are cleansing enemas, phosphate preparations, and oil retention enemas. The doctor orders the type of enema the patient is to receive.

A cleansing enema is usually given before surgery or a diagnostic procedure. For this enema 500 to 1000 ml of fluid is introduced into the rectum. The doctor may order a tap water, soapsuds (3 to 5 ml of castile soap in 500 to 1000 ml of tap water), or saline (1 to 2 teaspoons of table salt in 500 to 1000 ml of tap water) enema. Some doctors order that the enemas be given "until clear." This means that the enema is repeated until the return solution is clear and free of stool. Your charge nurse will tell you how many enemas to give to the patient.

A phosphate enema (Fleet) is a commercially prepared solution available in a 133-ml disposable plastic pouch with a pre-lubricated tip (Figure 21-2). It is often ordered for the relief of constipation or when the bowel does not need complete cleaning. Some facilities require that a licensed nurse give this type of enema.

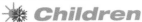

NOTES ON
Children

Infants and children do not usually receive tap water enemas.

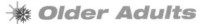

NOTES ON
Older Adults

The older patient tires more easily and is more likely to become dehydrated when enemas are administered until clear.

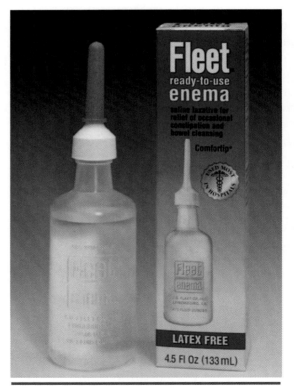

***Figure* 21-2** Commercially prepared enema.

An oil retention enema is a commercially prepared oil-based solution available in a 200- to 250-ml disposable plastic pouch with a pre-lubricated tip given to soften a fecal mass. Some facilities require that a licensed nurse give this type of enema.

Doctors may also order other types of solutions. Always check with your charge nurse before you give an enema.

Nursing assistants are not permitted to give enemas that contain medications.

Safety

Procedure
ADMINISTERING AN ENEMA

EQUIPMENT

- **Bath blanket**
- **Bed protector**
- **Enema kit (Figure 21-3) and intravenous (IV) pole or commercially prepared enema**
- **Toilet paper**
- **Bedpan or commode if needed**
- **Gloves**

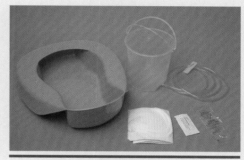

Figure 21-3

◆ **COMPLETE STANDARD BEGINNING STEPS (see inside front cover)**

1 Put on gloves.

2 If giving a cleansing enema, prepare the solution.

     a. Place the enema bag on the IV pole 12 inches above the height of the bed.

     b. Close the clamp on the tube.

     c. Fill the enema bag with the amount of water ordered at 105° F.

     d. Check the temperature of the water with a bath thermometer.

     e. Add salt or castile soap as the charge nurse instructs, and mix.

     f. Seal the bag, and take to the bedside.

Continued

Procedure
ADMINISTERING AN ENEMA—cont'd

3 Lower the side rail on the side of the bed nearest to you.

4 Lower the head of the bed.

5 Assist the patient into a left side-lying position (Figure 21-4).

6 Fanfold the covers to the foot of the bed, and cover the patient with a bath blanket.

7 Place a bed protector under the buttocks.

8 Expose the anal area (Figure 21-5).

9 If giving a cleansing enema:

   a. Place a bedpan behind the patient.
   b. Position the enema tube in the bedpan, and remove the cap.

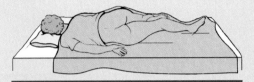

Figure 21-4 Step 5.

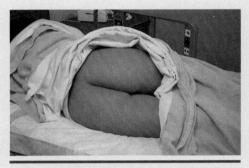

Figure 21-5 Step 8.

   c. Open the clamp on the tubing, and allow the solution to flow through the tubing to remove the air (Figure 21-6).
   d. Close the clamp.
   e. Lubricate 3 to 4 inches at the end of the enema tube.

10 If giving a commercially prepared enema, remove the cap from the enema tip (see Figure 21-2).

11 Separate the buttocks so that the anus is visible.

12 Ask the person to take a deep breath in through the mouth and to breathe out slowly.

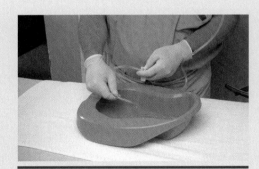

Figure 21-6 Step 9c.

Continued

Procedure

ADMINISTERING AN ENEMA—cont'd

13 Gently insert the enema tip 2 to 4 inches into the rectum as the person is breathing out. Stop if the person complains of pain or you feel resistance. When giving an enema to a child put the tip of the enema tube only 1 to 2 inches into the rectum to prevent injuring the child.

14 If giving a cleansing enema, open the clamp and slowly administer the amount of solution ordered (Figure 21-7). Clamp the tube if the person complains of abdominal cramping, expels the solution, or is unable to hold the solution. Unclamp the tubing, and complete the administration when the symptoms subside. Clamp the tubing before the tubing is empty to prevent air from entering the bowel.

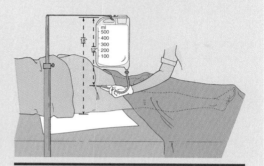

Figure 21-7   Step 14.

15 If giving a commercially prepared enema, squeeze and roll up the container to expel the contents into the rectum (Figure 21-8). Stop squeezing if the person complains of abdominal cramping, expels the solution, or is unable to hold the solution. Complete the administration when the symptoms subside.

16 Remove the tube from the anus, and replace the cap.

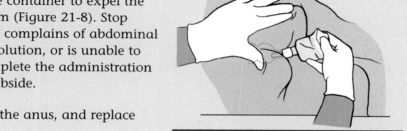

Figure 21-8   Step 15.

17 Help the patient to the bathroom or bedside commode or onto the bedpan with the head of the bed elevated (Figure 21-9).

18 Place the signal light within reach, and ask the patient to call when he has expelled the solution. Provide privacy as safety permits.

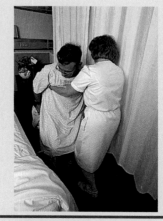

Figure 21-9   Step 17.

Continued

Procedure
ADMINISTERING AN ENEMA—cont'd

19 Discard all disposable items.

20 Remove your gloves and wash your hands.

21 Return when the patient signals he is finished.

22 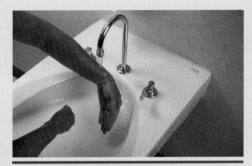 Wash your hands and put on gloves (Figure 21-10).

23 Look at the enema results for amount, color, and consistency.

24 Assist the patient with pericare and hand washing, if needed.

25 Empty, disinfect, and return all equipment to its proper place.

Figure 21-10 Step 22.

26 Return top linens, and remove the bath blanket.

27 Remove your gloves and wash your hands.

28 Report results to the charge nurse or document in the chart according to your facility's policy.

◆ **COMPLETE STANDARD ENDING STEPS (see inside front cover)**

Use of a Rectal Tube

A **rectal tube** is a tube inserted about 4 inches into the patient's rectum to relieve flatulence and abdominal bloating or distention. It can be left in place for up to 20 to 30 minutes.

A rectal tube is never used for a patient who has had rectal surgery.

The rectal tube may be connected to a bag or a container filled with water. Feces may be expelled along with the gas. Use of a rectal tube requires a doctor's order. Sometimes the doctor will order a **suppository**, a medication inserted into the rectum before inserting the rectal tube. The suppository is considered a medication and may not be given by the nursing assistant.

Safety

Procedure

INSERTING A RECTAL TUBE

EQUIPMENT
- **Bath blanket**
- **Bed protector**
- **Rectal tube and bag**
- **Water-soluble lubricant**
- **Gloves**

◆ **COMPLETE STANDARD BEGINNING STEPS (see inside front cover)**

1 Put on gloves.

2 Lower the side rail on the side of the bed nearest to you.

3 Lower the head of the bed.

4 Assist the patient into a left side-lying position (Figure 21-11).

5 Fanfold the covers to the foot of the bed, and cover the patient with a bath blanket.

6 Place a bed protector under the buttocks.

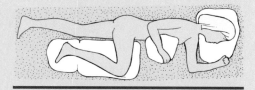

Figure 21-11 Step 4.

Continued

Procedure
INSERTING A RECTAL TUBE—cont'd

7 Expose the anal area (Figure 21-12).

8 Lubricate 4 inches of the rectal tube.

9 Separate the buttocks so that the anus is visible.

10 Ask the person to take a deep breath in through the mouth and to breathe out slowly.

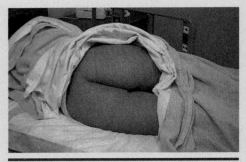

Figure 21-12 Step 7.

11 Gently insert the tube into the rectum as the person is breathing out. Stop if the person complains of pain or if you feel resistance (Figure 21-13).

12 Tape the rectal tube to the buttocks.

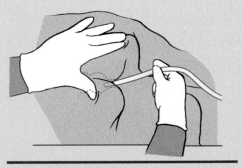

Figure 21-13 Step 11.

13 Position the bag so that it is on the bed protector (Figure 21-14). The rectal tube is inserted 4 inches into the adult rectum. The rectal tube is taped to the buttocks, and the bag is positioned so that it is on the bed protector.

14 Cover the person, and place the signal light within reach.

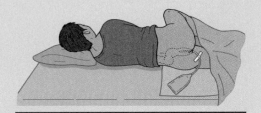

Figure 21-14 Step 13.

15 Raise the side rail if needed for safety.

16 Leave the tube in place for the amount of time the charge nurse requests but no more than 30 minutes.

17 Remove your gloves and wash your hands.

18 Return to the room when it is time to remove the tube.

Continued

Procedure

INSERTING A RECTAL TUBE—cont'd

19 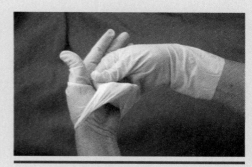 Wash your hands and put on gloves.

20 Remove the rectal tube, and assist the patient with pericare if needed.

21 Discard disposable items.

22 Remove your gloves and wash your hands (Figure 21-15).

23 Ask the patient about the amount of gas expelled, and report results to the charge nurse or document in the chart according to your facility's policy.

Figure 21-15 Step 22.

◆ COMPLETE STANDARD ENDING STEPS (see inside front cover)

How to Care for a Person With an Ostomy

An **ostomy** is a surgical procedure in which an opening is made to allow the passage of urine from the bladder or intestinal contents from the bowel to exit the body through a **stoma** or opening in the abdomen (Figure 21-15). A person may have an ostomy to correct a defect, to treat a disease such as cancer, or as the result of an injury such as a stab wound. The procedure is named for the location of the ostomy (Figure 21-16).

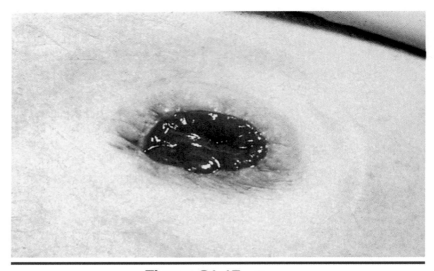

Figure 21-15 Stoma.

The person wears a pouch or bag over the stoma to collect the stool or urine (Figure 21-17). The bag has an adhesive back that is applied to clean, dry skin. Because there are no nerve endings in the stoma, this does not hurt the person. An elastic belt secures some bags. Many bags have a drain at the bottom that closes with a clip or clamp so that it can be easily emptied. Bags are usually changed 1 to 2 times a week or as desired by the person. Some people change their pouch or bag each day. There are many different types of ostomy products available (Figure 21-18). Your nurse will tell you what type the care plan lists for your patient.

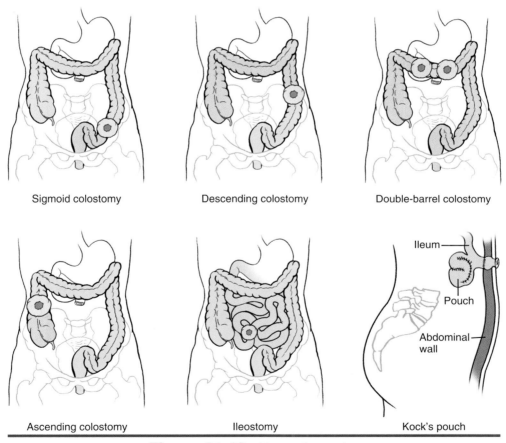

Sigmoid colostomy   Descending colostomy   Double-barrel colostomy

Ascending colostomy   Ileostomy   Kock's pouch

Ileum
Pouch
Abdominal wall

Figure **21-16**   Types of ostomies.

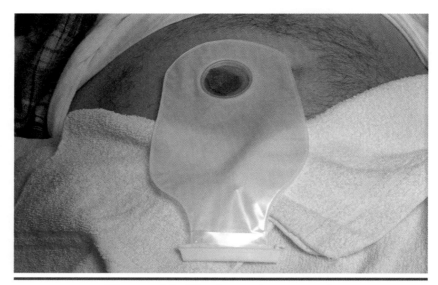

Figure **21-17**   Ostomy bag or pouch.

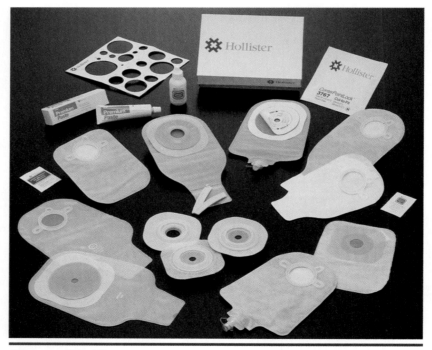

Figure **21-18**   There are many different types of ostomy products available.

The consistency of stool in a pouch depends on the location of the stoma (Table 21-1). Stools may be liquid to soft formed. The stool is irritating to the skin. Good skin care helps to prevent skin breakdown around the stoma. A skin barrier is usually used around the stoma to protect the skin.

Table 21-1

COMPARISON OF COLOSTOMIES AND ILEOSTOMY	
Type	Stool consistency
Ascending colostomy	Semi-liquid
Transverse colostomy	Semi-formed
Sigmoid colostomy	Formed
Ileostomy	Liquid to semi-liquid

Procedure
CHANGING AN OSTOMY BAG/POUCH

EQUIPMENT

- Bath blanket
- Bed protector
- Clean pouch/bag with skin barrier
- Basin of warm water
- Washcloth(s)
- Towel(s)
- Soap and soap dish
- Bedpan with cover
- Deodorant
- Clean belt, if worn
- Gloves

◆ **COMPLETE STANDARD BEGINNING STEPS** (**see inside front cover**)

1 Put on gloves.

2 Lower the side rail on the side of the bed nearest to you.

3 Lower the head of the bed, and raise the bed to a comfortable working height.

4 Assist the patient into a supine position.

5 Fanfold the covers to the foot of the bed, and cover the patient with a bath blanket.

Continued

Procedure
CHANGING AN OSTOMY BAG/POUCH—cont'd

6 Remove the old bag/pouch by gently pushing against the skin as you pull the pouch off.

7 Discard the old bag/pouch into the bedpan, and cover. Save the clip or clamp to re-use.

8 Clean the area around the stoma with warm water and soap, cleaning from the stoma outward.

9 Rinse well and pat dry.

10 Look at the skin around the stoma for redness or skin breakdown, and notify the charge nurse.

11 Add deodorant to the new pouch.

12 Remove the adhesive backing from the new pouch (Figure 21-19).

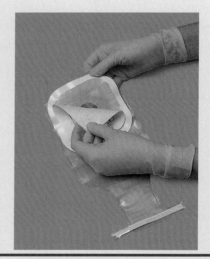

Figure 21-19   Step 12.

Procedure
CHANGING AN OSTOMY BAG/POUCH—cont'd

13 Center and apply the clean pouch over the stoma with the drain pointing downward (Figure 21-20).

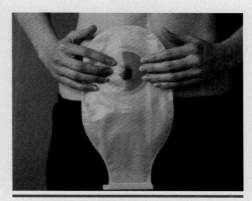

Figure **21-20**   Step 13.

14 Apply gentle pressure from the stoma outward to ensure a wrinkle-free seal between the adhesive and the skin (Figure 21-21).

15 Maintain pressure for 1 to 2 minutes.

16 Put a clean ostomy belt on the person, and connect to the bag if worn.

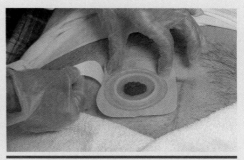

Figure **21-21**   Step 14.

17 Secure the end of the pouch with the clip or clamp (Figure 21-22).

18 Remove the bath blanket, and replace the covers.

19 Return the bed to its lowest position, and make the person comfortable.

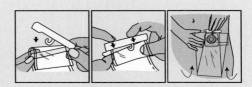

Figure **21-22**   Step 17.

20 Empty the pouch and bedpan into the toilet.

21 Dispose of the pouch according to facility policy.

22 Clean and return all equipment to its proper place.

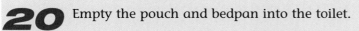

Continued

Procedure

CHANGING AN OSTOMY BAG/POUCH—cont'd

23 Remove your gloves and wash your hands.

24 Report completion of procedure to the charge nurse, or document in the chart according to facility policy.

 COMPLETE STANDARD ENDING STEPS (see inside front cover)

CHAPTER REVIEW

1. Define the following terms:
   Constipation
   Diarrhea
   Flatulence
   Impaction
   Incontinence

2. List 4 things the nursing assistant can do to help a patient maintain normal bowel function.

3. What is the purpose of a bowel re-training program?

4. What is an enema, and why is it used?

5. What should you do if the patient complains of abdominal cramping or is unable to hold the solution during the administration of an enema?

6. What is the purpose of a rectal tube?

7. How long is a rectal tube left in place?

8. How often should an ostomy bag or pouch be changed?

Circle the one BEST response.

9. What is the wavelike movement of the intestine called?
   a. Feces
   b. Stool
   c. Peristalsis
   d. Defecation

10. Which type of enema would be used as a cleansing enema before intestinal surgery?
    a. Phosphate enema
    b. Oil retention enema
    c. Soapsuds enema
    d. Commercial enema

11. What temperature of water is used when giving a tap water enema?
    a. 105° F
    b. 115° F
    c. 125° F
    d. 135° F

12. When providing ostomy care, how should the area around the stoma be cleaned?
    a. With disinfectant
    b. With a dry towel
    c. With cool water
    d. With warm water and soap

Answers are on page 709.

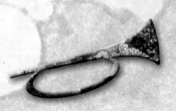

CHAPTER 22

Admission, Transfer, and Discharge

What you will learn

- The admission process
- How to prepare a patient room for an admission
- The role of the nursing assistant in the admission process
- The steps to transfer a patient to another unit within the facility
- The role of the nursing assistant in discharging a patient from a health care facility

KEY TERMS

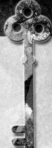

Admission The official entry of a person into a health care facility

AMA (against medical advice) discharge When the patient leaves the facility without the doctor's permission or against medical advice

Assessment Getting information about the patient's condition

Discharge The patient's release from the health care facility

Elective Done by choice

Emergency An event that calls for immediate action; a situation that is unplanned and threatens the life of the patient

Height How tall the patient is, usually in feet and inches

ID band Identification band applied to the patient's wrist that gives information that may include the patient's name, room number, patient number, doctor, and age

Intensive care unit A hospital unit that gives care to patients who need to be watched closely

Private room A room that has only 1 patient in it

Semi-private room A room that is shared with at least 1 other patient

Transfer To move a patient from one place to another in the facility

Vital signs Temperature, pulse, respiration, and blood pressure

Weight How much a patient weighs in pounds or kilograms

The Admission Process

An **admission** is the entry of a person into a health care facility. The patient may arrive from home, from the doctor's office, from the site of an accident or injury, or from another health care facility. Some admissions are **elective**. This means that the person chooses to enter the facility. Elective admissions are planned in advance. In some cases patients are admitted as an **emergency** admission. An emergency admission means that the person did not plan on being admitted to the hospital but became ill or was injured.

The patient's first impressions of the health care facility are important. When the patient and family have a positive first impression, the entire stay is more likely to be positive.

Being admitted to a health care facility can be stressful for both the patient and the family members. The patient is entering an unknown place and may be worried about illness or disease. Patients entering a nursing home may be upset about giving up their independence. Many patients feel unsafe and insecure in the health care facility.

Each facility has policies and procedures for admitting patients, but many procedures are similar. The nursing assistant plays an important role during the admission. Your professional and polite manner will help the patient to gain confidence in the facility and make the admission easier for the patient and his family.

Preparing a Room for a Patient Admission

The first step of the admission occurs before the patient even arrives on the nursing unit. A room is prepared for the patient as soon as the nursing unit is notified that someone is coming (Figure 22-1). It is usually the nursing assistant's job to prepare the room before the patient arrives. The way that the nursing assistant prepares the room varies from facility to facility. For example, some facilities may turn back the bed covers, and others do not. Your responsibilities in preparing the room will usually include:

- Making sure that the room is clean and odor free
- Making sure that the bed is made according to facility policy
- Placing clean towels and washcloths in the bathroom
- Providing an admission kit if used by your facility. This kit usually includes a bath basin, water glass and pitcher, and personal care supplies.

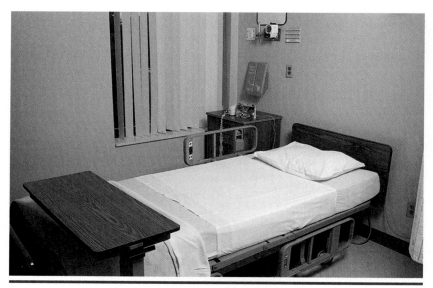

Figure 22-1   Room prepared for patient admission.

The Role of the Nursing Assistant in the Admission Process

The admission begins when patients enter the health care facility and lasts until they are settled in the room. An admitting clerk in the admitting office or emergency department gets general information about the patient and begins the admission. Patients admitted to a hospital are given an **ID (identification) band** that will be used to identify them for all procedures while they are in the hospital. Nursing homes may use ID bands or bracelets depending on the policy of the facility.

After check-in, the patient is brought to his room. The members of the health care team gather information about the patient. There is usually an admission form or checklist the nursing department completes that includes the following:

- Patient's temperature, pulse, respiration, and blood pressure
- Patient's **height** and **weight**
- Patient's physical condition on admission, including mental status, emotional state, disabilities, and complaints of pain

The nurse may ask you to assist in completing the admission form or checklist.

In many cases the nursing assistant is the first person patients see when they are admitted to their room (Figure 22-2). To make the patient feel welcome you should:

- Greet the patient by name, for example, Mr. Little or Ms. Henderson
- Introduce yourself to the patient and family
- Ask what name the patient prefers to be called
- Explain what you will be doing

NOTES ON
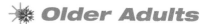
Older Adults

In some long-term care centers the residents are identified by a picture in the chart or on the door rather than with an ID bracelet.

Figure 22-2   Nursing assistant admitting a new patient.

NOTES ON
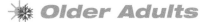 *Older Adults*

In a long-term care center or nursing home the resident is usually introduced to the roommate and given a tour of the facility.

NOTES ON
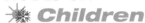 *Culture*

In some cultures the family is very involved in the patient's health care. Other cultures may prefer that the family leave the room while the patient is being admitted. Always ask your patients if they would like any family members to stay in the room or to step into the hallway during the admission.

NOTES ON
Children

When admitting a child, the parent(s) usually remains in the room.

- Make the patient comfortable in the bed or chair
- Show the patient how to operate the controls on the bed
- Show the patient how to call for help using the signal light or call light system
- Put the patient's belongings in the closet or drawers

You may need to repeat the information you give to the patient several times. People who are anxious or frightened may not hear or remember the information as well as they normally would. It is important to make the patient feel as comfortable as possible.

The nursing assistant should complete the portions of the admission form or checklist as the nurse instructs. Check the policies and procedures of your facility about which parts of the admission checklist you are responsible for. This usually includes obtaining the patient's **vital signs**, height, and weight (Chapter 13). It is the responsibility of the nurse to complete the **assessment** portion of the admission information (Figures 22-3 and 22-4). In some facilities the nursing assistant completes a list of the items the patient brought to the facility (Figure 22-5).

Text continued on p. 473

ADMISSION RECORD - SKILLED NURSING

Last Name	First Name	Middle Name	Date	Time
Attending Physician	Name, Relationship & Phone Number of primary family contact person:		Room & Bed #	Records #

Admitting Diagnosis | Height | Weight

Allergies | Temp | Pulse | Resp. | B/P

General physical appearance_____

Patient wears (circle): Dentures: upper lower partial   Glasses   Prosthesis (specify)_____

Brace or splint (specify)_____

Indicate on diagrams below all marks or deformities, e.g. bruises, scars, pressure areas, discolorations, amputations, malformations. Describe in detail in area provided.

Description:

Resident and family have been oriented to the following:

○ Use of call light   ○ Visiting hours/policies   ○ Meal times/procedures   ○ Room location   ○ Smoking policy   ○ Activity program   ○ Laundry done by (circle one) facility family

T.B. SCREENING

○ Chest X-ray Date:_____   ○ Mantoux Test Date:_____

○ NEGATIVE   ○ POSITIVE   ○ NEGATIVE   ○ POSITIVE

○ Copy of report in chart   ○ Copy of test document in chart

Sig. of Nurse verifying_____

CONTINENCE ASSESSMENT (circle below)

Continent Bowel Bladder   Incontinent Bowel Bladder   Catheter condom Foley suprapubic

Sig. of RN doing assessment: Date:

ADMISSION NOTES_____

Signature of Licensed Nurse (use back for additional notes if needed)

Figure 22-3   Sample long-term care center admission form.

Ashland Community Hospital

ADMIT FORM

Part I: Admission Routine		

		Temp.	Pulse	Resp.

Date   Time

Mode ☐ amb. ☐ gurney ☐ wc ☐ other   B/P

Via ☐ admitting ☐ ER ☐ other   Height   Actual Weight

Admitting Physician: **Family Physician:**

Admitting Diagnosis:

Most Recent Adm. (hosp./date/reason)

Patient's Statement (of present complaint)

Allergies:

Type of Reaction

Medications Patient's significant other understands purpose ☐ yes ☐ no   **Disposition of meds:**

Medication and strength	freq.	time last dose	Medication and strength	freq.	time last dose	
1.			6.			☐ did not bring
2.			7.			☐ patient has
3.			8.			☐ family has
4.			9.			☐ pharmacy
5.			10.			

Valuables List: (jewelry, clothing, etc.)

☐ glasses   ☐ contact lenses   ☐ dentures—   ☐ bridge/partial   ☐ other

Oriented to   ☐ room   ☐ bed   ☐ phone   ☐ call light/TV   ☐ visiting hours   ☐ safety/smoking policy
                    ☐ doctor's orders   ☐ armband

Part II: Patient/Family History		

Patient History (major illnesses/operations/major injuries) include endocrine history/problems—past pregnancies

1	4	7
2	5	8
3	6	9

Use of tobacco   ☐ no   ☐ yes   Type   Daily amount

Use of alcohol   ☐ no   ☐ yes   Type   Daily amount

Organ donor   ☐ no   ☐ yes   Living will ☐ no ☐ yes   If yes, copy at ACH ☐ no ☐ yes

Other pertinent information:

Family History   ☐ heart disease   ☐ stroke   ☐ hypertension   ☐ asthma   ☐ TB   ☐ diabetes   ☐ cancer
☐ kidney disease   ☐ allergy   ☐ epilepsy   ☐ blood disorder   ☐ mental disorder   ☐ other

Socio/Economic Religion: Marital status: ☐ single   ☐ married   ☐ divorced   ☐ widowed

Family   ☐ lives with   ☐ lives alone   ☐ no family   **Lives in**   ☐ house   ☐ apt.   ☐ other

Occupation   ☐ full time   ☐ part time   ☐ retired   ☐ other

ADL   ☐ independent   ☐ needs assist with (specify what kind of help is needed and who provides it)

Anticipated Discharge Needs: ☐ self care   ☐ community agency   ☐ discharge planner   ☐ other

Comments/plan:

Notify in emergency: relation   phone

Nearest relative: relation   phone

Info obtained from   ☐ patient   ☐ family   ☐ other   **Admitting Nurse:**

ACH 144

Figure 22-4 Sample hospital admission form.

Part III: System Assessment

Place an "X" in area of abnormality. If unable to assess, indicate reason.

Assess eyes, ears, nose, throat for abnormality. ☐ No problem

E E N T (other)

impaired vision	blind	pain	reddened	drainage	gums
hard of hearing	deaf	burning	edema	lesion	teeth

Explain: _____

Assess chest configuration, resp. rate, rhythm, depth, pattern, breath sounds, comfort. ☐ No problem

R E S P (other)

asymmetric	tachypnea	apnea	rales	cough	absent
barrel-chest	bradypnea	shallow	rhonchi	sputum	diminished
dyspnea	orthopnea	labored	wheezing	pain	cyanotic

Explain: _____

Assess heart sounds, rate rhythm, pulse, blood pressure, circulation, fluid retention, comfort. ☐ No problem

C V (other)

arrhythmia	tachycardia	rub	numbness	dimin. pulses	edema
irregular	bradycardia	murmur	tingling	absent pulses	
pain	S₃ or S₄	fatigue			

Explain: _____

Assess weight, abdomen, bowel habits, swallowing, bowel sounds, comfort. ☐ No problem

Home diet/food habits/caffeine amount—   stool color

G I (other)

weight loss	N or V	anorexia	diarrhea	distention	hypoactive BS	mass
obese	thirst	dysphagic	constipation	rigidity	hyperactive BS	pain

Explain: _____

Assess urine freq., control, color, consistency, odor, comfort/Gyn—bleeding, discharge, pregnancy. ☐ No problem

G U and G Y N (other)

Birth control method   last menses   last Pap smear

pain	hesitancy	oliguria	dysuria	urine color	vaginal bleeding	circumcised
frequency	incontinent	nocturia	hematuria	discharge	pregnancy	ø circumcised

Explain: _____

Assess motor function, sensation, LOC, strength, grip, gait, coordination, orientation, speech, vision. ☐ No problem

N E U R O (other)

weakness	numbness	headache	paralysis	stuporous	pupils
unsteady	tingling	seizures	lethargic	comatose	speech
vertigo	pain	tremors	confused	vision	grip

Explain: _____

Assess mobility, motion, gait, alignment, joint function/Skin color, texture, turgor, integrity. ☐ No problem

M S and S K I N

appliance	stiffness	itching	petechiae	hot	drainage
prosthesis	swelling	lesion	poor turgor	cool	
deformity	wound	rash	skin color	flushed	
atrophy	pain	eochymosis	diaphoretic	moist	

Explain: _____

Date: _____ Time: _____ R.N. Signature: _____

Figure 22-4, cont'd   Sample hospital admission form.

SAMPLE INVENTORY OF PERSONAL EFFECTS

INVENTORY OF PERSONAL EFFECTS

INSTRUCTIONS: Upon admission, identify the resident's personal belonging by indicating quantity of those items listed. Use the extra spaces to write in additional items as necessary. Keep the original copy in the resident's chart. Give the copy to the resident or resident representative. Update as necessary throughout the resident's stay by using the space provided. Upon discharge, use the "√" columns to indicate that all personal belongings are accounted for.

QTY.	ARTICLES	√	ITEMS OF SPECIFIC VALUE (JEWELRY, APPLIANCES, FURNITURE)			
			QTY.	DESCRIPTION	VALUE	√
	Belts				$	
	Blouses					
	Coats					
	Dresses					
	Gloves					
	Handkerchiefs					
	Hats					
	Housecoats/robes					
	Jackets					
	Nightgown/pajamas					
	Purses					
	Shaving kit					

	ITEMS ACQUIRED AFTER ORIGINAL ENTRY			√
	DATE	ITEM	HOW RECEIVED	INITIAL

QTY.	ARTICLES	√
	Shoes	
	Shorts	
	Slacks	
	Slippers	
	Slips	
	Shirts	
	Socks/hose	
	Suitcases	
	Suits	
	Suspenders	
	Sweaters	
	Ties	
	Undershirts	
	Underwear	

	USE THIS SPACE TO RECORD MISCELLANEOUS INFORMATION (LOST, STOLEN, RETURNED/GIVEN TO FAMILY, ETC.)		√
	DATE	DESCRIPTION/EXPLANATION	INITIAL

QTY.	ARTICLES	√
	Hearing aid	
	Dentures: Up Low Part	
	Eyewear	
	Cane	
	Walker	
	Wheelchair	
	Brace	
	Prosthetics	

CERTIFICATION OF RECEIPT

ON ADMISSION	ON DISCHARGE

Signed **X**_____
     Resident or resident representative   *Date*
Signed _____
     Facility representative   *Title*   *Date*
	Signed **X**_____
	     Resident or resident representative *Date*
	Signed _____
	     Facility representative *Title* *Date*

If resident unable to sign, state reason:	If resident unable to sign, state reason:

Signed _____
     Witness   *Date*
	Signed _____
	     Witness *Date*

Name - Last First Middle	Attending Physician Chart No.

(Adapted from Briggs Corporation, Des Moines, IA)

Figure 22-5 Patient inventory of personal effects.

Transferring a Patient to Another Unit Within the Facility

The term **transfer** means to move the patient from one place to another. Patients may be transferred from one room to another or from one unit or floor to another unit or floor within the facility. The patient or patient's family may request a transfer if the patient does not get along with his roommate or desires to move from a **semi-private** to a **private room.** Patients are also transferred when the type of care they require changes, such as moving from the **intensive care unit** to a regular nursing unit.

The transfer is done according to the policy of the health care facility. It is important that the transfer be as easy as possible for the patient and his family. If the purpose of the transfer is explained to the patient in advance, it is less likely to upset the patient.

In a long-term care center the resident must be notified of a transfer or room change before the transfer.

OBRA

The nurse will give you information about the transfer, including the room number and unit the patient will transfer to and the method of transfer (for example, bed, wheelchair, or stretcher). A time for the transfer is usually decided on between the nurse on the unit the patient is transferring from and the nurse on the unit the patient is transferring to. At the appropriate time the nursing assistant should:

- Explain or reinforce the nurse's explanation of the reason for the transfer
- Collect the patient's personal belonging and care items, and place them on a rolling cart
- Physically transfer the patient to the new room using the method the nurse indicates (for example, bed, wheelchair, or stretcher)
- Make the patient comfortable in the bed or chair
- Transfer the patient's belongings to the new room
- Introduce the patient to the staff on the new unit

In some facilities the nursing assistant will take the medical record to the new unit with the patient.

After returning to your unit, report to the nurse that the patient has been transferred and any observations you made during the transfer. Follow your facility's policy for cleaning the room after the patient has left.

HOW & WHY

To protect the patient's privacy, hand the medical record directly to the nurse on the new unit. *Do not leave it in the patient's room or at the nurses' station.*

Discharging a Patient From a Health Care Facility

A **discharge** is the patient's release from the health care facility. The doctor writes an order for the patient to be discharged. Patients leaving the facility may return home, go to the home of a friend or relative, or to another health care facility. Patients who leave the facility permanently are considered discharged. Patients and family members may be worried about the discharge. Many patients may not be sure of their ability to care for themselves after discharge. The entire health care team is involved in planning for the patient's discharge. The patient discharge plan includes instructions and arrangements for follow-up or home care, therapy, or other services the patient will need after discharge (Figure 22-6).

The nurse is responsible for the discharge and will give you the information you need to help the patient. Patients are discharged only with a doctor's order. To help with the discharge process the nursing assistant should:

- Make sure that the patient is clean and well groomed.
- Assist the patient with dressing in clothes appropriate to the weather. A family member may need to bring a coat or jacket if the weather is cold and the patient does not have one.
- Gather patients' personal belongings and pack them. If patients are able to do this on their own, check the dresser drawers and closets to make sure they have not forgotten anything. Some facilities have an inventory of patient belongings that must be checked to make sure that the patient has everything. Check with your facility regarding its policy.
- Make sure that the patient has items such as glasses, dentures, or hearing aids.
- Make sure that the patient and family have received care instructions and any paperwork or medications that are being sent with the patient at discharge. Do not remove the patient from the room until the nurse lets you know that it is all right to do so.
- If the patient is going to another health care facility, the nurse will complete a transfer form to provide information to the new facility (Figure 22-7). The nursing assistant should make sure that this form is sent with the patient.
- Assist the patient and family to the business office to complete any billing arrangements if necessary.
- If a patient's belongings were placed in a safe on admission, make sure the patient has these items before leaving the facility.

Barnes Hospital

PATIENT DISCHARGE SUMMARY

C-16

Addressograph Plate

Date _10/17/04_   Time _____1030_____

MEANS: ☐ Ambulatory ☒ Wheelchair ☐ Stretcher

METHODS: ☒ M.D. order ☐ AMA with release ☐ AMA with release

Afebrile 24 hours? ☒ Yes ☐ No   TPR _36^8-72-16_____   B/P _124/72_____

☐ Physician notified of irregularities

DISCHARGED TO: ☐ Home ☐ Nursing Home ☒ Home with Home Health Care ☐ Other

   If discharged to Nursing Home or other facility/service:

   Name _____   Address/Phone _____

☐ Release of information form signed ☐ Chart copied ☐ Transfer form completed ☐ Transportation Arranged

DISCHARGE CONSIDERATIONS:

☐ Valuables from cashier   ☐ PTA meds returned   ☐ Scripts given
☒ NA   ☒ NA   ☒ NA

DISCHARGE INSTRUCTIONS

FOR PROBLEMS OR FOLLOW-UP:

   Physician _Dr. Stan Jones_____   Phone _362-5000____   Appt. _10/24/04____

   Other: _____

   _____

Activity: __To remain in bed with Ⓛ foot elevated on two pillows. May be up only__
   __to go to the bathroom.__

Diet: _To follow 1800 calorie ADA diet as instructed by the dietitian. For questions__
   __about diet, call the dietitian (Sue Marlin) 362-3184.__

Medications: _To take usual dosage of 30 units NPH insulin and 8 units of regular__
   __insulin every morning before breakfast.__

Wound Care: ___Change dressings to Ⓛ foot daily using moistened fine mesh gauze__
   __with dry 4x4 gauze and wrap dressings with 4 kling gauze.__

Teaching Materials Given: _Copy of "Controlling Your Diabetes" and "Diabetic Menu__
   __Planning."__

Special Instructions: __Call doctor for increased pain, redness, swelling or drainage from__
   __Ⓛ foot wound. Barnes Home Health nurses will be visiting daily to change__
   __dressing to Ⓛ foot.__

My discharge instructions have been explained and a copy has been given to me.

Patient/Significant Other _*John Owens*_____   Relation ___HUSBAND____

Nurse _B. Rand, RN_____

Figure 22-6 Sample discharge summary.

INTERFACILITY TRANSFER AND ORDER FORM

PATIENT	BIRTHDATE	AGE	SEX	MARITAL STATUS S M W D SEP	RELIGION	HOSPITAL #

ADDRESS CITY	PHONE	ADM. DATE	DISCHARGE DATE

NEAREST RELATIVE OR FRIEND RELATIONSHIP PHONE	PHYSICIAN IN CHARGE AT TIME OF TRANSFER	PHONE

TRANSFERRED TO ADDRESS	PHONE	TRANSFERRED FROM	DISCHARGE COORD.

DISCHARGE DIAGNOSIS	SURGERY/DATE

Rehab Potential ❑ Good ❑ Fair ❑ Poor

Patient informed of condition ❑ Yes ❑ No If No/Why not?_____

Date of Chest X-ray or PPd _____ Results_____

Durable Power of Attorney: ❑ Yes ❑ No

Durable Power of Attorney For Health Care: ❑ Yes ❑ No

CPR Status ❑ Yes ❑ No

   Discussed with Family ❑ Yes ❑ No Discussed with Patient ❑ Yes ❑ No

Foley Catheter: ❑ Yes ❑ No   Catheter Size_____ Balloon Size_____

Reason for Catheter: ❑ Neurogenic ❑ Post Operative

❑ Other_____

Replace Foley Cath. Every 30 days and/or PRN non-patency ❑ Yes ❑ No

Diet:_____.

NG or G Tube: ❑ Yes ❑ No Give _____Cal_____cc

House Formula: or_____every 24 Hrs.

Flush tube with _____cc of water every_____Hrs. and post medication administration.

Replace NG tube when plugged, PRN. ❑ Yes ❑ No Routine Dental Care: ❑ Yes

Podiatry Care: q .3 mon. PRN (For mycotic/hypertrophic nails) ❑ Yes ❑ No

May participate in activity plan not in conflict with treatment plan.

"I certify that post-hospital ECF services are required on inpatient basis, because of individual need for skilled nursing care on a continuous basis for condition(s) for which patient was receiving inpatient hospital care".

REHABILITATIVE THERAPY

P.T. Evaluation ❑ Yes ❑ No Rx Plan:

Speech Evaluation ❑ Yes ❑ No Rx Plan:

OT Evaluation ❑ Yes ❑ No Rx Plan:

MOBILITY LEVEL: ❑ UP IN CHAIR ❑ UP AD LIB ❑ BED REST ❑ OTHER:_____

TREATMENT/WOUND AND SKIN CARE (SPECIFIC AREA TREATED): ISOLATION ❑ YES ❑ NO

RA ABG'S (COPY)	O2 (ROUTE) LPM	CONT.	PRN	CHANGE CANNULA, TUBING, HUMIDIFIER Q 5 DAYS
DIABETIC MONITORING:		DIALYSIS ❑		RADIATION THERAPY ❑

ALLERGIES:

MEDICATIONS	DOSAGE & FREQUENCY	DIAGNOSES (Every medication must have a diagnosis)

HISTORY AND PHYSICAL UPDATE ❑ YES ❑ NO   IF YES: PLEASE COMMENT.

PERIODIC LABS: (Any required to monitor meds)   FREQUENCY:

SIGNATURE_____ M.D. DATE_____

Figure 22-7 Sample inter-facility transfer form.

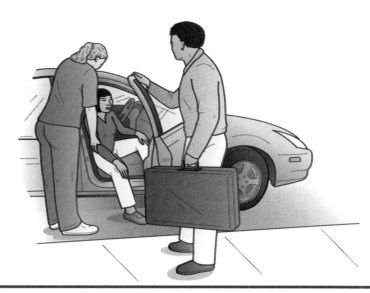

***Figure* 22-8**   Assist patients with putting their belongings in the car. The facility is responsible for patients until they are in the car with the door closed.

- Help the patient to the door and out of the building. The facility is responsible for patients until they are in the car with the door closed. Many facilities require that the patient use a wheelchair during discharge.
- Assist with putting the patient's belongings into the car (Figure 22-8).
- Report to the nurse that the discharge is complete.

Follow your facility's policy for cleaning the room after the patient has left.

Some patients may be unable to leave the facility in a car and must return home or move to a new facility in an ambulance. The nurse will tell you if there is anything special you need to know about the discharge.

Occasionally a patient will leave the facility without the doctor's permission. This is called an **AMA (against medical advice) discharge.** Let the nurse know right away if patients or family tells you that they plan on leaving.

Remember that the patient's last impressions are important to the relationship between the patient and the facility. The nursing assistant is usually the last employee to have contact with the patient. Make a special effort to tell the patient goodbye and to make this a good experience for the patient.

CHAPTER REVIEW

1. Who determines the time frame for a patient transfer?

2. List 4 responsibilities of the nursing assistant in preparing a room for an admission.

3. What is the purpose of an ID band?

4. When does the facility's responsibility for the care of the patient end?

Circle the one BEST response.

5. The official entry of the patient into the health care facility is called a(n)
   a. Admission
   b. Transfer
   c. Discharge
   d. AMA discharge

6. Patients entering a hospital or nursing home may feel
   a. Scared
   b. Upset
   c. Worried
   d. All of the above

7. The nursing assistant usually completes the part of the admission form that includes
   a. Height, weight, and vital signs
   b. Weight, medications, and patient history
   c. Vital signs, diagnosis, and doctor's name
   d. Insurance information, height, and age

8. Moving a patient from one place to another in the facility is called a(n)
   a. Admission
   b. Transfer
   c. Discharge
   d. AMA discharge

9. When taking the medical record to the new unit with the patient, the nursing assistant should
   a. Leave it on the counter in the nurses' station
   b. Place it in the patient's room
   c. Hand it to the nurse on the new unit
   d. Give it to the patient

10. The patient's authorized release from the facility is called a(n)
    a. Admission
    b. Transfer
    c. Discharge
    d. AMA discharge

11. If a patient tells you that he is planning on leaving without the doctor's permission, the nursing assistant should:
    a. Tell the patient that he is not allowed to leave
    b. Call the doctor immediately
    c. Notify the nurse
    d. Let the family know that the patient is leaving

Answers are on page 710.

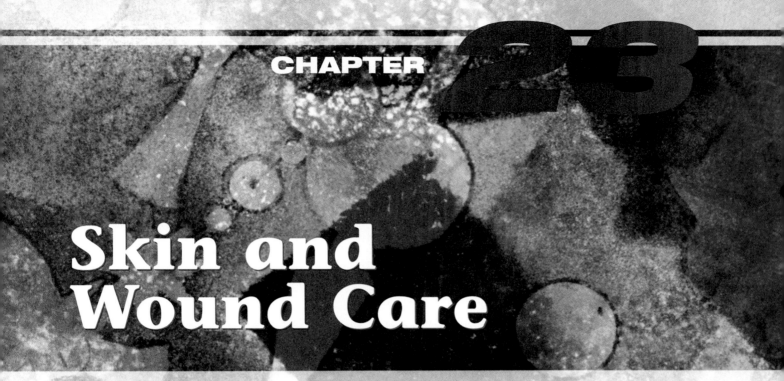

CHAPTER 23

Skin and Wound Care

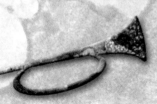

What you will learn

- Causes and stages of skin breakdown
- Methods for preventing skin breakdown
- How and why to give a back rub
- Care of pressure ulcers
- Care of circulatory ulcers
- How to apply elastic stockings
- Measures to promote wound healing
- Procedure to apply a dry, non-sterile dressing
- Use of abdominal binders

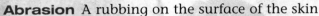

KEY TERMS

Abrasion A rubbing on the surface of the skin

Arterial Related to the arteries, the blood vessels that carry blood away from the heart

Blister A swelling on the skin filled with watery matter

Crater A cup-shaped opening

Diabetes A chronic disease caused by not enough production or use of insulin by the body

Edema Swelling, buildup of fluid in the tissues

Pressure ulcer An inflammation or sore that develops over areas where the skin and tissue underneath are injured due to a lack of blood flow and oxygen supply as a result of constant pressure

Shearing Pressure against the skin as tissues slide in the opposite direction from the underlying bones, such as when a patient slides down in bed

Skin tear A break in the skin that occurs when the top layer of the skin is separated from the underlying layers

Venous Related to the veins, the blood vessels that carry blood toward the heart

Wound Any physical injury involving a break in the skin

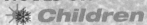

NOTES ON ❋ *Children*

Infants and toddlers are more likely to have to skin problems in the diaper area. It is important to clean the skin well with each diaper change and to notify your charge nurse if you notice signs of redness or a rash.

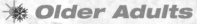

NOTES ON ❋ *Older Adults*

The skin of an older person is thinner and drier. The older person has less subcutaneous or fat tissue under the skin. Older people are more likely to develop skin tears than younger people.

Key Points of Skin Care

Skin care is an important part of daily grooming for the patient. Problems that appear on the skin can be a sign of a problem inside the body. Healthy skin can be maintained by keeping it clean and dry. Lotions can help keep skin from becoming too dry. A well-balanced diet and enough fluid intake also help to keep skin healthy. As you take care of the patient, look for any red or open areas on the patient's skin.

Causes of Skin Breakdown

There are different types of skin breakdown. A **skin tear** is a break in the skin that occurs when the top layer of the skin is separated from the underlying layers. It can be caused by holding a person's arm or leg too tightly or if the patient bumps an arm or leg against a hard surface such as a chair or bed rail. A skin tear is painful to the patient.

Shearing occurs when the body slides on a surface that moves the skin in one direction and the underlying bones in the opposite direction, such as when a patient slides down in bed (Figure 23-1). Tiny blood vessels are pinched or torn, and the supply of oxygen and other nutrients is cut off, leading to skin breakdown.

A **pressure ulcer** is an inflammation or sore that develops over areas where the skin and tissue underneath are injured due to a lack of blood flow and oxygen supply (Figure 23-2). The lack of circulation usually happens because of continuous pressure on the skin over a bony area. The way or length of time a patient is positioned can lead to pressure ulcers. Skin breakdown can occur after only 90 minutes of continuous pressure.

Most hospitals and nursing homes use a tool such as the Braden Scale to predict which patients are at risk for developing pressure ulcers (Figure 23-3). The Braden Scale uses a point system. Patients are given points in each of 6 areas. The points are added to get a total score. The nurse may ask for your help in filling out a tool such as the Braden Scale since the nursing assistant gives more hands-on care to the patient than any other member of the team. Patients who have a low number score are more likely to develop a pressure ulcer (Box 23-1).

Pressure ulcers develop in stages (Table 23-1).

HOW&**WHY**

Pressure ulcers are sometimes called bedsores, pressure sores, decubitus ulcers, and decubiti.

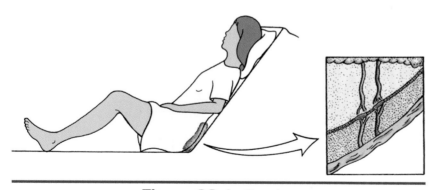

Figure 23-1 Shearing.

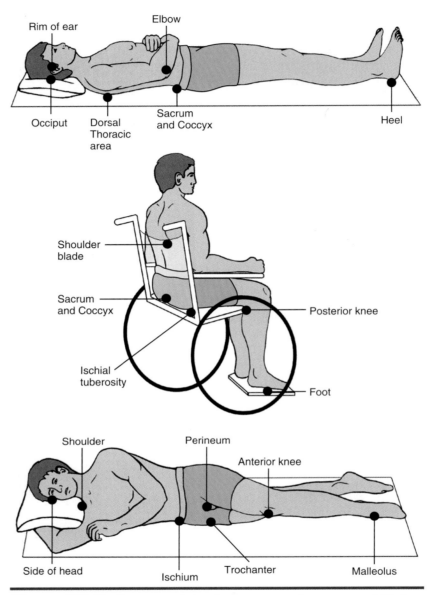

***Figure* 23-2** Pressure points where pressure ulcers are most likely to occur.

Braden Scale
FOR PREDICTING PRESSURE SORE RISK

Patient's Name _____ Evaluator's Name _____ Date of Assessment

SENSORY PERCEPTION ability to respond meaning-fully to pressure-related discomfort	**1. Completely limited:** Unresponsive (does not moan, flinch, or grasp) to painful stimuli, due to diminished level of con-sciousness or sedation. OR limited ability to feel pain over most of body surface.	**2. Very Limited:** Responds only to painful stimuli. Cannot communicate discomfort except by moaning or restlessness. OR has a sensory impairment which limits the ability to feel pain or discomfort over 1/2 of body.	**3. Slightly Limited:** Responds to verbal com-mands, but cannot always communicate discomfort or need to be turned. OR has some sensory impairment which limits ability to feel pain or discomfort in 1 or 2 extremities.	**4. No Impairment:** Responds to verbal com-mands. Has no sensory deficit which would limit ability to feel or voice pain or discomfort.
MOISTURE degree to which skin is exposed to moisture	**1. Constantly Moist:** Skin is kept moist almost constantly by perspiration, urine, etc. Dampness is detected every time patient is moved or turned.	**2. Very Moist:** Skin is often, but not always moist. Linen must be changed at least once a shift.	**3. Occasionally Moist:** Skin is occasionally moist, requiring an extra linen change approximately once a day.	**4. Rarely Moist:** Skin is usually dry, linen only requires changing at routine intervals.
ACTIVITY degree of physical activity	**1. Bedfast:** Confined to bed	**2. Chairfast:** Ability to walk severely limited or non-existent. Cannot bear own weight and/or must be assisted into chair or wheel-chair.	**3. Walks Occasionally:** Walks occasionally during day, but for very short distances, with or without assistance. Spends majority of each shift in bed or chair.	**4. Walks Frequently:** walks outside the room at least twice a day and inside room at least once every 2 hours during waking hours.
MOBILITY ability to change and control body position	**1. Completely Immobile:** Does not make even slight changes in body or extremity position without assistance.	**2. Very Limited:** Makes occasional slight changes in body or extremity position but unable to make frequent or significant changes independently.	**3. Slightly Limited:** Makes frequent though slight changes in body or extremity position independently.	**4. No Limitations:** Makes major and frequent changes in position without assistance.
NUTRITION usual food intake pattern	**1. Very Poor:** Never eats a complete meal. Rarely eats more than 1/3 of any food offered. Eats 2 servings or less of protein (meat or dairy products) per day. Takes fluids poorly. Does not take a liquid dietary supplement. OR is NPO and/or maintained on clear liquids or IV's for more than 5 days.	**2. Probably Inadequate:** Rarely eats a complete meal and generally eats only about 1/2 of any food offered. Protein intake includes only 3 servings of meat or dairy products per day. Occasion-ally will take a dietary supplement. OR receives less than optimum amount of liquid diet or tube feeding.	**3. Adequate:** Eats over half of most meals. Eats a total of 4 servings of protein (meat, dairy products) each day. Occasionally will refuse a meal, but will usually take a supplement if offered. OR is on a tube feeding or TPN regimen which probably meets most of nutritional needs.	**4. Excellent:** Eats most of every meal. Never refuses a meal. Usually eats a total of 4 or more servings of meat and dairy products. Occasionally eats between meals. Does not require supplementation.
FRICTION AND SHEAR	**1. Problem:** Requires moderate to maximum assistance in moving. Complete lifting without sliding against sheets is impossible. Frequently slides down in bed or chair, requiring frequent repositioning with maximum assistance. Spasticity, contractures or agitation leads to almost constant friction.	**2. Potential Problem:** Moves feebly or requires minimum assistance . During a move skin probably slides to some extent against sheets, chair, restraints, or other devices. Maintains relatively good position in chair or bed most of the time but occasion-ally slides down.	**3. No Apparent Problem:** Moves in bed and in chair independently and has sufficient muscle strength to lift up completely during move. Maintains good position in bed or chair at all times.	

At risk = 15-18; Moderate risk = 13-14; High risk = 10-12; Severe Risk = 9.   Total Score

Figure 23-3 Braden Scale for predicting pressure ulcer risk.

Box 23-1

PATIENTS AT RISK FOR PRESSURE ULCERS

Patients who are at risk for pressure ulcers are those who:
- Are unable to move because of paralysis, weakness, or coma
- Are unwilling to move because of severe pain, depression, or confusion
- Are unable to control bowel or bladder function
- Have poor food or fluid intake, are dehydrated
- Have poor circulation, especially patients with diabetes
- Are elderly, obese, or very thin
- Have casts, braces, or splints

Table 23-1

PRESSURE ULCER STAGES

Definition

Stage I

The skin is pale or red and does not return to its normal color when the pressure is relieved. Warmth or swelling may be present. The patient may complain of pain, burning, or tingling. This stage may be difficult to see in a patient with dark-colored skin. At this stage the skin damage can be reversed.

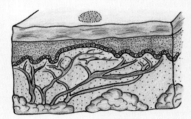 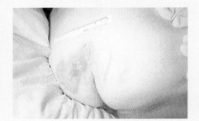

Stage II

Partial-thickness skin loss of the top layers of skin. May appear as a **blister, abrasion,** or shallow **crater.** The patient will usually complain of pain with a stage II ulcer.

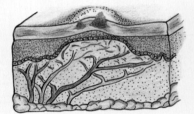 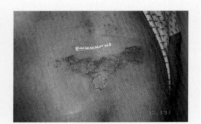

Stage III

Full-thickness skin loss with damage to fat tissue that may extend down to underlying muscle or bone. Appears as a deep crater, and drainage may be present.

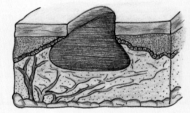 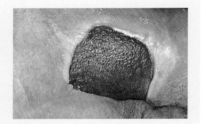

Stage IV

Full-thickness skin loss with extensive destruction; tissue death; damage to muscle, bone, tendons, or joints. Drainage is likely. At this stage, the patient does not generally feel pain at the site of the ulcer.

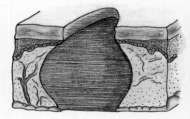 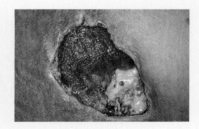

Preventing Skin Breakdown

Most pressure ulcers are preventable. It is more difficult and costly to treat a pressure ulcer than to prevent one. To prevent patients from developing pressure ulcers the nursing assistant should:

- Turn and reposition the patient at least every 2 hours. Follow your facility's policy regarding the use of a turning schedule individualized for each patient.
- Use pressure-relief devices such as pillows, cushions, and special mattresses as the nurse instructs and indicates on the care plan (Figures 23-4 to 23-7).
- Keep the skin clean and dry.
- Apply lotion to intact skin to prevent dry skin, such as during a back rub.
- Be gentle with the patient's skin when lifting or moving.
- Use a lift sheet to reposition the patient in the bed or chair. Do not slide or pull on the patient.
- Look at the skin when providing care to the patient, and report any areas of redness or breakdown to the nurse immediately.

OBRA requires that all residents of long-term care (LTC) centers receive skin care that prevents the development of pressure ulcers.

NOTES ON
☯ Culture

It may be harder to detect the early signs of a pressure ulcer in patients with dark skin tones. A stage I pressure ulcer may appear blue or purple in color rather than red. Dark skin that is damaged is more likely to appear shiny than skin that is lighter in color.

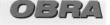

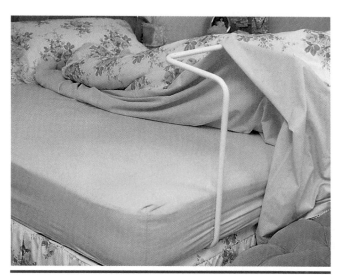

Figure 23-4   A bed cradle is a metal frame that is placed on the bed. The top linens are tucked in and mitered at the foot of the bed. The linens are brought over the top of the cradle to reduce pressure on the person's legs and feet.

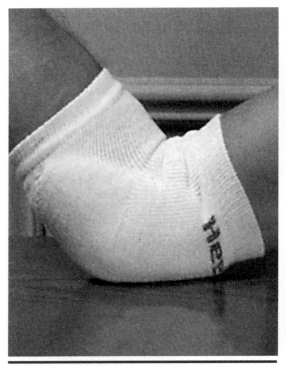

Figure 23-5 An elbow protector prevents the elbow from rubbing on the sheets.

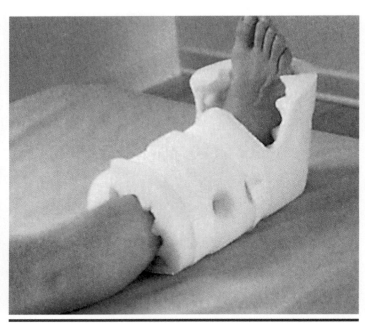

Figure 23-6 A heel elevator raises the heel off the mattress, reducing pressure.

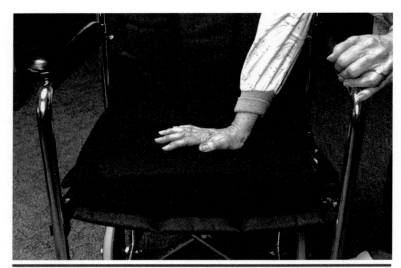

Figure 23-7 A flotation pad or mattress is filled with a gellike substance. It reduces pressure over bony areas when the person is in the bed or wheelchair. This photo shows a wheelchair flotation pad.

How and Why to Give a Back Rub

A back rub is usually given after the patient's bath or when he is repositioned in the bed. A back rub makes the patient more relaxed, eases muscle tension, and increases circulation. During a back rub, the nursing assistant has a chance to look at the skin for signs of redness or breakdown.

Procedure
GIVING A BACK RUB

EQUIPMENT

- Lotion
- Towel
- Gloves (if contact with blood) or body fluids is possible)

 COMPLETE STANDARD BEGINNING STEPS (see inside front cover)

1   Provide privacy for the patient.

2   Raise the bed to a comfortable working height.

3   Lower the side rail on the side nearest to you.

4   Assist the patient to a prone (lying on the stomach) or side-lying position with the back toward you.

5   Uncover the patient's back, and fold the covers down to the hips.

CAUTION

- If the skin is open or drainage is present, do not continue. Notify the nurse.

6   Put on gloves if needed.

7   If the skin is dirty, gently wash the back with soap and water; pat the skin dry (Figure 23-8).

8   Pour a small amount of lotion into your hand, and warm it by rubbing it between your hands.

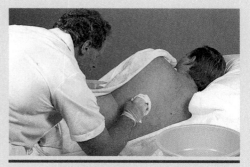

Figure 23-8   Step 7.

Continued

Procedure

GIVING A BACK RUB—cont'd

9 Begin by gently massaging the back in a circular motion, beginning at the sacral area (Figure 23-9).

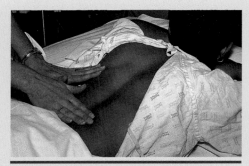

Figure 23-9   Step 9.

10 Using firm, smooth strokes, massage upward toward the shoulders, over the upper arms and back (Figure 23-10).

11 With long, smooth strokes, end the massage after 3 to 5 minutes, and remove excess lotion from the patient's back with a towel.

12 Retie the patient's gown.

13 Remove gloves if used and wash hands.

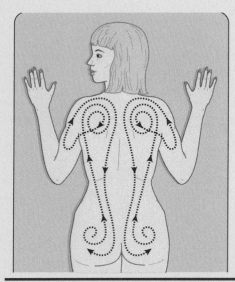

Figure 23-10   Step 10.

COMPLETE STANDARD ENDING STEPS **(see inside front cover)**

Care of Pressure Ulcers

When a patient has developed a pressure ulcer, the nurse will give you instructions about how to care for the wound. The nurse will follow the doctor's orders about what type of treatment to use with each patient. The nurse may ask the nursing assistant to help with the treatment.

The nursing assistant is NOT permitted to perform any treatments to open areas.

Safety

Remember to follow Standard Precautions when caring for a patient who has an open area on the skin.

Safety

The nursing assistant should observe the patient and report his observations to the nurse. Observations to make about pressure ulcers include:

- Location, such as "inside of the left ankle"
- Condition of the skin, such as "red and warm" or "open"
- Size—compare to familiar objects, such as "the size of a quarter"
- Drainage—report the amount and the color
- Odor if present
- Soiled or missing dressings

The nursing assistant is allowed to give pressure ulcer care to the patient who has a stage I pressure ulcer because the skin is not open.

Procedure

GIVING PRESSURE ULCER CARE TO THE PATIENT WITH A STAGE I PRESSURE ULCER

EQUIPMENT

- Lotion
- Basin of warm water
- Mild soap or body wash—per facility policy
- Washcloths
- Towels
- Dirty linen hamper
- Gloves (if contact with blood or body fluids is possible)

 COMPLETE STANDARD BEGINNING STEPS (see inside front cover)

1 Provide privacy for the patient.

2 Observe the reddened area.

CAUTION

- If the skin is open or drainage is present, do not continue and notify the nurse.

3 Put on gloves if needed.

4 Gently wash the area with soap and water if soiled; pat the skin dry (Figure 23-11).

5 Gently massage the skin *around* the reddened area with warm lotion.

6 Place clean linens on the bed if necessary.

7 Remove gloves if used and wash hands.

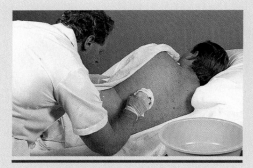

Figure 23-11 Step 4.

 COMPLETE STANDARD ENDING STEPS (see inside front cover)

Care of Circulatory Ulcers

Circulatory ulcers are caused by poor **venous** or **arterial** blood flow. Patients with poor venous circulation usually have swelling or **edema** in the lower leg (Figure 23-12). The skin on the foot and lower leg may be blue, gray, or brownish in color. The leg and foot may feel hard or cool to touch. Open areas are most common over the ankle (Figure 23-13). A venous or arterial ulcer looks very similar to a pressure ulcer. The doctor may place the patient on bedrest with the legs elevated or raised above the heart level. The doctor often orders drugs to decrease swelling and prevent infection. Venous ulcers are sometimes called stasis ulcers. Patients with varicose veins are at greater risk of having venous ulcers (Figure 23-14).

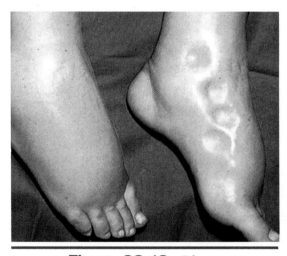

Figure 23-12   Edema.

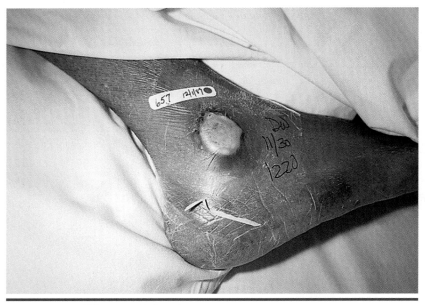

***Figure* 23-13** Ankle ulcer with dressing.

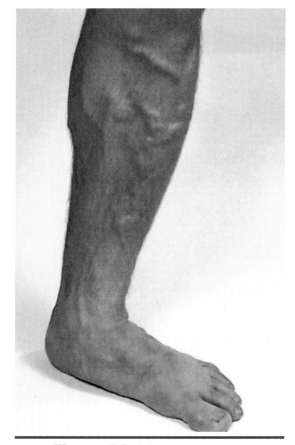

***Figure* 23-14** Varicose veins.

Patients who have poor arterial circulation usually complain of their feet and legs being cold. The color of the skin on the legs and feet will be darker than the rest of the skin and may appear reddish in color. The patient may complain of pain in the legs and feet at night or when resting. The pain is usually better if the patient stands or walks. Patients should be encouraged to wear well-fitting shoes and socks to prevent injury to the feet and lower legs. Patients with **diabetes** are at greater risk of having arterial ulcers.

Protective devices such as heel protectors or pillows that keep the heels and feet off the bed may be used. The doctor may order special elastic wraps or elastic stockings, sometimes called TED hose, to help the circulation in the lower legs.

Remove elastic stockings in the morning and evening, and give skin care to the legs. Some patients only wear their elastic stockings during the day while they are up. Other patients wear their stockings during the day and while they are sleeping. The nurse will order the stockings in the correct size and give you instructions about any special care required.

Wrinkles or twists in the stockings can cause skin irritation and breakdown.

Safety

The nursing assistant should observe the patient and report the observations to the nurse. Observations to make about circulatory ulcers are the same as those for pressure ulcers and include:

- Location, such as "inside of the left ankle"
- Condition of the skin, such as "red and warm" or "open"
- Size—compare to familiar objects such as "the size of a quarter"
- Drainage—report the amount and the color
- Odor if present
- Soiled or missing dressings

Procedure
APPLYING ELASTIC STOCKINGS

EQUIPMENT
* Elastic stockings

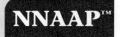

 COMPLETE STANDARD BEGINNING STEPS (see inside front cover)

1 Provide privacy for the patient.

2 Raise the bed to a comfortable working height.

3 Lower the side rail on the side nearest to you.

4 Assist the patient into a supine position, lying on her back.

5 Expose the legs by folding the linens up to the person's thigh.

6 Grasp the stocking at the top with both hands, and fold toward the toe end with the raised seams on the outside (Figure 23-15). (The manufacturer's instructions will give you information about the correct placement of the opening on the toe of the stocking.)

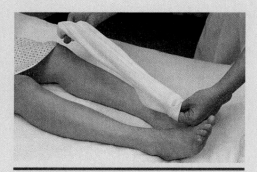

Figure 23-15   Step 6.

7 Adjust the toe of the stocking over the patient's toes (Figure 23-16).

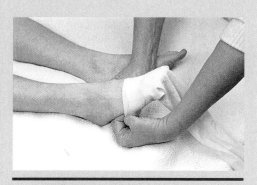

Figure 23-16   Step 7.

Continued

Procedure
APPLYING ELASTIC STOCKINGS—cont'd

8 Smooth the stocking up the leg, making sure that it is applied evenly and without wrinkles (Figure 23-17).

9 Repeat the procedure on the opposite leg.

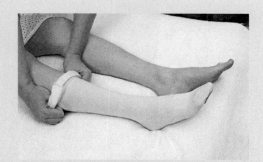

Figure 23-17 Step 8.

COMPLETE STANDARD ENDING STEPS (see inside front cover)

Promoting Wound Healing

A **wound** is any physical injury involving a break in the skin. An accident such as cutting the skin on the hand when using a kitchen knife causes a wound. An intentional act such as a surgical procedure also causes a wound. Figure 23-18 shows a surgical incision (wound) closed with staples. The edges of the incision are together, and there is no drainage from the site.

It may take anywhere from a few days to a year for a wound to heal, depending on the type of wound. For a wound to heal, the patient must have a well-balanced diet including adequate protein, carbohydrate, calorie, and fluid intake (Chapter 19). A patient who does not eat or drink enough will have a slower healing process. The wound must also be kept clean at all times. A wound that is not kept clean is more likely to become infected. Figure 23-19 shows an incision that has become infected. The edges of the incision are open, and there is yellow drainage present. In this photo the nurse is obtaining a sample of the drainage to check for infection. The nursing assistant should be aware of the signs of infection and report his observations to the nurse (Box 23-2).

Remember to follow standard precautions and the Bloodborne Pathogen Standard when caring for a patient who has an open area on the skin.

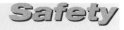

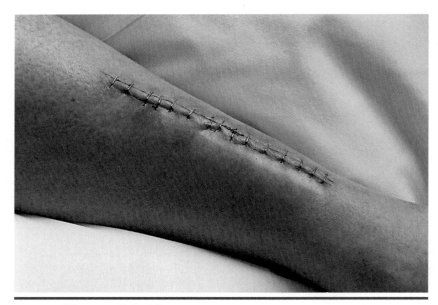

***Figure* 23-18**   Surgical incision closed with staples.

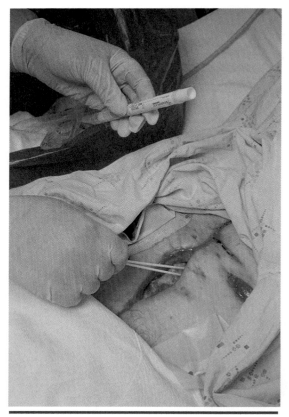

***Figure* 23-19**   The nurse is obtaining a
sample of the drainage to check for infection.

Box 23-2

SIGNS AND SYMPTOMS OF INFECTION

Signs and symptoms of infection can include:
- Redness
- Swelling
- Warmth
- Pain or tenderness
- Drainage, especially yellow, green, or brown
- Foul odor
- Increased body temperature

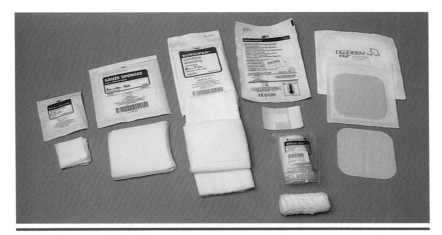

Figure 23-20 Examples of types of dressings available.

A clean, dry dressing may cover some wounds. There are many different types and sizes of dressings available (Figure 23-20). If your facility allows you to perform a non-sterile dressing change, the charge nurse will tell you what type of dressing to use.

Procedure
APPLYING A DRY NON-STERILE DRESSING

EQUIPMENT

- Clean dressing as directed by the nurse
- Tape
- Plastic bag
- Bath blanket
- Gloves and personal protective equipment as required

◆ **COMPLETE STANDARD BEGINNING STEPS (see inside front cover)**

1   Provide privacy for the patient.

2   Help the patient to a comfortable position.

3   Expose the affected body part, being careful to keep the patient covered as much as possible. Use a bath blanket to cover the patient if needed.

4   Put on gloves.

5   Remove the tape from the dressing by holding the skin down and pulling gently *toward* the wound.

6   Remove the old dressing, and place it in the plastic bag (Figure 23-21).

7   Look at the wound for signs of infection (see Box 23-2).

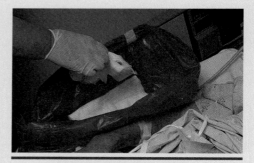

Figure 23-21   Step 6.

Procedure
APPLYING A DRY NON-STERILE DRESSING—cont'd

8 Remove gloves, and place them in the bag (Figure 23-22).

9 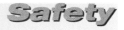 Wash your hands, and put on clean gloves.

10 Open the dressing package. Do not touch the dressing itself.

11 Apply the dressing as the nurse instructs.

12 Secure the dressing in place using tape.

13 Remove your gloves, and place them in the bag.

◆ **COMPLETE STANDARD ENDING STEPS (see inside front cover)**

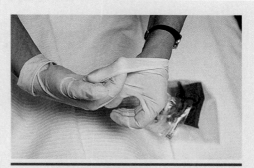

Figure 23-22   Step 8.

Use of Binders

Binders are used to support wounds and hold dressings in place. The most common type of binder is an elastic abdominal binder with a Velcro closure. Replace binders when they become wet or soiled. The abdominal binder should be released and re-wrapped every 4 hours or according to your facility's policy.

Wrinkles in the abdominal binder can cause pressure over the hipbones and may result in the formation of pressure ulcers. Make sure that the binder is wrinkle free.

Safety

Procedure
APPLYING AN ELASTIC ABDOMINAL BINDER

EQUIPMENT
- Abdominal binder
- Gloves (if contact with blood or body fluids is possible)

◆ **COMPLETE STANDARD BEGINNING STEPS** (see inside front cover)

1 Provide privacy for the patient.

2 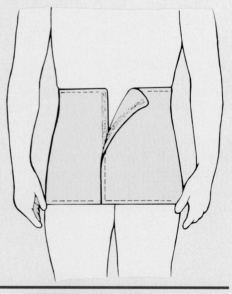 Put on gloves.

3 Help the patient to lie on his back (the supine position).

4 Ask the patient to raise his hips, and slide the binder under the patient with the top edge at the patient's waist.

5 Bring the edges of the binder around the patient, smooth the fabric, and secure by pressing the Velcro surfaces together (Figure 23-23).

6 The binder should provide firm support over the abdomen while still allowing the patient to breathe freely.

7 Remove your gloves and wash your hands.

Figure 23-23 Step 5.

◆ **COMPLETE STANDARD ENDING STEPS** (see inside front cover)

CHAPTER REVIEW

1. List 5 different types of patient conditions that put the person at risk for pressure ulcers.

2. At which stage is a pressure ulcer reversible?

3. Why is a back rub given?

4. What is the cause of circulatory ulcers?

5. Why are elastic stockings used?

6. List 7 signs or symptoms of a wound infection.

7. What is the purpose of an abdominal binder?

Circle the one BEST response.

8. An area of inflammation or a sore that develops over an area where the skin and tissue underneath are injured due to a lack of blood flow and oxygen supply is called a(n)
   a. Pressure ulcer
   b. Skin tear
   c. Abrasion
   d. Crater

9. A break in the skin that occurs when the top layer of the skin is separated from the underlying layers is called a(n)
   a. Pressure ulcer
   b. Skin tear
   c. Abrasion
   d. Crater

10. For a wound to heal the patient needs
    a. Good nutrition
    b. Adequate activity
    c. Medications
    d. Sterile dressings

11. When removing tape from a dressing you should
    a. Pull away from the wound
    b. Pull from top to bottom
    c. Pull towards the wound
    d. Pull from bottom to top

Answers are on page 710.

CHAPTER 24

Heat and Cold Applications

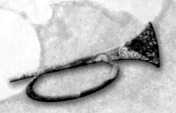

What you will learn

- Why heat and cold applications are ordered
- The effects of heat and cold applications
- Possible complications of heat and cold applications
- Types of heat and cold applications
- The procedures for using heat and cold applications
- Safety considerations in using heat and cold

KEY TERMS

Anal Pertaining to the opening at the end of the anal canal, the end portion of the large intestine

Constrict To reduce in size, to close

Dilate To enlarge or to widen

Perineal Pertaining to the part of the body between the pubic bone and the coccyx (tailbone)

Why Are Heat and Cold Applications Ordered?

Doctors order heat and cold applications for comfort and to help with healing. Some facilities allow only licensed nursing staff to perform heat and cold applications. In other facilities, the nursing assistant can perform the procedures while the licensed nurse supervises. It is important that you know your facility's policy and that you know how to use the equipment.

Information about the use of heat and cold is contained in the care plan. The nursing assistant should be familiar with the care plan and follow it when providing care to residents in long-term care (LTC) centers. Remember to explain what you are doing to residents and allow them to participate in their care as much as possible.

If you have a question about how to perform any procedure, always ask the charge nurse before you begin.

The Effects of Heat Applications

Heat applications are used to:
- Relax muscles
- Reduce pain
- Increase healing
- Decrease swelling
- Decrease joint stiffness
- Make the patient comfortable

When heat is applied to the skin, the blood vessels **dilate** or open wider. This allows more blood to flow to the tissues. The blood brings more oxygen and nutrients to the tissues to help them heal. If the patient has a buildup of fluid or swelling, the

NOTES ON
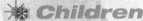
Children

The skin of children is more fragile and may be damaged by heat or cold more easily. Temperatures that are safe for a healthy adult may harm the skin of a child.

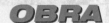
OBRA

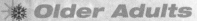
Safety

NOTES ON
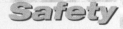
Older Adults

The skin of the elderly is more fragile and may be damaged by heat or cold more easily. Temperatures that are safe for a healthy adult may harm the skin of an elderly patient.

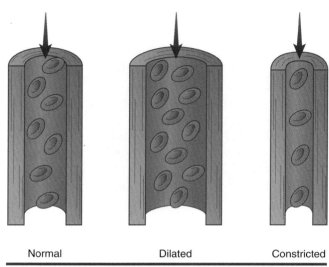

Normal   Dilated   Constricted

***Figure* 24-1** Blood vessels: Normal, dilated, and constricted.

extra blood flow helps to remove the fluids from the area (Figure 24-1).

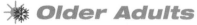

Caution: Temperatures over 115° F (46.1° C) may burn the skin. It is important to always check the temperature of any heat applications with a thermometer before applying the treatment.

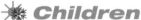

NOTES ON ❄ *Children*

Babies and young children have delicate skin and are more likely to be burned. Check the skin after 2 minutes and every 5 minutes until the treatment is complete.

NOTES ON ❄ *Older Adults*

Older patients have delicate skin and are more likely to be burned. Check the skin after 2 minutes and every 5 minutes until the treatment is complete.

Possible Complications of Heat Applications

There must be a doctor's order to use heat applications. High temperatures can cause burns. It is important that you check the patient's skin for redness or blisters. Some patients complain of pain if the skin is injured; others do not. Patients who are confused, paralyzed, or unconscious may not be able to tell you that the heat application is causing pain.

Types of Heat Applications

Heat applications may be moist heat, which means that there is water in contact with the skin. Examples of moist heat are:

- *Hot soaks or baths*—During a soak, some or all of the body is placed in water. To soak a small part of the body, a container is filled with hot water. A tub is used to soak a larger

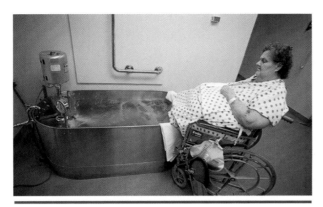

***Figure* 24-2** Hot soak or bath.

part or the entire body. The charge nurse will tell you what temperature of water to use, usually 105° F (41° C) (Figure 24-2).

- *Sitz bath*—During a sitz bath the patient's pelvic area is put into warm or hot water. This can be done in a regular bathtub with 10 to 12 inches of water. The charge nurse will tell you what temperature of water to use, usually 105° F (41° C). Some facilities have a specially designed tub for performing sitz baths. There are also portable sitz baths that can be used on the toilet in the patient's bathroom. Sitz baths are commonly used to clean and treat **anal** or **perineal** wounds (Figure 24-3).
- *Hot compresses*—A compress is a folded and moistened cloth or towel that is placed over a small area of the body (Figure 24-4). The compress is soaked in hot water and applied to the patient's skin for the amount of time ordered by the doctor, usually 15 to 30 minutes.

Moisture makes heat stronger, so moist heat works faster and feels hotter than dry heat. Because of this, the temperature of a moist heat application must be lower to prevent burning the skin.

Dry heat keeps the patient's skin dry during the application. Because water is not used, the temperature of a dry heat application must be hotter to work well. Burns can occur when the temperature of the application is higher. Examples of dry heat are:

- *Aquathermia/aquamatic pads*—These are heating pads that contain fluid-filled tubes or coils (Figure 24-5). An electric control unit or pump continually heats the liquid (usually distilled water) and moves it through the pad using plastic hoses. The unit must be kept at or above the level of the pad to work correctly. The temperature of the fluid is usually preset.

***HOW*&WHY**

Moisture in the air makes it feel hotter in climates that have a high humidity or moisture content in the air than it does at the same temperature in a dry climate.

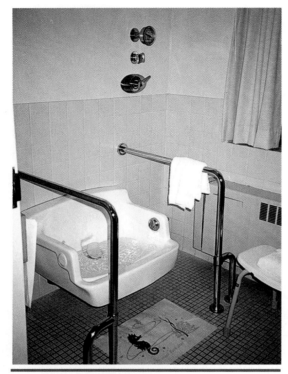

Figure 24-3   Built-in sitz bath.

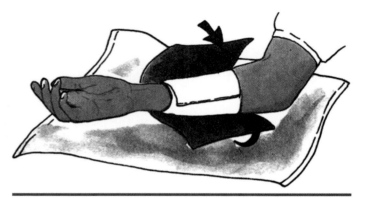

Figure 24-4   The compress is soaked in hot water and applied to the patient's skin for the amount of time ordered by the doctor.

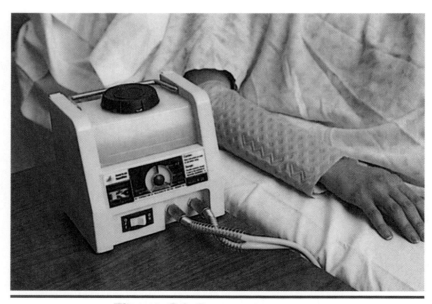

Figure 24-5   Aquathermia pad.

- *Hot packs*—Some facilities use hot packs that are filled with chemicals that become warm when you squeeze them (Figure 24-6). Be sure to follow the manufacturer's directions when using a chemical hot pack.
- *Heating pads*—Heating pads contains electric wires that produce heat when you plug them in (Figure 24-7). Hospitals and nursing homes do not use heating pads, but the nursing assistant in a home care setting may use them. Be sure to check with your supervising nurse for instructions before using a heating pad on any patient.
- *Hot water bottles/bags*—Hot water bottles/bags, like heating pads, are not commonly used in hospitals or nursing homes. A hot water bottle/bag is usually made of a rubber-like material and is filled with hot water (Figure 24-8, *A*). The bottle/bag must be covered with a towel or a specially made cover to protect the patient's skin from being burned (Figure 24-8, *B*). The nursing assistant in a home care setting may use the hot water bottle/bag. Always check with your supervising nurse for instructions before using a hot water bottle/bag on a patient.

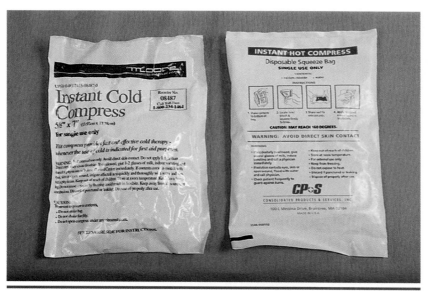

Figure 24-6 Chemical hot pack and chemical cold pack.

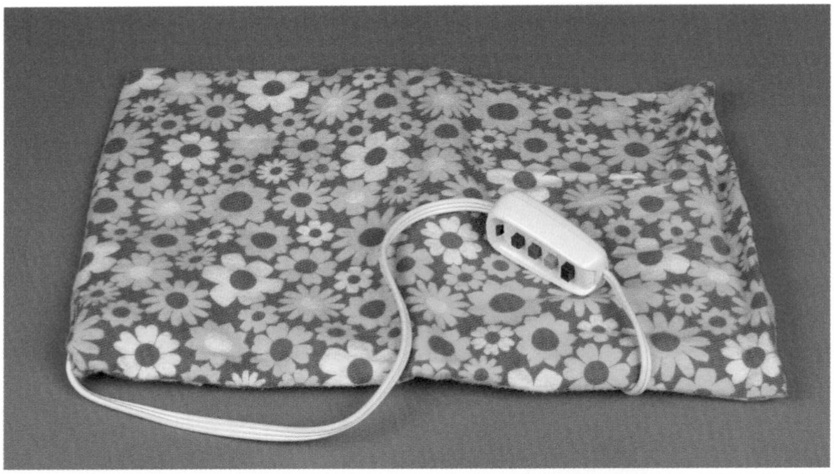

Figure 24-7   Heating pad.

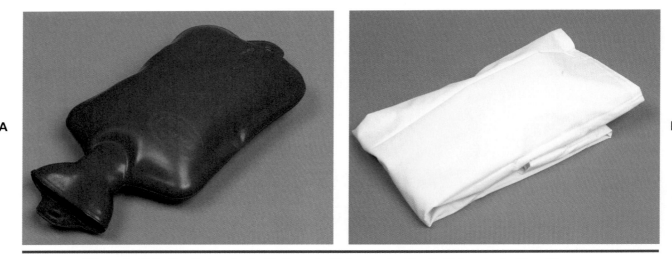

Figure 24-8   Hot water bottle/bag. **A,** Hot water bottle. **B,** Hot water bottle with cover.

Effects of Cold Applications

Cold applications are used to:
- Reduce pain
- Prevent swelling
- Decrease blood flow or bleeding
- Reduce a fever
- Decrease itching

When cold is applied to the skin, the blood vessels **constrict**, or become smaller, decreasing blood flow to the area. This also means that there is less oxygen and nutrients reaching the tissues. Cold applications are often used right after an injury to prevent swelling or to slow bleeding. Cold numbs the skin, so it also helps to reduce pain (see Figure 24-1).

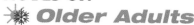

NOTES ON
Older Adults

Older patients are likely to be very sensitive to cold application and may find it uncomfortable or even painful. The length of the cold treatment may need to be shortened.

Possible Complications of Cold Applications

There must be a doctor's order to use cold applications. Cold temperatures can harm the skin just like heat. It is important that you check the patient's skin for redness, blisters, or **cyanosis** (bluish discoloration of the skin). Some patients will complain of pain if the skin is injured; others will not. Patients who are confused, paralyzed, or unconscious may not be able to tell you that the cold application is causing pain. Babies, young children, and older patients have delicate skin that is more likely to be damaged.

Types of Cold Applications

Just like heat applications, cold applications can be moist or dry. Examples of moist cold include:
- *Cold soaks*—During a soak, some or all of the body is placed in water. To soak a small part of the body, a container is filled with cold water. A tub is used to soak a larger part.
- *Cold compresses*—A compress is a folded and moistened cloth that is placed over a small area of the body. A pack is applied to larger areas of the body. The compress or pack is soaked in cold water and applied to the patient's skin for the amount of time ordered by the doctor, usually 15 to 30 minutes. A commercially prepared cold compress may also be used (Figure 24-9).
- *Sponge bath*—A sponge bath is given to reduce fever. Cool, moist washcloths are used to apply water to the patient's skin. The skin is allowed to air dry. As the water evapo-

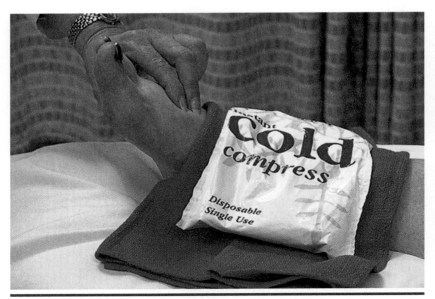

***Figure* 24-9** Cold compress.

rates, the skin is cooled. Sometimes alcohol is added to the water.

When the patient's skin remains dry during the procedure, it is considered a dry cold application. Examples of dry cold applications include:

- *Ice bags, ice collars, ice gloves, and cold packs*—Ice bags, gloves, and collars are devices filled with crushed ice. Some facilities use cold packs that are filled with chemicals that become cold when mixed together by squeezing. Be sure to follow the manufacturer's directions when using a chemical cold pack. Some devices have an outer covering. If not, the device is always placed in a covering or covered with a towel so that it is not directly on the patient's skin (Figure 24-10).

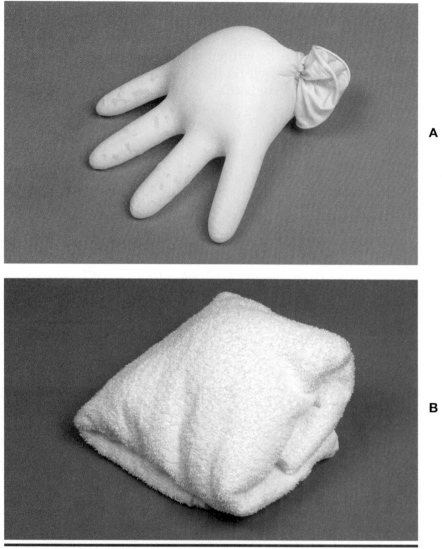

Figure 24-10   Ice bag. **A**, Ice glove. **B**, Ice glove with cover.

Cooling and Warming Blankets

Some facilities use cooling and warming blankets. A cooling blanket is used when the patient has a very high body temperature. A cooling blanket is usually made of plastic or rubber with fluid-filled tubing running through it. An electric pump cools the fluid and moves it through the tubes in the blanket. The cooling blanket is placed on the patient's bed and covered with a sheet. The patient is placed on top of the blanket. Some cooling blankets are large enough to also cover the patient. A warming blanket is used when the patient's body temperature is very low (Figure 24-11). It is very similar to the cooling blanket except that the fluid is heated before it is moved through the blanket. It is important to take the patient's temperature frequently while using the equipment to avoid excess cooling or warming.

Safety

Caution: It is important for your employer to teach you to use these pieces of equipment. There are many different types of cooling and warming blankets available. Be sure to follow the manufacturer's directions and your facility's policies and procedures when using a cooling or warming blanket.

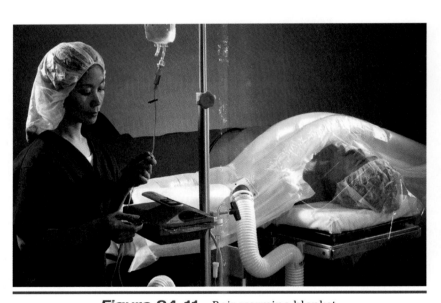

Figure 24-11 Bair warming blanket.

Safety Considerations When Using Heat and Cold

When you apply heat or cold it is important to:

- Provide privacy for the patient during the procedure. Expose only the body part being treated.
- Make sure the patient can reach the signal light during the procedure.
- Know how to use the equipment.
- Measure water temperature using a bath thermometer or follow facility policies to regarding measuring temperature.
- Follow facility policies for safe temperature ranges.
- Observe the skin for signs of problems during the procedure.
- Follow the doctor's order or instructions from the charge nurse about the length of time the treatment should remain in place.

Respect the resident's right to privacy. Keep the resident covered and expose only the area being treated.   **OBRA**

A hot bath or sitz bath increases the blood supply to the area being treated. This can cause the patient's blood pressure to drop and result in dizziness.   **Safety**

Make sure that the patient's signal light is within reach when applying hot or cold applications. This allows the patient to call for help if the treatment becomes uncomfortable.   **Safety**

When you apply a commercially prepared hot or cold pack, activate the pack according to the manufacturer's directions.   **Safety**

Procedure
PERFORMING A HOT OR COLD SOAK

EQUIPMENT
- Water basin, arm or foot bath
- Bath thermometer
- Bath blanket
- Waterproof pads
- Towels

◆ **COMPLETE STANDARD BEGINNING STEPS (see inside front cover)**

1 Position the patient for the procedure. Expose only the body part to be treated. Place the signal light within reach.

2 Place the waterproof pad under the part of the body to be soaked.

3 Fill the basin ½ full with hot or cold water as directed by the charge nurse. Using a bath thermometer, check the temperature of the water.

4 Gently lower the body part being treated into the basin (Figure 24-12). Make note of the time.

5 Cover the patient with a bath blanket for warmth.

6 Check the area for redness, cyanosis, or complaints of discomfort every 5 minutes. Stop the soak if any of these occur. Wrap the body part in a towel, and tell the charge nurse right away.

7 Check the temperature of the water every 5 minutes, and change the water as necessary. Wrap the part in a towel while changing the water.

8 At the end of the time ordered by the doctor, remove the body part from the water and pat dry.

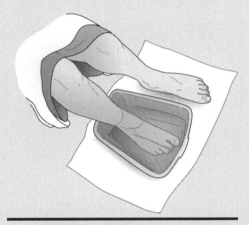

Figure 24-12 Step 4.

◆ **COMPLETE STANDARD ENDING STEPS (see inside front cover)**

Procedure
PERFORMING A HOT BATH OR SITZ BATH

EQUIPMENT
- Portable sitz bath if using
- Bath thermometer
- Bath blanket(s)
- Towels

◆ **COMPLETE STANDARD BEGINNING STEPS (see inside front cover)**

1 If using a portable sitz bath, position the device on the patient's toilet (Figure 24-13). If using a built-in sitz bath, transport the patient to the sitz bath room.

2 If providing a hot bath, transport the patient to the tub room.

3 Fill the sitz bath or tub ⅔ full of water at the ordered temperature.

4 Check the temperature of the water with the bath thermometer.

5 Assist the patient with undressing and into position in the tub or sitz bath. Note the time.

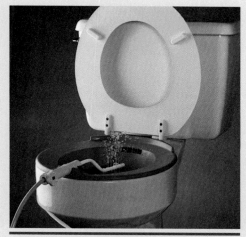

Figure 24-13   Step 1.

6 Cover the patient's shoulders with a bath blanket. If using a sitz bath, cover the patient's legs with a bath blanket. Make sure the signal light is within reach (Figure 24-14).

7 During the treatment, check the patient every 5 minutes for complaints of dizziness or weakness, redness, cyanosis, or complaints of discomfort. Stop the treatment if any of these occur, wrap the patient in a bath blanket, and tell the charge nurse right away.

8 At the end of the time ordered by the doctor, assist the patient from the tub or sitz bath and pat the skin dry.

9 Assist the patient with dressing, and transport her back to her room if needed.

10 Clean and store equipment according to facility policy.

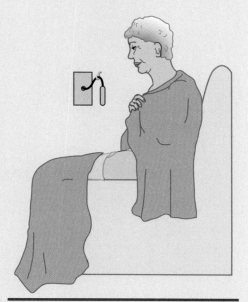

Figure 24-14   Step 6.

◆ **COMPLETE STANDARD ENDING STEPS (see inside front cover)**

Procedure

APPLYING A HOT OR COLD COMPRESS

EQUIPMENT

- Water basin
- Bath thermometer
- Bath blanket
- Waterproof pads
- Towels
- Small towels, washcloths, or gauze squares

◆ **COMPLETE STANDARD BEGINNING STEPS** **(see inside front cover)**

1 Position the patient for the procedure. Expose only the body part to be treated. Place the signal light within reach.

2 Place the waterproof pad under the part of the body to be treated.

3 Fill the basin $\frac{1}{2}$ to $\frac{2}{3}$ full with hot or cold water as directed by the charge nurse. Using a bath thermometer, check the temperature of the water.

4 Place the compress in the water.

5 Remove the compress from the water, and wring out excess water (Figure 24-15).

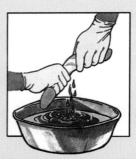

Figure 24-15 Step 5.

Procedure
APPLYING A HOT OR COLD COMPRESS—cont'd

6   Apply the compress to the area (Figure 24-16). Make note of the time.

7   Cover the patient with a bath blanket for warmth.

8   *For a warm compress,* wrap the compress with plastic wrap, a dry bath towel, and an aquamatic pad. (See procedure: *Using an Aquamatic or Aquathermia Pad,* p. 519.)

9   *For a cold compress,* wrap the compress with a dry bath towel. Check the temperature of the compress for warming every 5 minutes, and replace as needed.

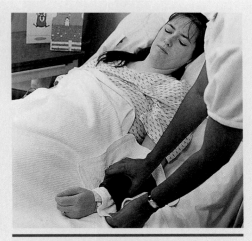

Figure 24-16   Step 6.

10   Check the area for redness, blistering, cyanosis, or complaints of discomfort every 5 minutes. Stop the compress if any of these occur, wrap the body part in a towel, and tell the charge nurse right away.

11   At the end of the time ordered by the doctor, remove the compress from the area and pat the skin dry.

◆ COMPLETE STANDARD ENDING STEPS **(see inside front cover)**

Procedure

APPLYING A HOT OR COLD PACK, ICE BAGS, ICE COLLARS, AND ICE GLOVES

EQUIPMENT
- Hot or cold pack, ice bag, ice collar or glove as ordered
- Bath blanket
- Flannel cover, towel, or pillowcase
- Paper towels
- Crushed ice for ice bag, collar, or glove

◆ **COMPLETE STANDARD BEGINNING STEPS** (see inside front cover)

1 When applying an ice bag, ice collar, or glove:

   a. Fill the device ½ to ⅔ full with crushed ice.
   b. Remove the air by gently squeezing the device (Figure 24-17).
   c. Secure the device with the stopper or cap.
   d. Check for leaks, and dry the device with the paper towels.
   e. Cover the device with a flannel cover, towel, or pillowcase.

2 Position the patient for the procedure. Expose only the body part to be treated.

3 Apply the treatment to the area. Make note of the time.

4 Cover the patient with a bath blanket for warmth, and place the signal light within reach.

5 Check the area for redness, cyanosis, or complaints of discomfort every 5 minutes. Stop the treatment if any of these occur, wrap the body part in a towel, and tell the charge nurse right away.

6 At the end of the time ordered by the doctor, remove the device from the area. Clean and store equipment according to facility policy.

7 Remove, clean, and store equipment according to facility policy.

◆ **COMPLETE STANDARD ENDING STEPS** (see inside front cover)

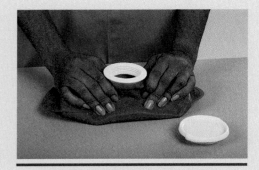

Figure 24-17   Step 1b.

Procedure
USING AN AQUAMATIC OR AQUATHERMIA PAD

EQUIPMENT
- Aquamatic and aquathermia pad and heating unit
- Distilled water
- Bath blanket
- Flannel cover, towel, or pillowcase

◆ **COMPLETE STANDARD BEGINNING STEPS (see inside front cover)**

1 Check the aquamatic or aquathermia pad to be sure the pad has no leaks and that the cord and plug are in good condition.

2 If needed, fill the unit to the fill line with distilled water.

3 Follow the manufacturer's directions and instructions from the nurse. Set the unit to the correct temperature if it was not preset, and plug in the unit.

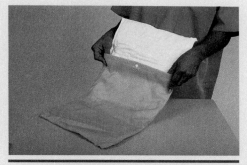

Figure 24-18 Step 4.

4 Make sure that the tubing is not twisted, and cover the pad with a pillowcase, towel, or flannel cover (Figure 24-18).

5 Position the patient for the procedure. Expose only the body part to be treated. Apply the aquathermia pad.

6 Position the unit on the nightstand or bedside table level with the pad (Figure 24-19).

7 Cover the patient for warmth, and place the signal light within reach.

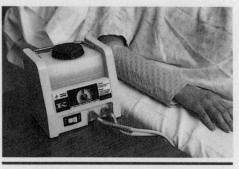

Figure 24-19 Step 6.

Continued

Procedure
USING AN AQUAMATIC OR AQUATHERMIA PAD—cont'd

8 Check the area for redness, blistering, cyanosis, or complaints of discomfort every 5 minutes. Stop the treatment if any of these occur, wrap the body part in a towel, and tell the charge nurse right away.

9 At the end of the time ordered by the doctor, remove the device from the area.

10 Remove, clean and store equipment according to facility policy.

◆ **COMPLETE STANDARD ENDING STEPS (see inside front cover)**

CHAPTER REVIEW

1. Why are heat and cold applications ordered?

2. Mr. Longwood has an order for an aquathermia pad to be placed on his left arm for 20 minutes each morning. You are not familiar with the equipment. What should you do?

Circle the one BEST response.

3. Heat applications are used to
   a. Prevent swelling
   b. Reduce a fever
   c. Decrease blood flow
   d. Decrease swelling

4. Cold applications are used to
   a. Relax muscles
   b. Decrease joint stiffness
   c. Decrease bleeding
   d. Increase healing

5. Which patient is at greatest risk of injury during a heat treatment?
   a. A patient who is conscious
   b. An elderly patient
   c. An alert patient
   d. An ambulatory patient

6. Which statement is correct regarding the use of heat and cold applications?
   a. Moisture decreases the effect of warm or cold applications.
   b. All heat and cold applications require a doctor's order.
   c. Infants and small children are usually less sensitive to heat and cold.
   d. Warm and cold applications are part of every nursing assistant's job.

7. How often should the temperature of a hot or cold application be checked?
   a. Every 5 minutes
   b. Every 10 minutes
   c. Every 15 minutes
   d. Every 20 minutes

8. When using an ice bag you should
   a. Fill the bag $\frac{3}{4}$ full with ice cubes
   b. Fill the bag $\frac{1}{2}$ full of ice and $\frac{1}{2}$ full of water
   c. Fill the bag $\frac{1}{2}$ to $\frac{2}{3}$ full of crushed ice
   d. Fill the bag $\frac{1}{4}$ full with crushed ice

Fill in the blank with the correct term.

9. A heating pad that contains tubes or coils that circulate heated fluid is called a(n) _____.

Answers are on page 710.

CHAPTER 25

Specimen Collection and Testing

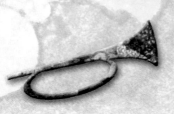

What you will learn

- How to collect and test urine specimens
- How to collect and test stool specimens
- How to collect sputum specimens

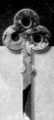

KEY TERMS

Sputum Mucus from the respiratory system that is spit or forced out of the mouth

Collecting and Testing Urine Specimens

Laboratory testing of urine gives information about how the urinary system is working. Urine also gives information about nutritional status and other diseases. Some tests require a single specimen of urine. Other tests require that the specimens of urine be obtained over several hours or days. Your supervisor may ask you, as a nursing assistant, to obtain a urine specimen from your patient. The most common types of specimens needed are:

- *Routine urine specimen*—a urine specimen free of feces and toilet tissue obtained in a non-sterile container.
- *Midstream (clean catch) urine specimen*—a specimen obtained in a sterile container after the patient has started to urinate. This type of specimen is frequently used to test for a urinary tract infection.
- *24-hour urine specimen*—urine collected during a 24-hour period and stored in the refrigerator or in a container of ice in the bathroom.

Never store specimens in a refrigerator that contains food or medications. Specimen refrigerators should be marked with an appropriate *BIOHAZARD* label (Figure 25-1).

Urine from patients with kidney stones is frequently "strained." The urine is poured through a mesh strainer that catches any stones or solids in the urine (Figure 25-3).

Occasionally you may be asked to test a patient's urine using a chemically treated "dipstick" (see Figure 25-14, p. 530). After you obtain a routine urine specimen (see procedure: *Collecting a Urine Specimen,* p. 525), the dipstick is dipped into the urine specimen. The small chemically treated squares will change color when they contact the chemicals in the urine. Each test has its own set of instructions to follow. Your supervisor will tell you how to do the test. Instructions for each test are also printed on the container.

Remember to follow Standard Precautions and the Bloodborne Pathogen Standard when obtaining specimens.

NOTES ON
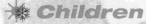
Children

A pediatric urine bag may be used to obtain a specimen from an infant or small child. The specimen is obtained from a sterile plastic bag that sticks firmly to the perineum (Figure 25-2). Your charge nurse will instruct you in the proper technique to use if a urine bag is required.

Safety

NOTES ON
Older Adults

When obtaining a specimen from an elderly patient, the nursing assistant may need to provide additional assistance with the procedure.

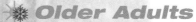
Safety

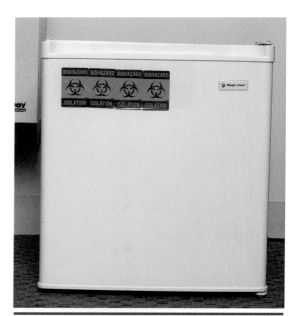

Figure 25-1 Specimen refrigerators should be marked with an appropriate *BIOHAZARD* label.

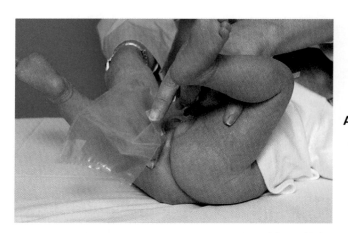

A

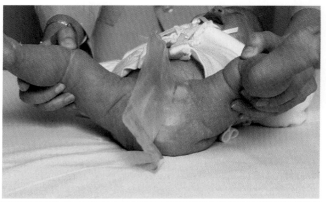

B

Figure 25-2 Pediatric urine bag. **A,** Adhesive portion is applied to the infant's perineum. **B,** Bag is securely attached to prevent leaks.

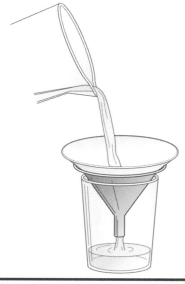

Figure 25-3 The urine is poured through a mesh strainer that catches any stones or solids in the urine.

Procedure
COLLECTING A URINE SPECIMEN

EQUIPMENT

- For all specimens
  - Washcloth
  - Towel
  - Soap and water
  - Specimen identification label
  - Completed laboratory requisition
  - Plastic bag for delivery of specimen
  - Gloves
- Random urine specimen
  - Clean collection container (specimen hat) (Figure 25-4) to place under toilet seat or urinal if needed

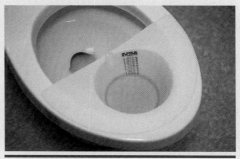

Figure 25-4   Specimen hat.

  - Non-sterile specimen container with lid (Figure 25-5)

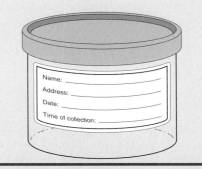

Figure 25-5   Specimen container with lid.

Continued

Procedure
COLLECTING A URINE SPECIMEN—cont'd

- Midstream (clean catch) urine specimen
  - Kit for midstream (clean catch) urine collection (Figure 25-6)

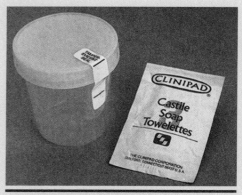

Figure 25-6 Midstream urine specimen kit.

- 24-hour urine collection
  - Large collection bottle with cap (obtained from lab)
  - Basin of ice or refrigerator to store urine (Figure 25-7)
  - Signs to remind patient/staff to save all urine
  - Clean collection container (specimen hat) to place under toilet seat or urinal

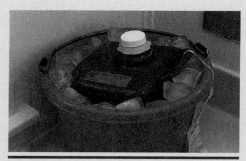

Figure 25-7 Twenty-four-hour urine collection container in a bucket of ice.

◆ **COMPLETE STANDARD BEGINNING STEPS (see inside front cover)**

1 Wash your hands and put on gloves.

2 Instruct or assist patient in cleansing the perineum using warm water and soap. Rinse well and pat dry.

Procedure
COLLECTING A URINE SPECIMEN—cont'd

3 Assist the patient to the bathroom, onto the commode, or to stand at the side of the bed to use the urinal.

4 Routine urine specimen

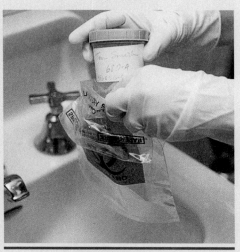

a. If the patient is independent, provide a non-sterile specimen container, and instruct the patient to urinate directly into the container.

b. If the patient needs assistance, allow the patient to urinate into a clean urinal or specimen hat. Pour 3 to 4 ounces of urine into the non-sterile specimen container.

c. Place the lid on the container without touching the inside of the container or the inside of the lid.

d. Attach completed identification label to the side of the container.

e. Place the urine container inside the plastic bag (Figure 25-8).

Figure 25-8   Step 4e.

f. Attach completed laboratory requisition form to the outside of the plastic bag.

g. Take the specimen to the lab, or place it in a specimen refrigerator for lab pickup.

5 Midstream (clean catch) urine specimen

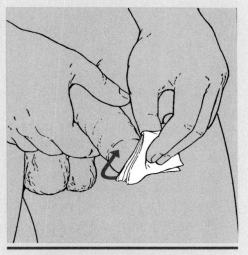

a. Open the specimen collection kit. Do not touch the inside of the container or the inside of the lid.

b. Instruct or assist the patient in cleansing the perineum using the antiseptic towelettes in the kit.

1) *Male:* Holding the penis in one hand, use the other hand to cleanse the penis with the antiseptic towelette using a circular motion, moving from the center to the outside (Figure 25-9).

Figure 25-9   Step 5b(1).

Continued

Procedure
COLLECTING A URINE SPECIMEN—cont'd

2) *Female:* Spread the labia with the fingers of one hand, and using the other hand, cleanse the area with the antiseptic towelette moving from front to back (Figure 25-10).

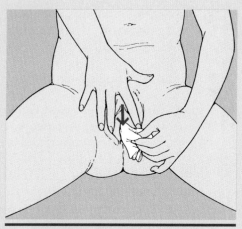

Figure 25-10   Step 5b(2).

c. While holding the penis or holding the labia apart, tell the patient to begin urinating (Figure 25-11).
d. After the patient has begun urinating, place the sterile specimen container under the stream of urine to collect 1 to 2 ounces of urine.
e. Remove the sterile specimen container before the patient stops urinating. The patient may continue urinating into the toilet.
f. Follow steps 4c to 4g.

 6   24-hour urine collection

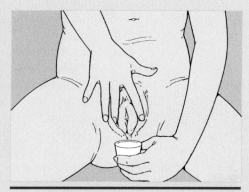

Figure 25-11   Step 5c.

a. Assist the patient to the bathroom or with using the urinal. Discard urine. Make a note of the time the patient urinated. This is the beginning of the 24-hour collection period.
b. Place collection bottle with cap in refrigerator or in a basin of ice on the bathroom floor.
c. Attach completed identification label to the side of the container.
d. Place a sign in the patient's bathroom showing the date and time urine collection started and date and time the 24-hour period will end.

Procedure
COLLECTING A URINE SPECIMEN—cont'd

e. Collect all urine for the next 24 hours. Pour urine into the bottle, and replace the cap every time after the patient urinates (Figure 25-12).

f. Keep collection bottle cold in the refrigerator, or keep replacing the ice in the basin to keep the bottle cool.

g. Five to 10 minutes before the end of the 24-hour collection period, ask the patient to urinate, and add the urine to the specimen bottle.

h. Place the urine container inside the plastic bag.

i. Attach a completed laboratory requisition form to the outside of the plastic bag.

j. Take the specimen to the lab, or place it in a specimen refrigerator for lab pickup.

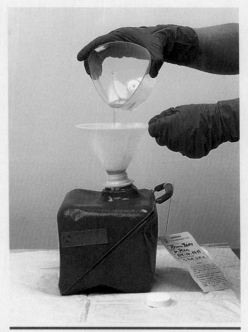

Figure 25-12   Step 6e.

7 After obtaining each urine specimen, remove your gloves and wash your hands.

8 Notify the charge nurse that the specimen has been obtained and the location of the specimen.

◆ COMPLETE STANDARD ENDING STEPS **(see inside front cover)**

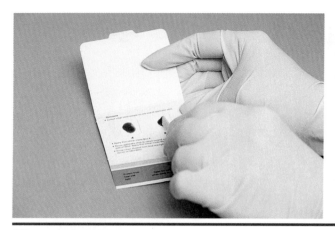
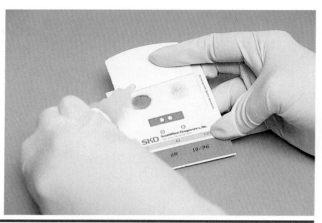

Figure 25-13 **A,** Apply stool to both spots on the cardboard slide. **B,** Apply the developing solution to the slide according to the manufacturer's directions.

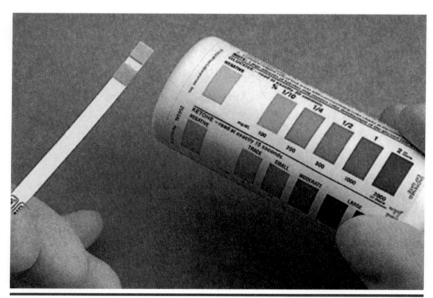

Figure 25-14 Compare the results on the dipstick with the chart on the container.

Collecting and Testing Stool Specimens

Laboratory testing of stool gives information about how the gastrointestinal system is working (Figures 25-13 and 25-14). The tests give information about infections, internal bleeding, and digestive problems. Your supervisor may ask you to obtain a stool specimen from your patient. The most common types of specimens needed are:

- *Stool for culture*—a specimen obtained with a sterile swab from a clean bedpan or container
- *Stool for other tests, including blood*—a specimen obtained by using tongue blades to put stool into a non-sterile container

Remember to follow Standard Precautions and the Bloodborne Pathogen Standard when obtaining specimens.

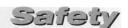

In some facilities your supervisor may ask you to obtain a stool specimen to check for the presence of blood. A stool specimen is obtained using the procedure *Collecting a Stool Specimen*. The charge nurse will give you instructions about the use of a specially prepared slide and developing liquid that finds blood in the stool.

Procedure
COLLECTING A STOOL SPECIMEN

EQUIPMENT
- Bedpan or clean collection container (specimen hat) to place under toilet seat
- Sterile swab and test tube for stool culture or non-sterile specimen container with lid
- Specimen identification label
- Completed laboratory requisition
- Plastic bag for delivery of specimen
- Gloves

◆ **COMPLETE STANDARD BEGINNING STEPS (see inside front cover)**

1   Wash your hands and put on gloves.

2   Assist the patient to the bathroom or onto the commode or bedpan.

3   Instruct the patient to urinate into the toilet or bedpan before defecating (moving his bowels). Discard urine.

Continued

Procedure
COLLECTING A STOOL SPECIMEN—cont'd

4 Provide the patient with a clean, dry bedpan or collection container (Figure 25-15).

5 Tell the patient to defecate into the bedpan or container.

6 If necessary, take the covered bedpan or container into the bathroom.

7 Obtain specimen.

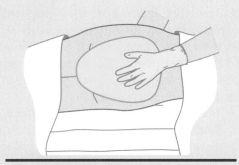

Figure 25-15 Step 4.

    a. *For culture:* Remove the sterile swab from the test tube. Gather a pea-sized sample of stool or soak the cotton with liquid stool. Return the swab to the test tube.

    b. *For other stool tests:* Obtain specimen by using tongue blades to transfer a portion of stool to the container (1 to $1\frac{1}{2}$ inches of formed stool or 15 ml of liquid stool) (Figure 25-16). Place lid on container without touching the inside of the container or the inside of the lid

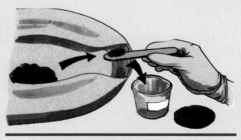

Figure 25-16 Step 7b.

8 Attach a completed identification label to the side of the container.

9 Place the specimen container inside the plastic bag.

10 Attach completed laboratory requisition form to the outside of the plastic bag.

11 Take the specimen to the lab, or place it in a specimen refrigerator for lab pickup.

12 Remove your gloves and wash your hands.

13 Notify the charge nurse that the specimen has been obtained and the location of the specimen.

◆ **COMPLETE STANDARD ENDING STEPS (see inside front cover)**

Collecting Sputum Specimens

Laboratory testing of **sputum** provides information about medical problems in the respiratory system. Information about infections such as tuberculosis and other diseases such as lung cancer can be obtained.

Remember to follow Standard Precautions and the Bloodborne Pathogen Standard when obtaining specimens.

Safety

It is important that you know how to collect each specimen in the correct way. If a specimen is not collected in the right way, the results will not help to diagnose the patient's problem. Label all specimens with the patient's name, patient ID number, room number, and the test to be performed. Follow your facility's policy regarding storing of specimens.

Remember, specimens are never stored in a refrigerator with food or medications.

Safety

It is important to protect the residents' privacy when collecting specimens. Allow as much privacy as possible by closing the door or pulling the privacy curtain. Explain the procedure to the residents so that they can participate in the process as much as possible. This enhances their quality of life and sense of self-esteem.

OBRA

Procedure
COLLECTING A SPUTUM SPECIMEN

EQUIPMENT
- Specimen container/sputum cup with lid
- Specimen identification label
- Completed laboratory requisition
- Plastic bag for delivery of specimen
- Gloves

◆ **COMPLETE STANDARD BEGINNING STEPS (see inside front cover)**

1 Wash your hands and put on gloves.

2 Assist the patient with sitting on the side of the bed, or raise the head of the bed to place the patient in a sitting position.

3 Help the patient to rinse her mouth with water.

Continued

Procedure
COLLECTING A SPUTUM SPECIMEN—cont'd

4 Tell the patient to take several deep breaths and then cough forcefully, coughing the sputum directly into the specimen container/sputum cup (Figure 25-17).

5 Repeat step 4 until you collect 2 to 3 teaspoons (5 to 10 ml) of sputum.
  NOTE: Do not collect saliva or oral secretions from the patient.

6 Place lid on container. Do not touch the inside of the container or the inside of the lid.

7 Attach completed identification label to the side of the container.

8 Place the sputum container inside the plastic bag.

9 Attach the completed laboratory requisition form to the outside of the plastic bag.

10 Take the specimen to the lab, or place it in a specimen refrigerator for lab pickup.

11 Remove your gloves and wash your hands.

12 Notify the charge nurse that the specimen has been obtained and the location of the specimen.

◆ **COMPLETE STANDARD ENDING STEPS (see inside front cover)**

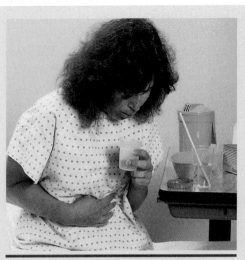

Figure 25-17 Step 4.

CHAPTER REVIEW

1. Why is urine testing done?

2. What is the purpose of stool testing?

3. Why is sputum testing performed?

Circle the one BEST response.

4. How should a 24-hour urine collection be stored until it is completed and taken to the lab?
   a. Keep the collection bottle cold in the refrigerator or by placing it on ice in a basin in the bathroom.
   b. Keep the collection bottle at the patient's bedside to allow for the addition of each specimen.
   c. Keep the collection bottle in the medicine room at the nurses' station until the test is completed.
   d. Keep the collection bottle in the lab during the test.

Mark T for true or F for false.

5. _____ Stool and urine specimens can be stored in the same refrigerator with food and medications.

Fill in the blank with the correct term.

6. When obtaining a stool or urine specimen, always wear _____.

Answers are on pages 710 to 711.

CHAPTER 26

Assisting With a Physical Examination

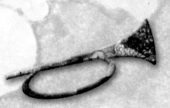

What you will learn

- Equipment needed for a physical exam
- How to prepare a person for a physical exam
- How to assist with a physical exam

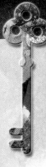

KEY TERMS

Cytobrush A small brush used to obtain a specimen for a Pap smear
Ophthalmoscope An instrument used to look at the eye
Otoscope An instrument used to look at the inside of the ear canal
Percussion hammer An instrument used to test reflexes
Sphygmomanometer An instrument used to measure blood pressure
Stethoscope An instrument that has two earpieces attached by flexible tubing to a
    diaphragm that is placed against the patient's skin to hear heart and lung sounds
Tuning fork A metal instrument used to test bone and air conduction of sound
Vaginal speculum A metal or plastic instrument used in an exam of the female
    genitalia

Physical Examination

A physical exam is performed as a routine procedure each year. It may also be done when applying for an insurance policy or before starting a new job. A physical exam is also done when a person is admitted to the hospital or nursing home.

Residents of long-term care (LTC) facilities have the right to know about the type of exam done, who performs the physical exam, and why the exam is done. You can respect the person's right to privacy by only exposing the part of the body being examined and remembering to close the door or privacy curtain during the exam.

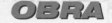

Preparing Equipment for a Physical Examination

Wash your hands before preparing the equipment needed for the physical exam. The equipment for the exam will vary depending upon how extensive the exam is. The doctor or nurse will tell you if you need special equipment in addition to the basic supplies (Figure 26-1). Check all equipment to make sure it is working before placing it in the exam room.

Basic equipment and supplies for a physical exam include:

- Eye chart
- Flashlight
- Forms (physical exam forms, laboratory requests, and so on)
- Gloves
- Gown (cloth or paper)

NOTES ON
⑤ Culture

People's culture affects their health-related behavior. It is important to respect each person's beliefs even when they are different from your own. People from some cultures may be very uncomfortable with the touching required during the physical exam.

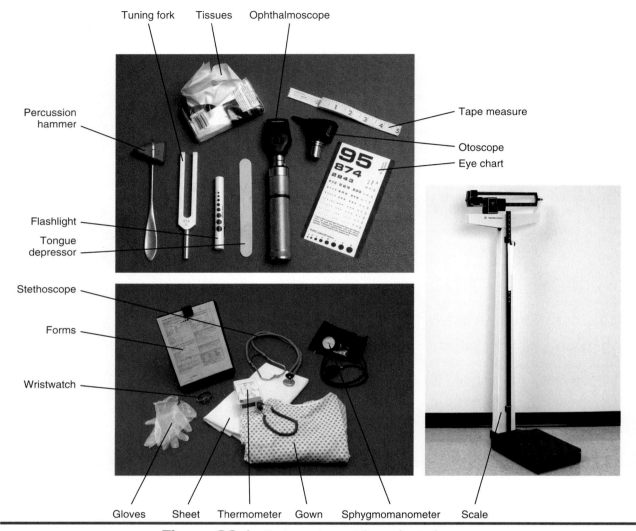

Tuning fork   Tissues   Ophthalmoscope

Percussion hammer

Tape measure

Otoscope

Eye chart

Flashlight

Tongue depressor

Stethoscope

Forms

Wristwatch

Gloves   Sheet   Thermometer   Gown   Sphygmomanometer   Scale

Figure 26-1   Basic equipment for a physical exam.

- **Ophthalmoscope** (an instrument used to view the eye)
- **Otoscope** (an instrument used to view the inside of the ear canal)
- **Percussion hammer** (an instrument used to test reflexes)
- Scale with height measurement rod
- Sheet(s) (cloth or paper)
- **Sphygmomanometer** and cuff (used to measure blood pressure)

- **Stethoscope**
- Tape measure
- Thermometer
- Tissues
- Tongue depressor
- **Tuning fork** (used to test hearing)
- Wristwatch or clock with a second hand

Special equipment and supplies needed for a physical exam may include:

- Cotton applicators
- **Cytobrush** (used to obtain a specimen for a Pap smear)
- Pap smear slides
- Specimen container(s)
- **Vaginal speculum**
- Water-soluble lubricant

It is important that you respect the patient's right to privacy during the physical exam. The exam may be performed in the person's home, a hospital room, or a doctor's office. The door to the room used for the exam should be closed. If the exam is performed in the patient's hospital or nursing home room, pull the privacy curtain around the bed.

Preparing a Person for a Physical Examination

It is important that the patient be comfortable during the physical exam. Before the exam begins, ask if the patient needs to use the bathroom. If a stool or urine specimen is needed, it can be obtained at this time (Chapter 25). Many people are nervous about the physical exam. A simple explanation about what you are doing and the reason for each step will make the person more comfortable. Ask the patient to undress and put on an exam gown. If the exam is limited to certain body parts, the patient may not need to remove all of the clothing. If a breast exam is to be performed on a female patient, she should wear the gown with the opening in the front. The nurse or doctor will tell you what part of the body will be examined. Give the patient plenty of time to change. Walking into the room while the patient is dressing or undressing can be embarrassing. If patients need assistance with changing clothes, give them the help that they need. After the person is undressed have the person sit or lie down on the exam table with the sheet over the lap or lower body.

Make sure that the patient is comfortable and that the room is warm enough so that the patient does not become chilled during the exam. If the room is cold, give the patient a warm blanket. Protect the patient from falls by assisting the patient on and off the exam table as needed.

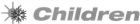

NOTES ON **Children**

Unless you are instructed otherwise, the child's parent(s) should remain in the room during the exam. This will help the child to feel more comfortable and the parent(s) can ask questions during the exam.

NOTES ON **Culture**

Remember to respect the cultural practices of your patients. Some patients may wish to have a family member present during the examination.

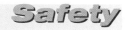

Assisting With the Physical Examination

The doctor or nurse may ask you to assist with the physical exam. You may be asked to take the patient's temperature, pulse, respirations, and blood pressure. You may also be asked to obtain an accurate height and weight (Chapter 13). During the exam you may need to help the patient into proper positions so that all of the body parts can be examined (Table 26-1).

Make sure that the patient stays covered with the gown and sheet as much as possible during the exam. This will keep the patient from getting cold or feeling embarrassed. The patient should be allowed to ask questions during the physical exam. Remember to follow Standard Precautions and the Bloodborne Pathogen Standards if there is a chance that you will have contact with blood, body fluids, mucous membranes, or non-intact skin.

When the physical exam is completed, help the patient up from the exam table and give the patient time to dress. If the doctor or nurse wishes to talk to the patient more, you may be asked to direct the patient to another office or room. Using Standard Precautions (Chapter 9), remove all equipment from the room. Clean re-usable equipment following your facility's policy. When you finish with the procedure, remember to wash your hands.

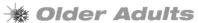

NOTES ON
Older Adults

Use special care when positioning older adults. They are more likely to have disabilities or find some positions to be very uncomfortable because of limited joint movement.

Table 26-1

POSITIONS FOR EXAMINATION

Position	Areas Assessed	Rationale	Limitations
Sitting	Head and neck, back, posterior thorax and lungs, anterior thorax and lungs, breasts, axillae, heart, vital signs, and upper extremities	Sitting upright provides full expansion of lungs and provides better visualization of symmetry of upper body parts.	Physically weakened client may be unable to sit. Examiner should use supine position with head of bed elevated instead.
Supine	Head and neck, anterior thorax and lungs, breasts, axillae, heart, abdomen, extremities, pulses	This is most normally relaxed position. It provides easy access to pulse sites.	If client becomes short of breath easily, examiner may need to raise head of bed.
Dorsal recumbent	Head and neck, anterior thorax and lungs, breasts, axillae, heart, abdomen	Position is used for abdominal assessment because it promotes relaxation of abdominal muscles.	Clients with painful disorders are more comfortable with knees flexed.
Lithotomy*	Female genitalia and genital tract	This position provides maximal exposure of genitalia and facilitates insertion of vaginal speculum.	Lithotomy position is embarrassing and uncomfortable, so examiner minimizes time that the client spends in it. Client is kept well draped.
Sims'*	Rectum and vagina	Flexion of hip and knee improves exposure of rectal area.	Joint deformities may hinder client's ability to bend hip and knee.
Prone	Musculoskeletal system	This position is used only to assess extension of hip joint.	This position is poorly tolerated in clients with respiratory difficulties.
Lateral recumbent	Heart	This position aids in detecting murmurs.	This position is poorly tolerated in clients with respiratory difficulties.
Knee-chest*	Rectum	This position provides maximal exposure of rectal area.	This position is embarrassing and uncomfortable.

*Clients with arthritis or other joint deformities may be unable to assume this position.

CHAPTER REVIEW

1. Why is a physical exam performed?

2. Match the instrument with the picture (Figure 26-2 on page 543).
   1. Eye chart
   2. Ophthalmoscope
   3. Otoscope
   4. Percussion hammer
   5. Sphygmomanometer and cuff
   6. Stethoscope
   7. Thermometer
   8. Tongue depressor
   9. Tuning fork
   10. Flashlight
   11. Watch
   12. Gloves
   13. Sheet
   14. Gown
   15. Scale
   16. Tissues
   17. Forms
   18. Tape measure

Circle the one BEST response.

3. How does the nursing assistant prepare patients for the physical exam?
   a. The nursing assistant should ask patients about their medications and document their answers on the medical record.
   b. The nursing assistant should ask patients if they need to use the bathroom and obtain a stool or urine specimen if needed.
   c. The nursing assistant should assist patients with undressing and place them in the lithotomy position before the doctor arrives.
   d. The nursing assistant should tell patients to remain dressed until the doctor arrives.

4. Which position should the patient be in when taking vital signs or listening to heart or lung sounds?
   a. Sitting
   b. Sims'
   c. Supine
   d. Prone

5. When assisting with the physical exam, the nursing assistant should
   a. Make sure the patient is comfortable and warm
   b. Explain what the doctor or nurse is doing as the exam is performed
   c. Keep the patient's body uncovered so that it can be fully examined
   d. Discourage the patient from asking questions during the exam

Answers are on page 711.

CHAPTER REVIEW

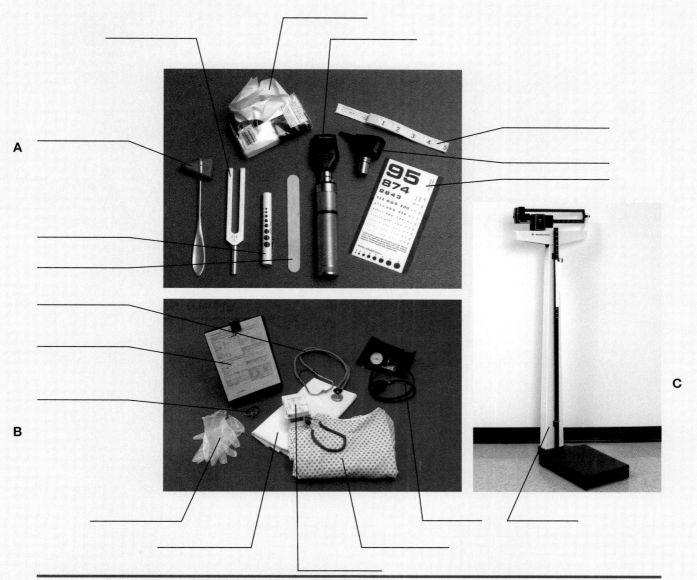

A

B

C

Figure 26-2 A, B, C, Basic equipment for a physical exam.

CHAPTER 27

Caring for the Person on Oxygen Therapy

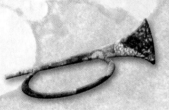

What you will learn

- Normal and abnormal respiratory function
- Measures to promote normal respiratory function
- How to perform deep breathing and coughing exercises
- How to care for the patient with special respiratory needs, including oxygen therapy

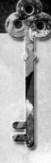

KEY TERMS

Cyanosis Change from the usual color to a bluish color

Expiration The act of breathing out

Hypoxia A condition in which the cells do not get enough oxygen

Incentive spirometer A device that measures the amount of air a person is able to take into the lungs

Inspiration The act of breathing in

Nasal cannula A small plastic tube with curved pieces that fits into the opening of the nose to provide oxygen

Pneumonia Inflammation/infection of the lungs

Pulse oximeter A device that measures the amount of oxygen in the blood through the skin

Respiration The cycle of breathing in and out

Normal and Abnormal Respiratory Function

The term **respiration** means breathing. Every cell in the body needs oxygen to live. Oxygen is an odorless, colorless gas. The respiratory system (Chapter 7) brings oxygen-rich air into the lungs during **inspiration**, or breathing in. As the body processes are carried out, waste products slowly increase and must be removed from the body. During **expiration**, or breathing out, air, carbon dioxide, and other waste products leave the lungs (see Figure 7-17). The oxygen is carried to the cells by the blood. Without oxygen, cells begin to die within minutes. Illness and injury can affect the amount of oxygen that reaches the cells.

A normal adult breathes 12 to 20 times a minute. Normal respirations are quiet and regular. During normal respirations, both sides of the chest will rise and fall evenly. Many factors can affect normal respirations, including:

- *Age*—The elderly have weaker respiratory muscles, and lung tissue is not as elastic. This makes coughing more difficult, and the patient can get **pneumonia**, or an inflammation/infection of the lungs.
- *Smoking*—Smoking damages the lungs, and the patient can get lung disease.
- *Diseases*—Emphysema, lung cancer, asthma, and allergies are diseases than can affect respiratory functioning.

- *Drugs*—Some medicines, especially pain medications, affect the part of the brain that controls respiration and can even cause a person to stop breathing.
- *Pain, fever, and exercise*—All of these increase the body's need for oxygen, so respiratory function is affected.

Measures to Promote Normal Respiratory Function

During normal respirations the person breathes quietly and easily. When the cells do not receive enough oxygen, they cannot function correctly. **Hypoxia** is a condition in which the cells do not get enough oxygen. The brain cells are very sensitive to even a slight decrease in the amount of oxygen available. Signs and symptoms of hypoxia that should be reported to the charge nurse immediately include:

- Restlessness
- Confusion
- Dizziness
- Feeling tired
- Behavior changes
- Personality changes
- Nervousness
- Increased pulse rate (Chapter 13)
- Fast or difficult breathing
- **Cyanosis** or a bluish discoloration of the lips, nail beds, and skin

Mucus and secretions in the respiratory tract are a common cause of abnormal respiratory functioning. The simplest method of clearing these secretions is through coughing. Deep breathing and coughing exercises help to prevent hypoxia and pneumonia by opening up the air passages to allow more oxygen-rich air into the lungs. Coughing helps by removing the secretions in the lungs. Deep breathing and coughing are important for the patient who has had surgery or a respiratory illness. Your charge nurse will instruct you in how often to perform the procedure.

NOTES ON
※ *Older Adults*
Confusion is often the first sign of respiratory problems in older adults.

Procedure
ASSISTING A PERSON TO DEEP BREATHE AND COUGH

EQUIPMENT
* Small pillow

◆ **COMPLETE STANDARD BEGINNING STEPS (see inside front cover)**

1 Assist the patient into a sitting position in a chair or on the side of the bed. If the patient cannot sit up, raise the head of the bed to Fowler's position (Chapter 11) (Figure 27-1).

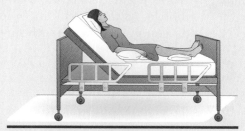

Figure 27-1   Step 1.

2 If the patient has had chest or abdominal surgery, place a small pillow over the incision and ask the patient to hold it firmly against her body (Figure 27-2).

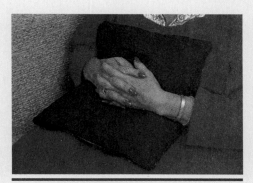

Figure 27-2   Step 2.

3 Instruct the patient to use the chest and abdominal muscles to:

a.   Breathe in slowly through the nose
b.   Hold each breath for 3 to 4 seconds
c.   Breathe out slowly through the mouth (Figure 27-3).

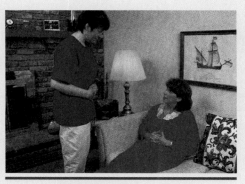

Figure 27-3   Step 3.

Continued

Procedure
ASSISTING A PERSON TO DEEP BREATHE AND COUGH—cont'd

4 Deep breathing exercises should be performed 5 to 10 times every 2 hours while the patient is awake.

5 For coughing exercises, follow steps 1 to 3 as above. As the patient breathes out, instruct her to cough with her mouth open.

6 Coughing exercises should be performed at least every 2 hours while the patient is awake.

7 If the patient is able to cough up secretions, she should dispose of them in a tissue. If the patient coughs up bloody, brown, yellow, or green secretions, tell the charge nurse.

◆ **COMPLETE STANDARD ENDING STEPS (see inside front cover)**

Caring for the Patient With Special Respiratory Needs, Including Oxygen Therapy

When a person is not able to keep enough oxygen in the body by breathing in room air, the doctor may prescribe oxygen therapy. Oxygen is considered a drug, and only a health care provider who is licensed or certified to give medications can give oxygen.

Safety   States differ on their laws about medications. It is important for you to know what the laws are in the state in which you are working.

Safety   An "Oxygen in Use" sign is put on the door of the patient's room to notify all staff members that the patient is receiving oxygen (Figure 27-4).

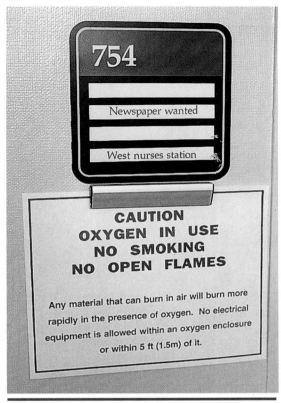

Figure 27-4 "Oxygen in Use" sign.

NOTES ON
☯ *Culture*

If patients or their family cannot read English, you will need to explain the purpose of the sign and tell them about safety factors. Some facilities use signs that provide information in more than one language.

The health care team develops a plan of care for each resident of a long-term care (LTC) facility. The nursing assistant should be familiar with the plan of care for each resident and follow it when providing care. Residents are encouraged to participate in developing the plan of care. LTC facilities are also required to provide a safe environment for their residents. You can help make the resident's home safe by being alert to the safety precautions required for residents receiving oxygen.

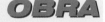

Oxygen can be administered by several different methods. The most common device used to administer oxygen is a **nasal cannula**, sometimes abbreviated NC (Figure 27-5, *A*). A nasal cannula consists of a small plastic tube with short, curved prongs that fit into the opening of the nose about $\frac{1}{4}$ inch to provide oxygen (Figure 27-5, *B*). The cannula is held in place by looping it over the ears and securing it under the person's chin (Figure 27-5, *C*). Figure 27-6 shows a woman with a nasal cannula receiving oxygen from a portable oxygen tank.

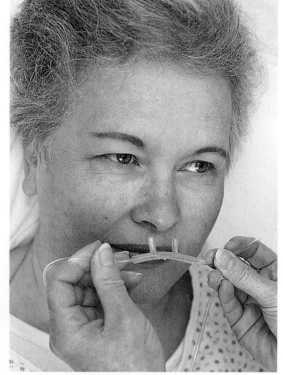

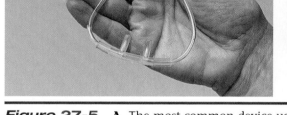

A   B

Figure 27-5 **A,** The most common device used to administer oxygen is a nasal cannula.
B, A nasal cannula consists of a small plastic tube with short curved prongs that fit into the
opening of the nose about $\frac{1}{4}$ inch to provide oxygen.

C

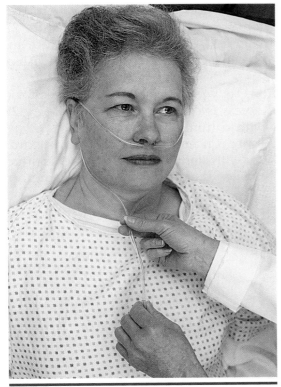

Figure **27-5, cont'd** **C**, The cannula is held in place by looping it over the ears and securing it under the person's chin.

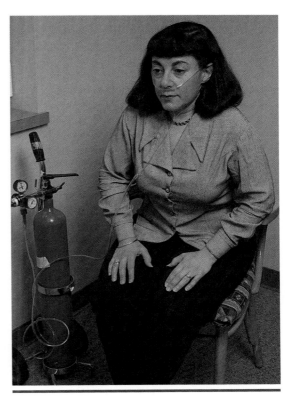

Figure **27-6** A woman with a nasal cannula receiving oxygen from a portable oxygen tank.

NOTES ON
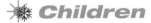
✳ *Children*

Oxygen tents or small oxygen hoods are still used for infants and children in some settings (Figure 27-9).

There are a variety of devices to administer oxygen, including masks, tracheostomy collars, and face tents (Figure 27-7). Figure 27-8 shows a patient receiving oxygen by face mask. Figure 27-9 shows oxygen being given to an infant using an oxygen hood.

In larger institutions, oxygen lines are in the walls for easy access. This type of access is called wall oxygen. Figure 27-10 shows wall oxygen with a humidifier jar attached. Oxygen is very drying and at higher concentrations may require extra humidity (moisture). A jar with sterile or distilled water is attached to the flowmeter to moisten the air the patient is breathing.

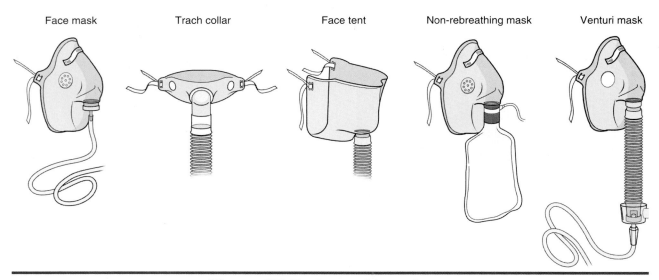

Face mask   Trach collar   Face tent   Non-rebreathing mask   Venturi mask

Figure 27-7 Oxygen delivery devices.

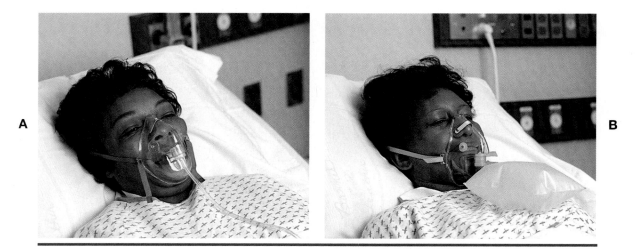

Figure 27-8 **A,** Face mask. **B,** Face mask with a reservoir bag.

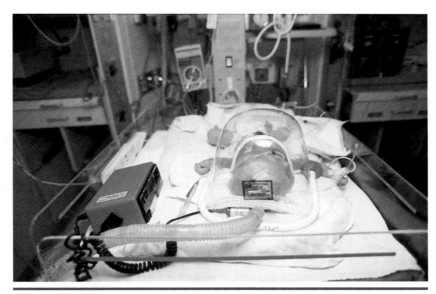

***Figure* 27-9**   Oxygen being given to an infant using an oxygen hood.

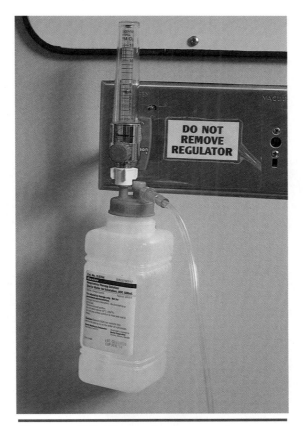

DO NOT REMOVE REGULATOR

***Figure* 27-10**   Wall oxygen with a humidifier jar attached.

In home or long-term care settings, oxygen concentrators are popular. An oxygen concentrator is an electric machine that collects and concentrates oxygen from room air (Figure 27-11). A flowmeter or gauge controls the amount of oxygen the patient gets from the tank, wall, or concentrator (Figure 27-12). The flowmeter or gauge is marked according to the number of liters per minute that will be delivered by the machine to the patient. A small plastic bead floats in the cylinder to indicate that amount at which the flowmeter is set. In Figure 27-12 the bead is centered on the line next to the 5. This means that the oxygen is set at 5 L/min. On a gauge, the needle points to the amount of oxygen being administered. The doctor will order the amount of oxygen the patient is to receive.

Safety   The nursing assistant should check that the flowmeter or gauge is at the correct setting but is NOT permitted to change the setting. Notify the charge nurse immediately if the flowmeter or gauge is not set at the correct level (Box 27-1).

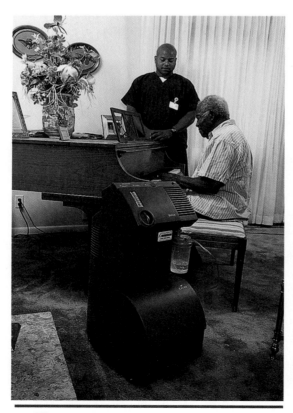

Figure 27-11 Oxygen concentrator.

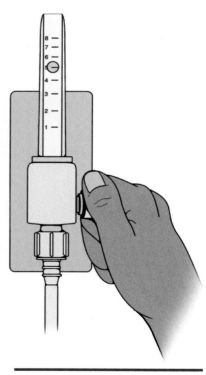

Figure 27-12 Oxygen flowmeter.

Box 27-1

SAFETY PRECAUTIONS FOR PATIENTS RECEIVING OXYGEN

- Never change the setting on an oxygen device.
- Check under nasal cannulas and oxygen masks for signs of irritation. Keep the skin under the device clean and dry.
- Make sure that there are no kinks in the oxygen tubing and that the patient is not lying or sitting on the tubing.
- Notify the nurse immediately if the flowmeter or gauge does not appear to be at the correct setting or if the humidifier bottle does not bubble or is low on water.
- Observe the patient for signs of hypoxia or respiratory distress as listed earlier in this chapter.
- Never allow open flames such as candles or smoking around oxygen.
- Avoid using electrical devices such as electric razors on patients who are receiving oxygen.
- Do not use flammable liquids such as nail polish remover on patients receiving oxygen.
- Each person has the right to be free from restraints.

Some patients require very little additional oxygen to supply their body with the oxygen necessary for it to function. The air you are breathing, known as room air, contains 21% oxygen. A patient who receives 1 L of oxygen per minute is breathing in 24% oxygen; 2 L provides 28% oxygen, 3 L provides 32% oxygen, and so on. To determine the amount of oxygen a patient needs, the doctor can request that blood be drawn from an artery to measure its oxygen content. This is both painful and costly.

Many doctors want patients to use a device called a **pulse oximeter.** The pulse oximeter measures the amount of oxygen in a person's blood through a sensor that is attached to a finger, toe, or earlobe (Figure 27-13). A beam of light on the sensor passes through the tissue of the body to the other side of the sensor and gives information about the patient's oxygen level. A pulse oximeter must be placed on an area of the body that has good blood flow. Nail polish, artificial nails, swollen areas, and open skin will all affect how the device gives information. The charge nurse may ask you to check the number on the pulse oximeter throughout your shift and report any alarms from the device (Figure 27-14).

NOTES ON
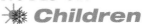 *Children*

Pulse oximeter sensors for infants and small children may be placed on the palm of the hand or bottom of the foot.

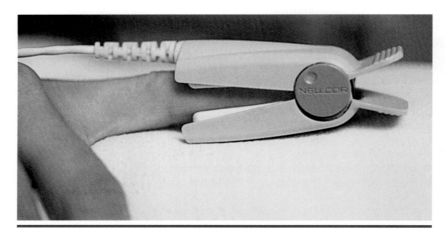

***Figure* 27-13** Pulse oximeter.

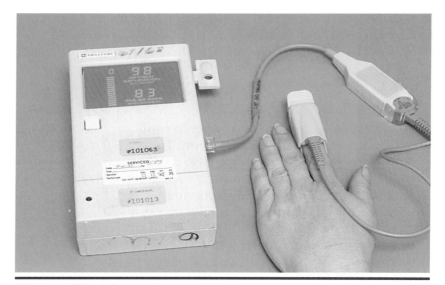

***Figure* 27-14** The pulse oximeter includes a probe that is connected by a cable to the oximeter. A digital readout provides information about the patient's oxygen saturation and pulse rate. In this photo the oxygen saturation is 98, and the pulse is 83.

An **incentive spirometer** measures the amount of air a person is able to inhale (Figure 27-15). When a person uses an incentive spirometer, the person breathes slowly and deeply through a mouthpiece until the balls or bars in the device reach a preset line. The person is able to see the movement of the balls or bars. The breath is held for 3 to 5 seconds to keep the balls floating or the bars at the upper level. The mouthpiece is removed from the person's mouth, and the person exhales slowly. This process frequently causes the person to cough because the lungs expand during the exercise. The charge nurse will tell you how often your patient should use the incentive spirometer. The nurse or respiratory therapist will set the desired level for the balls or bars.

In some settings patients use other types of equipment to provide adequate respiratory function. Artificial airways make an opening into the lungs (Figure 27-16). A tracheostomy is a surgical incision in the neck. A tube is inserted into the incision. This tube allows the patient to breathe (Figure 27-17). An Ambu-bag moves air into the lungs when the nurse squeezes it. Ambu-bags are frequently used in emergency situations when a

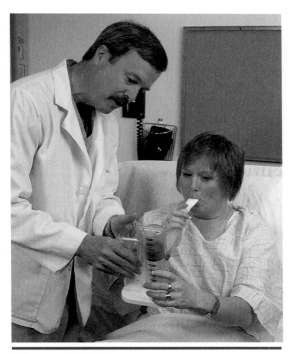

Figure 27-15   Patient using an incentive spirometer.

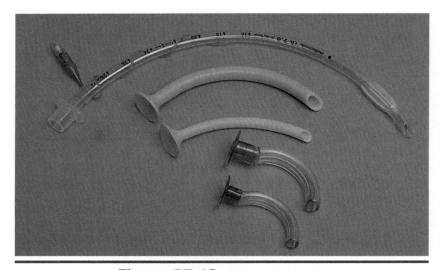

Figure 27-16 Types of airways.

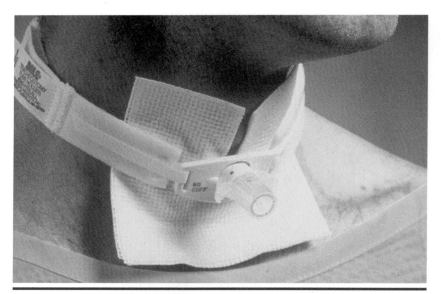

Figure 27-17 Patient with a tracheostomy tube.

patient is not breathing (Figure 27-18). A mechanical ventilator may be used. This device does the breathing for a patient who is unable to breathe on his own (Figure 27-19). A chest tube may be inserted into the area around the lungs after a surgical procedure or injury. The chest tube drains the fluid or air from the space around the lungs and allows the lung to work better. The chest tube is connected to a drainage system (Figure 27-20). When there are large amounts of secretions, the nurse may use

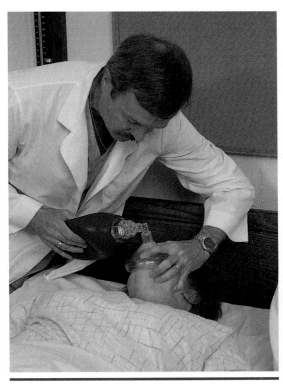

Figure 27-18   Ambu-bag being used.

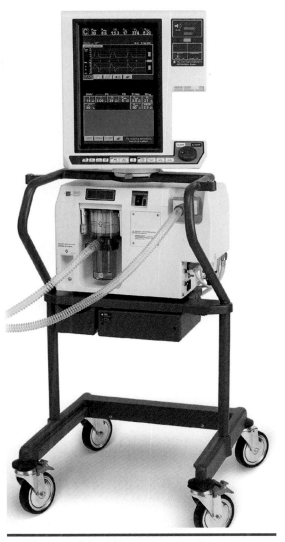

Figure 27-19   Mechanical ventilator.

a suction catheter to remove them (Figure 27-21). Patients who need to use this special equipment to maintain their respiratory function are extremely ill. You will have very little contact with these types of specialty equipment. Your charge nurse may ask you to help when the nurse provides care to a patient with the equipment.

It is important that you remember never to use equipment that you are not trained to use.

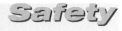

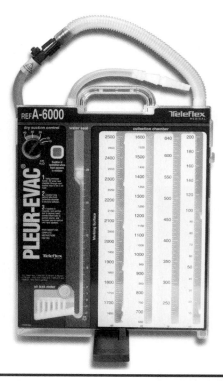

Figure 27-20 Chest tube and drainage system.

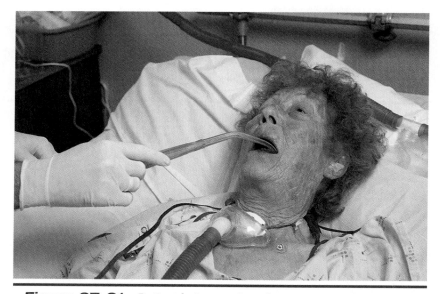

Figure 27-21 Patient being suctioned to remove oral secretions.

CHAPTER REVIEW

1. What does the term *respiration* mean?

2. List 3 factors that can affect respiratory functioning.

3. List 5 signs and symptoms of hypoxia.

4. What is a nasal cannula?

Circle the one BEST response.

5. How many times does the normal adult breathe per minute?
   a. 6 to 16
   b. 10 to 18
   c. 12 to 20
   d. 18 to 24

6. What is the simplest method of clearing secretions from the lungs?
   a. Oxygen therapy
   b. Coughing
   c. Suctioning
   d. Use of a ventilator

7. What position should the patient be in when performing deep breathing and coughing exercises?
   a. Side-lying
   b. Prone
   c. Standing
   d. Sitting

8. The device that controls the amount of oxygen released from an oxygen tank, wall oxygen unit, or concentrator for the patient is a/an
   a. Flowmeter
   b. Humidifier
   c. Concentrator
   d. Chest tube

Mark T for true or F for false.

9. _____ The nursing assistant is responsible for checking the setting on the oxygen flowmeter and adjusting it if necessary to provide the correct amount ordered by the doctor.

Answers are on page 712.

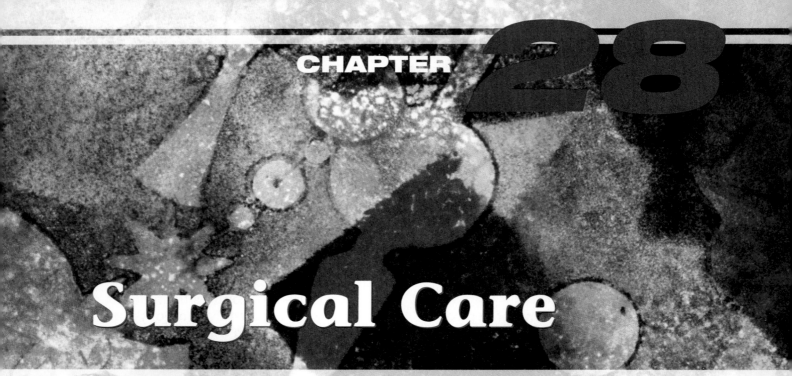

CHAPTER 28

Surgical Care

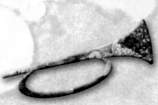

What you will learn

- How to prepare a patient for surgery
- Procedure for performing a surgical skin prep
- How to care for a patient after surgery
- Use of anti-embolism stockings

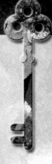

KEY TERMS

Anesthesiologist A doctor who specializes in providing medications (anesthesia) during surgery

Anti-embolism stockings Elastic stockings worn to prevent the formation of blood clots (embolism)

ECG or EKG (electrocardiogram) A recording of the electrical activity of the heart

NPO The abbreviation for "nothing by mouth"

How to Prepare a Patient for Surgery

People have surgery for many different reasons. Some operations, such as a hernia operation, are scheduled when the person wants to have it. Other operations must be done right away. For example, a person with a broken hip cannot wait several weeks for surgery. Doctors can do some minor surgeries, such as removing a mole, in their offices. People having minor surgery in a hospital or surgery center are admitted early the morning of the procedure and are discharged home later the same day. People who are having major surgery, such as heart surgery, may be admitted the day before the operation for tests.

Patients usually begin to prepare for surgery several days before the actual operation is scheduled. The admitting office calls patients to get insurance and billing information. The patients have blood and urine tests done to make sure that they are in good health. Patients who are over the age of 40 frequently have a chest x-ray film and an **ECG** or **EKG (electrocardiogram)**.

After the patient arrives at the hospital, the nurse will complete a nursing history and physical. You may help with the admission process by taking the patient's vital signs, measuring height and weight, helping the person with undressing and putting on a hospital gown, applying the identification bracelet, or obtaining a urine specimen. The surgeon will explain the procedure to the patient and obtain a signed consent form that gives the surgeon and the hospital permission to perform the operation.

A second doctor called an **anesthesiologist** will talk to the patient about medications that the patient will receive during the surgical procedure. Some patients prefer to be asleep for their surgery. This is called general anesthesia. Another type of

NOTES ON
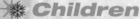 **Children**

The parents or guardian of a minor child sign the consent for surgery.

anesthesia numbs only the part of the body the doctor operates on. This is called regional or local anesthesia.

Food and fluids are usually limited for at least 6 to 8 hours before the surgery. A person who is admitted to the hospital the day before surgery will have an order to be **NPO** (nothing by mouth) after midnight. This means that the nursing assistant will remove the water glass and pitcher from the patient's bedside and remind the patient not to eat or drink anything until after surgery. In some facilities, a sign is posted over the bed to remind the patient, staff, and visitors that the person is NPO. Patients who are admitted to the hospital or surgery center the morning of surgery have to remember not to eat or drink anything after bedtime the night before the surgery. It is important that the patient's stomach be empty during surgery to prevent nausea and vomiting during the procedure. A surgical checklist is used to make sure that nothing is forgotten as the patient is prepared for surgery (Figure 28-1). You may be asked to help with the checklist. As a nursing assistant you can help the nurse by making sure that the patient is wearing a clean hospital gown and has removed all undergarments. The patient also must remove jewelry, glasses, contact lenses, hearing aids, and dentures.

NOTES ON
⑤ *Culture*

Information about the procedure and answers to questions that the patient has should be answered in a language the patient understands. This may involve asking a friend or family member to interpret the information. Many hospitals also have staff members who are bilingual (speak more than one language) who can translate the information for the patient. Many informational brochures in the hospitals are translated into several languages to help non–English-speaking patients to understand their care.

Safety

Check with your institution about the policy for storing valuables such as jewelry while the patient is in surgery. These items are usually given to a family member.

Sometimes the patient showers with a special soap the night before or the morning of surgery to remove as many germs as possible from the skin. Removing hair from the area to be operated on may also be done before the patient is moved to the operating room. (See procedure: *Surgical Skin Prep*, p. 567.) The nurse will talk to patients about what to expect when they return from surgery and will answer any questions patients have.

Safety

It is important to remember that the nurse or the doctor will answer all questions about the surgery.

Patients are asked to empty their bladder before the surgical procedure. Medication may be given to help patients to relax and prepare them for the surgery before they are moved to the operating room. The nurse will review the surgical checklist one last time before the patient moves to the operating room and sign the checklist to indicate that everything was completed.

A staff member from surgery will usually come to the patient's room to pick the patient up. You should help the patient with moving onto a stretcher if one is needed to transport the patient.

PRE-OP COMMUNICATION RECORD

Date of Interview: _____ Patient to Arrive at Hospital: (Time) _____

Patient's Language: ☐ English Out-Pt. Transportation Home: ☐ Yes ☐ No

☐ Spanish Overnight Caregiver: ☐ Yes ☐ No

☐ _____ Interpreter: _____
(name)

PATIENT PRE-OP EDUCATION & INSTRUCTION

☐ SDCC Booklet ☐ PCA Instructions ☐ Pre-op Bath/Shower

☐ In-Patient Surgery Booklet ☐ Epidural Pamphlet ☐ Enema

☐ Pediatric Coloring Book ☐ Community Resource Info ☐ Verbalizes Understanding

PATIENT HISTORY

☐ Pacemaker ☐ Seizure Disorder ☐ Diabetes ☐ Insulin Dependent ☐ Asthma

Communicable Disease Exposure? ☐ Yes ☐ No When/What?_____

Allergies: _____

Communication: _____

_____

_____ Interviewer's Signature _____

HT _____ BP _____ P _____ NPO for 8° ☐ Yes ☐ No Other _____

WT _____ T _____ R _____

Initial to Verify on Chart

_____ Operative Consent Signed _____ Urinalysis _____ EKG

_____ Special Consent Signed _____ Type and Crossmatch _____ MAR/PMFS

_____ History and Physical _____ Blood Consent Signed _____ IV Flow Sheet

_____ CBC _____ Chest X-Ray _____ Addressograph

Initial When Completed With Patient

_____ ID Band Checked _____ Jewelry ☐ Taped _____ Glasses/
Contacts ☐ Left In

_____ Patient Gown On ☐ Removed ☐ Removed

_____ Surgical Cap On Comments _____ Comments _____

_____ Bath Blanket On

_____ Voided (Time) _____ _____ Dentures ☐ Left In _____ Hearing Aids ☐ Left In

☐ Foley (Amt) _____ cc ☐ Removed ☐ Removed

Comments _____ Comments _____

Communication: _____

_____

_____

Pre-Op Diagnosis: _____

RN/LVN _____ O.R.RN _____

H7420-27 Addressograph

Figure 28-1 Sample pre-operative surgical checklist.

HOW & WHY

Any type of surgery can be frightening for patients and their family. You can help your patients to feel less afraid by remaining calm and explaining what you are doing as you prepare them for surgery.

Safety

Performing a Surgical Skin Prep

Hair may be removed from the surgical site. Germs stick to the hair and can cause an infection. Some doctors will order only a surgical scrub using a special soap. Other doctors will order a surgical skin prep, which includes washing the skin with a special soap and shaving the site to remove all hair. Figure 28-2 shows different areas of skin preparation for different types of surgery. In some facilities the surgical skin prep is completed by the nursing assistant before the patient is moved to the surgical area.

Remember to follow Standard Precautions and the Bloodborne Pathogen Standard when performing a surgical skin prep. Razors should be disposed of in an appropriate sharps container per facility policy.

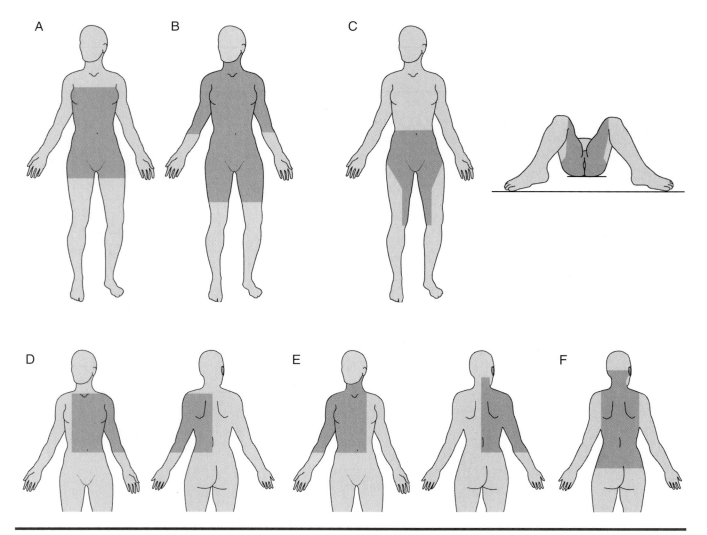

Figure 28-2 Areas of skin prep for different types of surgery. **A,** Abdominal surgery prep. **B,** Heart surgery prep. **C,** Perineal surgery prep. **D,** Chest or thoracic surgery prep. **E,** Breast surgery prep. **F,** Cervical spine surgery prep.

Procedure
SURGICAL SKIN PREP

EQUIPMENT

- Razor
- Bath basin
- Soap or skin wash
- Antibacterial solution if ordered
- Bed protector
- Gauze squares
- Towel
- Gloves

◆ **COMPLETE STANDARD BEGINNING STEPS (see inside front cover)**

1 Place the bed protector under the area to be prepped.

2 Fill the basin ½ full with warm water and soap.

3 Put on gloves.

4 Wet the gauze squares with the soap and water solution, and work up a good lather on the area to be shaved.

5 With the razor in your dominant hand, shave hair, moving away from the incision site (Figure 28-3).

6 Use firm, steady strokes, and shave a small area at a time.

7 Wash all hair off the site with gauze squares.

8 Apply the antibacterial solution with clean gauze squares or a sponge applicator.

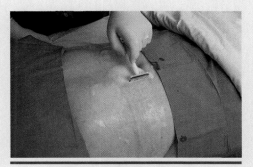

Figure 28-3 Step 5.

Continued

Procedure
SURGICAL SKIN PREP—cont'd

9 Begin at the incision site and work in a circular motion, moving away from the incision site (Figure 28-4).

10 Scrub with the antibacterial solution for 2 to 3 minutes.

11 Rinse the area with clean warm water, and dry with clean gauze squares.

12 Assist patient into a clean gown.

13 Remove, clean, and store equipment according to facility policy. Dispose of razor in a sharps container.

14 Remove your gloves and wash your hands.

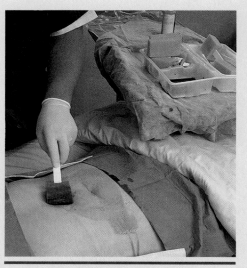

Figure 28-4 Step 9.

◆ **COMPLETE STANDARD ENDING STEPS (see inside front cover)**

How to Care for a Patient After Surgery

While patients are in surgery, you should prepare the room for their return. Make the bed with fresh linens. (See procedure: *Making a Surgical Bed,* p. 317.) Leave the bed in the high position to make it easier to transfer patients into the bed from the stretcher when they return to their room (Figure 28-5). Place any supplies or equipment needed in the room (Figure 28-6). These include:

- Intravenous (IV) pole
- Thermometer
- Stethoscope and sphygmomanometer
- Emesis basin
- Tissues
- Incentive spirometer (if ordered) (Chapter 27)

When patients returns to their room, the nurse will complete a postoperative assessment of patients. The nurse may ask you to help with the assessment by taking vital signs or measuring urine output. While each institution has its own routine, vital signs are usually taken every 15 minutes for the first hour, every 30 minutes for 2 hours, and then every hour for 4 hours. If the vital signs are within normal limits, they are taken every 4 hours for the next 1 to 3 days, depending on the type of surgery performed. Vital signs are an important part of post-surgery care. Any abnormal vital signs should be reported to the nurse im-

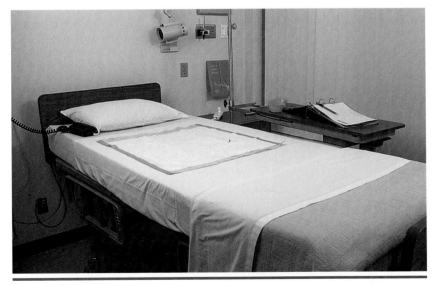

***Figure* 28-5**   Surgical bed prepared for patient returning from surgery.

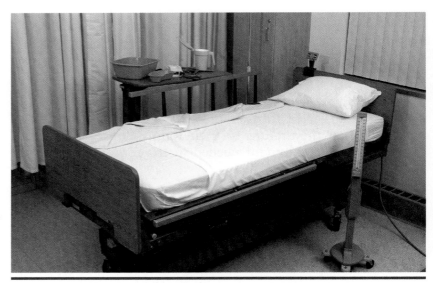

Figure 28-6 Room prepared for patient returning from surgery.

NOTES ON
✳ *Older Adults*

The elderly patient is more likely to become confused after surgery than a younger patient. The older person may be more sensitive to the medications given by the anesthesiologist. The older person is also more likely to have problems with postural hypotension after surgery (Chapter 13).

mediately. Some facilities use a postoperative checklist similar to Figure 28-7 to document the patient's condition.

If your institution uses an electronic blood pressure monitoring device, make sure you know how to use it and are comfortable with the equipment.

The doctor will provide written orders about patients' diet and activity level after the surgery. The nurse will instruct you in how to care for patients when they return to their room based on these doctor's orders.

POSTOPERATIVE RECORD

Department: _____

Date: _____ Time Received on Unit _____

Type of Surgery: _____

INITIAL POST-OP ASSESSMENT (Circle Appropriate Response)

CONSCIOUSNESS:	Awake	Arousable	Unconscious	Other: _____
AIRWAY:	None	Oral	Nasal	Endotracheal
RESPIRATION:	Deep	Shallow	Regular	Irregular
OXYGEN THERAPY:	_____ liter.	None Cannula mask Vent Tent		Other: _____
COLOR:	WNL	Pale	Cyanotic	Other: _____

PULSES: Location: _____
          Strong   Weak   Regular   Irregular

SKIN: Warm   Dry   Cool   Moist   Other: _____

DRESSINGS: None   Location: _____
              Dry   Serous   Bloody   Other: _____

DRAINS: None   Location: _____ Type: _____
                      Location: _____ Type: _____

ORTHOPEDIC: None   Cost: Location: _____ Dry   Moist
                 Splint: Location: _____
            Traction: Type: _____ # of weight: _____
                 PAS   TEDS

GI: Nausea   Emesis

GU: Foley   Suprapubic   Other: _____

                       RECEIVED BY: _____ R.N.

(See 24 Hours Patient Care Flow Sheet and Nurses Documentation Notes for Ongoing Assessment Date)

	Initial*	15"	30"	1 Hr.	1.5 Hrs.	2.5 Hrs.	3.5 Hrs.			
Actual Time										
Temp.										
B.P.										
Pulse										
Resp. *										
C.M.S.										
TCDB										
Dressing										
Voided/Amt.										
Fluids										
Fundus/Lochia										
Initials										

* Received from PAR

Initials	Signature
_____	_____
_____	_____
_____	_____
_____	_____
_____	_____

Addressograph

H8720-59 (05/02/94) G.e65

Figure 28-7   Postoperative checklist/record.

Applying Anti-embolism Stockings

Many doctors order some type of **anti-embolism stockings** (elastic stockings) for their patients after major surgery. The stockings come in three lengths: knee high, thigh high, and full length. The nurse will measure the patient's legs and order the correct size of stockings. The stockings increase the circulation in the legs (Chapter 23). (See procedure: *Applying Elastic Stockings*, p. 494.) If a patient is at high risk for blood clots in the legs, the doctor may order a device that alternately squeezes and releases the lower legs to improve circulation (Figure 28-8). There are different names for this type of device. They may be called pneumatic stockings or pneumatic boots. They may also be called compression stockings or compression boots.

Safety   The nurse will show you how to use this type of equipment if it is permitted in your job description. Never use a piece of equipment that you have not been trained to used.

Anti-embolism stockings should be removed each shift to check for skin breakdown or redness. Stockings may be washed using a mild soap and warm water. Rinse thoroughly, squeeze out excess water, and roll in a dry towel. Allow the stockings to hang to air dry. A second pair of stockings should be ordered so that the patient is not without the stockings for more than 30 minutes twice a day.

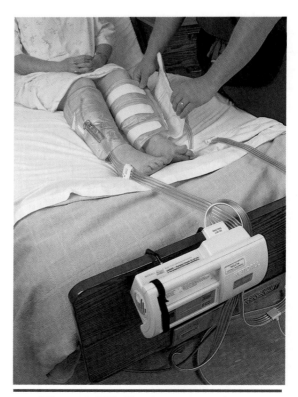

***Figure* 28-8**   Compression boots.

CHAPTER REVIEW

1. List 3 things the nursing assistant can do to assist in preparing the patient for surgery.

2. What does the abbreviation NPO mean?

3. Why are patients NPO before their surgery?

4. What is the purpose of a surgical skin prep?

5. What kind of equipment is usually needed to care for patients after they return from their surgery?

6. How often are vitals signs normally taken when a patient returns from surgery?

7. How often should anti-embolism stockings be removed and why?

Circle the one BEST response.

8. Mr. Smithton is an 84-year-old patient scheduled for hernia surgery. What types of tests should he expect to have done before the procedure?
   a. ECG
   b. Chest x-ray film
   c. Blood tests
   d. All of the above

Answers are on page 712.

CHAPTER 29

Rehabilitation and Restorative Care

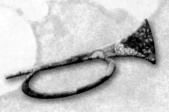

What you will learn

- The goals of rehabilitation and restorative care
- Types of therapy services available
- The role of team members
- Assisting with rehabilitation and restorative care

KEY TERMS

Acute Short term or sudden

Chronic Long-lasting or ongoing

Contractures Joints that do not have a normal shape, which is caused by shortening of the muscle

Disability A lost physical or mental function

Pneumonia Inflammation/infection of the lungs

The Goals of Rehabilitation and Restorative Care

The terms *rehabilitation* and *restorative care* are sometimes used to mean the same thing. It is the process of helping injured or ill people return to their highest possible level of wellness. It also refers to care that helps people regain their health, independence, and strength after an injury or illness.

All residents of long-term care (LTC) facilities must receive restorative care that helps them to return to their highest level of functioning and helps to prevent the loss of present functioning.

OBRA

Illness, injury, and surgery can affect the body's ability to function. The term **disability** is used to describe a lost physical or mental function. A disability may be either a physical or a mental loss. The inability to walk after a stroke is an example of a physical disability. The inability to think clearly or use good judgment due to Alzheimer's disease is an example of a mental disability. Some disabilities last only a short time and are called **acute** disabilities. If you broke your hand and it was placed in a cast for 4 weeks, you would have an acute disability. Your lost physical function would last only as long as you had the cast on your hand. A **chronic** disability is a problem that lasts for a long time or even permanently. People who have had their leg amputated (removed) due to medical problems of diabetes have a chronic disability.

There are 3 main reasons to provide rehabilitation or restorative care:

1. To keep present function
2. To restore or regain lost function after illness, injury, or surgery
3. To prevent the complications of immobility such as **contractures**, **pneumonia**, and blood clots

Types of Therapy Services Available

The type of services people need depends on the type of disability they have. Any disability, illness, or injury affects people's physical, emotional, and social well-being. For example, people who have had a stroke may need services to help them with eating, dressing, bathing, walking, and speaking. Three types of therapy services are available:

1. *Physical therapy* (PT) treats disabilities using physical methods, including heat, massage, physical exercises, and whirlpool therapy.
2. *Occupational therapy* (OT) treats disabilities by providing adaptive equipment and activities to improve function.
3. *Speech therapy* (ST) treats speech and language disorders and swallowing problems.

Doctors will order a consult with the therapy department for their patient. A therapist from each type of therapy evaluates the patient to determine the best way to give restorative or rehabilitative care. Each therapist makes recommendations to the doctor, who approves them and gives the OK for the therapy to begin.

The Role of Team Members

Providing restorative care is a team approach (Figure 29-1). Members of the team share their thoughts and ideas about the rehabilitation. Together the team members put together a plan with specific goals. The team meets frequently to discuss the plans and to decide if the team is meeting its goals. The patient or resident is the "team captain" and is the most important member of the team. Patients' goals are the most important, and the team has to listen to their opinions. If the goals of the team are not the same as the goals of the patient, everyone will be unhappy with the end result. For example, if walking without help is the most important goal to the patient, but the rest of the team feels that working on speech is more important, the patient is less likely to be motivated and may even give up.

OBRA

The development of a plan of care that focuses on the resident and promotes physical, emotional, and psychological well-being is an OBRA requirement. OBRA also requires that all LTC facilities provide restorative or rehabilitation services. Some LTC facilities have a contract with an outside therapy service to provide its rehabilitation or restorative services. The facility is still responsible for making sure the resident receives the care required.

Successful rehabilitation depends on positive attitudes. The staff must always be supportive of patients and focus on their abilities, not their disabilities. Even when progress is slow and

The Rehabilitation Team

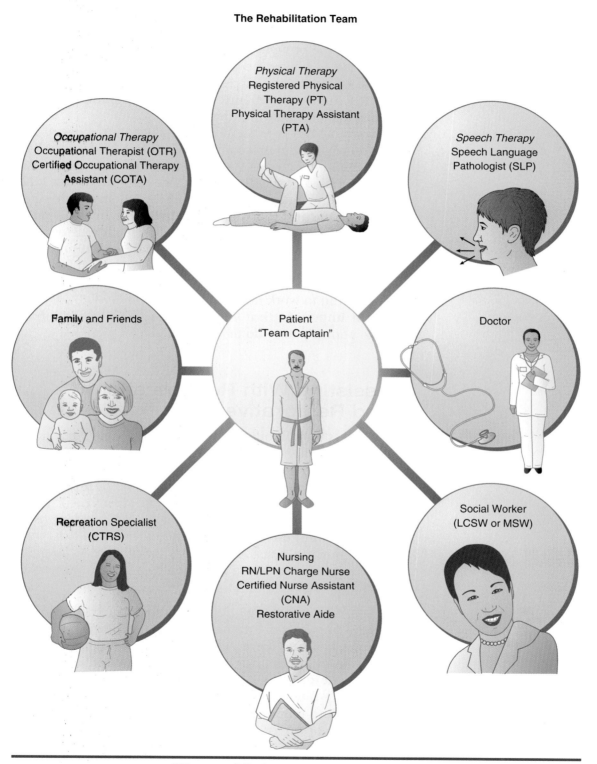

Figure 29-1 The rehabilitation team.

NOTES ON
☯ *Culture*

The role of the patient's family and friends in the restorative process varies with different cultures.

the patient is discouraged, a positive attitude will help the patient to move forward. The team must also think about the attitude of the patient. If patients are unwilling to do the therapy activities or have a negative attitude, it will be much more difficult for them to be successful and to reach their goals. The support of family and friends can help keep patients motivated to participate in their therapy.

Some health care facilities use restorative aides to help with the rehabilitation process. The restorative aide is usually a nursing assistant who has been given more training in physical, occupational, and speech therapy. The restorative aide follows the plan of care and works with the patient. Some states offer a separate certification for the restorative aide. In some states there are no specific requirements and each facility determines what the role of the restorative aide will be. Becoming a restorative aide is considered a promotion, and the position is offered to individuals who show excellent communication skills and who are willing to work hard.

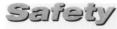

It is important that you know what the regulations in your state permit you to do or not do.

Assisting With Rehabilitation and Restorative Care

Successful rehabilitation improves people's quality of life. Even if people have a disability that cannot be cured, helping them to become as independent and healthy as possible will help them to feel better about themselves. Your participation in the rehabilitation process will help people succeed. Your job focuses on encouraging people to be as independent as possible and to prevent any further decline in their abilities.

OBRA

The nursing assistant provides rehabilitation or restorative care according to the OBRA guidelines by following the recommendations in Box 29-1.

Safety

If you have any questions about assistive devices, splints, or braces, always ask the therapist or the charge nurse for direction before using them.

While many therapy services are provided in a hospital or nursing home setting, therapy can also be provided to patients in an outpatient therapy center or in their home. The principles of providing rehabilitation or restorative services are the same regardless of where the services are provided.

Box 29-1

ROLE OF THE NURSING ASSISTANT IN REHABILITATION AND RESTORATIVE CARE

- Following the care plan to help people be able to do what they want
- Providing emotional support and encouragement
- Focusing on people's abilities, not their disabilities
- Treating people with dignity and respect
- Trying to understand people's feelings if they are discouraged or sad
- Allowing as much time as people need to complete their activities of daily living such as bathing, dressing, and grooming
- Providing assistive devices as indicated on the care plan and assisting people with using them correctly (Figures 29-2 to 29-9)

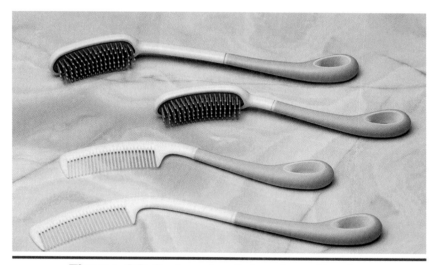

Figure 29-2   Long-handled combs and brushes.

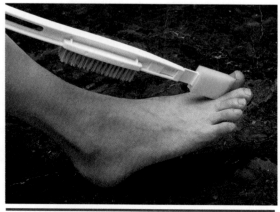

Figure 29-3   Long-handled brush for bathing.

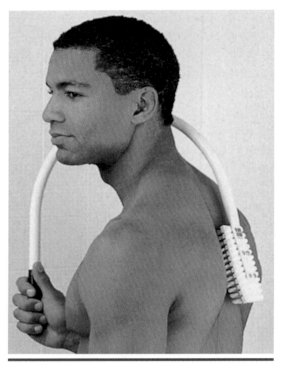

Figure 29-4 Brush with curved handle to assist with bathing.

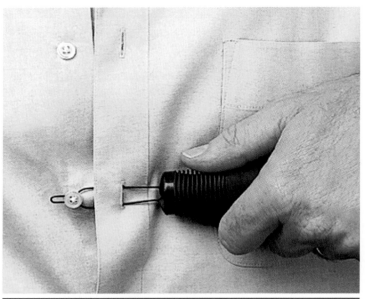

Figure 29-5 Button hook for buttoning shirts and blouses.

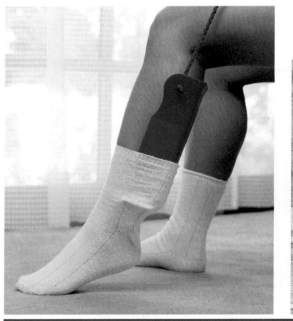

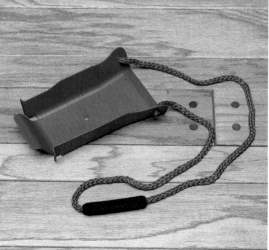

Figure 29-6 Sock assist is used to pull on socks or stockings.

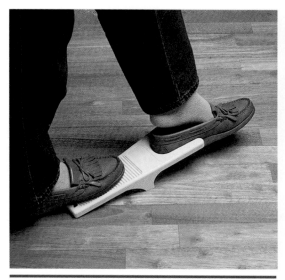

Figure 29-7 Shoe remover assists with removing shoes.

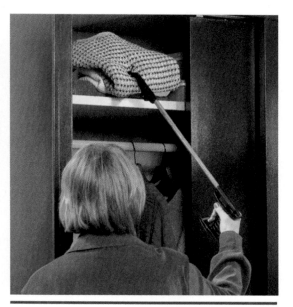

Figure 29-8 Reachers help when picking items up off the floor or reaching for items above the person's head.

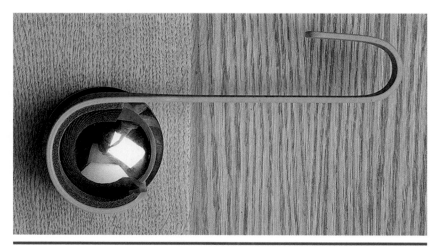

Figure 29-9 Door knob turner increases leverage and makes knobs easier to turn.

CHAPTER REVIEW

1. What is rehabilitation or restorative care?

2. What are the 3 main reasons to provide rehabilitation or restorative care?

3. Who is the most important member of the rehabilitation team?

4. How can you help with the process of rehabilitation or restorative care?

Circle the one BEST response.

5. A problem that lasts a short period of time is called
   a. Acute
   b. Chronic
   c. Disability
   d. Functional

6. Which type of therapy treats disabilities by providing adaptive equipment and activities to improve function?
   a. Occupational therapy
   b. Physical therapy
   c. Respiratory therapy
   d. Speech therapy

Answers are on page 712 to 713.

CHAPTER 30

Confusion, Dementia, and Other Mental Health Disorders

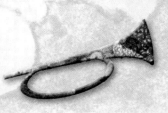

What you will learn

- Caring for a confused person
- Caring for a person with dementia or Alzheimer's disease
- Caring for persons with other mental health disorders

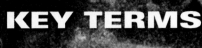

KEY TERMS

Alzheimer's disease (AD) A disease of the brain cells that control memory, thinking, judgment, language, behavior, and personality. It is the most common form of dementia

Catastrophic reaction When people with dementia are unable to control their behavior and react to the frustration they feel by showing too much emotion in a situation. During a catastrophic reaction people may try to hit people because they are angry or afraid

Confusion A mental state in which people do not know who the people around them are, where they are, or what time period they are in. Both memory and thinking are affected

Delirium Confusion that is temporary and can come on suddenly. Delirium is likely to be the side effect of a medication, an illness, or an infection

Dementia Confusion caused by an injury to the brain or a long-term lack of blood flow to the brain. The confusion starts slowly, gets worse over time, and is permanent

Hallucinations Seeing, hearing, or feeling something that is not real

Reality orientation Helping people to know and remember people around them and the place and time they are in

Sundowning Behavior problems that get worse in the late afternoon or evening as the sun goes down

Validation therapy A method of talking with someone that allows confused people to talk about their thoughts and feel safe and accepted

Caring for a Confused Person

The term **confusion** refers to a mental state in which people do not understand what is happening around them or who the people around them are. Both memory and thinking are affected. There are many causes of confusion, such as:

- Dehydration
- Infections
- Constipation in an elderly person
- Medications
- Hearing or vision loss
- Depression
- New surroundings

Some confusion is temporary and can come on suddenly. This type of confusion, called **delirium**, is likely to be the side effect of a medication, an illness, or an infection. When the person stops taking the medication or the illness or infection is treated, the confusion goes away.

When caring for a person with confusion, the nursing assistant should:

- Follow the person's care plan so that the care is the same from day to day.
- Call the person by name and identify yourself.
- Explain what you are doing and why as you assist with care.
- Provide a clock, calendar, and familiar objects to help the person to become familiar with the surroundings (Figure 30-1). This is called **Reality orientation.**
- Keep a calm, quiet environment where there is no noise and confusion.

Confused people may not know their family members and may not know where they are. Some people are unable to remember how to perform their daily grooming when they become confused. The person who is confused may become angry, frightened, or withdrawn.

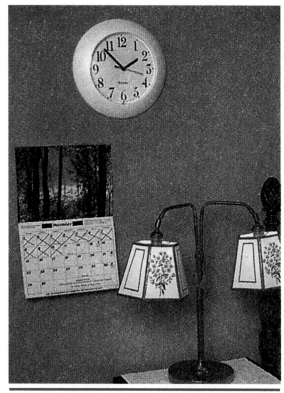

***Figure* 30-1**   Clocks and calendars help the person to stay oriented to time.

Caring for a Person With Dementia or Alzheimer's Disease

When confusion is caused by an injury to the brain or a long-term lack of blood flow to the brain, the confusion starts slowly and gets worse. This type of confusion is called **dementia** and is permanent. Dementia can be caused by several diseases or conditions, including:

- Alzheimer's disease
- Acquired immunodeficiency syndrome (AIDS)
- Brain tumors
- Stroke
- Pick's disease
- Huntington's disease
- Syphilis
- Head injury

The most common form of dementia is Alzheimer's disease. **Alzheimer's disease (AD)** is a disease of the brain cells that control memory, thinking, judgment, language, behavior, and personality. The person with AD begins to have problems with work, family, and social relationships. There is a steady loss of memory and thinking ability. Over 3 to 20 years, people with AD lose more and more of their ability until they must depend on others for their care.

Stages of Alzheimer's Disease

Alzheimer's disease is described in 3 stages based on the person's symptoms.

STAGE 1. At this stage people are usually able to live at home and look normal (Figure 30-2). Symptoms of stage 1 include:

- Difficulty concentrating
- Gradual loss of ability to remember recent events such as what they ate for breakfast
- Easily becoming annoyed or unhappy
- Poor judgment
- Decreased interest in social events
- Saying that others are responsible for their mistakes and problems

STAGE 2. The person continues to be in good physical health, but the memory loss is more severe (Figure 30-3). Symptoms during this stage begin to cause problems and include:

- Not understanding time
- Loses personal belongings
- May be very restless and be moving around an area without a place to go (wandering)
- Forgets normal routines and needs help with grooming

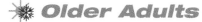

NOTES ON
Older Adults

Alzheimer's disease is most commonly seen in people over the age of 65.

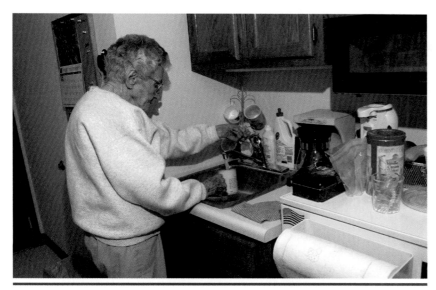

***Figure* 30-2**   The person with stage 1 Alzheimer's disease is usually able to remain in her home.

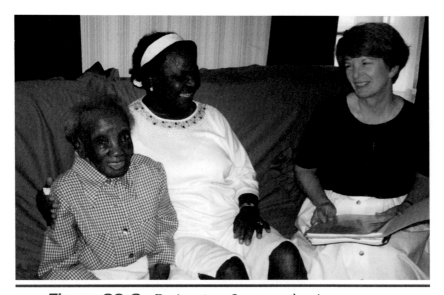

***Figure* 30-3**   During stage 2 memory loss is more severe.

- May become incontinent
- Begins to have problems talking with others
- Difficulty walking or walk without lifting their feet off the ground
- Sleep problems
- **Hallucinations**—seeing, hearing, or feeling something that is not real

- Inability to control behavior, sudden powerful expression of anger
- **Sundowning**—behavior problems that get worse in the late afternoon or evening as the sun goes down

During stage 2 many families will require help caring for the person with Alzheimer's disease. Home health care or nursing home placement may be required.

STAGE 3. During stage 3 of Alzheimer's disease the person becomes totally dependent on a caregiver (Figure 30-4). The person continues to decline mentally and physically with symptoms including:

- Inability to recognize friends or family
- Inability to speak
- Cannot swallow
- Little or no response to surroundings
- Severe weight loss
- Inability to walk
- Total incontinence

The person with stage 3 Alzheimer's becomes totally bed bound and eventually becomes comatose and dies.

Caring for people with dementia takes patience. People with dementia may have trouble dealing with the stress of day-to-day living. Imagine how you would feel if you did not know who you were and did not understand the things going on around you. People with dementia are unable to control their

NOTES ON
☯ Culture

People with Alzheimer's disease may go back to speaking their native language during the second and third stage of the disease even though they have been speaking English for many years.

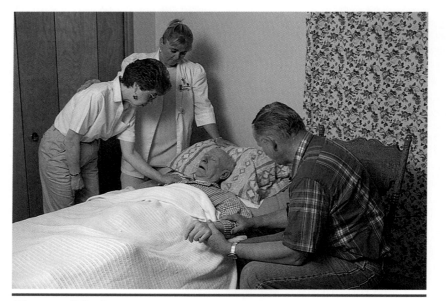

***Figure* 30-4** During stage 3 the person becomes totally dependent on the caregiver.

behavior and may show too much emotion in situations. This is called a **catastrophic reaction.** During a catastrophic reaction people may hit others because they are angry or afraid. It is important for you to create a calm, low-stress environment for the person with dementia. You can do this by:

- Looking for signs that the person is getting upset
- Treating the person with respect; do not argue with the person
- Using **validation therapy**—a way of talking to people that allows confused people to talk about their thoughts and to feel safe and accepted
- Speaking calmly and quietly (Figure 30-5)
- Speaking to the person in short simple sentences
- Knowing the person as an individual, including the person's likes and dislikes
- Providing rest periods throughout the day (Figure 30-6)
- Assisting the person with using the bathroom at least every 2 to 3 hours
- Maintaining a constant routine from day to day
- Maintaining a calm, quiet environment where there is no noise and confusion
- Providing a safe area for the person to walk around freely (Figure 30-7)

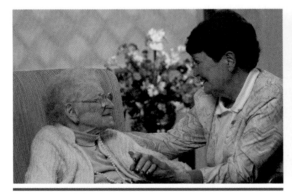

***Figure* 30-5**   Speak calmly and quietly to the patient with Alzheimer's disease.

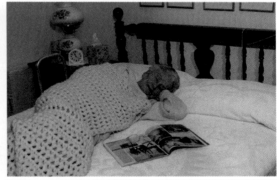

***Figure* 30-6**   Rest periods throughout the day help prevent the person from being overly tired.

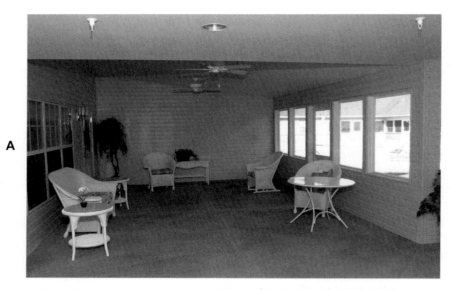

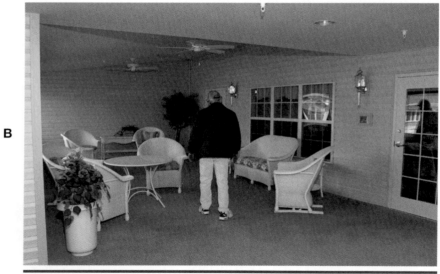

Figure 30-7 A, B, Providing a safe environment is important when caring for patients who wander.

The concept of using validation therapy instead of reality orientation when caring for patients with dementia is based on the work of social worker Naomi Feil. For many years caregivers tried to reorient patients with dementia to their environment using the traditional methods of reminding patients of the day, date, and time, as well as who and where they were. In most cases it did not work, and patients became more agitated or withdrawn.

Validation therapy was developed to help the older person with dementia. It is believed that the elderly person may be trying to "tie up loose ends." By careful listening, eye contact, and touch the caregiver can build a sense of mutual respect and trust with the elder. Most important, feelings can be understood. When recent memory fails, such as with Alzheimer's disease, patients may try to restore balance to their life by reliving the past. Validation therapy allows disoriented people to express their feelings in a safe environment (Box 30-1).

Some facilities provide a special unit to care for people with Alzheimer's disease and dementia. Staff members on the special unit receive training to help them better understand the needs of their patients. There are medications available to treat some of symptoms of AD, but at this time there is no cure.

Box 30-1

USING VALIDATION THERAPY

Esther is a 91-year-old patient with stage 2 Alzheimer's disease. She is a resident in a long-term care facility. When Esther wanders the halls calling for her mother, the staff reminds her that she is 91 years old, lives in a nursing home, and her mother has died. This causes Esther to become very upset and even violent with the staff. If asked, Esther thinks that she is in her 40s and needs to return home to care for her mother, who is ill.

By using validation therapy, the nursing staff would be better able to meet Esther's needs. Instead of forcing Esther to become reoriented to reality, the nursing assistant can talk to Esther about her mother, asking questions and making statements such as "You must miss your mother" and "Can you tell me about your mother? What was her name?"

The nursing assistant is honest with Esther and does not tell her things that are untrue. But she does not force Esther to acknowledge that she is old, she is living in a nursing home, and her mother has died. Esther tells the nursing assistant about her mother and admits that she misses her. Esther feels safe talking to the nursing assistant, who is kind and allows her to talk about her feelings. It is even possible that Esther will remember that her mother has died. Esther is calm and allows the nursing assistant to redirect her to the dining room for lunch.

OBRA
All employees who care for confused residents must receive special training so that residents receive care that makes their quality of life better.

OBRA
When a long-term care (LTC) resident is placed on a secured unit, a safe environment where the residents can be active must be provided.

Safety
Safety is a major concern when working with patients who are confused or mentally ill. These patients may not be able to make good decisions and may act in ways that are unsafe and put them at risk for injury.

Caring for Persons With Other Mental Health Disorders

Mental health disorders can affect people's physical health, as well as their social and spiritual well-being. Mental health disorders can be caused by:

- Chemical imbalances
- Genetic factors
- Social or cultural factors
- Drug or alcohol abuse

Mental health disorders may also be called mental illness, psychiatric disease, or emotional problems. It is important that you remember that people with a mental health disorder are ill. Just like people with heart disease or diabetes, they did not choose to have a disease. Commonly seen mental health disorders include:

- *Anxiety disorders*—People with an anxiety disorder experience an intense feeling of nervousness and cannot relax when they are in a stressful situation. Symptoms can include dry mouth, sweating, nausea, diarrhea, rapid pulse and respirations, increased blood pressure, difficulty sleeping, and loss of appetite.
- *Panic disorder*—A panic disorder is the highest level of anxiety. During a panic attack the person has an intense and sudden feeling of fear or terror. During a panic attack the person cannot function. A panic attack can last for a few minutes or several hours.
- *Phobic disorders*—The person with a phobia has a strong fear of a situation or an object. Examples of phobias include fear of water, flying, heights, public places, insects, or strangers. A person can have a strong fear of almost anything.
- *Obsessive-compulsive disorder (OCD)*—People with OCD have a constant thought or idea and feel that they have to do some action again and again. Fear of dirt and constant hand washing is an example of an OCD.
- *Schizophrenia*—People with schizophrenia do not see reality correctly. They may believe that they are someone else, hear or see things that do not exist, or think that people around them are trying to do something bad to them.
- *Bipolar disorder*—In bipolar disorder people have severe mood swings. Their mood changes from a high (mania) to low feeling (depression). During the manic phase people are full of energy and are very excited and busy. During the depressive phase, they feel sad, lonely, or that they have no good qualities.
- *Depression*—With depression people feel very sad. They may not want to perform the tasks of daily living, may have problems sleeping or paying attention to things, and may even think about suicide (killing themselves).
- *Personality disorders*—People with a personality disorder may have trouble functioning in society. They will deal with daily stresses in negative ways such as by becoming violent, using cruel words, thinking that other people are trying to do something bad to them, or getting angry and arguing with others.

NOTES ON
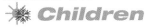
Mental health disorders are also seen in children.

NOTES ON

☯ Culture

In some cultures mental illness is seen as a "weakness." Some cultures also view the person who is mentally ill as dangerous or evil.

You should talk to your charge nurse and review the care plan for guidance in caring for a patient with a mental health disorder. A person who is admitted to a health care facility for a physical problem such as a fractured hip or diabetes may also have a diagnosed mental health disorder but will be admitted to a general medical or surgical unit. If people are being admitted specifically for treatment of a mental health disorder, they are usually admitted to a special area of the hospital called a psychiatric or mental health unit. Treatment of mental health disorders can include medications and psychotherapy that helps people to think and talk about their thoughts or feelings.

CHAPTER REVIEW

1. What is confusion?

2. List 4 possible causes of confusion.

3. List 3 things you can do when caring for the confused person.

4. What is dementia?

5. What is the most common form of dementia?

6. Mr. Henderson has a hard time remembering recent events, has become moody, and is having a hard time concentrating. Which stage of Alzheimer's disease do you think he is in?

7. What is a hallucination?

8. What is a catastrophic reaction?

9. How can you create a low-stress environment for the person with dementia?

Circle the one BEST response.

10. Mental health disorders can be caused by
    a. Chemical imbalances
    b. Genetic factors
    c. Social or cultural factor
    d. Drug or alcohol abuse
    e. All of the above

11. Mrs. Lewis has a strong fear of spiders This is a called a(n)
    a. Anxiety disorder
    b. Panic disorder
    c. Phobic disorder
    d. Personality disorder

12. Dry mouth, sweating, nausea, diarrhea, rapid pulse and respirations, increased blood pressure, difficulty sleeping, and loss of appetite due to stress are symptoms of
    a. Anxiety disorder
    b. Panic disorder
    c. Phobic disorder
    d. Personality disorder

Fill in the blank with the correct term.

13. Some confusion is temporary and can come on suddenly. This type of confusion is called _____.

Answers are on page 713.

CHAPTER 31

Care of the Dying Person

What you will learn

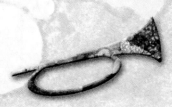

- Cultural and individual attitudes toward death
- Advance directives
- Stages of death and dying
- Caring for the dying person
- Hospice care
- Signs of death
- Providing postmortem care

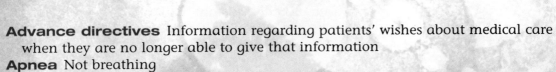

KEY TERMS

Advance directives Information regarding patients' wishes about medical care when they are no longer able to give that information

Apnea Not breathing

Cheyne-Stokes respiration An irregular breathing pattern with slowing of respiration with periods of not breathing

Coroner A person with the legal power to pronounce the patient dead

DNR ("Do Not Resuscitate") order An order written by the doctor when the patient does not want any life-prolonging treatment such as cardiopulmonary resuscitation (CPR)

Hospice A type of care that provides support for the patient and family during the dying process

Palliative care When the goal of medical and nursing care is to keep the person as comfortable as possible rather than to cure the disease

Postmortem care Care of the person after death

Rigor mortis A temporary stiffening of the muscles after death, which occurs shortly after death

Cultural and Individual Attitudes Toward Death

As a nursing assistant, you will provide care to patients during the final stage of their lives. In all cultures and religions there are customs and beliefs to help us deal with death and dying. Your feelings about death may be affected by your own personal experiences, your culture, your religion, and the age of the person involved. To help your patients and their families cope with the dying process, you must better understand your own feelings. For example, in some cultures the body must be buried, and in other cultures cremation (burning the body) is preferred. If your own beliefs or customs are different from those of your patients, you may feel uncomfortable carrying out their wishes. If the person who is dying is very old, it may be easier to accept than the death of a child. Regardless of the beliefs of the caregiver, all dying patients have certain rights, including:

- The right to be treated as a living person until the time of their death
- The right to be as pain free and comfortable as possible
- The right to honest answers and information about medical conditions

- The right to competent and compassionate care
- The right to express emotions freely without being judged
- The right to die with dignity
- The right to respectful treatment of the body after death

As a nursing assistant, you are responsible for providing the best possible care for your dying patients.

Advance Directives

Advance directives give information about patients' wishes about medical care when they are no longer able to give that information. When developing an advance directive, patients decide what are important to them and what types of care are life-prolonging versus comfort measures. The patient's decisions regarding tube feedings, cardiopulmonary resuscitation (CPR), and ventilators are written down in a legal record. The patient can give another person durable power of attorney for health care. This means that this person makes decisions about a patient's medical treatment if he is unable to do so. A copy of the patient's advance directive is placed in the medical record so that all caregivers know the patient's wishes.

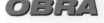

There is much discussion in health care today regarding end-of-life decisions. Residents have the right to accept or refuse any medical care. Residents may decide that if their condition is terminal, they do not want to receive life-prolonging treatment such as CPR. When this happens, the doctor will write a **DNR** (**"Do Not Resuscitate"**) **order.** As a health care provider, you must deal with your own feelings and values and respect the feelings and values of your residents when they are different from your own.

Stages of Death and Dying

During the 1960s a psychiatrist named Dr. Elisabeth Kübler-Ross began working with people with terminal illnesses. During this time she identified 5 different stages that people go through during the loss and grieving process. A person's family and friends may also feel the stages of loss and grieving. These stages are denial, anger, bargaining, depression, and acceptance (Box 31-1). Some people stay in one stage until their death. Others move back and forth between the stages. As a nursing assistant, you may also feel the stages of grieving and loss when caring for the dying person.

A person may be in the stage of acceptance when you arrive on duty and become angry by lunchtime. Since the nursing assistant provides most of the hands-on care to patients, you need

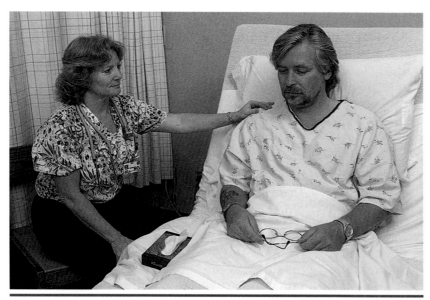

Figure 31-1 Take time to listen and talk to your patient.

Box 31-1

DR. ELISABETH KÜBLER-ROSS'S 5 STAGES OF GRIEVING

1. *Denial*—"No, not me!" People refuse to believe that they are dying. They may get other opinions or believe that the doctor is wrong.
2. *Anger*—"Why me?" People become angry with the people around them and often blame the doctor or nursing staff for their illness.
3. *Bargaining*—"OK, me but . . . ." People try to get more time by bargaining with their health care providers or God.
4. *Depression*—"This is hopeless." People become very sad and mourn over things they did not do or the people they will leave behind.
5. *Acceptance*—"I'm ready to die." People find a sense of peace and accept their death. This stage does not mean that death is near. Many older people accept their own death a long time before they actually die.

to be aware of the stage the patient is experiencing at that time (Figure 31-1).

Families will also go through these stages and may need your support as much as your patient does. Some patients may not be comfortable talking to their family members about dying but will share their thoughts and feelings with you, the nursing assistant.

Caring for the Dying Person

Nursing care for the dying patient is not very different from the care you provide to all of your patients each day. It is important to encourage all patients to make as many decisions about their care as possible. This is also true with the dying patient. For many dying patients the focus is on "care" rather than on "cure." This means that the goal of medical and nursing care is to keep the person as comfortable as possible, not to cure the disease. This is called **palliative care.** Things that you can do to make the dying person as comfortable as possible include:

- Tell the charge nurse about all complaints of pain. With the medications available, it is not necessary for the patient to suffer. Some people may not "complain" of pain, so you will have to ask them how they feel.
- Continue to give food and fluids to the patient that the doctor orders. Some diseases and medications can cause nausea or a loss of appetite. Allow these patients to decide what they would like to eat or drink, and give small, frequent meals if patients want them. Provide good oral hygiene.
- If the person is spending a lot of time in bed, skin care is more important than normal. Make sure the person's skin is clean and dry, and help your patient to turn and reposition at least every 2 hours to avoid skin breakdown.
- Speak in a normal tone of voice to these patients, and remember that even if they cannot respond to you, they may be able to understand what you are saying to them. Explain what you are doing, and be careful what you say in front of the patient. Many people believe that hearing is the last sense to leave the body when a person dies.
- Allow for frequent rest periods when providing care. Bathing and grooming can make the person feel tired or "worn out." Dying patients gets weaker and weaker and may need more help with their hygiene needs. Allow the patients to do as much as possible for themselves, but do not make them do more than they feel they can.
- Take time to listen to your patient. We all need to feel that our life has had meaning. Dying patients may want to tell you their life story as they work through the stages of grieving. Show an interest in what the patient is telling you.

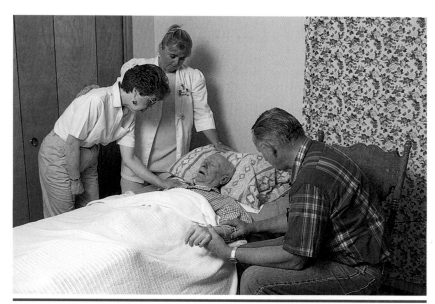

Figure **31-2**   In hospice care, care is provided to the family as well as the patient, such as with a patient in the last stage of Alzheimer's disease.

Hospice Care

Hospice is a type of care that gives support to the patient and family during the dying process. It is provided to a person who has a life expectancy of 6 months or less. The idea behind hospice care is that death is a natural part of the life cycle. Hospice care encourages the patient to make each day the best it can be. Hospice care can be provided in a hospital, nursing home, or the patient's home because it is a way of providing care, not a place (Figure 31-2). The goals of hospice care include:

- Controlling pain so that the people are active in their life until the day that they die
- Providing emotional, spiritual, physical, and social support to the patient and the family, including follow-up with the family after the person has died
- Helping the patient and family to make decisions about legal and financial issues
- Using a team approach that includes doctors, nurses, social workers, clergy, and volunteers to support the patient and family

All patients have the right to appropriate and competent care and to be treated with dignity and respect. Some staff members may not be comfortable caring for dying patients and may not give them the care they need. This violates the patient's rights.

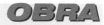

Signs of Death

It is impossible to predict when death will actually occur. Sometimes patients who appear to be near death will improve and live additional days, weeks, or months. We do know that as a person nears death the body systems slow down and the person becomes weaker. The dying person tends to sleep more and may have little or no desire for food or fluids. As the person moves closer to death, other signs may include:

- Decreased urine output and/or incontinence may occur.
- Decreased blood pressure may occur.
- Skin may become cool, pale, or gray.
- An irregular breathing pattern with slowing of respiration with periods of not breathing (**apnea**) called **Cheyne-Stokes respiration** may occur.
- Body temperature may rise even though the arms and legs are cool to the touch.
- Pulse is fast, weak, and irregular.
- Mucus may collect in the back of the throat, causing a "death rattle."

Death occurs when the patient is not breathing and does not have a pulse or a blood pressure. The heart may continue to beat for a few minutes even after the person has stopped breathing.

Providing Postmortem Care

Postmortem care is the care of the person after death. Postmortem care is provided as soon as possible after the person dies. **Rigor mortis**, a temporary stiffening of the muscles after death, occurs shortly after death. It is harder to give postmortem care after rigor mortis occurs. Your facility will have a policy and procedure for caring for your patients after their death. Depending on the circumstances of the death, a doctor may be required to see the patient to pronounce the patient dead and complete a death certificate. In other settings a person with the legal power to pronounce the patient dead may do this. This person is called a **coroner.** It is important to be familiar with the policies of your institution. If you are not familiar with the postmortem care policies and procedures, ask your charge nurse or supervisor for direction.

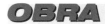

Even after the person has died, the body should be treated with respect. Do not expose the body more than is necessary to provide care. Remember to close the door and the privacy curtain when giving postmortem care. The patient also has the right to privacy regarding a medical condition. Questions about a person's illness or cause of death should be referred to the charge nurse.

In some cases the family may be asked if they wish to donate the organs of the person who has died. Some families will wish to the view the body of the person who has died. Other families want the body transported to the morgue or a funeral home. Basic postmortem care is similar in most facilities. Some patients donate their bodies to medical schools or research facilities to help doctors learn how to cure diseases. Your charge nurse will let you know if there is anything special you need to do when providing postmortem care.

Remember to follow Standard Precautions and the Bloodborne Pathogen Standard when providing postmortem care.

NOTES ON
☯ Culture

Some cultures and religions have rituals that must be performed after the person has died. It is important to respect each patient's cultural beliefs.

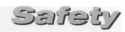

Procedure
PROVIDING POSTMORTEM CARE (CARE AFTER DEATH)

EQUIPMENT

- Basin of warm water
- Towels
- Washcloths
- Comb or brush
- Denture cup if needed
- Bags for valuables
- Gloves

◆ **COMPLETE STANDARD BEGINNING STEPS (see inside front cover)**

1 Raise the bed to a comfortable working height, and place the overbed table next to the bed.

2 Ask the nurse to remove any tubes or dressings.

3 Wash your hands and put on gloves.

4 Place the person in the supine position with a pillow under the head.

5 Raise the head of the bed 30 degrees to prevent discoloration of the face (Figure 31-3).

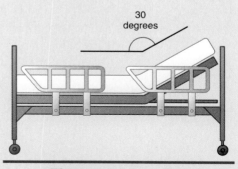

30 degrees

Figure 31-3   Step 5.

Continued

Procedure
PROVIDING POSTMORTEM CARE
(CARE AFTER DEATH)—cont'd

6   If the eyes are open, close the eyes

7   Following the procedure for bathing in Chapter 15, wash any soiled areas of the body and pat dry.

8   Following the procedure in Chapter 18, put a clean gown on the person.

9   Follow your facility's policy if the person has dentures. Some facilities require that the dentures be placed in the person's mouth. Other facilities require that the dentures be placed in a denture cup marked with the person's name.

10   Comb or brush the hair.

11   Place all belongings and valuables in a bag, and give it to the charge nurse to be returned to the family per facility policy.

12   Arrange linens neatly by bringing the top sheet up to the person's chest and folding it back once to make a cuff.

13   Straighten the room, and remove all medical equipment.

14   Provide privacy for the family if they wish to view the body.

15   Remove your gloves and wash your hands.

◆ **COMPLETE STANDARD ENDING STEPS (see inside front cover)**

CHAPTER REVIEW

1. List 4 things that may affect your attitudes about death.

2. What are advance directives?

3. What are the 5 stages people go through when dealing with death or loss, according to Dr. Elisabeth Kübler-Ross?

4. What is hospice care?

5. List 3 signs of death.

6. What is postmortem care?

Circle the one BEST response.

7. Which of the following should the nursing assistant do when caring for a dying person?
   a. Make sure the person spends a lot of time out of bed.
   b. Provide large meals to ensure good nutrition.
   c. Be as quiet as possible when providing care.
   d. Allow for frequent rest periods.

Answers are on page 713 to 714.

CHAPTER 32

Care of Mothers and Infants

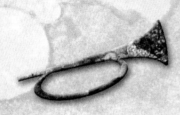

What you will learn

- How to provide postpartum care
- Basic infant care and feeding
- Safety and security for mothers and infants

KEY TERMS

Cesarean section (C-section) A surgical procedure in which the baby is delivered through an incision in the abdomen rather than through the vagina, or birth canal

Episiotomy A surgical incision made to enlarge the vaginal opening for delivery

Fundus The top of the uterus

Lochia Discharge that flows from the vagina after childbirth

Postpartum care Care of the new mother and her baby for 6 weeks after delivery

The birth of a child is a time of change for the family, but especially for the mother. During the first day or two after delivery, the woman needs rest and food that will help her stay healthy. For the first few days after delivery, some women may have difficulty sleeping or feel sad and feel like they want to cry. This may be caused by being tired, hormonal changes, and the emotional changes that come with a new baby. If this is the woman's first child, she may feel that she does not know what to do and ask a lot of questions about caring for her infant.

For many women the hospital stay for a regular delivery is 12 to 48 hours. Your care can help the new mother be more comfortable when she is discharged from the hospital.

Providing Postpartum Care

The term **postpartum care** is used to describe the care of the new mother and her baby for 6 weeks after delivery. During this time the mother returns to her pre-pregnant state. She makes physical and mental changes after the birth of her child. The physical changes that occur with childbirth affect the reproductive organs and other body systems.

After the baby is born, the uterus begins the process of healing. The top of the uterus, called the **fundus,** can be felt at the midline of the abdomen level with the umbilicus (belly button). Over the next 2 weeks the uterus shrinks and the top of the uterus, or fundus, moves down in the pelvis approximately $\frac{1}{2}$ inch or 1 finger width per day (Figure 32-1). By the time the baby is 5 to 6 weeks old, the uterus returns to its normal size.

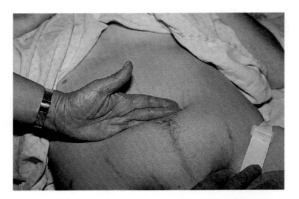

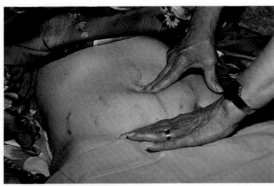 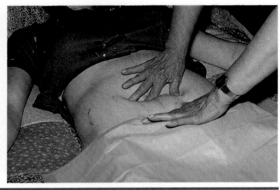

***Figure* 32-1** The fundus can be felt at the midline of the abdomen. Over the first 2 weeks after delivery, the uterus shrinks and returns to its normal size by the time the baby is 5 to 6 weeks old.

As the uterus heals, the woman has a vaginal discharge similar to a menstrual flow. This discharge is called **lochia.** For the first 3 to 4 days after delivery the discharge is dark red and may contain some small clots. This discharge is called lochia rubra. From the fourth through the tenth day after delivery, the discharge becomes pink in color and is called lochia serosa. As the healing process continues, the amount of blood in the discharge decreases. As the discharge becomes more yellow in color it is called lochia alba. Lochia alba will continue for 1 to 2 weeks more. The total amount of discharge or lochia is about 1 cup or 8 ounces over a 3- to 4-week period.

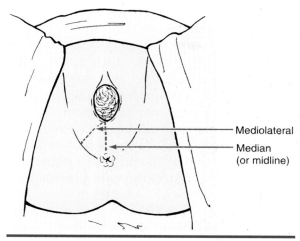

Mediolateral

Median
(or midline)

Figure 32-2   Types of episiotomies.

Discharge that is heavy, contains large clots, or smells bad may be a sign of complications and should be reported to the charge nurse.

As you work with the patients in the postpartum area, you will become more familiar with what is normal and abnormal during this time.

During the early postpartum period, the soft tissue of the perineum may be swollen and bruised. Many women will have an **episiotomy**, or a surgical incision made to enlarge the vaginal opening for delivery (Figure 32-2). This incision is done to prevent the tissue from tearing as the baby is born. After delivery the episiotomy is repaired by stitching the edges of the incision together. If the woman has had an episiotomy, the edges of the incision should be drawn together. The area around the episiotomy may be swollen and bruised as well.

After delivery the skin and muscles of the abdomen may appear loose and soft. Stretch marks caused by the stretching of the elastic fibers of the skin are red or purplish in color. There may be swelling and bruising around the bladder and urethra after delivery. This can cause pressure on the uterus, causing abnormal uterine bleeding. The swelling can also make it difficult to empty the bladder and can lead to urinary tract infections.

During the first few hours after birth the woman may have some orthostatic hypotension (Chapter 13). This will cause her to have a lower blood pressure while she is sitting than while lying in bed. You should take your patient's blood pressure with her lying on her back with her arm at her side each time you check vital signs.

After-birth pains are caused by uterine contractions. They feel like severe cramps and are more common in women who have had more than one pregnancy. They are also more common in women who deliver multiple babies such as twins or triplets.

A **cesarean section** (C-section) is a surgical procedure in which the baby is delivered through an incision in the abdomen rather than through the vagina or birth canal. The woman who delivers her baby by C-section will usually remain in the hospital 3 to 5 days after delivery since she is recovering from major abdominal surgery, as well as the birth of a baby. She will need to receive postpartum care and the care provided to a patient after surgery (Chapter 28).

The doctor will write orders for each patient's care. Most hospitals have specific procedures to care for patients on the postpartum unit. These orders and procedures will provide guidance in caring for your patients. Your charge nurse will tell you if there are other things you need to do. Routine care for the postpartum patient includes:

- Vital signs, usually every 4 hours
- Helping the patient to the bathroom
- Observing for excessive bleeding or bad-smelling vaginal discharge (lochia)
- Ice packs to the episiotomy or perineum if ordered
- Emotional support

Basic Infant Care and Feeding

Most of us think of a normal pregnancy as 9 months (Figure 32-3). On average a full-term pregnancy can last from 38 to 42 weeks. Babies born before 38 weeks or after 42 weeks are more likely to have problems than babies who are considered full term.

For the first 28 days after birth a newborn is adjusting from life inside of the uterus to life outside of the uterus. The infant must begin breathing immediately after birth. In the mother's uterus the oxygen was supplied through the circulation in the umbilical cord. The normal newborn respiratory rate is 30 to 60 breaths per minute. A newborn breathes through the nose, so it is important to keep the nose and throat clear of mucus or obstructions.

There are also changes in the function of the heart after the baby is born. The average resting heartbeat for the first week of life is 110 to 150 beats per minute. An apical pulse taken for 1 full minute will provide the most accurate pulse rate.

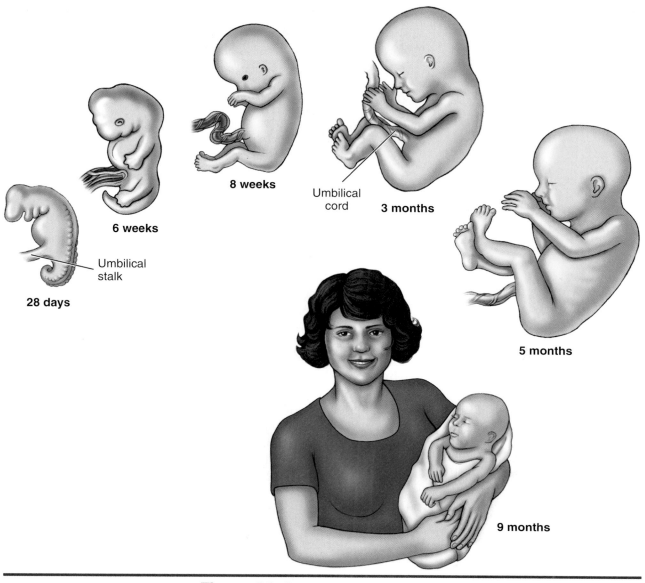

28 days

Umbilical stalk

6 weeks

8 weeks

Umbilical cord

3 months

5 months

9 months

Figure 32-3　Development of embryo.

Keeping a stable body temperature can be difficult for a newborn. A full-term infant loses about 4 times the amount of heat that an adult loses. This is because of the large amount of skin surface compared to the baby's small body weight. If an infant is wet or is in a cold room, his body temperature is more likely to drop than that of an older child or an adult. Temperature can be taken axillary (under the arm) or tympanic (ear), or it can be taken using a continuous skin probe that provides a constant

Box 32-1

AVERAGE NEWBORN

Respiratory rate: 30 to 60 breaths per minute
Resting heartbeat: 110 to 150 beats per minute
Body temperature: 97.7° to 98.6° F
Birth weight: 7 pounds, 8 ounces
Length: 18 to 22 inches
Head circumference: 12.5 to 14.5 inches
Chest circumference: 10.5 to 12.5 inches

digital readout of the baby's temperature. The average body temperature for a full-term infant is 97.7° to 98.6° F.

A normal full-term infant has an average birth weight of 7 pounds, 8 ounces and is 18 to 22 inches long. Both the head and chest are measured when the baby reaches the nursery. A newborn baby's head is large, about $\frac{1}{4}$ of the baby's body size. The average measurement around the baby's head is 12.5 to 14.5 inches, and the average chest circumference is 10.5 to 12.5 inches (Box 32-1).

When working with newborns, you may be asked to obtain a weight, length, head and chest measurements, and vital signs. Babies are usually weighed each day they are in the hospital. Vital signs are taken on admission to the nursery and usually every 4 hours for the first day of life. The nurse will do a complete assessment of the baby when the baby is admitted to the nursery (Figure 32-4).

Safety

Learning to pick up a baby safely is an important skill for both the nursing assistant and the new parents to learn. Slide one hand under the baby's neck, head, and shoulders and the other hand under the buttocks. This method provides support for the newborn's head. Newborns are unable to support their head until they are at least 3 to 4 months old (Figure 32-5).

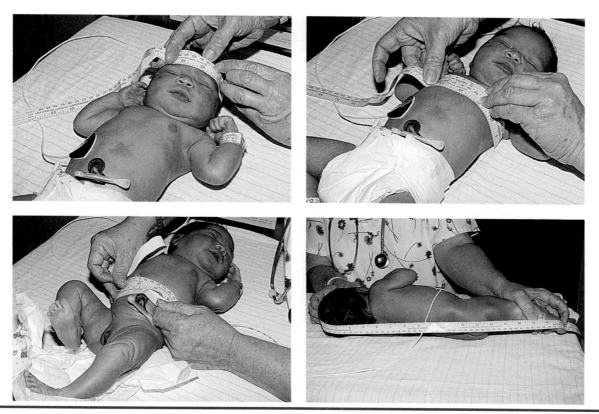

Figure 32-4   The infant is measured on admission to the nursery.

To decrease the risk of sudden infant death syndrome (SIDS), infants should be placed in the crib on their back or side. Never leave infants alone unless they are in the crib. Because newborn babies frequently spit up, a bulb syringe should be close at hand (Figure 32-6). The bulb syringe allows for easy suctioning of the mouth and nose.

For many parents, feeding their new baby is both exciting and frightening. A woman chooses to breast-feed or bottle-feed. Either way, babies will get the food they need to live and be healthy.

Some medical conditions may affect a mother's ability to breast-feed. A doctor may tell women with acquired immunodeficiency syndrome (AIDS) or breast cancer not to breast-feed. Many medications pass into breast milk and are passed on to the baby and can cause harm. For the woman who chooses bottle-feeding, there are many types of infant formula available. The baby's doctor can tell the parents which formula is right for each child (Figures 32-7 and 32-8).

**NOTES ON
☯ Culture**

Culture and society influence a woman's decisions about feeding her child.

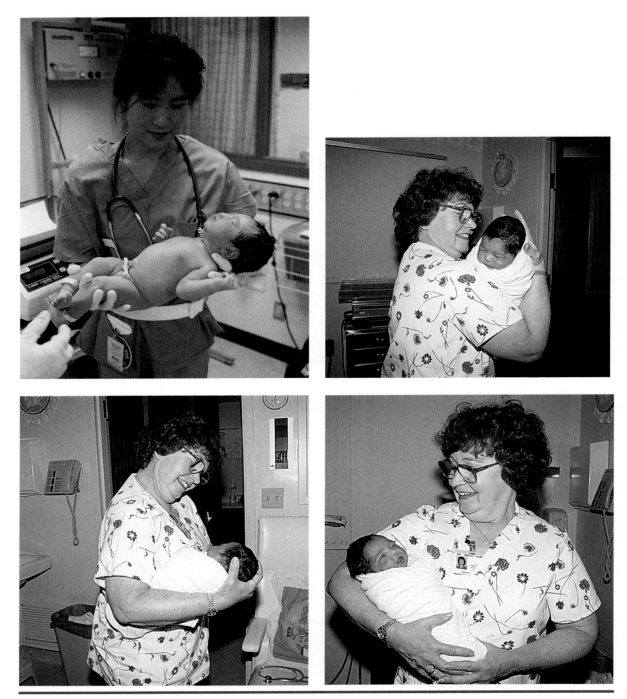

Figure 32-5 Correctly holding the newborn to support the head and neck.

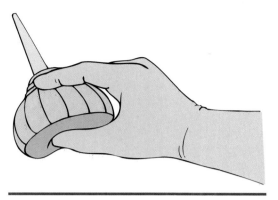

Figure **32-6**　Bulb syringe.

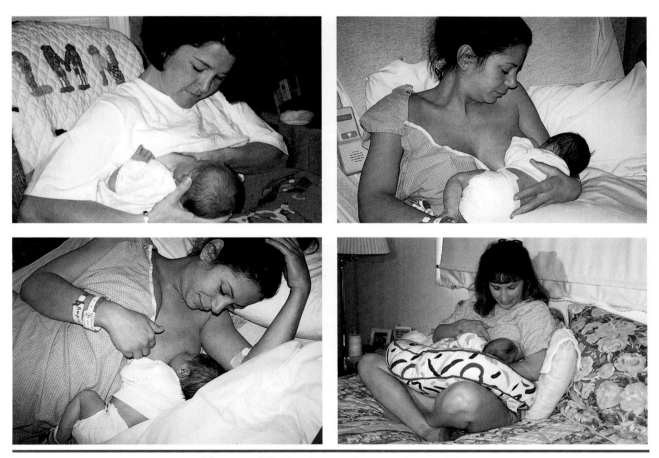

Figure **32-7**　Some infants are breast-fed.

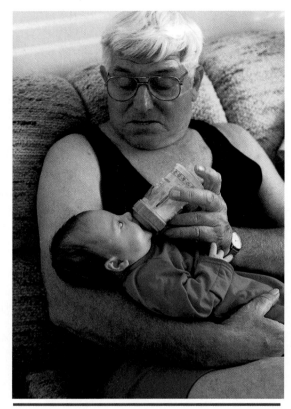

Figure 32-8   Some infants are bottle-fed.

As a nursing assistant, you may be responsible for infant care. It is important that you know the basics, including:

1. Watch for excessive mucus and spitting up. Use a bulb syringe to remove secretions.
2. Place babies on their back or side to sleep.
3. Normal urine is a light yellow color. Expect 6 to 10 wet diapers a day if a baby is taking in enough fluids.
4. Normal stool changes from thick, dark green to pale yellow/gold. A bottle-fed baby will normally have 1 or 2 stools a day, whereas a breast-fed baby may have 6 or more.
5. Keep the umbilical cord (belly button) clean and dry. Clean the cord and the skin around it with each diaper change. Fold diapers below the cord to allow it to air dry (Figure 32-9).
6. The cord should be dark and dry. Later, it will fall off. Never pull on the umbilical cord.
7. If a male infant has been circumcised, rinse the penis with water and pat dry. Apply a small amount of petroleum jelly with each diaper change, and fasten the diaper loosely over the penis.

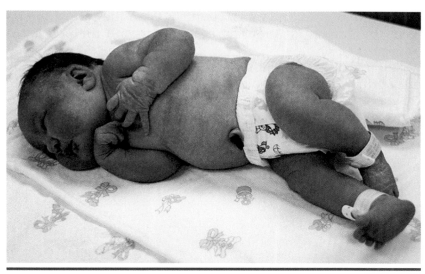

***Figure* 32-9**   Diapers should be folded below the cord to allow it to air dry.

8. Clean the baby's skin with warm water or baby wipes with each diaper change. Check the baby frequently to help avoid diaper rash.

Safety and Security for Mothers and Infants

There is a growing concern about the safety and security of infants in institutional settings. When the baby is born, identification bands with matching numbers are placed on each mother and her infant. The bands contain the name of the mother, the doctor's name, and the baby's sex. When staff members take babies to their mother, they must check the numbers on the baby's ID band and the band of the mother. This is to make sure that each woman receives the correct infant.

It is important that mothers do not leave their babies alone while the babies are in the mother's room. A baby could choke or be taken from the mother's room while she is in the bathroom or shower. If the mother is unable to see her baby, the baby should be returned to the nursery. Many women are choosing "rooming in." This means that the baby spends most of the time in the mother's room, both day and night. The mother, not the nursing staff, cares for the infant. When the nurse cares for the infant, she does so in the mother's room and not in the nursery. Some hospitals encourage the father, grandparents, and other children to participate in the care of the infant. It is important that you be familiar with the policies at your facility.

Safety

Many facilities now limit the people who can enter the nursery and postpartum areas. Visitors are screened to make sure they are allowed to enter the area. Staff may be required to wear a special badge that identifies them as a member of the care team for the new mother. Many of these security measures have been added because of recent infant abductions. As a nursing assistant, it is your responsibility to follow your facility policies and help to protect your patients and their babies from any possible harm.

CHAPTER REVIEW

1. What does the term *postpartum care* mean?

2. How long after delivery does to take the uterus to return to its normal size?

3. What is lochia?

4. What is an episiotomy?

5. What is a cesarean section?

6. Why does the staff compare the numbers on the mother's ID bracelet with those of the baby?

Circle the one BEST response.

7. Which of the following are routine types of care you would expect to provide to the postpartum patient?
   a. Vital signs
   b. Observing for bleeding
   c. Emotional support
   d. All of the above

8. The normal resting heart rate for a newborn is
   a. 60 to 80 beats per minute
   b. 800 to 110 beats per minute
   c. 110 to 150 beats per minute
   d. 130 to 180 beats per minute

Fill in the blanks with the correct term.

9. To decrease the risk of sudden infant death syndrome (SIDS), an infant should be placed in the crib on his _____ or _____.

Answers are on page 714.

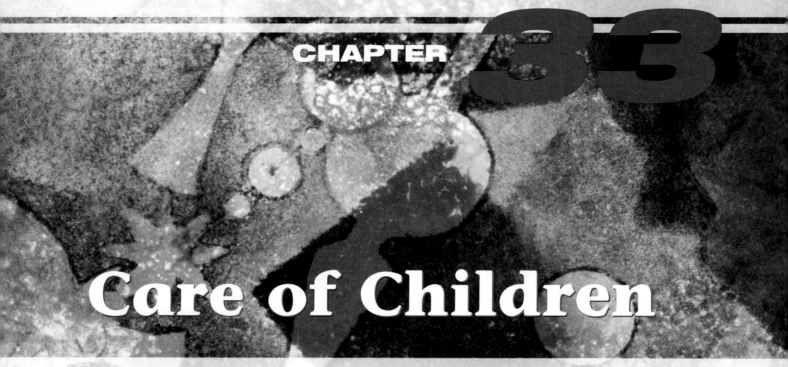

CHAPTER 33

Care of Children

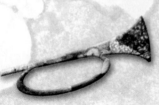

What you will learn

- Children as patients in a health care setting
- Understanding and meeting the needs of the pediatric patient
- Vital sign variations in children

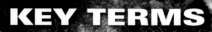

KEY TERMS

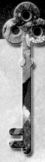

Development Changes in psychological and social functioning; how people act or behave at different ages of their life

Growth Series of physical changes that occur as a person ages

Pediatric patient A child 18 years old or under

Children as Patients in a Health Care Setting

When taking care of the child in a health care setting, it is important to understand that a child is not like an adult. We usually consider patients to be children or **pediatric patients** if they are 18 years old or under. Children have special physical, social, and emotional needs that are different from those of an adult. Children of various age-groups are very different from each other. For example, a 3-year-old child has different needs than a 13-year-old.

Children are very dependent upon the adults in their lives, usually their parents or guardians. When caring for a child, you are really caring for the entire family unit. As children get older, they become less dependent on their parents and family. This is normal as children move toward becoming young adults. Health care for all age-groups is moving toward preventing illness. This is especially true of pediatric health care. It is important to provide care for a child together with the family. This means that you will be a role model for the family members.

Understanding and Meeting the Needs of the Pediatric Patient

As you may remember from Chapter 4, as a nursing assistant you provide care to the "whole" person. A person is not a disease or a condition to be treated. A person is a unique individual with physical, social, emotional, and spiritual needs. Chapter 4 also discussed how a person's culture and beliefs affect him. In Chapter 5 you learned about normal growth and development. When we talk about **growth**, we are talking about the physical growth we see as children move through the years. When we talk about **development**, we are talking about how people act or behave at different ages of their life. This chapter will discuss how children's culture and upbringing affect their needs. Refer to Chapters 4 and 5 for additional information.

Culture

People's culture is different from their race or ethnic background. A culture is made of people with similar values, beliefs, language, dress, diet, and acceptable behaviors. For example, a white person from the United States is from a different culture than a white person from Europe or South America, even though they may look similar.

What is considered normal can be different in each culture. Behaviors that are unacceptable in one culture may be accepted in another. For example, the father in a Vietnamese family is the head of the family and deals with issues outside of the family such as health care. Asking health care questions of the mother in this family could be considered incorrect. It is important that you remember that you will work with people from many different cultures in your job as a nursing assistant.

Ethnicity and Race

Some groups of people are more likely to get certain diseases than others. For example, African-Americans are more likely to have sickle cell anemia than people of other ethnic backgrounds. People of different ethnic groups can belong to the same culture, even though they look very different.

Religious Beliefs

Religious beliefs are important in health care as well. For example, Christian Scientist parents may not believe that their child is ill. They may refuse to allow the child to be treated with drugs or other types of therapies. The parents may rely on spiritual not medical ways to heal their child. If a nurse tries to give this child medication, the parents might not want the child to take the medicine. It is almost as important to remember that even though patients may belong to a certain religion, they may not adhere to all of the beliefs of that religion.

Nutritional Needs

Good nutrition is important to everyone. It is especially important for children. Children need a well-balanced diet to provide their bodies with the energy needed to grow and develop properly (Chapter 19). Younger children need the same variety of foods as older children but may need fewer calories and

NOTES ON Culture

The values and beliefs of a culture are not with us at birth. Our families teach our values and beliefs to us.

NOTES ON Culture

Even though you may not understand other people's culture, try to learn as much about it as you can and be respectful of their wishes.

smaller servings. A 3-year-old does not eat the same amount of food as a 10-year-old. It is important that children have at least 2 cups of milk per day, and adolescents need at least 3 cups (Boxes 33-1 and 33-2). If children do not have the correct type of nutrition, their height, weight, and brain development can be negatively affected.

Safety and Security Needs

All people have a need to feel safe and secure. This is especially important for children. When children are hospitalized, they will experience many new things. One of the most important things you can do to help your young patient feel secure is to involve the parent/guardian as much as possible in the child's care. With an infant, the parent should remain where the child can see the parent whenever possible. With the toddler or preschool-age child, a simple explanation of what you are

---

Box 33-1

SAMPLE MENU FOR SCHOOL-AGE CHILDREN BASED ON FOOD GUIDE PYRAMID*

Breakfast	2 four-inch waffles
	2 tablespoons syrup
	½ cup orange juice
Lunch	1 four-ounce cheeseburger and bun
	½ cup raw carrot sticks
	¾ cup apple juice
Snack	1 cup frozen yogurt *or*
	1 cup unsweetened cereal with low-fat milk
Dinner	1 cup spaghetti with tomato sauce
	1 piece garlic bread
	Green salad with romaine lettuce and dressing
	½ cup broccoli
	1 banana
	1 cup low-fat milk
Snack	2 cups plain popcorn

Total Servings

Bread, cereal, rice, pasta	6-7
Vegetable	3
Fruit	3
Milk, yogurt, cheese	3
Meat, poultry, fish, dried beans, nuts	2

*Use fats, oils, and sweets sparingly. Increase fluids with servings of water.

Serving sizes are minimums for nutritional adequacy. Many children eat more.

Box 33-2

FOOD GUIDE PYRAMID: SAMPLE SERVING SIZES

Bread, Cereal, Rice, and Pasta Group

1 slice of bread
1 ounce of ready-to-eat cereal
½ cup of cooked cereal, rice, or pasta

Vegetable Group

1 cup of raw leafy vegetable
½ cup of another vegetable, cooked or chopped raw
¾ cup of vegetable juice

Fruit Group

1 medium apple, banana, or orange
½ cup of chopped, cooked, or canned fruit
¾ cup of fruit juice

Milk, Yogurt, and Cheese Group

1 cup of milk or yogurt
1½ ounces of natural cheese
2 ounces of processed cheese

Meat, Poultry, Fish, Dry Beans, Eggs, and Nuts Group

2 to 3 ounces of cooked lean meat, poultry, or fish
½ cup of cooked dry beans, 1 egg, or 2 tablespoons of peanut butter count as 1 ounce of lean meat

doing and the parent's presence decreases the child's fear. School-age and adolescent children are able to understand basic medical terms and should be given as much control over their care as possible. Allowing the older child to decide when a procedure such as drawing blood is done gives them a sense of control. Even routine procedures such as measuring blood pressure or obtaining a urine specimen can frighten a child. When you have a good relationship with the child and the parent, the child will begin to trust you. When this occurs, the child feels safer and is usually more cooperative.

Safety

It is important to pay special attention to providing a safe environment when you care for children. For example, it would be reasonable to expect adults to know that it is not safe to put their finger into an electrical outlet, but a child may be curious and not think about how dangerous this is.

Emotional and Social Needs

Relationships with others is an important emotional need for children. The mothering person is the single most important person during early childhood. As children mature, they turn to teachers, friends, and other relatives for comfort. The school-age child and adolescent turn to people their own age to help meet their emotional and social needs. Pets can also play an important role by providing love and companionship. The single most important emotional need of children is to feel loved and accepted by the people who are important in their lives. When children feel secure in this love, they are able to deal with the stresses of growing up. Most pediatric facilities have liberal policies about visitors. Brothers, sisters, and friends are encouraged to spend time with the patient. Watching movies and playing age-appropriate games allows children to interact with others their own age.

Developmental Needs

A child's physical growth is easy to see. Developmental changes or changes in the child's personality and level of maturity are not easy to see. To determine if growth and development are taking place, a child can be compared to other children of similar ages from similar backgrounds. Because each child is an individual, this is only a general guideline.

Childhood is usually broken up into 4 different periods:

- *Infancy period*—birth to 12 months of age (Figure 33-1). During this time children have a basic trust in the world based on their activities with their caregivers. This trust will make it possible for the child to have a good life.
- *Early childhood*—1 to 6 years of age. This group is sometimes broken down further into:
  - *Toddlers*—1 to 3 years of age (Figure 33-2)
  - *Preschoolers*—3 to 6 years of age (Figure 33-3)

  During this stage children learn to talk and develop their personalities. There are more social activities with others, and the child learns some self-control. There is also a move toward becoming more independent.
- *Middle childhood, also commonly called the school-age period* (Figure 33-4)—6 to 12 years of age. At this time children spend more time away from the family and have more relationships with other children their own age. These children develop more social skills and a sense of who they are.
- *Later childhood, also called adolescence*—12 to 18 years of age (Figure 33-5). During this stage children move from childhood into young adulthood after graduation from high school. They begin to focus on their individual identity.

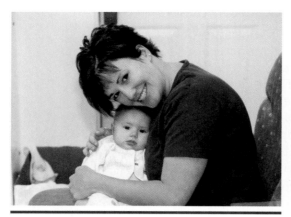

Figure **33-1** Infants develop trust based on interaction with their caregivers.

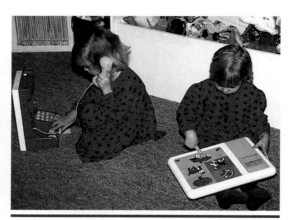

Figure **33-2** The toddler becomes more social and independent.

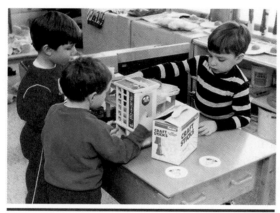

Figure **33-3** Social interaction and self-control are seen in the preschool years.

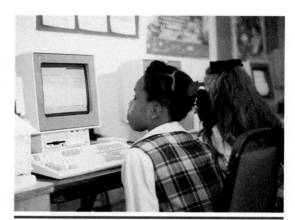

Figure **33-4** The school-age child spends more time away from the family.

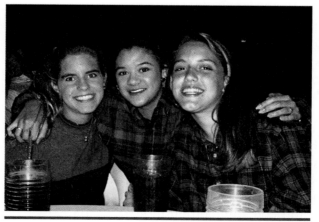

Figure **33-5** Between ages 12 and 18 the child begins to focus on his personal identity.

Vital Sign Variations in Children

To know when a child's vital signs are *abnormal,* you will need to know the *normal* vital signs for different ages of children. Table 33-1 provides the normal ranges in temperature, pulse, respiration, and blood pressure for children from birth to 15 years of age.

Always report any abnormal vital signs to your charge nurse right away. Variations in vital signs can be a symptom of a serious problem.

When you care for a child, you are really taking care of the whole family, including brothers and sisters, parents, grandparents, and even aunts and uncles in large families. One of the most important things you can do when caring for a child is to respect the values of the family.

NOTES ON
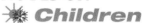
Children

When taking a blood pressure on a child, a smaller cuff called a pediatric cuff should be used for an accurate reading.

Table 33-1

NORMAL RANGES			
Age	Resting pulse	Respiratory rate	Blood pressure
Newborn	100-180	33-60	70-100/50-65
6 months	120-160	25-50	87-105/53-66
2 years	80-150	18-35	90-106/55-67
5 years	80-110	17-27	94-109/56-69
10 years	70-110	15-23	102-117/62-75
15 years	55-100	10-23	105-128/66-80

CHAPTER REVIEW

1. What is a person's culture?

2. What can you do to help your young patients to feel more safe and secure?

3. What is the most important emotional need of children?

4. Jasmine is a 24-month-old female patient admitted to your division. Which developmental period is she in based on the information provided in this chapter?

5. While caring for Jasmine, you notice that she gets angry when you do things for her such as feeding her or helping her to get dressed. Is this normal or abnormal for her age-group?

Mark T for true or F for false.

6. ____ The needs of the adult and child patient are the same.

7. ____ There is no difference in the normal vitals signs for children of different age-groups.

Answers are on page 714.

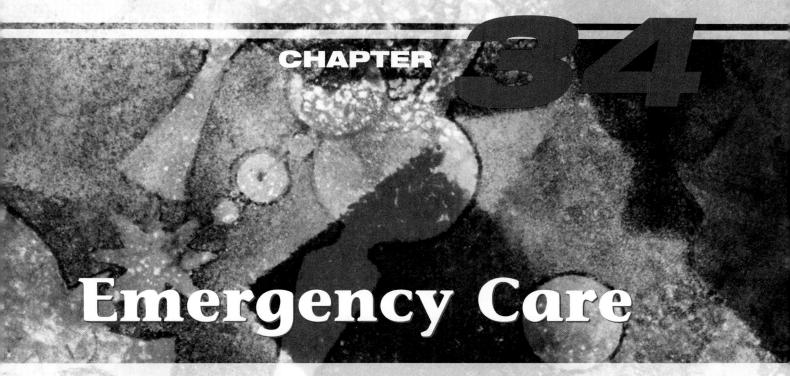

CHAPTER 34

Emergency Care

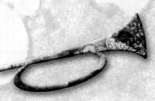

What you will learn

- General guidelines for providing emergency care
- How to care for people with:
  - Fainting
  - Bleeding emergencies
  - Shock
  - Seizures
  - Heat injuries and burns
  - Bites, stings, and poisoning
  - Sprains and strains
  - Respiratory and cardiac emergencies

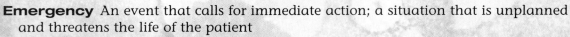

KEY TERMS

Emergency An event that calls for immediate action; a situation that is unplanned and threatens the life of the patient

Fainting Short-term loss of consciousness

First aid Care given to an injured or ill person until professional help arrives

Hemorrhage A large amount of sudden uncontrolled bleeding

Poison Any substance that causes illness or death when taken into the body

Seizure (convulsion) Sudden uncontrolled muscle contraction resulting from abnormal brain activity

Shock Abnormal condition of the body in which there is not enough blood supply to the body's tissues

General Guidelines for Providing Emergency Care

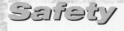

An **emergency** is an event that calls for immediate action. Emergencies happen everywhere. Knowing what to do can save a person's life. **First aid** is the care given to an injured or ill person before professional medical help arrives.

Because you never know when an emergency will occur, the best thing you can do is to be prepared.

Emergencies can occur in the home, community, and workplace. You are encouraged to take a first aid course so that you are familiar with the correct actions to take in an emergency. This chapter outlines the basics of emergency care in the health care setting. It should NOT be considered the same as certification. Your instructor or employer should be able to provide you with information about first aid courses such as those offered through the American Red Cross. Many employers require that all staff members be certified in basic life support or cardiopulmonary resuscitation (CPR). In some settings the training is provided at your place of employment. There are many agencies that provide CPR training at a reasonable cost, including the American Red Cross and the American Heart Association.

Every health care institution has procedures to follow in the event of an emergency. In a hospital there will be doctors and nurses available to provide the emergency care needed. In extended care facilities such as group homes or nursing homes, you will need to contact the emergency medical service (EMS). In most areas of the United States, dialing 911 on a telephone can activate EMS. This will put you in contact with an EMS operator who can send the police, fire department, and paramedics. In some rural areas it may be necessary to contact the service you need by dialing directly. It is important that you know how to reach EMS in your area.

The phone number for EMS should be posted on the telephone.

When calling EMS, you need to be prepared to tell the operator:

1. Your name
2. The phone number and address you are calling from
3. The type of assistance that is needed
4. The number and types of injuries involved

For example, the operator would not send the fire department to an accident that involves a fall or bleeding. The operator would send an ambulance, paramedics, and the local police. Also, it would not be necessary to send paramedics to the scene of a small brush fire if no one were injured.

Remember to stay on the phone until the EMS operator tells you to hang up.

During an emergency you may come in contact with blood or body fluids. Remember to follow Standard Precautions and the Bloodborne Pathogen Standard when providing emergency care.

Safety

Safety

Safety

Fainting

Fainting is a short-term loss of consciousness. Someone who faints may pass out for a few seconds or longer.

There are many reasons people faint, including:
- Low blood sugar
- Anemia or lack of iron in the blood
- Any condition in which there is a rapid loss of blood
- Heart and circulatory problems such as heart attack or stroke
- Prolonged exposure to extreme heat
- A sudden change in body position such as standing up too quickly (postural hypotension)
- Severe pain
- Sudden emotional stress, fright, or anxiety
- Taking some medications

If your patient faints, you should:
- Call for help as you assist the person.
- Help the person lie down with the legs elevated 10 to 12 inches (Figure 34-1). If a person who is about to faint can lie down right away, the person may not lose consciousness.
- Loosen any tight clothing.
- Apply moist towels to the person's face and neck.
- Stay with the person until help arrives.
- Follow the directions of your charge nurse.

NOTES ON
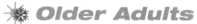 *Older Adults*

Postural hypotension is more common in the elderly (Chapter 13).

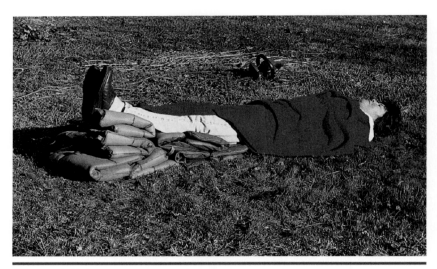

***Figure* 34-1** Help the person lie down with the legs elevated 10 to 12 inches.

Bleeding Emergencies

The term **hemorrhage** refers to sudden uncontrolled bleeding. Bleeding can be either internal (inside the body) or external (outside of the body). If the person is bleeding externally, you should:

- Call for help as you assist the person.
- Apply firm pressure to the bleeding area with a gloved hand (Figure 34-2).
- If the person is standing, assist the person to a sitting or lying position in case the person faints.
- If the injury is to an arm or a leg, raise the limb higher than the level of the heart to slow the bleeding.
- Stay with the person until help arrives.
- *Never apply a tourniquet!*
- Follow the directions of your charge nurse.

It is difficult to know if a person is bleeding internally. Symptoms of internal bleeding include decreased blood pressure; pale, cold skin; and rapid or weak pulse. If you suspect internal bleeding, you should:

- Call for help as you assist the person.
- If the person is standing, assist the person to a sitting or lying position in case the person faints.
- Stay with the person until help arrives.
- Follow the directions of your charge nurse.

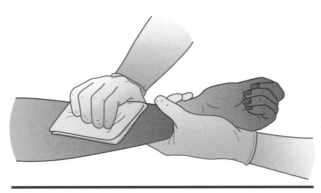

Figure **34-2** Apply firm pressure with a gloved hand to the bleeding area.

Shock

Shock is an abnormal condition of the body in which there is not enough blood supply to the body's tissues. Shock can occur due to complications of diabetes, medication allergies, severe infection, and hemorrhage. Shock can be life threatening and should be treated as an emergency situation. Symptoms include:

- Low blood pressure
- Weak, rapid pulse
- Rapid respirations
- Pale, cold, clammy skin
- Confusion

Shock can be caused by many things, including:

- Heart attack
- Sudden blood loss
- Blood poisoning from major infections
- Exposure to extreme heat or cold for too long
- Fractures of a large bone
- A severe allergic reaction
- Very low blood sugar such as occurs with diabetes
- Drug overdose

If the person does not receive medical treatment, the shock can get worse and the person will lose consciousness. If you suspect shock, you should:

- Call for help as you assist the person
- If the person is standing, assist the person to a sitting or lying position in case the person faints.
- Stay with the person until help arrives.
- Follow the directions of your charge nurse.

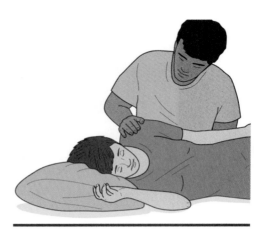

Figure **34-3** Cushion the person's head with a soft towel or article of clothing to prevent injury during a seizure.

Seizures

A **seizure** is a sudden uncontrolled muscle contraction due to abnormal brain activity. Drugs, head injuries, or brain tumors can cause seizures. Seizures may be very mild with very little noticeable muscle movement. They may also be very violent and result in injury to the patient. If your patient has a seizure, you should:

- Call for help as you assist the person.
- If the person is standing, assist the person to a lying position.
- Loosen any tight clothing.
- Remove any objects that could cause injury to the person during a seizure, such as furniture that is close to the person.
- Put a soft towel or article of clothing under the person's head (Figure 34-3).
- Stay with the person until help arrives.
- Follow the directions of your charge nurse.

NOTES ON
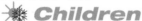 *Children*

Infants and small children are more likely to die as a result of a burn injury.

NOTES ON
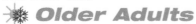 *Older Adults*

Elderly people are more likely to die as a result of a burn injury.

Heat Injuries and Burns

Fire, hot liquids, electricity, and chemicals can cause burns. Some burns are mild, and others are severe. The severity of the burn depends on the amount of skin burned and the depth of the injury (Figures 34-4 to 34-6). Burns on the face, hands, and feet are usually more severe than burns on the arms and legs.

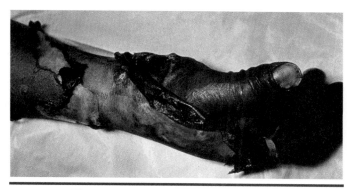

Figure 34-4 Full-thickness burn.

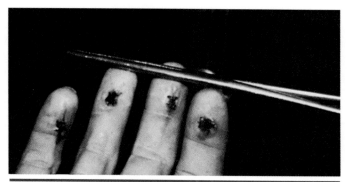

Figure 34-5 In this electrical burn the current entered through the hand.

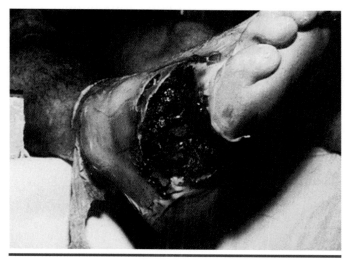

Figure 34-6 The electrical current exited through the foot and burned both areas of the body.

To provide emergency care to a person who has been burned:
- Call for help as you assist the person.
- Do not touch the person if he is in contact with an electrical source such as an electric wire.
- Remove the person from the fire or source of the burn.
- If the person is standing, assist the person to a sitting or lying position in case the person faints.
- Do not remove the burned clothing.
- Cover the burns with a sterile dressing if possible.
- Stay with the person until help arrives.
- Follow the directions of your charge nurse.

Bites, Stings, and Poisoning

The most common animal bites are from dogs and cats. Less commonly, wild animals, snakes, and spiders may bite humans. Some bites such as those from snakes and spiders may be poisonous. Warm-blooded animals can carry a disease called rabies that affects the nervous system and can be fatal.

Insects that sting include bees, hornets, wasps, and yellow jackets. After an insect stings someone, the person will usually experience pain, swelling, itching, and redness on the body part where the person was stung.

Some people have severe allergic reactions to bites and insect stings. Symptoms of a severe allergic reaction can include:
- Severe swelling, all over and/or of the face, tongue, lips
- Weakness, dizziness
- A difficult time breathing or swallowing
- Death due to airway obstruction or shock

These symptoms may happen right after the person is bitten or stung or within the next 30 to 60 minutes. If your patient develops a severe allergic reaction to a bite or sting, you should:
- Call for help as you assist the person.
- If possible, remove the stinger with a pair of tweezers.
- Keep the limb of the bite site level with or just below the level of the heart.

- Clean the area with soapy water, and put a cold compress on the area for 15 to 20 minutes.
- Follow the directions of your charge nurse.

A **poison** is any substance that causes illness or death when taken into the body. Poisons can affect every organ of the body.

The best way to decrease the risk of poisoning is to keep all dangerous chemicals in a place where the patient cannot get them. This means that many chemicals need to be kept in a locked cabinet. There are treatments available for some types of poisons.

The phone number for your local poison control center should be posted close to the telephone so that it is easy to find.

Sprains and Strains

The most common causes for sprains and strains are falls, twisting, and sports injuries. Both sprains and strains result in pain and swelling. Treatment for sprains and strains depends on how much damage there is to the limb or joint. For mild sprains or strains, treatment usually includes:

- Resting the injured area for a day or two
- Ice packs or cold compresses for 5 to 20 minutes every hour for the first 2 to 3 days or until the area no longer looks or feels hot
- Elevating the area to reduce swelling

Severe sprains may require professional medical treatment. Some sprains require a cast or splint, and others may need surgery if the person tore tissue.

Respiratory and Cardiac Emergencies

Many people have trouble breathing because of asthma and allergies. Some people are allergic to foods such as nuts. Other people are allergic to things such as insect stings. A person who has severe breathing difficulty requires emergency care. Causes of respiratory emergencies include:

- Severe allergic reactions
- Face, head, nose, or lung injuries
- Carbon monoxide poisoning
- Choking (see p. 638)
- Drug overdose
- Poisoning
- Respiratory diseases such as asthma, emphysema, or pneumonia

NOTES ON

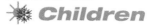 *Children*

Children are more likely to be victims of poisoning by chemicals in the home.

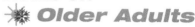 *Safety*

NOTES ON

Older Adults

In the long-term care setting, a confused person or a person with poor vision may mistake a chemical such as a cleaning solution for his favorite beverage.

- Congestive heart failure
- Heart attack
- Blood clot in a lung

If your patient is having difficulty breathing you should:

- Call for help as you assist the person.
- Help the person lie down.
- Loosen any tight clothing.
- Stay with the person until help arrives.
- Follow the directions of your charge nurse.

If your patient is choking, you will need to act quickly to assist the person. The proper action to take depends on the age of the victim. This text provides information about caring for a choking adult. Your actions are also based on whether the person is conscious or unconscious.

Safety

Remember, these guidelines are for information and are not a substitute for taking a course in basic life support.

Care of the Choking Victim

If the victim is conscious:

- Choking is usually indicated by hands clutching the throat (Figure 34-7).

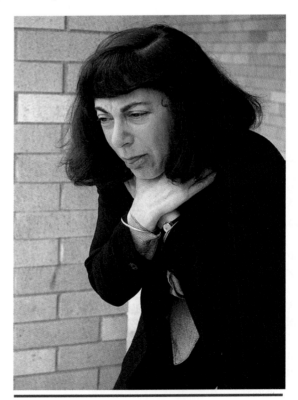

Figure 34-7   Hands clutching the throat is the universal sign of choking.

- Call for help as you assist the person.
- Ask if the victim can speak.
- If the victim can speak, cough, or breathe, do not interfere.
- If the victim cannot speak, cough, or breathe, give abdominal thrusts.
- Stand behind the victim.
- Reach around the victim's waist.
- Position your closed fist, thumb side in, above the navel below the rib cage.
- Grasp the closed fist with other hand (Figure 34-8).
- With a backward and upward motion, press the closed fist into the person's abdomen.
- Continue until the obstruction is relieved, the person becomes unconscious, or help arrives.

If the victim becomes unconscious, position the victim on the back, arms by sides.

- Open the airway with a head-tilt/chin-lift movement (Figure 34-9).

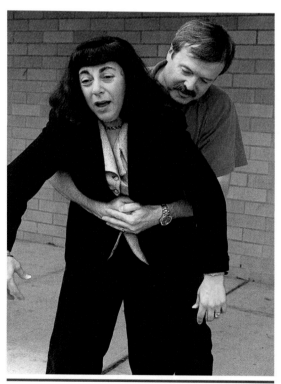

Figure 34-8 Stand behind the victim, and wrap your arms around her waist. Position your closed fist, thumb side in, above the naval below the rib cage. Grasp the closed fist with your other hand. With a backward and upward motion, give quick thrusts into the abdomen.

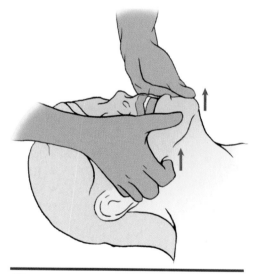

Figure 34-9 Open the airway using a head-tilt/chin-lift movement.

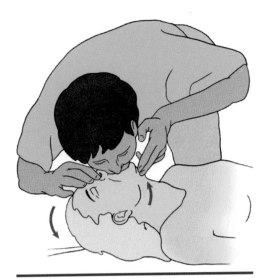

***Figure* 34-10** Give 2 rescue breaths.

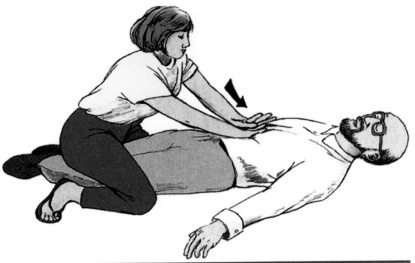

***Figure* 34-11** Straddle the victim's hips, and provide abdominal thrusts.

- Look, listen, and feel for breathing.
- Perform finger sweep to try to remove the foreign body.
- Give 2 rescue breaths (Figure 34-10).
- If unsuccessful, reposition the head and attempt to give 2 rescue breaths.
- Provide abdominal thrusts.
- Straddle the patient at the hip level (Figure 34-11).
- Position the heel of one hand on the patient's abdomen at the midline between the naval and the rib cage with the fingers pointing toward the patient's head.
- Place your other hand over the hand on the abdomen with your shoulders directly over the patient's abdomen.
- Press your hands down and up toward the patient's upper back.
- Repeat 5 times.
- Open the airway with a head-tilt/chin-lift movement.
- Look, listen, and feel for breathing.
- Perform finger sweep to try to remove the foreign body.
- Give 2 rescue breaths; if unsuccessful, continue with abdominal thrusts and breathing cycle until the obstruction is removed or help arrives.
- Stay with the person until help arrives.
- Follow the directions of your charge nurse.

Cardiac emergencies can be caused by things such as:
- Irregular heartbeat
- Heart attack (Figure 34-12)

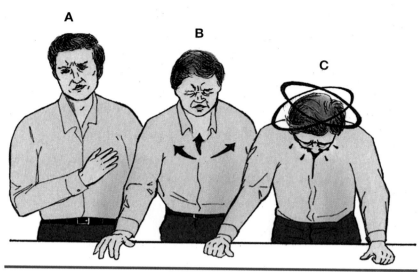

Figure 34-12 Signs of a heart attack. A, Feeling of pressure in the chest. B, Pain in the chest, neck, and/or down the left arm. C, Dizziness and sweating.

- Heart failure
- Medications
- Electrocution

The most important thing you can do for a person having a cardiac emergency is to call for help and stay with the person until help arrives.

If the person has a cardiac arrest and you have taken a CPR class, you will be able to provide basic life support until the paramedics arrive.

It is important that you know when to perform CPR and when NOT to perform CPR. Never attempt CPR if you have not been properly trained. Performing CPR on a person who has just fainted or is not in cardiac arrest can be life threatening.

Automated external defibrillators (AEDs) are becoming very common in public areas. An AED unit allows an untrained person to assist a victim of sudden cardiac arrest (SCA). Statistics show that if victims of SCA receive treatment including defibrillation within 2 minutes of the arrest, their chance of surviving the incident increases from less than 5% to better than 90%. Organizations that provide training in CPR can also provide information about AED units. In some facilities, use of the AED is included in the annual safety training program.

OBRA requires that all residents of long-term care (LTC) facilities be provided with a safe environment. Being alert to possible dangers and being prepared in case of an emergency helps you to provide a safe environment.

Safety

Safety

OBRA

CHAPTER REVIEW

1. What is an emergency?

2. How is EMS activated in your community?

3. When calling EMS, what do you need to be prepared to tell the operator?

4. What is fainting?

5. List 3 reasons a person might faint.

6. What is a hemorrhage?

7. What are 3 causes of shock?

8. What ages of patients are most likely to die from burn injuries?

9. How long after being stung do symptoms of an allergic reaction appear?

10. What is a poison?

11. List 3 causes of respiratory emergencies.

12. List 3 causes of cardiac emergencies.

Circle the one BEST response.

13. How are mild sprains and strains usually treated?
    a. Rest, cold compresses, and elevating the area
    b. Rest, warm compresses, and walking
    c. Exercise, ice packs, and TED hose
    d. Exercise, ice packs, and elevating the area

14. Sudden uncontrolled muscle contraction due to abnormal brain activity is a
    a. Hemorrhage
    b. Poison
    c. Seizure
    d. Shock

Answers are on page 714 to 715.

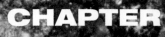

CHAPTER 35

Professional Skills

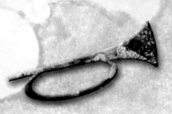

What you will learn

- Career planning
- How to write a résumé, cover letter, and job application
- Do's and dont's in an interview
- How to write a resignation letter
- Importance of continuing education
- How to keep certification

KEY TERMS

Employee evaluation A review of the employee's work
Employment agency An agency that helps job seekers find employers
Interview A meeting between 2 or more people
Networking An informal way to find out about job openings
Personnel policies A set of rules for employees
Reference A statement about your abilities given by another person, usually a previous employer
Résumé A summary of your education and work experience
Staffing agency An agency that hires health care workers and provides staff to facilities that need help on a temporary basis

Career Planning

Training to become a nursing assistant takes time and energy and so does finding the right job. Each person wants different things from a job. You will spend almost $\frac{1}{3}$ of your life working, so you will want to work for an organization that meets your needs. As you begin to look for a job, there are several things you can do to make the search easier and more productive.

Step 1: Self-Evaluation

The first step is a self-evaluation, an honest look at your strengths and weaknesses. Fold a sheet of paper in half lengthwise to make 2 columns. On the left side of the paper write down your strengths, the things that you enjoy doing or do well. On the right side of the paper write down your weaknesses, things that you do not like to do or do not do especially well (Figure 35-1).

On the back of the folded sheet of paper, make 2 more lists. On the left side of the paper write down the things that you feel are the most important to you when looking for a job. These are the things that you need the most. On the right side write down things that would be nice but are not necessary in a job. These are things that you want from a job but that you do not need (Figure 35-2).

Put your lists away, and review them in a day or two. You may want to add or change the things on your list. You can begin this step before you even finish with your class work if you want to. You may ask friends, family members, or other stu-

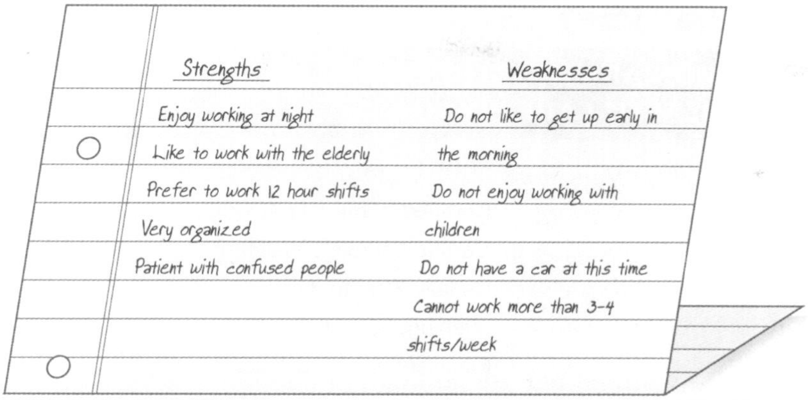

Figure 35-1   Strengths and weaknesses list.

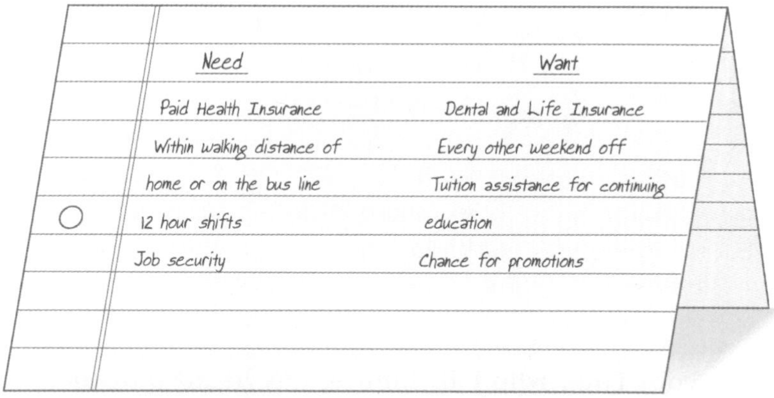

Strengths	Weaknesses
Enjoy working at night	Do not like to get up early in the morning
Like to work with the elderly	Do not enjoy working with children
Prefer to work 12 hour shifts	Do not have a car at this time
Very organized	Cannot work more than 3-4 shifts/week
Patient with confused people	

Figure 35-2   Needs versus wants list.

Need	Want
Paid Health Insurance	Dental and Life Insurance
Within walking distance of home or on the bus line	Every other weekend off
12 hour shifts	Tuition assistance for continuing education
Job security	Chance for promotions

dents what they think your strengths and weaknesses are. When you are satisfied that you know what you are looking for in a job, you are ready to take the next step in your job search.

Step 2: Finding a Job Opening

There are many different ways that you can find out about jobs that might be right for you. **Networking** is an informal way to find out about job openings. Tell your friends, family, and classmates that you are looking for a job. Some employers do not advertise and depend on their employees to refer people who are looking for a job.

For example, Roberto has just completed the nursing assistant program at the local technical school. His cousin Paul works at the regional hospital in the maintenance department.

Table 35-1

COMMON ABBREVIATIONS USED IN ADVERTISEMENTS FOR HEALTH CARE POSITIONS	
Abbreviation	Meaning
CHHA	Certified home health aide
CNA	Certified nursing assistant
Days	Usually 7 AM to 3 PM
Eves	Evenings, usually 3 to 11 PM
Exc.	Excellent, such as "exc. benefits"
Exp.	Experience, such as "6 mos exp."
FT	Full time, usually 36 to 40 hours per week
HCA	Home care aide
HHA	Home health aide
M-F	Monday through Friday
NA	Nursing assistant
Nites	Usually 11 PM to 7 AM
PT	Part time, usually less than 36 to 40 hours per week
Req.	Required, such as "experience req."
W/E	Weekend(s)

Roberto calls Paul, who tells him he has heard that there are openings for nursing assistants in the hospital. Paul also tells Roberto that he is happy working for the hospital and that his benefits and salary are good. Roberto applies for a nursing assistant position at the hospital and is hired.

Another way to find out about job opportunities is in the classified advertisements in your local newspapers. Start by circling the ads for positions that seem to be the most similar to your "needs" list. Some newspapers list all of the positions in health care together under either the "medical" section or "health care" section. Most newspapers use abbreviations in their classified ads. You will need a basic understanding of the abbreviations used when reading the ads (Table 35-1).

It is not a good use of your time to apply for positions that do not meet your needs. For example, if you do not have a car, it would not be a good use of your time to apply for a position that requires you to travel between different patients' homes.

A third way to find out about job openings is employment agencies. **Employment agencies** are agencies that match a person who is looking for a job with employers. The employer usually pays the agency if the employer finds the right person for the job. Some agencies charge the job seeker a fee as well. It is important to understand any contracts an agency asks you to sign. Another type of agency is a staffing agency. A **staffing agency** hires health care workers and provides staff to facilities that need temporary help. As an employee of the agency, you can decide if you want to accept an assignment. Agency employees are frequently paid more per hour than facility employees because there are no benefits such as insurance, and the employee is not guaranteed a set number of work hours per week. Some people enjoy the flexibility and variety of working for a staffing agency. Other people need the security of working for a facility that will give them full-time employment.

The facility where you did your clinical training is another possible source of employment. Many facilities will offer students jobs when they have completed their training programs. Depending on the regulations in your state, you may be permitted to work before you complete your training and become certified. Your instructor will be able to tell you when you can work as a nursing assistant in your state. There are advantages to working at the facility where you did your clinical training. You are already familiar with the facility and have had a chance to see if the employees work well as a team. You also know if the location is convenient and easy to get to.

Jobs may also be posted on the Internet. Some employers routinely post all openings on their website. You will have to send your résumé electronically when you apply for a job using the Internet. This means you will need to keep a copy of your résumé as an electronic file.

Preparing a Résumé and Cover Letter

A **résumé** is a summary of your education and work experience (Figure 35-3). The résumé gives the employer information about you and helps you to get an appointment for an **interview** or meeting with the person who is hiring for the position. Your résumé should give enough information about you so that the employer will want to take the time to meet with you for an interview. There are many formats you can use when putting together a résumé. Your instructor or a counselor at your school should be able to help you with your résumé. Your instructor can tell you if the facility you apply to wants you to send a résumé.

The résumé should be accurate and neatly prepared, preferably typed. Your résumé should include:

1. Your name, address (with zip code), and telephone number.
2. Your objective—the title of the job you are seeking.
3. Your educational background, starting with your most recent training.

Jorges Ortiz
456 Bridge Street
Any Town, NJ 01234
Phone—555-678-9012

OBJECTIVE: To obtain a position as a nursing assistant

PROFILE

- Certified Nursing Assistant
- Graduate of Any Town County Technical School, Nursing Assistant Program
- Fluent in Spanish and English
- Career oriented; dedicated to superior patient care
- Punctual, reliable, and hard working
- Enjoy working with patients of all ages
- Special ability to communicate easily with patients

EDUCATION

Graduate, October, 2004, Any Town Technical School, Nursing Assistant Program,
Any Town, NJ; received "Most Caring Student" Award
Graduate, 2001, Riverview High School, Riverview, NJ

SKILLS AND EXPERIENCE
Acquired at Any Town Technical School

- Giving patients personal care: Bathing, grooming, dressing, feeding, transfers, and walking
- Preventing infection, medical asepsis, and bloodborne pathogen training
- Observing, recording, and reporting information, including vital signs
- Performing special procedures and specimen collection
- Clinical experience

WORK HISTORY

Waiter	Seafood Buffet Restaurant	Atlantic Beach, NJ 2002-2003

Selected "Best Waiter of the Summer" in competition 2001 and 2002

Retail Sales Associate	Ralph's Tall Mens Shop	Nearby, PA 2001-2002

OTHER ACTIVITIES
Member, Any Town Rescue Squad, beginning volunteer, certified in CPR, 2004

References furnished on request

Figure **35-3** Sample résumé.

4. Your work history over at least the last 5 years. List your most recent employer first.

5. Any special skills or experience that you have that are necessary for the job for which you are applying.

6. References are optional. You may use the statement "References available on request." A **reference** is a statement about your abilities given by another person, usually a previous employer. If references are not listed on your résumé, prepare a separate sheet listing 3 references. List each person's full name, title, address, and telephone number. *You must have people's permission to use them as a reference.* Select people who know you well enough to give a good recommendation about you and your work habits.

Remember, this is your chance to sell yourself to a potential employer. If your résumé is longer than 1 page, the employer may lose interest before finishing reading it. It is important to use correct grammar and spelling on your résumé to present yourself as a professional. White unlined paper is generally used for a résumé.

Some facilities want you to send your résumé to them by mail, fax, or e-mail. When you send a résumé, you will need to include a cover letter (Figure 35-4). Other facilities want you to apply in person. When you apply in person, a cover letter is not necessary.

When you prepare a cover letter, use business letter style and unlined white paper. Remember to:

- Address the letter to the correct person. If you are not sure who to send the letter to, call the facility and ask for the name and spelling of the person to whom the letter should be addressed.
- Clearly state the job you are interested in and the reason you are interested in working for the facility.
- Briefly state why you should be considered for the position.
- Ask for an interview, making sure your address and phone number are included in the letter.
- Sign the letter.

When you mail a résumé and a cover letter, place the documents in a 9 × 12 addressed envelope and attach proper postage.

Completing a Job Application

Classified advertisements may request that you apply in person. A specific time when the facility will accept applications may be included in the ad (Figure 35-5).

Some employers will send you an application in the mail, but most prefer that you fill out the application in their office. Many times you will be interviewed immediately after you complete

546 Bridge Street
Any Town, NJ 01235
October 28, 2004

Ms. Arlene Weller
Personnel Manager
ABC Community Hospital
99 Elm Drive
Any Town, NJ 01235

Dear Ms. Weller:

The nursing assistant position with ABC Community Hospital, listed in the classified ads section of the October 27, 2004 edition of *The Gazette*, interests me very much. Please consider me an applicant for the position.

As shown in the enclosed resume, I have completed the Nursing Assistant program at Any Town Technical School and am a Certified Nursing Assistant. Also, I have had extensive experience working with people of all ages. I understand the importance of good communication and working as a team member. My patient care skills, along with my work experience, have given me the abilities needed to be successful as a nursing assistant.

I would like to discuss the possibility of employment with you at your convenience. You may contact me at the above address or by phone to arrange for an interview. I look forward to hearing from you.

Sincerely,

Jorges Ortiz

Jorges Ortiz

Enclosure

Figure 35-4   Sample cover letter.

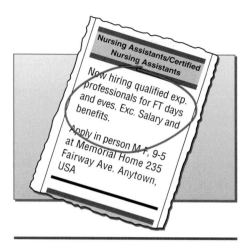

Figure 35-5   Example of a classified ad.

the application. From the minute you walk in the door, you are being evaluated as a potential employee. This means that you will need to be appropriately dressed even if you do not have an interview scheduled. (See interviewing do's and don'ts.) Be prepared to complete the entire application form. Information/items you will need to have when you complete the application include:

1. Social Security card
2. State picture ID or driver's license
3. A copy of your nursing assistant certification or proof of enrollment in the nursing assistant training program at your school
4. Name and location of all schools attended, including dates of attendance
5. Name, title, address, and phone number for at least 3 references
6. Employment information for at least the last 5 years, including phone numbers, addresses, and supervisors' names
7. A copy of your résumé
8. A pen

When you complete the application, print clearly so that the information can be read (Figure 35-6). Be truthful on the application. Giving false information can prevent you from getting the job or result in termination at a later date. Provide a copy of your résumé with the completed application. The employer may ask you to stay for an interview, so schedule some time for this. Be prepared for the interview process when you go to a facility to complete a job application.

APPLICATION FOR EMPLOYMENT
(Please print clearly)

Personal Information

Date: _____

Name _____
Last   First   Middle

Address _____
Street   City   State   Zip Code

Telephone _____ Social Security No. _____
Area Code   Number

If under 18 years of age, do you have work permit? ❑ Yes ❑ No

If not a U.S. citizen, do you have the right to remain permanently and work in the U.S.A.? ❑ Yes ❑ No

       Alien Reg. No. _____

Employment Desired

Position applied for: _____

Shift you can work: ❑ Day ❑ Evening ❑ Either   Hours desired: ❑ Full time ❑ Part time ❑ Temporary

How did you learn of this opening? _____

Date you can start: _____
Month   Day   Year

Have you ever applied to this company before? ❑ Yes ❑ No When _____

Have you ever worked for this company before? ❑ Yes ❑ No

When _____ Supervisor _____

Reason for leaving _____
_____

Education

	1 2 3 4 5 6 7 8	9 10 11 12	1 2 3 4
Highest grade completed (circle):	Grade School	High School	College

Name and location of last school attended _____

Vocational or trade training _____

Extracurricular
activities while in school _____

Area of specialization
or major interest _____

Professional organization memberships, honors received, volunteer or community service or other qualifications you have which you feel are related to the position for which you are applying:

_____
_____
_____
_____

Form 3290R BRIGGS, Des Moines, IA 50306 (800) 247-2343 PRINTED IN U.S.A.   Rev. 4/92

Figure **35-6** Job application.   *Continued*

References

List three persons who know you well. Do not include relatives or former employers.

Name	Address	Phone	Years Acquainted With You

Former Employers

List below your work experience, starting with your present or last place of employment.

Date Employed	Name and Address of Employer	Name of Supervisor	Position(s) Held
from _____			start _____
to _____			finish _____
from _____			start _____
to _____			finish _____
from _____			start _____
to _____			finish _____
from _____			start _____
to _____			finish _____
from _____			start _____
to _____			finish _____

May we contact your present employer at this time?   ❏ Yes   ❏ No

Employment Understanding (Please Read and Sign)

This institution does not discriminate in hiring or any other decision on the basis of race, color, sex, citizenship, national origin, ancestry, Vietnam era veteran status, or on the basis of age or physical or mental disability unrelated to the ability to perform the work required. No question on this application is intended to secure information to be used for such discrimination.

I voluntarily give this institution the right to make a thorough investigation of my past employment and activities, agree to cooperate in such investigation and release from all liability or responsibility all persons, companies or corporations supplying such information. I consent to take the physical examination, and such future physical examinations as may be required by this institution at such times and places as the institution shall designate. I understand that an offer of employment may be contingent on passing the physical examination which relates to the essential duties I would be required to perform.

I understand that my employment is at will, and that either party is free to terminate the employment relationship at any time without cause. I also understand that my employment may be terminated for any misstatement or omission of fact appearing on this application form.

If employed, I will be required to complete an Employment Verification Form (1-9), and within three days show satisfactory evidence of identity and eligibility for employment.

_____   _____
Applicant's Signature   Date

Figure 35-6, cont'd Job application.

Do's and Don'ts to Follow During an Interview

The interview is your opportunity to sell yourself to a potential employer. Not only is the employer interviewing you as a possible employee, but this is also your opportunity to decide if the position will meet your needs as well.

If they have asked you to make an appointment for an interview, make sure to arrive a few minutes before your scheduled appointment. This will allow you to relax and do your best. Do's and don'ts for an interview include:

Do's

1. Know the name of the interviewer and his position in the company.

2. Know as much about the organization as possible. This may require you to look for information about the organization at the library. For example, if you are not interested in working with the elderly, it would be important to know that the facility provides mostly geriatric care.

3. Have all of the information required to complete your application available. Some interviewers will ask you questions and compare your answers to what you wrote on your application or résumé. It is acceptable to look at your notes for dates of employment if necessary.

4. Be neat, clean, and well groomed for the interview.

5. Wear appropriate clothing for the position for which you are applying. A clean uniform is generally considered acceptable when applying for a position in which a uniform is worn. For other positions business attire is required (Figure 35-7 and Box 35-1).

6. Shake hands firmly with the interviewer when introduced. Call the interviewer by the correct title and name. For example, "Good morning Mr. Henderson."

7. Wait to sit down until invited to do so.

8. Place all of your personal belongings such as a purse or brief case on the floor next to your chair. Make sure you have a paper and pencil in case you need to take notes.

9. Be positive and enthusiastic during the interview. Sit straight in the chair with your hands in your lap and both feet on the floor.

10. Take time to think about each question before answering it.

11. Give clear, short answers.

12. Answer all questions honestly, but do not volunteer personal information during the interview. If you do not know the answer to a question, it is fine to say so.

13. Be prepared to answer a variety of questions during the interview (Box 35-2).

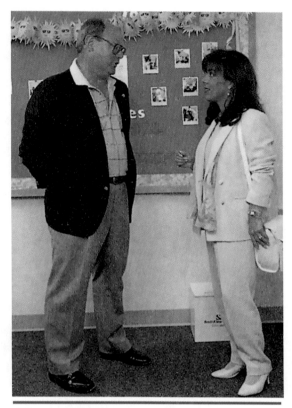

Figure 35-7　Appropriate interview dress.

Box 35-1

BUSINESS ATTIRE

Men

- Navy or black dress pants and dress shirt with a collar or a suit.
- A tie makes a good impression but is not required for entry-level positions.
- Dress shoes (polished) and socks.
- A watch and wedding ring are the only jewelry that should be worn.

Women

- Dress/suit or nice skirt and blouse.
- Navy or black dress pants and a nice blouse are also acceptable.
- Stockings and dress shoes (polished).
- A watch, wedding ring, and small earrings are the only jewelry that should be worn.

Box 35-2

POTENTIAL INTERVIEW QUESTIONS

- Tell me about yourself.
- What are your career goals?
- Why are you applying for this position?
- Why are you leaving your current employer, or why did you leave your previous employer?
- What skills do you have that would be useful to the facility?
- What are your strengths?
- What are your weaknesses?
- What other types of jobs have you done in the past?
- What makes you a good nursing assistant?

Box 35-3

POTENTIAL QUESTIONS TO ASK AT THE END OF AN INTERVIEW

- What is included in the job description for the position?
- Are there opportunities for growth with this position?
- What are the hours of work?
- What is the dress code for the position?
- What are the personnel policies or rules to be followed by employees that apply to this position?
- Is additional on-the-job training or in-service training available to employees?
- How is the employee evaluation, a review of the employee's work, done?
- If the interviewer has not discussed salary and benefits with you, ask what the salary range and benefit package includes.

14. Look at the interviewer while speaking with the person.
15. After the interviewer has finished asking his questions and telling you about the position, you can ask questions (Box 35-3).
16. When the interview is complete, thank the interviewer for the time and firmly shake the interviewer's hand. Ask when a decision regarding the position will be made.
17. Leave the building immediately after the interview is complete.

Sending a thank-you note by mail after the interview will help the interviewer to remember you (Figure 35-8).

546 Bridge Street
Any Town, NJ 01235
November 18, 2004

Ms. Arlene Weller
Personnel Manager
ABC Community Hospital
99 Elm Drive
Any Town, NJ 01235

Dear Ms. Weller:

Thank you for the opportunity to interview for the nursing assistant position on November 15, 2004. I appreciate the time spent with me during the interview and the tour of the agency's offices.

I believe that the skills and knowledge gained from the nursing assistant program at Any Town County Technical School, my present and past work experience, and certification as a nursing assistant make me an excellent and qualified applicant for this entry-level position in the health field.

I look forward to hearing from you soon and am grateful for your consideration.

Sincerely,

Jorges Ortiz
Jorges Ortiz

Figure 35-8   Sample thank-you note.

Don'ts
1. Don't arrive late or more than 5 minutes early for your appointment.
2. Do not chew gum or eat candy after arriving at the facility.
3. Avoid smoking for at least 15 to 20 minutes before you arrive for your interview. Smelling like smoke does not give a good first impression.
4. Avoid clothing that is short, tight, low cut, or very brightly colored or patterned (Figure 35-9).

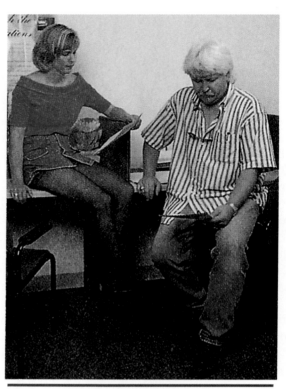

Figure 35-9 Avoid clothing that is short, tight, low cut, or very brightly colored or patterned.

5. Avoid jewelry other than a wedding ring, small earrings, and a watch. Multiple earrings or large dangling bracelets are distracting and unprofessional.
6. A small amount of cologne or perfume is OK; do not use strong scents.
7. Don't keep moving your hands and feet or squirm during the interview. Habits such as nail biting and hair twirling during the interview are distracting.
8. Don't bring children, friends, or pets to the interview with you.
9. Don't use foul language or slang terms or make racial comments during the interview.
10. Don't use the interview to share negative comments about a previous employer. It is much better to say that you left your previous employment because you were unable to grow professionally than to say that your boss would not give you a chance to be promoted and held you back.
11. Don't brag about yourself or talk too much or too long.

After completing the application and interview, you will need to decide if you will accept the job if it is offered to you. There are positives and negatives to every position. Take time to write down the pros and cons of the position and compare them to the lists you made earlier. Does the job meet all of your needs and at least some of your wants? Does this position allow you to use your strengths?

Looking back at the examples given earlier, a job in a geriatric facility that would permit the person to work three 12-hour night shifts a week, is on a major bus line, and provides health insurance would meet the person's needs and allow him to use his strengths (see Figure 35-1).

If the position involved every weekend and did not provide health insurance, even though the salary was a little higher, it would not be a good match.

When deciding to accept a job, you need to look at the entire picture rather than focusing only on the hourly salary.

How to Complete a Resignation Letter

There may come a time in your career when you decide to accept a new position with another organization. It is important to leave your present employer under positive circumstances. Many facilities address the resignation process in the personnel policies. Generally it is expected that you will give the facility notice that you will be leaving 2 weeks before your last day. The correct way to resign your position is with a letter of resignation (Figure 35-10). You should put your notice of resignation in writing, as well as informing your supervisor or director of nursing in person whenever possible. Your letter of resignation is given to your employer before telling your co-workers that you are leaving and should include:

- The date the letter was written
- The date your resignation is effective
- Your signature

Your letter of resignation may be typed or handwritten.

Date

Mark Henderson, RN
Director of Nursing
Happy Acres Rest Home
123 Oak Street
Anytown, USA 12345

Dear Mr. Henderson;

Please accept this letter as notice of my resignation. I have
enjoyed working with the staff and residents at Happy Acres
Rest Home. My last day of work will be (date).

Sincerely,

Employee name
Address
City, state, zip code
Phone number

***Figure* 35-10**   Letter of resignation.

Importance of Continuing Education

Continued professional growth is an important part of your
job as a nursing assistant. Many organizations require that you
attend a specific number of continuing education or in-service
programs each year.

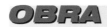

OBRA requires that all nursing assistants who work in long-
term care participate in a minimum of 12 hours of in-service
training per year.

In-service programs may include:
- State and federal guidelines that affect your job performance
- Facility policies and procedures
- Updates on infection control and safety issues

Your place of employment may hold education or in-service
programs. Some facilities will give you the opportunity to attend programs held offsite at other health care facilities or
schools.

The more you learn, the better you will be able to perform
your job and care for your patients.

Maintaining Certification

Becoming certified as a nursing assistant is only the beginning. As a professional, you are responsible for making sure that you meet the requirements of both your employer and the state where you work.

The world of health care is constantly changing. New procedures, types of equipment, and ways of providing care are constantly being evaluated. If you are unemployed for a long period of time, your skills and knowledge will not remain current.

According to the OBRA guidelines, a nursing assistant who has not worked for 24 months (2 years) must complete a new competency evaluation before being allowed to work in a long-term care facility.

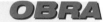

Your instructor can provide you with information about the requirements for recertification in your state. If you move to another state, that state may have requirements that are different.

CHAPTER REVIEW

1. What are some ways that you can find out about jobs that might be right for you?

2. List 3 things that should be included when writing a cover letter.

3. What information/items will you need to complete the application process?

Circle the one BEST response.

4. What is a résumé?
   a. A meeting between 2 or more people
   b. A review of the employee's performance
   c. An agency that helps job seekers find employers
   d. A summary of your education and work experience

5. Which of the following would be an appropriate outfit to wear for an interview?
   a. A pair of dark colored dress pants and a nice blouse or shirt with a collar
   b. A pair of shorts and a print T-shirt
   c. A pair of dress jeans and a sweatshirt
   d. A pair of dark colored pants and a T-shirt

6. Which of the following is *unprofessional* behavior during an interview?
   a. Arriving 5 minutes before the scheduled time
   b. Being clean and well groomed
   c. Making eye contact with the interviewer during the interview process
   d. Smoking a cigarette immediately before the interview

7. How many hours of in-service/continuing education does OBRA require for nursing assistants working in long-term care?
   a. 4 hours per year
   b. 8 hours per year
   c. 12 hours per year
   d. 16 hours per year

8. If nursing assistants do not work in health care for 2 years, OBRA requires that they must:
   a. Re-take the entire CNA course before returning to work
   b. Complete a competency evaluation before returning to work
   c. Submit a fee/fine to the state before returning to work
   d. Do nothing before returning to work

Fill in the blank with the correct term.

9. Generally it is expected that you will give the facility notice that you will be leaving _____ before your last day.

Answers are on page 715.

APPENDIXES

Appendix

Numeric Identifier_____

MINIMUM DATA SET (MDS) — *VERSION 2.0*
FOR NURSING HOME RESIDENT ASSESSMENT AND CARE SCREENING

BASIC ASSESSMENT TRACKING FORM

SECTION AA. IDENTIFICATION INFORMATION

1.	RESIDENT NAME⊙	
		a. (First) b. (Middle Initial) c. (Last) d. (Jr/Sr)

2.	GENDER⊙	1. Male 2. Female

3.	BIRTHDATE⊙	Month — Day — Year

4.	RACE/⊙ ETHNICITY	1. American Indian/Alaskan Native 4. Hispanic 2. Asian/Pacific Islander 5. White, not of 3. Black, not of Hispanic origin Hispanic origin

5.	SOCIAL SECURITY⊙ AND MEDICARE NUMBERS⊙ [C in 1st box if non med. no.]	a. Social Security Number b. Medicare number (or comparable railroad insurance number)

6.	FACILITY PROVIDER NO.⊙	a. State No. b. Federal No.

7.	MEDICAID NO. ["+" if pending, "N" if not a Medicaid recipient]⊙	

8.	REASONS FOR ASSESS-MENT	[Note—Other codes do not apply to this form] **a.** Primary reason for assessment 1. Admission assessment (required by day 14) 2. Annual assessment 3. Significant change in status assessment 4. Significant correction of prior full assessment 5. Quarterly review assessment 10. Significant correction of prior quarterly assessment 0. *NONE OF ABOVE* **b. *Codes for assessments required for Medicare PPS or the State*** *1. Medicare 5 day assessment* *2. Medicare 30 day assessment* *3. Medicare 60 day assessment* *4. Medicare 90 day assessment* *5. Medicare readmission/return assessment* *6. Other state required assessment* *7. Medicare 14 day assessment* *8. Other Medicare required assessment*

9. Signatures of Persons who Completed a Portion of the Accompanying Assessment or Tracking Form

I certify that the accompanying information accurately reflects resident assessment or tracking information for this resident and that I collected or coordinated collection of this information on the dates specified. To the best of my knowledge, this information was collected in accordance with applicable Medicare and Medicaid requirements. I understand that this information is used as a basis for ensuring that residents receive appropriate and quality care, and as a basis for payment from federal funds. I further understand that payment of such federal funds and continued participation in the government-funded health care programs is conditioned on the accuracy and truthfulness of this information, and that I may be personally subject to or may subject my organization to substantial criminal, civil, and/or administrative penalties for submitting false information. I also certify that I am authorized to submit this information by this facility on its behalf.

Signature and Title	Sections	Date
a.		
b.		
c.		
d.		
e.		
f.		
g.		
h.		
i.		
j.		
k.		
l.		

GENERAL INSTRUCTIONS

Complete this information for submission with all full and quarterly assessments (Admission, Annual, Significant Change, State or Medicare required assessments, or Quarterly Reviews, etc.)

⊙ = Key items for computerized resident tracking

☐ = When box blank, must enter number or letter   [a.] = When letter in box, check if condition applies

MDS 2.0 September, 2000

MDS Basic Assessment Tracking Form

Resident _____ Numeric Identifier _____

MINIMUM DATA SET (MDS) — *VERSION 2.0*
FOR NURSING HOME RESIDENT ASSESSMENT AND CARE SCREENING

BACKGROUND (FACE SHEET) INFORMATION AT ADMISSION

SECTION AB. DEMOGRAPHIC INFORMATION

1.	DATE OF ENTRY	*Date the stay began. Note — Does not include readmission if record was closed at time of temporary discharge to hospital, etc. In such cases, use prior admission date* ☐☐ — ☐☐ — ☐☐☐☐ Month · Day · Year
2.	ADMITTED FROM (AT ENTRY)	1. Private home/apt. with no home health services 2. Private home/apt. with home health services 3. Board and care/assisted living/group home 4. Nursing home 5. Acute care hospital 6. Psychiatric hospital, MR/DD facility 7. Rehabilitation hospital 8. Other
3.	LIVED ALONE (PRIOR TO ENTRY)	0. No 1. Yes 2. In other facility
4.	ZIP CODE OF PRIOR PRIMARY RESIDENCE	☐☐☐☐☐
5.	RESIDEN-TIAL HISTORY 5 YEARS PRIOR TO ENTRY	(***Check all settings** resident **lived in** during 5 years prior to date of entry given in item AB1 above*) Prior stay at this nursing home — a. Stay in other nursing home — b. Other residential facility—board and care home, assisted living, group home — c. MH/psychiatric setting — d. MR/DD setting — e. *NONE OF ABOVE* — f.
6.	LIFETIME OCCUPA-TION(S) [Put "/" between two occupations]	☐☐☐☐☐☐☐☐☐☐☐☐☐☐☐☐☐
7.	EDUCATION (*Highest Level Completed*)	1. No schooling 5. Technical or trade school 2. 8th grade/less 6. Some college 3. 9-11 grades 7. Bachelor's degree 4. High school 8. Graduate degree
8.	LANGUAGE	(*Code for correct response*) **a.** Primary Language 0. English 1. Spanish 2. French 3. Other **b. If other, specify** ☐☐☐☐☐☐☐☐
9.	MENTAL HEALTH HISTORY	Does resident's RECORD indicate any history of mental retardation, mental illness, or developmental disability problem? 0. No 1. Yes
10.	CONDITIONS RELATED TO MR/DD STATUS	(***Check all conditions** that are related to MR/DD status that were manifested before age 22, and are likely to continue indefinitely*) Not applicable—no MR/DD (Skip to AB11) — a. MR/DD with organic condition Down's syndrome — b. Autism — c. Epilepsy — d. Other organic condition related to MR/DD — e. MR/DD with no organic condition — f.
11.	DATE BACK-GROUND INFORMA-TION COMPLETED	☐☐ — ☐☐ — ☐☐☐☐ Month · Day · Year

SECTION AC. CUSTOMARY ROUTINE

1.	CUSTOMARY ROUTINE (*In year prior to DATE OF ENTRY to this nursing home, or year last in community if now being admitted from another nursing home*)	(***Check all that apply.** If all information UNKNOWN, check last box only.*)

CYCLE OF DAILY EVENTS

Stays up late at night (e.g., after 9 pm)	a.
Naps regularly during day (at least 1 hour)	b.
Goes out 1+ days a week	c.
Stays busy with hobbies, reading, or fixed daily routine	d.
Spends most of time alone or watching TV	e.
Moves independently indoors (with appliances, if used)	f.
Use of tobacco products at least daily	g.
NONE OF ABOVE	h.

EATING PATTERNS

Distinct food preferences	i.
Eats between meals all or most days	j.
Use of alcoholic beverage(s) at least weekly	k.
NONE OF ABOVE	l.

ADL PATTERNS

In bedclothes much of day	m.
Wakens to toilet all or most nights	n.
Has irregular bowel movement pattern	o.
Showers for bathing	p.
Bathing in PM	q.
NONE OF ABOVE	r.

INVOLVEMENT PATTERNS

Daily contact with relatives/close friends	s.
Usually attends church, temple, synagogue (etc.)	t.
Finds strength in faith	u.
Daily animal companion/presence	v.
Involved in group activities	w.
NONE OF ABOVE	x.
UNKNOWN—Resident/family unable to provide information	y.

SECTION AD. FACE SHEET SIGNATURES

SIGNATURES OF PERSONS COMPLETING FACE SHEET:

a. Signature of RN Assessment Coordinator   Date

I certify that the accompanying information accurately reflects resident assessment or tracking information for this resident and that I collected or coordinated collection of this information on the dates specified. To the best of my knowledge, this information was collected in accordance with applicable Medicare and Medicaid requirements. I understand that this information is used as a basis for ensuring that residents receive appropriate and quality care, and as a basis for payment from federal funds. I further understand that payment of such federal funds and continued participation in the government-funded health care programs is conditioned on the accuracy and truthfulness of this information, and that I may be personally subject to or may subject my organization to substantial criminal, civil, and/or administrative penalties for submitting false information. I also certify that I am authorized to submit this information by this facility on its behalf.

Signature and Title	Sections	Date
b.		
c.		
d.		
e.		
f.		
g.		

☐ = When box blank, must enter number or letter   ☐a. = When letter in box, check if condition applies

MDS 2.0   September, 2000

Resident _____   Numeric Identifier_____

MINIMUM DATA SET (MDS) — *VERSION 2.0*
FOR NURSING HOME RESIDENT ASSESSMENT AND CARE SCREENING
FULL ASSESSMENT FORM
(Status in last 7 days, unless other time frame indicated)

SECTION A. IDENTIFICATION AND BACKGROUND INFORMATION

1. RESIDENT NAME
a. (First)   b. (Middle Initial)   c. (Last)   d. (Jr/Sr)

2. ROOM NUMBER

3. ASSESSMENT REFERENCE DATE
a. Last day of MDS observation period
Month   Day   Year
b. Original (0) or corrected copy of form (enter number of correction)

4a. DATE OF REENTRY
Date of reentry from most recent temporary discharge to a hospital in last 90 days (or since last assessment or admission if less than 90 days)
Month   Day   Year

5. MARITAL STATUS
1. Never married   3. Widowed   5. Divorced
2. Married   4. Separated

6. MEDICAL RECORD NO.

7. CURRENT PAYMENT SOURCES FOR N.H. STAY
(Billing Office to indicate; check all that apply in last 30 days)
Medicaid per diem   a.
Medicare per diem   b.
Medicare ancillary part A   c.
Medicare ancillary part B   d.
CHAMPUS per diem   e.
VA per diem   f.
Self or family pays for full per diem   g.
Medicaid resident liability or Medicare co-payment   h.
Private insurance per diem (including co-payment)   i.
Other per diem   j.

8. REASONS FOR ASSESSMENT
[Note—If this is a discharge or reentry assessment, only a limited subset of MDS items need be completed]
a. Primary reason for assessment
1. Admission assessment (required by day 14)
2. Annual assessment
3. Significant change in status assessment
4. Significant correction of prior full assessment
5. Quarterly review assessment
6. Discharged—return not anticipated
7. Discharged—return anticipated
8. Discharged prior to completing initial assessment
9. Reentry
10. Significant correction of prior quarterly assessment
0. NONE OF ABOVE
b. Codes for assessments required for Medicare PPS or the State
1. Medicare 5 day assessment
2. Medicare 30 day assessment
3. Medicare 60 day assessment
4. Medicare 90 day assessment
5. Medicare readmission/return assessment
6. Other state required assessment
7. Medicare 14 day assessment
8. Other Medicare required assessment

9. RESPONSIBILITY/ LEGAL GUARDIAN
(Check all that apply)
Legal guardian   a.
Other legal oversight   b.
Durable power of attorney/health care   c.
Durable power attorney/financial   d.
Family member responsible   e.
Patient responsible for self   f.
NONE OF ABOVE   g.

10. ADVANCED DIRECTIVES
(For those items with supporting documentation in the medical record, check all that apply)
Living will   a.
Do not resuscitate   b.
Do not hospitalize   c.
Organ donation   d.
Autopsy request   e.
Feeding restrictions   f.
Medication restrictions   g.
Other treatment restrictions   h.
NONE OF ABOVE   i.

SECTION B. COGNITIVE PATTERNS

1. COMATOSE
(Persistent vegetative state/no discernible consciousness)
0. No   1. Yes   (If yes, skip to Section G)

2. MEMORY
(Recall of what was learned or known)
a. Short-term memory OK—seems/appears to recall after 5 minutes
0. Memory OK   1. Memory problem
b. Long-term memory OK—seems/appears to recall long past
0. Memory OK   1. Memory problem

3. MEMORY/ RECALL ABILITY
(Check all that resident was normally able to recall during last 7 days)
Current season   a.
Location of own room   b.
Staff names/faces   c.
That he/she is in a nursing home   d.
NONE OF ABOVE are recalled   e.

4. COGNITIVE SKILLS FOR DAILY DECISION-MAKING
(Made decisions regarding tasks of daily life)
0. INDEPENDENT—decisions consistent/reasonable
1. MODIFIED INDEPENDENCE—some difficulty in new situations only
2. MODERATELY IMPAIRED—decisions poor; cues/supervision required
3. SEVERELY IMPAIRED—never/rarely made decisions

5. INDICATORS OF DELIRIUM—PERIODIC DISORDERED THINKING/ AWARENESS
(Code for behavior in the last 7 days.) [Note: Accurate assessment requires conversations with staff and family who have direct knowledge of resident's behavior over this time].
0. Behavior not present
1. Behavior present, not of recent onset
2. Behavior present, over last 7 days appears different from resident's usual functioning (e.g., new onset or worsening)
a. EASILY DISTRACTED—(e.g., difficulty paying attention; gets sidetracked)
b. PERIODS OF ALTERED PERCEPTION OR AWARENESS OF SURROUNDINGS—(e.g., moves lips or talks to someone not present; believes he/she is somewhere else; confuses night and day)
c. EPISODES OF DISORGANIZED SPEECH—(e.g., speech is incoherent, nonsensical, irrelevant, or rambling from subject to subject; loses train of thought)
d. PERIODS OF RESTLESSNESS—(e.g., fidgeting or picking at skin, clothing, napkins, etc; frequent position changes; repetitive physical movements or calling out)
e. PERIODS OF LETHARGY—(e.g., sluggishness; staring into space; difficult to arouse; little body movement)
f. MENTAL FUNCTION VARIES OVER THE COURSE OF THE DAY—(e.g., sometimes better, sometimes worse; behaviors sometimes present, sometimes not)

6. CHANGE IN COGNITIVE STATUS
Resident's cognitive status, skills, or abilities have changed as compared to status of 90 days ago (or since last assessment if less than 90 days)
0. No change   1. Improved   2. Deteriorated

SECTION C. COMMUNICATION/HEARING PATTERNS

1. HEARING
(With hearing appliance, if used)
0. HEARS ADEQUATELY—normal talk, TV, phone
1. MINIMAL DIFFICULTY when not in quiet setting
2. HEARS IN SPECIAL SITUATIONS ONLY—speaker has to adjust tonal quality and speak distinctly
3. HIGHLY IMPAIRED/absence of useful hearing

2. COMMUNICATION DEVICES/ TECHNIQUES
(Check all that apply during last 7 days)
Hearing aid, present and used   a.
Hearing aid, present and not used regularly   b.
Other receptive comm. techniques used (e.g., lip reading)   c.
NONE OF ABOVE   d.

3. MODES OF EXPRESSION
(Check all used by resident to make needs known)
Speech   a.
Writing messages to express or clarify needs   b.
American sign language or Braille   c.
Signs/gestures/sounds   d.
Communication board   e.
Other   f.
NONE OF ABOVE   g.

4. MAKING SELF UNDERSTOOD
(Expressing information content—however able)
0. UNDERSTOOD
1. USUALLY UNDERSTOOD—difficulty finding words or finishing thoughts
2. SOMETIMES UNDERSTOOD—ability is limited to making concrete requests
3. RARELY/NEVER UNDERSTOOD

5. SPEECH CLARITY
(Code for speech in the last 7 days)
0. CLEAR SPEECH—distinct, intelligible words
1. UNCLEAR SPEECH—slurred, mumbled words
2. NO SPEECH—absence of spoken words

6. ABILITY TO UNDERSTAND OTHERS
(Understanding verbal information content—however able)
0. UNDERSTANDS
1. USUALLY UNDERSTANDS—may miss some part/intent of message
2. SOMETIMES UNDERSTANDS—responds adequately to simple, direct communication
3. RARELY/NEVER UNDERSTANDS

7. CHANGE IN COMMUNICATION/ HEARING
Resident's ability to express, understand, or hear information has changed as compared to status of 90 days ago (or since last assessment if less than 90 days)
0. No change   1. Improved   2. Deteriorated

☐ = When box blank, must enter number or letter   a. = When letter in box, check if condition applies

MDS 2.0 September, 2000

Resident _____ Numeric Identifier _____

SECTION D. VISION PATTERNS

1.	VISION	(Ability to see in adequate light and with glasses if used)
		0. ADEQUATE—sees fine detail, including regular print in newspapers/books 1. IMPAIRED—sees large print, but not regular print in newspapers/books 2. MODERATELY IMPAIRED—limited vision; not able to see newspaper headlines, but can identify objects 3. HIGHLY IMPAIRED—object identification in question, but eyes appear to follow objects 4. SEVERELY IMPAIRED—no vision or sees only light, colors, or shapes; eyes do not appear to follow objects
2.	VISUAL LIMITATIONS/ DIFFICULTIES	Side vision problems—decreased peripheral vision (e.g., leaves food on one side of tray, difficulty traveling, bumps into people and objects, misjudges placement of chair when seating self) a.
		Experiences any of following: sees halos or rings around lights; sees flashes of light; sees "curtains" over eyes b.
		NONE OF ABOVE c.
3.	VISUAL APPLIANCES	Glasses; contact lenses; magnifying glass 0. No 1. Yes

SECTION E. MOOD AND BEHAVIOR PATTERNS

1.	INDICATORS OF DEPRESSION, ANXIETY, SAD MOOD	(Code for indicators observed in last 30 days, irrespective of the assumed cause) 0. Indicator not exhibited in last 30 days 1. Indicator of this type exhibited up to five days a week 2. Indicator of this type exhibited daily or almost daily (6, 7 days a week)

VERBAL EXPRESSIONS OF DISTRESS

a. Resident made negative statements—e.g., "Nothing matters; Would rather be dead; What's the use; Regrets having lived so long; Let me die"

b. Repetitive questions—e.g., "Where do I go; What do I do?"

c. Repetitive verbalizations—e.g., calling out for help, ("God help me")

d. Persistent anger with self or others—e.g., easily annoyed, anger at placement in nursing home; anger at care received

e. Self deprecation—e.g., "I am nothing; I am of no use to anyone"

f. Expressions of what appear to be unrealistic fears—e.g., fear of being abandoned, left alone, being with others

g. Recurrent statements that something terrible is about to happen—e.g., believes he or she is about to die, have a heart attack

h. Repetitive health complaints—e.g., persistently seeks medical attention, obsessive concern with body functions

i. Repetitive anxious complaints/concerns (non-health related) e.g., persistently seeks attention/reassurance regarding schedules, meals, laundry, clothing, relationship issues

SLEEP-CYCLE ISSUES

j. Unpleasant mood in morning

k. Insomnia/change in usual sleep pattern

SAD, APATHETIC, ANXIOUS APPEARANCE

l. Sad, pained, worried facial expressions—e.g., furrowed brows

m. Crying, tearfulness

n. Repetitive physical movements—e.g., pacing, hand wringing, restlessness, fidgeting, picking

LOSS OF INTEREST

o. Withdrawal from activities of interest—e.g., no interest in long standing activities or being with family/friends

p. Reduced social interaction

2.	MOOD PERSISTENCE	One or more indicators of depressed, sad or anxious mood were not easily altered by attempts to "cheer up", console, or reassure the resident over last 7 days 0. No mood indicators 1. Indicators present, easily altered 2. Indicators present, not easily altered
3.	CHANGE IN MOOD	Resident's mood status has changed as compared to status of 90 days ago (or since last assessment if less than 90 days) 0. No change 1. Improved 2. Deteriorated
4.	BEHAVIORAL SYMPTOMS	(A) Behavioral symptom frequency in last 7 days 0. Behavior not exhibited in last 7 days 1. Behavior of this type occurred 1 to 3 days in last 7 days 2. Behavior of this type occurred 4 to 6 days, but less than daily 3. Behavior of this type occurred daily

(B) Behavioral symptom alterability in last 7 days
0. Behavior not present OR behavior was easily altered
1. Behavior was not easily altered   (A)   (B)

a. WANDERING (moved with no rational purpose, seemingly oblivious to needs or safety)

b. VERBALLY ABUSIVE BEHAVIORAL SYMPTOMS (others were threatened, screamed at, cursed at)

c. PHYSICALLY ABUSIVE BEHAVIORAL SYMPTOMS (others were hit, shoved, scratched, sexually abused)

d. SOCIALLY INAPPROPRIATE/DISRUPTIVE BEHAVIORAL SYMPTOMS (made disruptive sounds, noisiness, screaming, self-abusive acts, sexual behavior or disrobing in public, smeared/threw food/feces, hoarding, rummaged through others' belongings)

e. RESISTS CARE (resisted taking medications/ injections, ADL assistance, or eating)

5.	CHANGE IN BEHAVIORAL SYMPTOMS	Resident's behavior status has changed as compared to status of 90 days ago (or since last assessment if less than 90 days) 0. No change 1. Improved 2. Deteriorated

SECTION F. PSYCHOSOCIAL WELL-BEING

1.	SENSE OF INITIATIVE/ INVOLVEMENT	At ease interacting with others	a.
		At ease doing planned or structured activities	b.
		At ease doing self-initiated activities	c.
		Establishes own goals	d.
		Pursues involvement in life of facility (e.g., makes/keeps friends; involved in group activities; responds positively to new activities; assists at religious services)	e.
		Accepts invitations into most group activities	f.
		NONE OF ABOVE	g.
2.	UNSETTLED RELATIONSHIPS	Covert/open conflict with or repeated criticism of staff	a.
		Unhappy with roommate	b.
		Unhappy with residents other than roommate	c.
		Openly expresses conflict/anger with family/friends	d.
		Absence of personal contact with family/friends	e.
		Recent loss of close family member/friend	f.
		Does not adjust easily to change in routines	g.
		NONE OF ABOVE	h.
3.	PAST ROLES	Strong identification with past roles and life status	a.
		Expresses sadness/anger/empty feeling over lost roles/status	b.
		Resident perceives that daily routine (customary routine, activities) is very different from prior pattern in the community	c.
		NONE OF ABOVE	d.

SECTION G. PHYSICAL FUNCTIONING AND STRUCTURAL PROBLEMS

1.	(A) ADL SELF-PERFORMANCE—(Code for resident's PERFORMANCE OVER ALL SHIFTS during last 7 days—Not including setup)

0. INDEPENDENT—No help or oversight —OR— Help/oversight provided only 1 or 2 times during last 7 days

1. SUPERVISION—Oversight, encouragement or cueing provided 3 or more times during last 7 days —OR— Supervision (3 or more times) plus physical assistance provided only 1 or 2 times during last 7 days

2. LIMITED ASSISTANCE—Resident highly involved in activity; received physical help in guided maneuvering of limbs or other nonweight bearing assistance 3 or more times — OR—More help provided only 1 or 2 times during last 7 days

3. EXTENSIVE ASSISTANCE—While resident performed part of activity, over last 7-day period, help of following type(s) provided 3 or more times:
— Weight-bearing support
— Full staff performance during part (but not all) of last 7 days

4. TOTAL DEPENDENCE—Full staff performance of activity during entire 7 days

8. ACTIVITY DID NOT OCCUR during entire 7 days

(B) ADL SUPPORT PROVIDED—(Code for MOST SUPPORT PROVIDED OVER ALL SHIFTS during last 7 days; code regardless of resident's self-performance classification)

0. No setup or physical help from staff
1. Setup help only
2. One person physical assist   8. ADL activity itself did not occur during entire 7 days
3. Two+ persons physical assist

			(A) SELF-PERF	(B) SUPPORT
a.	BED MOBILITY	How resident moves to and from lying position, turns side to side, and positions body while in bed		
b.	TRANSFER	How resident moves between surfaces—to/from: bed, chair, wheelchair, standing position (EXCLUDE to/from bath/toilet)		
c.	WALK IN ROOM	How resident walks between locations in his/her room		
d.	WALK IN CORRIDOR	How resident walks in corridor on unit		
e.	LOCOMOTION ON UNIT	How resident moves between locations in his/her room and adjacent corridor on same floor. If in wheelchair, self-sufficiency once in chair		
f.	LOCOMOTION OFF UNIT	How resident moves to and returns from off unit locations (e.g., areas set aside for dining, activities, or treatments). If facility has only one floor, how resident moves to and from distant areas on the floor. If in wheelchair, self-sufficiency once in chair		
g.	DRESSING	How resident puts on, fastens, and takes off all items of street clothing, including donning/removing prosthesis		
h.	EATING	How resident eats and drinks (regardless of skill). Includes intake of nourishment by other means (e.g., tube feeding, total parenteral nutrition)		
i.	TOILET USE	How resident uses the toilet room (or commode, bedpan, urinal); transfer on/off toilet, cleanses, changes pad, manages ostomy or catheter, adjusts clothes		
j.	PERSONAL HYGIENE	How resident maintains personal hygiene, including combing hair, brushing teeth, shaving, applying makeup, washing/drying face, hands, and perineum (EXCLUDE baths and showers)		

Resident _____   Numeric Identifier _____

2.	BATHING	How resident takes full-body bath/shower, sponge bath, and transfers in/out of tub/shower (EXCLUDE washing of back and hair.) **Code for most dependent** *in self-performance and support.* (A) BATHING SELF-PERFORMANCE codes appear below	(A)	(B)
		0. Independent—No help provided		
		1. Supervision—Oversight help only		
		2. Physical help limited to transfer only		
		3. Physical help in part of bathing activity		
		4. Total dependence		
		8. Activity itself did not occur during entire 7 days *(Bathing support codes are as defined in **Item 1, code B above**)*		

3.	TEST FOR BALANCE (see training manual)	*(Code for ability during test in the **last 7 days**)* 0. Maintained position as required in test 1. Unsteady, but able to rebalance self without physical support 2. Partial physical support during test; or stands (sits) but does not follow directions for test 3. Not able to attempt test without physical help	
		a. Balance while standing	
		b. Balance while sitting—position, trunk control	

4.	FUNCTIONAL LIMITATION IN RANGE OF MOTION (see training manual)	*(Code for limitations during **last 7 days** that interfered with daily functions or placed resident at risk of injury)* (A) *RANGE OF MOTION* (B) *VOLUNTARY MOVEMENT* 0. No limitation 0. No loss 1. Limitation on one side 1. Partial loss 2. Limitation on both sides 2. Full loss	(A)	(B)
		a. Neck		
		b. Arm—Including shoulder or elbow		
		c. Hand—Including wrist or fingers		
		d. Leg—Including hip or knee		
		e. Foot—Including ankle or toes		
		f. Other limitation or loss		

5.	MODES OF LOCOMOTION	*(**Check all that apply** during **last 7 days**)*			
		Cane/walker/crutch	a.	Wheelchair primary mode of locomotion	d.
		Wheeled self	b.		
		Other person wheeled	c.	*NONE OF ABOVE*	e.

6.	MODES OF TRANSFER	*(**Check all that apply** during **last 7 days**)*			
		Bedfast all or most of time	a.	Lifted mechanically	d.
		Bed rails used for bed mobility or transfer	b.	Transfer aid (e.g., slide board, trapeze, cane, walker, brace)	e.
		Lifted manually	c.	*NONE OF ABOVE*	f.

7.	TASK SEGMENTATION	Some or all of ADL activities were broken into subtasks during **last 7 days** so that resident could perform them 0. No 1. Yes	

8.	ADL FUNCTIONAL REHABILITATION POTENTIAL	Resident believes he/she is capable of increased independence in at least some ADLs	a.
		Direct care staff believe resident is capable of increased independence in at least some ADLs	b.
		Resident able to perform tasks/activity but is very slow	c.
		Difference in ADL Self-Performance or ADL Support, comparing mornings to evenings	d.
		NONE OF ABOVE	e.

9.	CHANGE IN ADL FUNCTION	Resident's ADL self-performance status has changed as compared to status of **90 days ago** (or since last assessment if less than 90 days) 0. No change 1. Improved 2. Deteriorated	

SECTION H. CONTINENCE IN LAST 14 DAYS

1. CONTINENCE SELF-CONTROL CATEGORIES *(**Code for resident's PERFORMANCE OVER ALL SHIFTS**)*

0. *CONTINENT*—Complete control *[includes use of indwelling urinary catheter or ostomy device that does not leak urine or stool]*

1. *USUALLY CONTINENT*—BLADDER, incontinent episodes once a week or less; BOWEL, less than weekly

2. *OCCASIONALLY INCONTINENT*—BLADDER, 2 or more times a week but not daily; BOWEL, once a week

3. *FREQUENTLY INCONTINENT*—BLADDER, tended to be incontinent daily, but some control present (e.g., on day shift); BOWEL, 2-3 times a week

4. *INCONTINENT*—Had inadequate control BLADDER, multiple daily episodes; BOWEL, all (or almost all) of the time

a.	BOWEL CONTINENCE	Control of bowel movement, with appliance or bowel continence programs, if employed	
b.	BLADDER CONTINENCE	Control of urinary bladder function (if dribbles, volume insufficient to soak through underpants), with appliances (e.g., foley) or continence programs, if employed	

2.	BOWEL ELIMINATION PATTERN	Bowel elimination pattern regular—at least one movement every three days	a.	Diarrhea	c.
				Fecal impaction	d.
		Constipation	b.	*NONE OF ABOVE*	e.

3.	APPLIANCES AND PROGRAMS	Any scheduled toileting plan	a.	Did not use toilet room/ commode/urinal	f.
		Bladder retraining program		Pads/briefs used	g.
		External (condom) catheter	b.	Enemas/irrigation	h.
			c.	Ostomy present	i.
		Indwelling catheter	d.	*NONE OF ABOVE*	j.
		Intermittent catheter	e.		

4.	CHANGE IN URINARY CONTINENCE	Resident's urinary continence has changed as compared to status of **90 days ago** (or since last assessment if less than 90 days) 0. No change 1. Improved 2. Deteriorated	

SECTION I. DISEASE DIAGNOSES

Check only those diseases that have a relationship to current ADL status, cognitive status, mood and behavior status, medical treatments, nursing monitoring, or risk of death. (Do not list inactive diagnoses)

1. DISEASES *(If none apply, **CHECK the NONE OF ABOVE box**)*

ENDOCRINE/METABOLIC/ NUTRITIONAL		Hemiplegia/Hemiparesis	v.	
Diabetes mellitus	a.	Multiple sclerosis	w.	
Hyperthyroidism	b.	Paraplegia	x.	
Hypothyroidism	c.	Parkinson's disease	y.	
HEART/CIRCULATION		Quadriplegia	z.	
Arteriosclerotic heart disease (ASHD)	d.	Seizure disorder	aa.	
Cardiac dysrhythmias	e.	Transient ischemic attack (TIA)	bb.	
Congestive heart failure	f.	Traumatic brain injury	cc.	
Deep vein thrombosis	g.	**PSYCHIATRIC/MOOD**		
Hypertension	h.	Anxiety disorder	dd.	
Hypotension	i.	Depression	ee.	
Peripheral vascular disease	j.	Manic depression (bipolar disease)	ff.	
Other cardiovascular disease	k.	Schizophrenia	gg.	
MUSCULOSKELETAL		**PULMONARY**		
Arthritis	l.	Asthma	hh.	
Hip fracture	m.	Emphysema/COPD	ii.	
Missing limb (e.g., amputation)	n.	**SENSORY**		
Osteoporosis	o.	Cataracts	jj.	
Pathological bone fracture	p.	Diabetic retinopathy	kk.	
NEUROLOGICAL		Glaucoma	ll.	
Alzheimer's disease	q.	Macular degeneration	mm.	
Aphasia	r.	**OTHER**		
Cerebral palsy	s.	Allergies	nn.	
Cerebrovascular accident (stroke)	t.	Anemia	oo.	
Dementia other than Alzheimer's disease	u.	Cancer	pp.	
		Renal failure	qq.	
		NONE OF ABOVE	rr.	

2. INFECTIONS *(If none apply, **CHECK the NONE OF ABOVE box**)*

Antibiotic resistant infection (e.g., Methicillin resistant staph)	a.	Septicemia	g.	
		Sexually transmitted diseases	h.	
Clostridium difficile (c. diff.)	b.	Tuberculosis	i.	
Conjunctivitis	c.	Urinary tract infection **in last 30 days**	j.	
HIV infection	d.	Viral hepatitis	k.	
Pneumonia	e.	Wound infection	l.	
Respiratory infection	f.	NONE OF ABOVE	m.	

3.	OTHER CURRENT OR MORE DETAILED DIAGNOSES AND ICD-9 CODES	a. _____			•	
		b. _____			•	
		c. _____			•	
		d. _____			•	
		e. _____			•	

SECTION J. HEALTH CONDITIONS

1. PROBLEM CONDITIONS *(**Check all problems present** in **last 7 days** unless other time frame is indicated)*

INDICATORS OF FLUID STATUS		Dizziness/Vertigo	f.	
		Edema	g.	
Weight gain or loss of 3 or more pounds within a 7 day period	a.	Fever	h.	
		Hallucinations	i.	
Inability to lie flat due to shortness of breath	b.	Internal bleeding	j.	
		Recurrent lung aspirations in **last 90 days**	k.	
Dehydrated; output exceeds input	c.	Shortness of breath	l.	
		Syncope (fainting)	m.	
Insufficient fluid; did **NOT** consume all/almost all liquids provided during **last 3 days**	d.	Unsteady gait	n.	
		Vomiting	o.	
OTHER		*NONE OF ABOVE*	p.	
Delusions	e.			

MDS 2.0 September, 2000

Resident _____   Numeric Identifier _____

2.	PAIN SYMPTOMS	(Code the **highest level of pain** present in the **last 7 days**)			
		a. FREQUENCY with which resident complains or shows evidence of pain 0. No pain (**skip to J4**) 1. Pain less than daily 2. Pain daily		**b. INTENSITY** of pain 1. Mild pain 2. Moderate pain 3. Times when pain is horrible or excruciating	
3.	PAIN SITE	(If pain present, **check all sites** that apply in **last 7 days**)			
		Back pain	a.	Incisional pain	f.
		Bone pain	b.	Joint pain (other than hip)	g.
		Chest pain while doing usual activities	c.	Soft tissue pain (e.g., lesion, muscle)	h.
		Headache	d.	Stomach pain	i.
		Hip pain	e.	Other	j.
4.	ACCIDENTS	(**Check all that apply**)			
		Fell in **past 30 days**	a.	Hip fracture in **last 180 days**	c.
		Fell in **past 31-180 days**	b.	Other fracture in **last 180 days**	d.
				NONE OF ABOVE	e.
5.	STABILITY OF CONDITIONS	Conditions/diseases make resident's cognitive, ADL, mood or behavior patterns unstable—(fluctuating, precarious, or deteriorating)			a.
		Resident experiencing an acute episode or a flare-up of a recurrent or chronic problem			b.
		End-stage disease, 6 or fewer months to live			c.
		NONE OF ABOVE			d.

SECTION K. ORAL/NUTRITIONAL STATUS

1.	ORAL PROBLEMS	Chewing problem	a.
		Swallowing problem	b.
		Mouth pain	c.
		NONE OF ABOVE	d.
2.	HEIGHT AND WEIGHT	Record (**a.**) height in inches and (**b.**) weight in pounds. Base weight on most recent measure in **last 30 days**; measure weight consistently in accord with standard facility practice—e.g., in a.m. after voiding, before meal, with shoes off, and in nightclothes **a.** HT (in.) ___ **b.** WT (lb.) ___	
3.	WEIGHT CHANGE	**a. Weight loss**—5 % or more in **last 30 days**; or 10 % or more in **last 180 days** 0. No 1. Yes	
		b. Weight gain—5 % or more in **last 30 days**; or 10 % or more in **last 180 days** 0. No 1. Yes	
4.	NUTRI-TIONAL PROBLEMS	Complains about the taste of many foods	a.	Leaves 25% or more of food uneaten at most meals	c.
		Regular or repetitive complaints of hunger	b.	NONE OF ABOVE	d.
5.	NUTRI-TIONAL APPROACH-ES	(**Check all that apply in last 7 days**)			
		Parenteral/IV	a.	Dietary supplement between meals	f.
		Feeding tube	b.	Plate guard, stabilized built-up utensil, etc.	g.
		Mechanically altered diet	c.	On a planned weight change program	h.
		Syringe (oral feeding)	d.	NONE OF ABOVE	i.
		Therapeutic diet	e.		
6.	PARENTERAL OR ENTERAL INTAKE	(**Skip to Section L if neither 5a nor 5b is checked**)	
		a. Code the proportion of **total calories** the resident received through parenteral or tube feedings in the **last 7 days** 0. None 3. 51% to 75% 1. 1% to 25% 4. 76% to 100% 2. 26% to 50%	
		b. Code the average **fluid intake** per day by IV or tube in **last 7 days** 0. None 3. 1001 to 1500 cc/day 1. 1 to 500 cc/day 4. 1501 to 2000 cc/day 2. 501 to 1000 cc/day 5. 2001 or more cc/day	

SECTION L. ORAL/DENTAL STATUS

1.	ORAL STATUS AND DISEASE PREVENTION	Debris (soft, easily movable substances) present in mouth prior to going to bed at night	a.
		Has dentures or removable bridge	b.
		Some/all natural teeth lost—does not have or does not use dentures (or partial plates)	c.
		Broken, loose, or carious teeth	d.
		Inflamed gums (gingiva); swollen or bleeding gums; oral abcesses; ulcers or rashes	e.
		Daily cleaning of teeth/dentures or daily mouth care—by resident or staff	f.
		NONE OF ABOVE	g.

SECTION M. SKIN CONDITION

			Number at Stage
1.	ULCERS (Due to any cause)	(Record the number of ulcers at each ulcer stage—regardless of cause. If none present at a stage, record "0" (zero). Code all that apply during **last 7 days**. Code 9 = 9 or more.) **[Requires full body exam.]**	
		a. Stage 1. A persistent area of skin redness (without a break in the skin) that does not disappear when pressure is relieved.	
		b. Stage 2. A partial thickness loss of skin layers that presents clinically as an abrasion, blister, or shallow crater.	
		c. Stage 3. A full thickness of skin is lost, exposing the subcutaneous tissues - presents as a deep crater with or without undermining adjacent tissue.	
		d. Stage 4. A full thickness of skin and subcutaneous tissue is lost, exposing muscle or bone.	
2.	TYPE OF ULCER	(For each type of ulcer, **code for the highest stage in the last 7 days** using scale in item M1—i.e., 0=none; stages 1, 2, 3, 4)	
		a. Pressure ulcer—any lesion caused by pressure resulting in damage of underlying tissue	
		b. Stasis ulcer—open lesion caused by poor circulation in the lower extremities	
3.	HISTORY OF RESOLVED ULCERS	Resident had an ulcer that was resolved or cured in **LAST 90 DAYS** 0. No 1. Yes	
4.	OTHER SKIN PROBLEMS OR LESIONS PRESENT	(**Check all that apply** during **last 7 days**)	
		Abrasions, bruises	a.
		Burns (second or third degree)	b.
		Open lesions other than ulcers, rashes, cuts (e.g., cancer lesions)	c.
		Rashes—e.g., intertrigo, eczema, drug rash, heat rash, herpes zoster	d.
		Skin desensitized to pain or pressure	e.
		Skin tears or cuts (other than surgery)	f.
		Surgical wounds	g.
		NONE OF ABOVE	h.
5.	SKIN TREAT-MENTS	(**Check all that apply** during **last 7 days**)	
		Pressure relieving device(s) for chair	a.
		Pressure relieving device(s) for bed	b.
		Turning/repositioning program	c.
		Nutrition or hydration intervention to manage skin problems	d.
		Ulcer care	e.
		Surgical wound care	f.
		Application of dressings (with or without topical medications) other than to feet	g.
		Application of ointments/medications (other than to feet)	h.
		Other preventative or protective skin care (other than to feet)	i.
		NONE OF ABOVE	j.
6.	FOOT PROBLEMS AND CARE	(**Check all that apply** during **last 7 days**)	
		Resident has one or more foot problems—e.g., corns, callouses, bunions, hammer toes, overlapping toes, pain, structural problems	a.
		Infection of the foot—e.g., cellulitis, purulent drainage	b.
		Open lesions on the foot	c.
		Nails/calluses trimmed during **last 90 days**	d.
		Received preventative or protective foot care (e.g., used special shoes, inserts, pads, toe separators)	e.
		Application of dressings (with or without topical medications)	f.
		NONE OF ABOVE	g.

SECTION N. ACTIVITY PURSUIT PATTERNS

1.	TIME AWAKE	(**Check appropriate time periods over last 7 days**)			
		Resident awake all or most of time (i.e., naps no more than one hour per time period) in the:			
		Morning	a.	Evening	c.
		Afternoon	b.	NONE OF ABOVE	d.
	(If resident is comatose, skip to Section O)				
2.	AVERAGE TIME INVOLVED IN ACTIVITIES	(**When awake and not receiving treatments or ADL care**)			
		0. Most—more than 2/3 of time 2. Little—less than 1/3 of time 1. Some—from 1/3 to 2/3 of time 3. None			
3.	PREFERRED ACTIVITY SETTINGS	(**Check all settings** in which activities are **preferred**)			
		Own room	a.		
		Day/activity room	b.	Outside facility	d.
		Inside NH/off unit	c.	NONE OF ABOVE	e.
4.	GENERAL ACTIVITY PREFER-ENCES (adapted to resident's current abilities)	(**Check all PREFERENCES** whether or not activity is currently available to resident)			
		Cards/other games	a.	Trips/shopping	g.
		Crafts/arts	b.	Walking/wheeling outdoors	h.
		Exercise/sports	c.	Watching TV	i.
		Music	d.	Gardening or plants	j.
		Reading/writing	e.	Talking or conversing	k.
		Spiritual/religious activities	f.	Helping others	l.
				NONE OF ABOVE	m.

MDS 2.0 September, 2000

Resident _____   Numeric Identifier _____

5.	PREFERS CHANGE IN DAILY ROUTINE	*Code for resident preferences in daily routines* 0. No change 1. Slight change 2. Major change	
		a. Type of activities in which resident is currently involved	
		b. Extent of resident involvement in activities	

SECTION O. MEDICATIONS

1.	NUMBER OF MEDICA-TIONS	(*Record the number of different medications used in the last 7 days;* enter "0" if none used)	
2.	NEW MEDICA-TIONS	(*Resident currently receiving medications that were initiated during the last 90 days*) 0. No 1. Yes	
3.	INJECTIONS	(*Record the number of DAYS injections of any type received during the last 7 days;* enter "0" if none used)	

4.	DAYS RECEIVED THE FOLLOWING MEDICATION	(*Record the number of DAYS during last 7 days;* enter "0" if not used. Note—enter "1" for long-acting meds used less than weekly)	
		a. Antipsychotic	**d.** Hypnotic
		b. Antianxiety	**e.** Diuretic
		c. Antidepressant	

SECTION P. SPECIAL TREATMENTS AND PROCEDURES

1. SPECIAL TREATMENTS, PROCEDURES, AND PROGRAMS

a. SPECIAL CARE—*Check treatments or programs received during the last 14 days*

TREATMENTS		PROGRAMS	
		Ventilator or respirator	l.
Chemotherapy	a.	**PROGRAMS**	
Dialysis	b.	Alcohol/drug treatment program	m.
IV medication	c.		
Intake/output	d.	Alzheimer's/dementia special care unit	n.
Monitoring acute medical condition	e.	Hospice care	o.
Ostomy care	f.	Pediatric unit	p.
Oxygen therapy	g.	Respite care	q.
Radiation	h.	Training in skills required to return to the community (e.g., taking medications, house work, shopping, transportation, ADLs)	r.
Suctioning	i.		
Tracheostomy care	j.		
Transfusions	k.	NONE OF ABOVE	s.

b. THERAPIES - *Record the number of days and total minutes each of the following therapies was administered (for at least 15 minutes a day) in the last 7 calendar days (Enter 0 if none or less than 15 min. daily)*
[Note—count only post admission therapies]
(A) = # of days administered for **15 minutes or more**
(B) = total # of minutes provided in last 7 days

	DAYS (A)	MIN (B)
a. Speech - language pathology and audiology services		
b. Occupational therapy		
c. Physical therapy		
d. Respiratory therapy		
e. Psychological therapy (by any licensed mental health professional)		

2.	INTERVEN-TION PROGRAMS FOR MOOD, BEHAVIOR, COGNITIVE LOSS	(**Check all interventions or strategies used in last 7 days**—no matter where received)	
		Special behavior symptom evaluation program	a.
		Evaluation by a licensed mental health specialist in **last 90 days**	b.
		Group therapy	c.
		Resident-specific deliberate changes in the environment to address mood/behavior patterns—e.g., providing bureau in which to rummage	d.
		Reorientation—e.g., cueing	e.
		NONE OF ABOVE	f.

3.	NURSING REHABILITA-TION/RESTOR-ATIVE CARE	*Record the NUMBER OF DAYS each of the following rehabilitation or restorative techniques or practices was **provided to the resident for more than or equal to 15 minutes per day in the last 7 days** (Enter 0 if none or less than 15 min. daily.)*	
		a. Range of motion (passive)	**f.** Walking
		b. Range of motion (active)	**g.** Dressing or grooming
		c. Splint or brace assistance	**h.** Eating or swallowing
		TRAINING AND SKILL PRACTICE IN:	**i.** Amputation/prosthesis care
		d. Bed mobility	**j.** Communication
		e. Transfer	**k.** Other

4.	DEVICES AND RESTRAINTS	(*Use the following codes for **last 7 days**:*) 0. Not used 1. Used less than daily 2. Used daily	
		Bed rails	
		a. — Full bed rails on all open sides of bed	
		b. — Other types of side rails used (e.g., half rail, one side)	
		c. Trunk restraint	
		d. Limb restraint	
		e. Chair prevents rising	
5.	HOSPITAL STAY(S)	Record number of times resident was admitted to hospital with an overnight stay **in last 90 days** (or since last assessment if less than 90 days). (*Enter 0 if no hospital admissions*)	
6.	EMERGENCY ROOM (ER) VISIT(S)	Record number of times resident visited ER without an overnight stay **in last 90 days** (or since last assessment if less than 90 days). (*Enter 0 if no ER visits*)	
7.	PHYSICIAN VISITS	In the **LAST 14 DAYS** (or since admission if less than 14 days in facility) how many days has the physician (or authorized assistant or practitioner) examined the resident? (*Enter 0 if none*)	
8.	PHYSICIAN ORDERS	In the **LAST 14 DAYS** (or since admission if less than 14 days in facility) how many days has the physician (or authorized assistant or practitioner) changed the resident's orders? *Do not include order renewals without change. (Enter 0 if none)*	
9.	ABNORMAL LAB VALUES	Has the resident had any abnormal lab values during the **last 90 days** (or since admission)? 0. No 1. Yes	

SECTION Q. DISCHARGE POTENTIAL AND OVERALL STATUS

1.	DISCHARGE POTENTIAL	**a.** Resident expresses/indicates preference to return to the community 0. No 1. Yes	
		b. Resident has a support person who is positive towards discharge 0. No 1. Yes	
		c. Stay projected to be of a short duration— discharge projected **within 90 days** (do not include expected discharge due to death) 0. No 2. Within 31-90 days 1. Within 30 days 3. Discharge status uncertain	

2.	OVERALL CHANGE IN CARE NEEDS	Resident's overall self sufficiency has changed significantly as compared to status of **90 days ago** (or since last assessment if less than 90 days)
		 0. No change 1. Improved—receives fewer 2. Deteriorated—receives
		                      supports, needs less more support
		                       restrictive level of care	

SECTION R. ASSESSMENT INFORMATION

1.	PARTICIPA-TION IN ASSESS-MENT	a. Resident: 0. No 1.Yes	
		b. Family: 0. No 1.Yes 2. No family	
		c. Significant other: 0. No 1. Yes 2. None	

2. SIGNATURE OF PERSON COORDINATING THE ASSESSMENT:

a. Signature of RN Assessment Coordinator (sign on above line)

b. Date RN Assessment Coordinator signed as complete		—		—		
	Month		Day		Year	

Resident _____

Numeric Identifier _____

SECTION T. THERAPY SUPPLEMENT FOR MEDICARE PPS

1.	SPECIAL TREAT- MENTS AND PROCE- DURES	**a. RECREATION THERAPY**—*Enter number of days and total minutes of recreation therapy administered (**for at least 15 minutes a day**) in the **last 7 days** (Enter 0 if none)*	DAYS (A)	MIN (B)
		(A) = **# of days** administered for 15 minutes or more		
		(B) = **total # of minutes** provided in last 7 days		

Skip unless this is a Medicare 5 day or Medicare readmission/ return assessment.	
b. ORDERED THERAPIES—*Has physician ordered any of following therapies to begin in FIRST 14 days of stay—physical therapy, occupational therapy, or speech pathology service?* 0. No 1. Yes	
If not ordered, skip to item 2	
c. Through day 15, provide an estimate of the number of days when at least 1 therapy service can be expected to have been delivered.	
d. Through day 15, provide an estimate of the number of therapy minutes (across the therapies) that can be expected to be delivered?	

2.	WALKING WHEN MOST SELF SUFFICIENT	*Complete item 2 if ADL self-performance score for TRANSFER (G.1.b.A) is 0,1,2, or 3 AND at least one of the following are present:*
		• Resident received physical therapy involving gait training (P.1.b.c)
		• Physical therapy was ordered for the resident involving gait training (T.1.b)
		• Resident received nursing rehabilitation for walking (P.3.f)
		• Physical therapy involving walking has been discontinued within the past 180 days

Skip to item 3 if resident did not walk in last 7 days

(FOR FOLLOWING FIVE ITEMS, BASE CODING ON THE EPISODE WHEN THE RESIDENT WALKED THE FARTHEST WITHOUT SITTING DOWN. INCLUDE WALKING DURING REHABILITATION SESSIONS.)

a. Furthest distance walked without sitting down during this episode.

0. 150+ feet   3. 10-25 feet
1. 51-149 feet   4. Less than 10 feet
2. 26-50 feet

b. Time walked without sitting down during this episode.

0. 1-2 minutes   3. 11-15 minutes
1. 3-4 minutes   4. 16-30 minutes
2. 5-10 minutes   5. 31+ minutes

c. Self-Performance in walking during this episode.

0. *INDEPENDENT*—No help or oversight
1. *SUPERVISION*—Oversight, encouragement or cueing provided
2. *LIMITED ASSISTANCE*—Resident highly involved in walking; received physical help in guided maneuvering of limbs or other nonweight bearing assistance
3. *EXTENSIVE ASSISTANCE*—Resident received weight bearing assistance while walking

d. Walking support provided associated with this episode (code regardless of resident's self-performance classification).

0. No setup or physical help from staff
1. Setup help only
2. One person physical assist
3. Two+ persons physical assist

e. Parallel bars used by resident in association with this episode.

0. No   1. Yes

3.	CASE MIX GROUP	Medicare	State

MDS 2.0 September, 2000

SECTION V. RESIDENT ASSESSMENT PROTOCOL SUMMARY

Numeric Identifier _____

Resident's Name:	Medical Record No.:

1. Check if RAP is triggered.

2. For each triggered RAP, use the RAP guidelines to identify areas needing further assessment. Document relevant assessment information regarding the resident's status.

- Describe:
  — Nature of the condition (may include presence or lack of objective data and subjective complaints).
  — Complications and risk factors that affect your decision to proceed to care planning.
  — Factors that must be considered in developing individualized care plan interventions.
  — Need for referrals/further evaluation by appropriate health professionals.

- Documentation should support your decision-making regarding whether to proceed with a care plan for a triggered RAP and the type(s) of care plan interventions that are appropriate for a particular resident.

- Documentation may appear anywhere in the clinical record (e.g., progress notes, consults, flowsheets, etc.).

3. Indicate under the Location of RAP Assessment Documentation column where information related to the RAP assessment can be found.

4. For each triggered RAP, indicate whether a new care plan, care plan revision, or continuation of current care plan is necessary to address the problem(s) identified in your assessment. The Care Planning Decision column must be completed within 7 days of completing the RAI (MDS and RAPs).

A. RAP PROBLEM AREA	(a) Check if triggered	Location and Date of RAP Assessment Documentation	(b) Care Planning Decision—check if addressed in care plan
1. DELIRIUM			
2. COGNITIVE LOSS			
3. VISUAL FUNCTION			
4. COMMUNICATION			
5. ADL FUNCTIONAL/ REHABILITATION POTENTIAL			
6. URINARY INCONTINENCE AND INDWELLING CATHETER			
7. PSYCHOSOCIAL WELL-BEING			
8. MOOD STATE			
9. BEHAVIORAL SYMPTOMS			
10. ACTIVITIES			
11. FALLS			
12. NUTRITIONAL STATUS			
13. FEEDING TUBES			
14. DEHYDRATION/FLUID MAINTENANCE			
15. DENTAL CARE			
16. PRESSURE ULCERS			
17. PSYCHOTROPIC DRUG USE			
18. PHYSICAL RESTRAINTS			

B.

1. Signature of RN Coordinator for RAP Assessment Process

2. ☐☐ — ☐☐ — ☐☐☐☐
   Month   Day   Year

3. Signature of Person Completing Care Planning Decision

4. ☐☐ — ☐☐ — ☐☐☐☐
   Month   Day   Year

MDS 2.0 September, 2000

MDS Resident Assessment Protocol Summary

RESIDENT ASSESSMENT PROTOCOL TRIGGER LEGEND FOR REVISED RAPS (FOR MDS VERSION 2.0)

Key:
- ● = One item required to trigger
- ❷ = Two items required to trigger
- ★ = One of these three items, plus at least one other item required to trigger
- @ = When both ADL triggers present, maintenance takes precedence

> **Proceed to RAP Review once triggered**

Trigger columns (left to right): Delirium · Cognitive Loss/Dementia · Visual Function · Communication · ADL‑Rehabilitation Trigger A @ · ADL‑Maintenance Trigger B @ · Urinary Incontinence and Indwelling Catheter · Psychosocial Well‑Being · Mood State · Behavioral Symptoms · Activities Trigger A · Activities Trigger B · Falls · Nutritional Status · Feeding Tubes · Dehydration/Fluid Maintenance · Dental Care · Pressure Ulcers · Psychotropic Drug Use · Physical Restraints

MDS ITEM		CODE	Delirium	Cognitive Loss/Dementia	Visual Function	Communication	ADL‑Rehab A @	ADL‑Maint B @	Urinary Incont./Catheter	Psychosocial Well‑Being	Mood State	Behavioral Symptoms	Activities A	Activities B	Falls	Nutritional Status	Feeding Tubes	Dehydration/Fluid Maint.	Dental Care	Pressure Ulcers	Psychotropic Drug Use	Physical Restraints
B2a	Short term memory	1		●																		
B2b	Long term memory	1		●																		
B4	Decision making	1,2,3		●																		
B4	Decision making	3					●															
B5a to B5f	Indicators of delirium	2	●																		●	
B6	Change in cognitive status	2	●																		●	
C1	Hearing	1,2,3				●																
C4	Understood by others	1,2,3				●																
C6	Understand others	1,2,3		●		●																
C7	Change in communication	2																			●	
D1	Vision	1,2,3			●																	
D2a	Side vision problem	√			●																	
E1a to E1p	Indicators of depression, anxiety, sad mood	1,2									●											
E1n	Repetitive movement	1,2																			●	
E1o	Withdrawal from activities	1,2								●												
E2	Mood persistence	1,2									●											
E3	Change in mood	2	●																		●	
E4aA	Wandering	1,2,3											●									
E4aA - E4eA	Behavioral symptoms	1,2,3										●										
E5	Change in behavioral symptoms	1										●										
E5	Change in behavioral symptoms	2	●																		●	
F1d	Establishes own goals	√								●												
F2a to F2d	Unsettled relationships	√								●												
F3a	Strong id, past roles	√								●												
F3b	Lost roles	√								●												
F3c	Daily routine different	√								●												
G1aA - G1jA	ADL self‑performance	1,2,3,4					●															
G1aA	Bed mobility	2,3,4,8																		●		
G2A	Bathing	1,2,3,4					●															
G3b	Balance while sitting	1,2,3																		●		
G6a	Bedfast	√																		●		
G8a,b	Resident, staff believe capable	√					●															
H1a	Bowel incontinence	1,2,3,4																		●		
H1b	Bladder incontinence	2,3,4							●													
H2b	Constipation	√																			●	
H2d	Fecal impaction	√																			●	
H3c,d,e	Catheter use	√							●													
H3g	Use of pads/briefs	√							●													
I1i	Hypotension	√																●				
I1j	Peripheral vascular disease	√																		●		
I1ee	Depression	√																			●	
I1jj	Cataracts	√			●																	
I1ll	Glaucoma	√			●																	
I2j	UTI	√																				
I3	Dehydration diagnosis	276.5																●				
J1a	Weight fluctuation	√																●				
J1c	Dehydrated	√																●				
J1d	Insufficient fluid	√																●				
J1f	Dizziness	√													●						●	
J1h	Fever	√																●				
J1i	Hallucinations	√																			●	
J1j	Internal bleeding	√																●				
J1k	Lung aspirations	√																			●	
J1m	Syncope	√																			●	

MDS 2.0 September, 2000

MDS Resident Assessment Protocol Trigger Legend for Revised RAPS

RESIDENT ASSESSMENT PROTOCOL TRIGGER LEGEND FOR REVISED RAPS (FOR MDS VERSION 2.0)

Key:
- ● = One item required to trigger
- ❷ = Two items required to trigger
- ★ = One of these three items, plus at least one other item required to trigger
- @ = When both ADL triggers present, maintenance takes precedence

Proceed to RAP Review once triggered

MDS ITEM	Description	CODE	Delirium	Cognitive Loss/Dementia	Visual Function	Communication	ADL-Rehabilitation Trigger A @	ADL-Maintenance Trigger B @	Urinary Incontinence and Indwelling Catheter	Psychosocial Well-Being	Mood State	Behavioral Symptoms	Activities Trigger A	Activities Trigger B	Falls	Nutritional Status	Feeding Tubes	Dehydration/Fluid Maintenance	Dental Care	Pressure Ulcers	Psychotropic Drug Use	Physical Restraints	
J1n	Unsteady gait	√																			●		J1n
J4a,b	Fell	√													●						●		J4a,b
J4c	Hip fracture	√																			●		J4c
K1b	Swallowing problem	√																			●		K1b
K1c	Mouth pain	√																	●				K1c
K3a	Weight loss	1														●							K3a
K4a	Taste alteration	√														●							K4a
K4c	Leave 25% food	√														●							K4c
K5a	Parenteral/IV feeding	√														●	●						K5a
K5b	Feeding tube	√															●	●					K5b
K5c	Mechanically altered	√														●							K5c
K5d	Syringe feeding	√														●							K5d
K5e	Theraputic diet	√														●							K5e
L1a,c,d,e	Dental	√																	●				L1a,c,d,e
L1f	Daily cleaning teeth	Not √																	●				L1f
M2a	Pressure ulcer	2,3,4														●							M2a
M2a	Pressure ulcer	1,2,3,4																		●			M2a
M3	Previous pressure ulcer	1																		●			M3
M4e	Impaired tactile sense	√																		●			M4e
N1a	Awake morning	√											❷										N1a
N2	Involved in activities	0											❷										N2
N2	Involved in activities	2,3												●									N2
N5a,b	Prefers change in daily routine	1,2												●									N5a,b
O4a	Antipsychotics	1-7																			★		O4a
O4b	Antianxiety	1-7													●						★		O4b
O4c	Antidepressants	1-7													●						★		O4c
O4e	Diuretic	1-7																●					O4e
P4c	Trunk restraint	1,2													●							●	P4c
P4c	Trunk restraint	2																		●			P4c
P4d	Limb restraint	1,2																				●	P4d
P4e	Chair prevents rising	1,2																				●	P4e

Activity intolerance
Risk for **Activity** intolerance
Impaired **Adjustment**
Ineffective **Airway** clearance
Latex **Allergy** response
Risk for latex **Allergy** response
Anxiety
Death **Anxiety**
Risk for **Aspiration**
Risk for impaired parent/infant/child **Attachment**
Autonomic dysreflexia
Risk for **Autonomic** dysreflexia
Disturbed **Body** image
Risk for imbalanced **Body** temperature
Bowel incontinence
Effective **Breastfeeding**
Ineffective **Breastfeeding**
Interrupted **Breastfeeding**
Ineffective **Breathing** pattern
Decreased **Cardiac** output
Caregiver role strain
Risk for **Caregiver** role strain
Impaired verbal **Communication**
Readiness for enhanced **Communication**
Decisional **Conflict**
Parental role **Conflict**
Acute **Confusion**
Chronic **Confusion**
Constipation
Perceived **Constipation**
Risk for **Constipation**
Defensive **Coping**
Ineffective **Coping**
Ineffective community **Coping**
Readiness for enhanced **Coping**
Readiness for enhanced community **Coping**
Defensive **Coping**
Compromised family **Coping**
Disabled family **Coping**
Readiness for enhanced family **Coping**
Ineffective **Denial**
Impaired **Dentition**
Risk for delayed **Development**

Diarrhea
Risk for **Disuse** syndrome
Deficient **Diversional** activity
Disturbed **Energy** field
Impaired **Environmental** interpretation syndrome
Adult **Failure** to thrive
Risk for **Falls**
Dysfunctional **Family** processes: alcoholism
Family processes
Readiness for enhanced **Family** processes
Interrupted **Family** processes
Fatigue
Fear
Readiness for enhanced **Fluid** balance
Deficient **Fluid** volume
Excess **Fluid** volume
Risk for deficient **Fluid** volume
Risk for imbalanced **Fluid** volume
Impaired **Gas** exchange
Anticipatory **Grieving**
Dysfunctional **Grieving**
Delayed **Growth** and development
Risk for disproportionate **Growth**
Ineffective **Health** maintenance
Health-seeking behaviors
Impaired **Home** maintenance
Hopelessness
Hyperthermia
Hypothermia
Disturbed personal **Identity**
Functional urinary **Incontinence**
Reflex urinary **Incontinence**
Stress urinary **Incontinence**
Total urinary **Incontinence**
Urge urinary **Incontinence**
Risk for urge urinary **Incontinence**
Disorganized **Infant** behavior
Risk for disorganized **Infant** behavior
Readiness for enhanced organized **Infant** behavior
Ineffective **Infant** feeding pattern
Risk for **Infection**
Risk for **Injury**

Risk for perioperative-positioning **Injury**
Decreased **Intracranial** adaptive capacity
Deficient **Knowledge**
Readiness for enhanced **Knowledge**
Risk for **Loneliness**
Impaired **Memory**
Impaired bed **Mobility**
Impaired physical **Mobility**
Impaired wheelchair **Mobility**
Nausea
Unilateral **Neglect**
Noncompliance
Imbalanced **Nutrition**: less than body requirements
Imbalanced **Nutrition**: more than body requirements
Readiness for enhanced **Nutrition**
Risk for imbalanced **Nutrition**: more than body requirements
Impaired **Oral** mucous membrane
Acute **Pain**
Chronic **Pain**
Impaired **Parenting**
Readiness for enhanced **Parenting**
Risk for impaired **Parenting**
Risk for **Peripheral** neurovascular dysfunction
Risk for **Poisoning**
Post-trauma syndrome
Risk for **Post-trauma** syndrome
Powerlessness
Risk for **Powerlessness**
Ineffective **Protection**
Rape-trauma syndrome
Rape-trauma syndrome: compound reaction
Rape-trauma syndrome: silent reaction
Relocation stress syndrome
Risk for **Relocation stress syndrome**
Ineffective **Role** performance
Bathing/hygiene **Self-care** deficit
Dressing/grooming **Self-care** deficit
Feeding **Self-care** deficit
Toileting **Self-care** deficit
Readiness for enhanced **Self-Concept**
Chronic low **Self-esteem**
Situational low **Self-esteem**
Risk for situational low **Self-esteem**

Self-mutilation
Risk for **Self-mutilation**
Disturbed **Sensory** perception (specify)
Sexual dysfunction
Ineffective **Sexuality** patterns
Impaired **Skin** integrity
Risk for impaired **Skin** integrity
Sleep deprivation
Disturbed **Sleep** pattern
Readiness for enhanced **Sleep**
Impaired **Social** interaction
Social isolation
Chronic **Sorrow**
Spiritual distress
Risk for **Spiritual** distress
Readiness for enhanced **Spiritual** well-being
Risk for **Suffocation**
Risk for **Suicide**
Delayed **Surgical** recovery
Impaired **Swallowing**
Effective **Therapeutic** regimen management
Ineffective **Therapeutic** regimen management
Readiness for enhanced **Therapeutic** regimen management
Ineffective community **Therapeutic** regimen management
Ineffective family **Therapeutic** regimen management
Ineffective **Thermoregulation**
Disturbed **Thought** processes
Impaired **Tissue** integrity
Ineffective **Tissue** perfusion (specify)
Impaired **Transfer** ability
Risk for **Trauma**
Impaired **Urinary** elimination
Readiness for enhanced **Urinary** elimination
Urinary retention
Impaired spontaneous **Ventilation**
Dysfunctional **Ventilatory** weaning response
Risk for other-directed **Violence**
Risk for self-directed **Violence**
Impaired **Walking**
Wandering

NANDA International: *NANDA nursing diagnoses: definitions and classification 2003-2004,* Philadelphia, 2002, NANDA.

Useful Spanish Words

English	Spanish	Pronunciation
Abdomen	Abdomen	Ahb-doh-mehn
Abnormal	Anormal	Ah-nohr-mahl
Above	Arriba	Ah-ree-bah
Abuse	Abuso	Ah-boo-soh
Accident	Accidente	Ahk-see-dehn-teh
Activities	Actividades	Ahk-tee-bee-dah-dehs
Administration	Administracion	Ahd-meh-nees-trah-see-ohn
Adults	Adultos	Ah-dool-tohs
After	Después de	Dehs-poo-ehs deh
Aggressive	Agresivo	Ah-greh-see-boh
Air	Aire	Ah-ee-reh
Air conditioning	Aire acondicionado	Ah-ee-reh ah-kohn-dee-see-oh-nah-doh
Airway	Vía aérea	Bee-ah ah-eh-reh-ah
Alert	Avisele	Ah-bee-seh-leh
Allergies	Alergias	Ah-lehr-hee-ahs
Allergy	Alérgico	Ah-lher-hee-ahs
Allergy	Alergia	Ah-lher-hee-ah
Amputation	Amputación	Ahm-poo-tah-see-ohn
Amputee	Amputado	Ahm-poo-tah-doh
Analgesic	Analgésicos	Ah-nahl-heh-see-kohs
Anaphylactic shock	Choque anafilático	Choh-keh ah-nah-fee lah-tee-koh
Anemia	Anemia	Ah-neh-mee-ah
Anesthesia	Anestesia	Ah-nehs-teh-see-ah
Aneurysm	Aneurisma	Ah-neh-oo-rees-mah
Anger	Enojo	Eh-noh-hoh
Angina	Angina	Aahn-hee-nah
Ankle	Tobillo	Toh-bee-yoh
Anxiety	Ansiedad	Ahn-see-eh-dahd
Anxious	Ansioso	Ahn-see-oh-soh
Arm	El brazo	???
Armpit/axilla	La axilla/el sobaco	???
Arrest	Arresto	Ah-rehs-toh
Arthritis	Arthritis	Ahr-tree-tees
Assessment	Avalúo	Ah-bah-loo-oh
Asthma	Asma	Ahs-mah
Baby	Bebé	Beh-beh
Bacteria	Bacteria	Bahk-teh-ree-ah
Bad	Mal	Mahl
Balanced	Balanceada	Bah-lahn-seh-ah-dah
Basin	Lavabo	Lah-bah-boh

English	Spanish	Pronunciation
Bathroom	Baño	Bah-nyoh
Bed	Cama	Kah-mah
Bed cover	Colcha	Kohl-chah
Bed rails	Barandal	Bah-rahn-dahl
Bedpan	Bacín	Bah-seen
Bedroom	Recamara	Reh-kahm-ah-rah
Bedspread	Colcha	Kohl-cha
Before	Antes de	Ahn-tehs deh
Behavior	Conducta	Kohn-dook-tah
Bell(s)	Campana/timbre	Kahm-pah-nah/teem-breh
Below	Abajo	Ah-bah-hoh
Bend	Doblar	Doh-blahr
Blanket	Frazada/covertor	Frah-sah-dah/koh-behr-tohr
Bleeding	Sangrado	Sahn-grah-doh
Blood	Sangre	Sahn-greh
Blood flow	Circulación sanguínea	Seer-koo-lah-see-ohn
Blouse	Blusa	Bloo-sah
Bottle	Botella	Boh-teh-yah
Bowel	Intestino	Een-tehs-tee-noh
Bradycardia	Bradicardia	Brah-dee-kahr-dee-ah
Breathe!	¡Respire!	Rehs-pee-reh
Broken bone	Hueso roto	Oo-eh-soh roh-toh
Bronchitis	Bronquitis	Brohn-kee-tees
Brother	Hermano	Ehr-mah-noh
Bruises/ecchymosis	Moretones/equimosis	Moh-reh-toh-nehs/eh-kee-moh-sees
Burns	Quemaduras	Keh-mah-doo-rahs
Burp	Repetir/eructar	Reh-peh-teer/eh-rook-tahr
Button	Botón	Boh-tohn
By mouth	Por la boca	Pohr lah boh-kah
Café (coffee)	Café	Kah-feh
Call (for/name)	Llamar	Yah-mahr
Call-bell	Campana/timbre	Kahm-pah-nah/teem-breh
Cancer	Cáncer	Kahn-sehr
Canes	Bastones	Bahs-toh-nehs
Cardiac	Cardíaco	Kahr-dee-ah-koh
Cardio-pulmonary	Cardio-pulmonar	Kahr-dee-oh-pool-moh-nahr
Care	Cuidado	Koo-ee-dah-doh
Carotid	Carótida	Kah-roh-tee-dah

English	Spanish	Pronunciation
Cast	Yeso	Yeh-soh
Cataract	Catarata	Kah-tah-rah-tah
Cavity	Cavidad	Kah-bee-dahd
Cereal (cooked)	Cereal/cocido	Seh-reh-ahl/koh-see-doh
Cereal (dry)	Cereal/seco	Seh-reh-ahl/ seh-koh
Chairs	Sillas	See-yahs
Chaplain/priest	Capellán/sacerdote/cura	Kah-peh-yahn/sah-sehr-doh-teh/koo-rah
Cheek	Mejilla	Meh-hee-yah
Chest	Pecho	Peh-choh
Chest pain	Dolor de pecho	Doh-lohr deh peh-choh
Chest/breast	Pecho/seno/la teta	Peh-choh
Child	Niño(a)	Nee-nyoh(-nyah)
Choking	Ahogar	Ah-oh-gahr
Clean	Limpiar	Leem-peahr
Cognitive	Cognoscitivo	Kohg-noh-see-tee-boh
Cold	Frío	Free-oh
Cold water	Agua fría	Ah-goo-ah free-ah
Color	Color	Koh-lohr
Comatose	Comatose	Koh-mah-toh-soh
Comb	Peine	Peh-ee-neh
Communicate	Comunicar	Koh-moo-nee-kahr
Communication	Comunicación	Koh-moo-nee-kah-see-ohn
Complete	Completa	Kohm-pleh-tah
Complete dentures	Dentadura completa	Dehn-tah-doo-rah kohm-pleh-tah
Complications	Complicaciones	Kohm-plee-kah-see-ohn-ehs
Complications (major)	Complicaciones mayors	Kohm-plee-kah-see-oh-nes mah-yoh-rhes
Compound fractures	Fracturas compuestas	Frahk-too-rahs kohm-poo-ehs-tahs
Confuse	Confundir	Kohn-foon-deer
Consciousness	Conocimiento	Koh-noh-see-mee-ehn-toh
Constipation	Constipación/estreñimiento	Kohns-tee-pah-see-ohn/ehs- treh-nyee-mee-ehn-toh
Coping	Sobrellevando	Soh-breh-yeh-bahn-doh
Cough	Toser	Toh-sehr
Cry	Llorar	Yoh-rahr
Cubic centimeter	Centímetro cúbico	Sehn-tee-meh-troh koo-bee-koh

English	Spanish	Pronunciation
Cup	Tasa	Tah-sah
Cut	Cortar	Kohr-tahr
Dad	Papá	Pah-pah
Daughter	Hija	Ee-hah
Dehydrated	Deshidratado	Deh-see-drah-tah-doh
Dehydration	Deshidratación	Deh-see-drah-tah-see-ohn
Delirious	Delirio	Deh-lee-ree-oh
Demented	Demente	Deh-mehn-teh
Dementia	Demencia	Deh-mehn-see-ah
Dentist	Dentista	Dehn-tees-tah
Dentures	Dentadura	Dehn-tah-doo-rah
Deodorant	Desodorante	Deh-soh-doh-rahn-teh
Dependence	Dependencia	Deh-pehn-dehn-see-ah
Dependent	Dependiente	Deh-pehn-dehn-dee-ehn-teh
Depressed	Deprimido	Deh-pree-mee-doh
Develop	Desarrollar	Deh-sah-roh-yahr
Development	Desarrollo	Deh-sah-roh-yoh
Diabetes	Diabetes	Dee-ah-beh-tees
Diabetic	Diabética(o)	Dee-ah-beh-tee-kah
Diagnosis	Diagnóstico	Dee-ahg-nohs-tee-koh
Diaper	Pañal	Pah-nyahl
Diarrhea	Diarrea	Dee-ah-rreh-ah
Diet(s)	Dieta(s)	Dee-eh-tah(s)
Different	Diferente	Dee-feh-rehn-teh
Dizzy	Mareado	Mah-reh-ah-doh
Dizzy spell	Desmayo/mareo	Dehs-mah-yoh/mah-reh-oh
Doctor	Doctor(a)/medico(a)	Dohk-tohr(-toht-ah)/meh-dee-koh(-kah)
Doctor's office	Oficina/consultorio	Oh-fee-see-nah/kohn-sool-toh-ree-oh
Don't move!	¡No se mueva!	Noh seh moo-eh-bah
Door	Puerta	Poo-her-tah
Dress	Vestír	Behs-teer
Dress	Vestido	Behs-tee-doh
Dresser	Aparador	Ah-pah-rah-dohr
Drink	Beber/tomar	Beh-behr/toh-mahr
Drinking glass	Vidrio/vaso	Bee-dree-oh/bah-soh
Dry	Seca	Seh-kah
Ear	Oreja/el oído	Oh-reh-hah
Eat	Comer	Koh-mehr
Eat breakfast	Desayunar	Deh-sah-yoo-nahr
Eczema	Eczema	Ehk-seh-mah
Eight	Ocho	Oh-choh
Eighty	Ochenta	Oh-chehn-tah
Elbow	Codo	Koh-doh

English	Spanish	Pronunciation
Elder	Anciana (feminine)	Ahn-see-ah-nah
Elderly	Anciano	Ahn-see-ah-noh
Electrocardiogram	Electro cardiograma	Eh-lehk-troh-kahr-dee-oh-grah-mah
Embolism	Embolia	Ehm-boh-lee-ah
Embolism	Embolismo	Ehm-boh-lees-moh
Emergencies	Emergencias	Eh-mehr-hehn-see-ahs
Emergency	Emergencia	Eh-mehr-hehn-see-ah
Enema	Enema/sonda	Eh-neh-mah/sohn-dah
Epilepsy	Epilepsia	Eh-pee-lehp-see-ah
Examinations	Exámenes	Ehx-ah-meh-nehs
Exercise	Ejercicio	Eh-hehr-see-see-oh
Eye	Ojo	Oh-hoh
Facial	Facial	Fah-see-ahl
Familiar	Familiar	Fah-mee-lee-ahr
Family	Familia	Fah-mee-lee-ah
Father	Padre	Pah-dreh
Fear	Miedo	Mee-eh-doh
Feel	Sentír	Sehn-teer
Fever	Fiebre	Fee-eh-breh
Fifteen	Quince	Keen-she
Fifty	Cincuenta	Seen-koo-ehn-tah
Five	Cinco	Seen-koh
Fluid	Fluído	Floo-ee-doh
Foods	Comidas	Koh-mee-dahs
Fork	Tenedor	The-neh-dohr
Formula	Formula	Fohr-moo-lah
Forty	Cuarenta	Koo-ah-rehn-tah
Four	Cuatro	Koo-ah-troh
Fracture (pelvic)	Fractura pélvica	Frahk-too-rah pehl-bee-kah
Fractures	Fracturas	Frahk-too-rahs
Friday	Viernes	Bee-ehr-nehs
Fungus	Hongos	Ohn-gohs
Gallbladder	Vesicular biliar/hiel	Beh-see-koo-lah bee-lee ahr/ee-ehl
Gangrene	Gangrena	Gahn-greh-nah
Glass	Vaso	Bah-soh
Glaucoma	Glaucoma	Glah-oo-koh-mah
Gloves	Guantes	Goo-ahn-tehs
Goals	Metas	Meh-tahs
Gout	Gota	Goh-tah
Gown	Bata/vestido	Bah-tah/behs-tee-doh
Grandmother	Abuela	Ah-boo-eh-lah
Grief	Pena	Peh-nah
Grieve	Sufrir	Soo-freer
Grieving	Afligir	Ah-flee-heer
Groin	Ingle	Een-gleh
Growth	Crecimiento	Kreh-see-mee-ehn-toh
Guilt	Culpa	Kool-pah

English	Spanish	Pronunciation
Gynecologist	Ginecólogo	Hee-neh-koh-loh-goh
Hairbrush	Cepillo de pelo	Seh-pee-yoh deh peh-loh
Hazard	Peligro	Peh-lee-groh
Headache	Dolor de cabeza	Doh-lohr deh kah-beh-sah
Heal	Sano	Sah-noh
Healing	Curación	Koo-rah-see-ohn
Health	Salud	Sah-lood
Health (mental)	Salud mental	Sah-lood mehn-tahl
Heart(s)	Corazón (corazones)	Koh-rah-sohn/koh-rah-sohn-ehs
Hematoma	Hematoma	Eh-mah-toh-mah
Hemorrhage	Hemorragia	Eh-moh-rah-hee-ah
Hepatitis	Hepatitis	Eh-pah-tee-tees
Hernia	Hernia	Ehr-nee-ah
Hip	Cadera	Kah-deh-rah
Hip fracture	Fractura de cadera	Frahk-too-rah deh kah-deh-rah
Hope	Esperanza	Ehs-peh-rahn-sah
Hose/stockings	Medias	Meh-dee-ahs
Hot water	Agua caliente	Ah-goo-ah kah-lee-ehn-teh
Hours (visiting)	Horas de visita	Oh-rahs deh bee-see-tah
Husband	Esposo	Ehs-poh-soh
Hypertension	Hipertensión	Ee-pehr-tehn-see-ohn
Hypertension (pulmonary)	Hipertensión pulmonar	Ee-pehr-tehn-see-ohn pool-moh-nahr
Hyperthermia	Hipertermia	Ee-pehr-tehr-mee-ah
Hypoglycemia	Hipoglucemia	Ee-poh-gloo-seh-mee-ah
Identification	Identificacíon	Ee-dehn-tee-fee-kah-see-ohn
Illness	Enfermedad	Ehn-fehr-meh-dahd
Incision	Incisión	Een-see-see-ohn
Independence	Independencia	Een-deh-pehn-dehn-see-ah
Indigestion	Indigestión	Een-dee-hehs-tee-ohn
Infection	Infección	Een-fehk-see-ohn
Infections	Infecciones	Een-fehk-see-oh-nehs
Inflammation	Inflamación	Een-flah-mah-see-ohn
Internal	Interior	Een-teh-ree-ohr
Irritable	Irritable	Ee-ree-tah-bleh
Jacket	Chaqueta	Chah-keh-tah
Juice(s)	Jugo(s)	Hoo-goh(s)
Knee	La rodilla	Roh-dee-yah
Knife	Cuchillo	Koo-chee-yoh
Laboratory	Laboratorio	Lah-boh-rah-toh-ree-oh

English	Spanish	Pronunciation	English	Spanish	Pronunciation
Lamp	Lámpara	Lahm-pah-rah	No smoking	No se permite fumar	Noh she pehr-mee-the foo-mahr
Laxative(s)	Laxante(s)/ purgante(s)	Lahx-ahn-teh(s)/ poor-gahn-teh(s)	Normal	Normal	Nohr-mahl
Left	Izquierda	Ees-kee-ehr-dah	Nose	Nariz	Nah-rees
Leg	Pierna	Pee-her-nah	Nurse	Enfermero(a)	Ehn-fehr-meh-roh(-rah)
Linen	Lino	Lee-noh	Nutrition	Nutrición	Noo-tree-see-ohn
Liquid	Líquida	Lee-kee-dah	Obesity	Obesidad	Oh-beh-see-dahd
Loneliness	Soledad	Soh-leh-dahd	Observe	Observe	Ohb-sehr-beh
Lose	Perder	Pehr-dehr	Obstruction	Obstrucción	Ohb-strook-see-ohn
Loss	Pérdida	Pehr-dee-dah	Office	Oficina	Oh-fee-see-nah
Love	Amor	Ah-mohr	Older	Mayors	Mah-yoh-rehs
Low cholesterol	Poco colesterol	Poh-koh koh-lehs-teh-rohl	One	Uno	Oo-noh
			One hundred	Cien	See-ehn
Low cholesterol	Colesterol bajo	Koh-lehs-teh-rohl bah-hoh	Open!	¡Abra!	Ah-brah
			Ophthalmic	Oftálmico	Ohf-tahl-mee-koh
Low fat	Poca grasa	Poh-kah grah-sah	Oral	Oral	Oh-rahl
Low sodium	Baja en sal/ poca sal	Bah-hah ehn sahl/ poh-kah sahl	Organ(s)	Órgano(s)	Ohr-gah-noh(s)
			Ounces	Onzas	Ohn-sahs
Lunch	Comida	Koh-mee-dah	Oxygen	Oxígeno	Ohx-ee-heh-noh
Lungs	Pulmones	Pool-moh-nehs	Pacemaker	Marcapasos	Mahr-kah-pah-sohs
Management	Manejo	Mah-neh-hoh	Pain	Dolor	Doh-lohr
Mattress	Colchón	Kohl-chohn	Pajama	Pijama	Pee-hah-mah
Measures	Medidas	Meh-dee-dahs	Pancreas	Páncreas	Pahn-kreh-ahs
Mechanisms	Mecanismos	Meh-kah-nees-mohs	Panic	Pánico	Pah-nee-koh
Medical	Médico	Meh-dee-koh	Pants/slacks	Pantalones	Pahn-tah-loh-nehs
Memory	Memoria	Meh-moh-ree-ah	Paralysis	Parálisis	Pah-rah-lee-sees
Meningitis	Meningitis	Meh-neen-hee-tees	Pathogen	Patogénico	Pah-toh-heh-nee-koh
Mental retardation	Retraso mental	Reh-trah-soh mehn-tahl	Patient (mental)	Enfermo mental	Eehn-fehr-moh mehn-tahl
Milk	Leche	Leh-cheh	Patient walkers	Pacientes con andadera	Pah-see-ehn- tehs kohn ahn-dah-deh-rah
Minerals	Minerals	Mee-neh-rah-lees			
Mirror	Espejo	Ehs-peh-hoh			
Miss	Señorita	Seh-nyoh-ree-tah	Patient(s)	Paciente(s)	Pah-see-ehn-the(s)
Mom	Mamá	Mah-mah	Pelvis	Pelvis	Pehl-bees
Monday	Lunes	Loo-nehs	People	Gente	Hehn-teh
Monitor	Monitor	Moh-nee-tohr	Permission	Permiso	Pehr-mee-soh
Mother	Madre	Mah-dreh	Person	Persona(s)	Pehr-soh-nah(s)
Mouth	Boca/oral	Boh-kah/oh-rahl	Personal	Personales	Pehr-soh-nah-lehs
Move!	¡Mueva!	Moo-eh-bah	Personality	Personalidad	Pehr-soh-nah-lee-dahd
Mr.	Señor	Seh-nyohr			
Mrs.	Señora	Seh-nyoh-rah	Phone	Teléfono	Teh-leh-foh-noh
Napkin	Servilleta	Sehr-bee-yeh-tah	Physician(f)	Médica-doctora	Meh-dee-kah/ dohk-toh-rah
Nasal	Nasal	Nah-sahl			
Nausea	Náusea	Nah-oo-seh-ah	Physician(m)	Médico/doctor	Meh-dee-koh/ dohk-tohr
Navel	Ombligo	Ohm-blee-goh			
Nervous	Nervioso	Nehr-bee-oh-soh	Physicians	Los medicos	Lohs meh-dee-kohs
Nightgown/ gown	Camisa de dormir/bata	Kah-mee-sah deh dohr-meer/bah-tah	Pillow	Almohada	Ahl-moh-ah-dah
			Pillowcase	Funda	Foon-dah
Nine	Nueve	Noo-eh-beh	Plate	Platón	Plah-tohn
Ninety	Noventa	Noh-behn-tah	Pneumonia	Pulmonía/ neumonía	Pool-moh-nee-ah/ neh-oo-moh-nee-ah
No salt	Sin sal	Seen sahl			

English	Spanish	Pronunciation
Polydipsa	Polidipsia	Poh-lee-deep-see-ah
Polyphagia	Polifagia	Poh-lee-fah-hee-ah
Polyuria	Poliuria	Poh-lee-oo-ree-ah
Postoperative	Postoperatorio	Pohst-oh-peh-rah-toh-ree-oh
Potential	Posibles	Poh-see-blehs
Practice	Práctica	Prahk-tee-kah
Precaution	Precaución	Preh-kah-oo-see-ohn
Pregnant	Embarazada	Ehm-bah-rah-sah-dah
Preoperative	Preoperatorio	Preh-oh-peh-rah-toh-ree-oh
Preparation	Preparación	Preh-pah-rah-see-ohn
Prepare (to)	Preparar	Preh-pah-rahr
Priest	Sacerdote	Sah-sehr-doh-the
Problem	Problema(s)	Proh-bleh-mah(s)
Procedure(s)	Procedimiento(s)	Proh-seh-dee-mee-ehn-toh(s)
Psoriasis	Soriasis	Soh-ree-ah-sees
Pubic	Púbico	Poo-bee-koh
Pulse	Pulso	Pool-soh
Pureed	Puré	Poo-reh
Purpose	Propósito	Proh-poh-see-toh
Question(s)	Pregunta(s)	Preh-goon-tah(s)
Razor/shave	Navaja/máquina de afeitar	Nah-bah-hah/mah-kee-nah deh ah-feh-ee-tahr
Reach	Alcanzar	Ahl-kahn-sahr
Reassurance	Asegurar	Ah-seh-goo-rahr
Recognize	Reconocer	Reh-koh-noh-sehr
Recommendations	Recomendaciones	Reh-koh-men-dah-see-ohn-es
Rectal	Rectal	Rehk-tahl
Rectum	El recto	Rehk-toh
Recuperating	Recuperando	Reh-koo-peh-rahn-doh
Regular	Regular	Reh-goo-lahr
Rehabilitation	Rehabilitación	Reh-ah-bee-lee-tah-see-ohn
Relation	Relación	Reh-lah-see-ohn
Relax	Descansa/relaja	Dehs-kahn-sah/reh-lah-hah
Remain	Quedese	Keh-deh-seh
Remember	Recordar/acordarse	Reh-kohr-dahr/ah-kohr-dahr-seh
Respiratory arrest	Paro respiratorio	Pah-roh rehs-pee-rah-toh-ree-oh
Response	Contestación	Kohn-tehs-tah-see-ohn
Responsibilities	Respon sabilidades	Rehs-pohn-sah-bee-lee-dah-dehs
Rest	Reposo	Reh-poh-soh
Restless	Inquieto	Een-kee-eh-toh

English	Spanish	Pronunciation
Restroom	Cuarto de baño	Koo-ahr-toh deh bah-nyoh
Rib(s)	Costilla(s)	Kohs-tee-yah(s)
Right	Derecha	Deh-reh-chah
Rigidity	Rigidez	Ree-hee-dehs
Room (operating)	Cuarto de cirugía quirófano	Koo-ahr-toh deh see-roo-hee-ah/kee-roh-fah-noh
Saliva	Saliva	Sah-lee-bah
Salt	Sal	Sahl
Sample	Muestra	Moo-ehs-trah
Saturday	Sábado	Sah-bah-doh
Scratch	Raspón	Rahs-pohn
Sebaceous	Sebásceo	She-bah-seh-oh
Semi-solid	Semisólido	Seh-mee-soh-lee-doh
Seven	Siete	See-eh-teh
Seventy	Setenta	Seh-tehn-tah
Sheets	Sábanas	Sah-bah-nahs
Shirt	Camisa	Kah-mee-sah
Shoes	Zapatos	Sah-pah-tohs
Shoulder	Hombro	Ohm-broh
Shower	Regadera/ducha	Reh-gah-deh-rah/doo-chah
Sign	Firme/letrero	Feer-meh/leh-treh-roh
Signs	Signos/señales	Seeg-nohs/seh-nyah-lehs
Similar	Similares	See-mee-lah-rhes
Sister	Hermana	Ehr-mah-nah
Sit!	¡Siéntese!	See-ehn-teh-seh
Six	Seis	Seh-ees
Sixty	Sesenta	Seh-sehn-tah
Skin	Piel	Pee-ehl
Skirt	Falda	Fahl-dah
Skull	El cráneo	???
Sleep	Sueño	Soo-eh-nyoh
Sneeze	Estornudo	Ehs-tohr-noo-doh
Soap	Jabón	Hah-bohn
Social	Social	Soh-see-ahl
Social worker	Trabajadora social	Trah-bah-hah-doh-rah soh-see ahl
Sociocultural	Sociocultural	Soh-see-oh-kool-too-rahl
Socks	Calcetines/calcetas	Kahl-seh-tee-nehs/kahl-seh-tahs
Soft	Suave	Soo-ah-beh
Son	Hijo	Ee-hoh
Speak	Hablar	Ah-blahr
Specimen	Muestra	Moo-ehs-trah
Sternum	Esternón	Ehs-tehr-nohn
Stethoscope	Estetoscopio	Ehs-teh-tohs-koh-pee-oh

English	Spanish	Pronunciation	English	Spanish	Pronunciation
Stockings	Medias	Meh-dee-ahs	To breathe	Respirar	Rehs pee-rahr
Subcutaneous	Subcutáneo	Soob-koo-tah-neh-oh	To change	Cambiar	Kahm-bee-ahr
Sugar	Azúcar	Ah-soo-kahr	To communicate	Comunicar	Koh-moo-nee-kahr
Sunday	Domingo	Doh-meen-goh			
Suppository	Supositorio	Soo-poh-see-toh-ree-oh	To complain	Quejar	Keh-hahr
			To cure	Curar	Koo-rahr
Surgeon	Cirujano	See-roo-hah-noh	To dress	Vestír	Behs-teer
Surgery	Cirugía	See-roo-hee-ah	To drink	Beber/tomar	Beh-behr/toh-mahr
Surgical	Quirúrgico	Kee-roor-hee-koh	To eat	Comer	Koh-mehr
		sahn-gee-neh-ah	To eat breakfast	Desayunar	Deh-sah-yoo-nahr
Sutures	Suturas/puntos	Soo-too-rahs/poon-tohs	To examine	Examinar	Ex-ah-mee-nahr
Sweater	Chamarra/suéter	Chah-mah-rah/soo-eh-tehr	To feel	Sentír	Sehn-teer
			To get better	Mejorar	Meh-hoh-rahr
Swelling	Hinchazón	Een-chah-sohn	To get up/raise	Levanter	Leh-bahn-tahr
Swollen	Hinchado	Een-chah-doh			
Symptoms	Síntomas	Seen-toh-mahs	To go out	Salir	Sah-leer
Systole	Sístole	Sees-toh-leh	To go to bed	Acostarse	Ah-kohs-tahr-she
Table (overnight)	Mesa de noche	Meh-sah deh noh-cheh	To hear me	Oirme	Oh-eer-meh
			To hear/listen	Escuchar/oír	Ehs-koo-chahr/oh-eer
Table(s)	Mesa(s)	Meh-sah(s)	To hurt	Doler	Doh-lehr
Tablespoon	Cuchara/cucharada	Koo-chah-rah/koo-chah-rah-dah	To lie down	Acostar/dormir	Ah-kohs-tahr/dorh-meer
Taste	Gusto	Goos-toh	To leave	Dejar	Deh-hahr
Tea	Té	Teh	To listen	Oir	Oh-eer
Teaspoon	Cucharita/cucharadita	Koo-chah-ree-tah/koo-chah-rah-dee-tah	To point	Señalar	She-nyah-lahr
			To raise	Levanter	Leh-bahn-tahr
Teeth	Dientes	Dee-ehn-tehs	To reach	Alcanzar	Ahl-kahn-sahr
Television	Televisor	The-leh-bee-sohr	To remember	Acordar/recordar	Ah-kohr-dahr/reh-kohr-dahr
Temperature	Temperatura	Tehm-peh-rah-too-rah			
Temporal	Temporal	Tehm-poh-rahl	To sit	Sentar	Sehn-tahr
Ten	Diez	Dee-ehs	To sleep	Dormir	Dohr-meer
Tense	Tenso	Tehn-soh	To speak	Hablar	Ah-blahr
Terminal	Terminal	Tehr-mee-nahl	To suffer	Sufrir	Soo-freer
Thank you	Gracias	Grah-see-ahs	To vomit	Vomitar	Boh-mee-tahr
The family	La familia	Lah fah-mee-lee-ah	To walk	Caminar	Kah-mee-nahr
Theories	Teorías	Teh-oh-ree-ahs	To wash	Lavar	Lah-bahr
Thermometer	Termómetro	Tehr-muh-meh-troh	Toes	dedos	Deh-dos
Thirty	Treinta	Treh-een-tah	Toilet	Excusado/inodoro	Ex-koo-sah-doh/ee-noh-doh-roh
Three	Tres	Trehs			
Thrombus	Coágulo	Koh-ah-goo-loh	Toothache	Dolor de muelas	Doh-lor deh moo-eh-lahs
Thursday	Jueves	Hoo-eh-behs			
Tissue (muscle)	Tejido	The-hee-doh	Toothbrush	Cepillo de dientes	Seh-pee-yoh deh dee-ehn-tehs
Tissues	Tisues	Tee-sooh(ehs)	Toothpaste	Pasta de dientes	Pahs-tah deh dee-ehn-tehs
Tisue damage	Daño del tejido	Dah-nyoh dehl teh-hee-doh			
			Topical	Topical/tópico	Toh-pee-kahl/toh-pee-koh
To bathe	Bañar	Bah-nyahr			
To become ill	Enfermar	Ehn-fehr-mahr	Towel	Toalla	Too-ah-yah
To bleed	Sangrar	Sahn-grahr	Traumatic	Traumático	Trah-oo-mah-tee-koh
To break	Romper	Rohm-pehr	Treatment	Tratamiento	Trah-tah-mee-ehn-toh

English	Spanish	Pronunciation
Trust	Confianza	Kohn-fee-ahn-sah
Tuesday	Martes	Mahr-tehs
Tumor	Tumor	Too-mohr
Turn!	¡Voltée!	Bohl-the-eh
Twenty	Viente	Beh-een-teh
Two	Dos	Dohs
Ulcer(s)	Úlcera(s)	Ool-seh-rah(s)
Ultrasound	Ultrasonido	Ool-trah-soh-nee-doh
Underwear	Ropa interior	Roh-pah een-teh-ree-ohr
Universal	Universal	Oo-nee-behr-sahl
Urinal	Pato	Pah-toh
Urine	Orina	Oh-ree-nah
Use	Usar	Oo-sahr
Uterus	Útero	Oo-the-roh
Vaginal	Vaginal	Bah-hee-nahl
Vein	Vena	Beh-nah
Vitamins	Vitaminas	Bee-tah-mee-nahs
Vomit	Vómito	Boh-mee-toh
Vomiting	Vomitando	Boh-mee-tahn-doh
Waist	La cintura	???
Warning	Advertencia	Ahd-behr-tehn-see-ah
Wednesday	Miércoles	Mee-ehr-koh-lehs
Wife	Esposa	Ehs-poh-sah
Worker	Trabajador	Trah-bah-hah-dohr
Wound	Herida	Eh-ree-dah
Wrist	Muñeca	Moo-nveh-kah
X-rays	Rayos-x	Rah-yohs eh-kiss
Young	Jovenes	Hoh-beh-nehs

Useful Spanish Phrases

English	Spanish	Pronunciation
A bowel movement.	Hacer del baño.	Ah-sehr dehl ban-nyoh
A glass of juice?	Un vaso de jugo?	Oon bah-soh deh hoo-goh
A heart.	Un corazón.	Oon koh-rah-sohn
About your baby.	En cuanto a su bebé.	Ehn koo-ahn-toh ah soo beh-beh
Activities are part of the plan while you are here.	Las actividades son parte del plan de su tratamiento minetras esté aquí.	Lahs ahk-tee-bee-dah-dehs sohn pahr-teh dehl plahn deh soo trah-tah-mee-ehn-toh mee-ehn-trahs ehs-teh ah-kee
After meals.	Después de las comidas.	Dehs-poo-ehs deh lahs koh-mee-dahs
Any questions?	¿Alguna pregunta?	Ahl-goo-nah preh-goon-tah
Are you allergic to anything?	¿Es alérgico a alguna cosa?	Ehs ah-lehr-hee-koh ah ahl-goo-nah koh-sah
Are you allergic to foods?	¿Es alérgico a comidas?	Ehs ah-lehr-hee-koh ah koh-mee-dahs
Are you cold?	¿Tiene frío?	Tee-eh-neh free-oh
Are you comfortable?	¿Está cómoda?	Ehs-tah koh-moh-dah
Are you constipated?	¿Está estreñido?	Ehs-tah ehs-treh-nyee-doh
Are you diabetic?	¿Es diabética?	Ehs dee-ah-beh-tee-kah
Are you dizzy?	¿Tiene mareos?	Tee-eh-neh mah-reh-ohs
Are you employed?	¿Trabaja usted?	Trah-bah-hah oos-tehd

English	Spanish	Pronunciation	English	Spanish	Pronunciation
Are you having problems breathing?	¿Tiene problemas al respirar?	Tee-eh-neh proh-bleh-mahs ahl rehs-pee-rahr	Bend your knee!	¡Doble su rodilla!	Doh-bleh soo roh-dee-yah
Are you hot?	¿Tiene calor?	Tee-eh-neh kah-lohr	Bend your shoulder.	Dobla tu hombro.	Doh-bleh too ohm-broh
Are you hungry?	¿Tiene hambre?	Tee-eh-neh ahm-breh	Bend your toes.	Dobla tus dedos.	Doh-blah toos deh-dohs
Are you hurting?	¿Tiene dolor?	Tee-eh-neh doh-lohr	Breast-feed or give a bottle every 3 hours.	Déle pecho o biberón cada tres horas.	Deh-leh peh-choh oh bee-beh-rohn kah-dah trehs oh-ras
Are you nauseated?	¿Tiene náuseas?	Tee-eh-neh nah-oo-seh-ahs	Breast-feeding?	¿Tomando pecho?	Toh-mahn-doh peh-choh
Are you okay?	¿Está bien/Se siente bien?	Ehs-tah bee-ehn/seh see-ehn-the bee-ehn	Breathe deeply; let it out slowly.	Respira hondo; déjalo ir despacio.	Rehs-pee-rah oon-doh; deh-hah-loh eer dehs-pah-see-oh
Are you sleepy?	¿Tiene sueño?	Tee-eh-neh soo-eh-nyoh	Breathe deeply!	¡Respire hondo/profundo!	Rehs-pee-reh ohn-doh/ proh-foon-doh
Are you thirsty?	¿Tiene sed?	Tee-eh-neh sehd	Breathe in.	Respire.	Rehs-pee-reh
At bedtime.	Al acostarse/hora de dormir.	Ahl ah-kohs-tahr-seh/oh-rah deh dohr-meer	Breathe out.	Saque el aire.	Sah-keh ehl ah-ee-reh
At eleven thirty.	A las once y media.	Ah lahs ohn-seh ee meh-dee-ah	Brush your teeth!	¡Cepíllese los dientes!	Seh-pee-yeh-seh lohs dee-ehn-tehs
At five PM.	A las cinco de la tarde.	Ah lahs seen-koh deh lah tahr-deh	Call if you need help.	Llame sí necesita ayuda.	Yah-meh see neh-seh-see-tah ah-yoo-dah
At what time do you get up?	¿A qué hora se levanta?	Ah keh oh-rah seh leh-bahn-tah	Can you breathe?	¿Puede respirar?	Poo-eh-deh rehs-pee-rahr
At what time do you go to bed?	¿A qué hora se acuesta?	Ah keh oh-rah seh ah-koo-ehs-tah	Can you feed yourself?	¿Puede alimentarse?	Poo-eh-deh ah-lee-mehn-tahr-seh
Before/after meals.	Antes/después de las comidas.	Ahn-tehs/ dehs-poo-ehs deh lahs koh-mee-dahs	Can you get out of bed?	¿Puede salir de la cama?	Poo-eh-deh sah-leer deh lah kah-mah
Bend the elbow.	Doble el codo.	Doh-bleh-ehl koh-doh	Can you hear me?	¿Puede oírme?	Poo-eh-deh oh-eer-meh
Bend the wrist.	Dobla la muñeca.	Doh-blah lah moo-nyeh-kah	Can you move in bed?	¿Puede moverse en la cama?	Poo-eh-deh moh-behr-seh ehn lah kah-mah
Bend your hip.	Dobla su cadera.	Doh-bleh soo kah-deh-rah			

English	Spanish	Pronunciation	English	Spanish	Pronunciation
Can you sit up?	¿Puede sentarse?	Poo-eh-deh sehn-tahr-seh	Do not smoke in the room when the oxygen is being used.	No fume en el cuarto donde se usa el oxígeno.	Noh foo-meh ehn ehl koo-ahr-toh dohn-deh seh oo-sah ehl ohx-ee-heh-noh
Can you talk?	¿Puede hablar?	Poo-eh-deh ah-blahr			
Change into this gown.	Póngase esta bata.	Pohn-gah-seh ehs-tah bah-tah	Do you dribble?	¿Se orina sin sentir?	Seh oh-ree-nah seen sehn-teer
Chest pain?	¿Dolor en el pecho?	Doh-lohr ehn ehl peh-choh	Do you feel all right?	¿Se siente bien?	She see-ehn-the bee-ehn
Close your mouth.	Cierre la boca.	See-eh-reh lah boh-kah	Do you feel dizzy?	¿Se siente mareado?	Seh see-ehn-teh mah-reh-ah-doh
Cough deeply.	Tosa más fuerte.	Toh-sah mahs foo-her-teh			
Cough!	¡Tosa!	Toh-sah	Do you feel nauseated?	¿Siente náuseas?	See-ehn-teh nah-oo-seh-ahs
Daily.	Diariamente./ Una por día./Cada día.	Dee-ah-ree-ah-mehn-teh/Oo-nah pohr dee-ah/Kah-dah dee-ah	Do you feel weak?	¿Se siente débil?	Seh see-ehn-teh deh-beel
			Do you have a pacemaker?	¿Tiene marcapasos?	Tee-eh-neh mahr-kah-pah-sohs
Did you bring a hearing aid?	¿Trajo un aparato para oír?	Trah-hoh oon ah-pah-rah-toh pah-rah oh-eer	Do you have allergies?	¿Tiene alergias?	Tee-eh-neh ah-lehr-ghee-ahs
Did you bring an artificial eye?	¿Trajo un ojo artificial?	Trah-hoh oon oh-hoh ahr-tee-fee-see-ahl	Do you have any questions?	¿Tiene preguntas?	Tee-eh-neh preh-goon-tahs
Did you bring dentures?	¿Trajo una dentadura postiza?	Trah-hoh oon-ah dehn-tah-doo-rah pohs-tee-sah	Do you have any symptoms: nausea, dizziness, other unusual feelings?	¿Tiene algún síntoma como: náuseas, vértigo, otra sensación rara?	Tee-eh-neh ahl-goon seen-toh-mah koh-moh nah-oo-seh-ahs, behr-tee-goh, oh-trah sehn-sah-see-ohn rah-rah
Did you bring glasses?	¿Trajo anteojos/ lentes?	Trah-hoh ahn-the-oh-hohs/ lehn-tehs			
Did you faint?	¿Se desmayó?	Seh dehs-mah-yoh			
Did you have a bowel movement?	¿Hizo del baño/ caca/evac-uró?	Ee-soh dehl bah-nyoh/ kah-kah/eh-bah-koo-oh	Do you have chest pain?	¿Tiene dolor en el pecho?	Tee-eh-neh doh-lohr ehn ehl peh-choh
Did you see blood in the urine?	¿Vio sangre en la orina?	Bee-oh sahn-greh ehn lah oh-ree-nah	Do you have diarrhea?	¿Tiene diarrea?	Tee-eh-neh dee-ah-reh-ah
Difficulty in swallow-ing . . .	Dificultad al tragar . . .	Dee-fee-kool-tahd ahl trah-gahr	Do you have hesitancy (when urinating)?	¿Se corta el chorro de la orina?	She kohr-tah ehl choh-roh deh lah oh-ree-nah

English	Spanish	Pronunciation	English	Spanish	Pronunciation
Do you have problems with starting to urinate?	¿Tiene dificultad para empezar a orinar?	Tee-eh-neh dee-fee-kool-tahd pah-rah ehm-peh-sahr ah oh-ree-nahr	Do you want the toast with butter?	¿Quiere el pan tostado con mantequilla?	Kee-eh-reh ehl pahn tohs-tah-doh kohn mahn-teh-kee-yah
Do you have problems with your teeth?	¿Tiene(s) problemas con los dientes?	Tee-eh-neh(s) proh-bleh-mahs kohn lohs dee-ehn-tehs	Do you want water?	¿Quiére agua?	Kee-eh-reh ah-goo-ah
Do you have questions?	¿Tiene dudas?	Tee-eh-neh doo-dahs	Do you want: A glass of water?	¿Quiere: Un vaso de agua?	Kee-eh-reh: Oon bah-soh deh ah-goo-ah
Do you have respiratory problems?	¿Tiene problemas respiratorios?	Tee-eh-neh proh-bleh-mahs rhes-pee-rah-toh-ree-ohs	Do you want: Something to eat?	¿Quiere: Algo de comer?	Kee-eh-reh: Ahl-goh deh koh-mehr
			Do you wear glasses?	¿Usas anteojos/ lentes?	Oo-sahs ahn-teh-oh-hohs/lehn-tehs
Do you know the day of the week?	¿Sabe el día de la semana?	Sah-beh ehl dee-ah deh lah seh-mah-nah	Do you wish to have a bowel movement?	¿Quiere evacuar/ hacer del baño?	Kee-eh-reh eh-bah-koo-ahr/ah-sehr dehl bah-nyoh
Do you know the day?	¿Qué día es hoy?	Keh dee-ah ehs oh-ee	Do you wish to pass urine?	¿Quiére orinar?	Kee-eh-reh oh-ree-nahr
Do you know where you are?	¿Sabe dónde está?	Sah-beh dohn-deh ehs-tah	Do you wish/want something to eat?	¿Quiére algo de comer?	Kee-eh-reh ahl-goh deh koh-mehr
Do you need help?	¿Necesita ayuda?	Neh-she-see-tah ah-yoo-dah			
Do you need more pillows?	¿Necesita más almohadas?	Neh-seh-see-tah mahs ahl-moh-ah-dahs	Do you wish/want to drink?	¿Quiére tomar/ beber?	Kee-eh-reh toh-mahr/ beh-behr
Do you speak English?	¿Habla ingles/Habla usted ingles?	Ah-blah een-glehs/Ah-blah oos-tehd een-glehs	Does the pain move from one place to another?	¿El dolor se mueve de un lugar a otro?	Ehl doh-lohr seh moo-eh-beh deh oon loo-gahr ah oh-troh
Do you take a special diet?	¿Toma dieta especial?	Toh-mah dee-eh-tah ehs-peh-see-ahl	Don't walk barefoot.	No camine descalzo.	Noh kah-mee-neh dehs-kahl-soh
Do you understand?	¿Entiende?	Ehn-tee-ehn-deh	Don't worry!	¡No se preocupe!	Noh seh preh-oh-koo-peh
Do you use sugar in the coffee?	¿Usa azúcar en el café?	Oo-sah ah-soo-kahr ehn ehl kah-feh	Drink.	Beba./Tome.	Beh-bah/ Toh-meh
Do you want the bedpan?	¿Usa azúcar en el café?	Kee-eh-reh ehl pah-toh/ehl bah-seen	Eat!	¡Coma!	Koh-mah
			Eight o'clock.	Las ocho.	Lahs oh-choh
			Eight o'clock (mil).	Las viente horas.	Lahs beh-een-teh oh-rahs
			Eleven o'clock.	Las once.	Lahs ohn-seh

English	Spanish	Pronunciation
Eleven o'clock (mil).	Las veintitrés horas.	Lahs beh-een-tee-trehs oh-rahs
Every time you go to the bathroom to void, you must place the urine in the container.	Cada vez que vaya al baño a orinar, debe poner la orina en el recipiente.	Kah-dah behs keh bah-yah ahl bah-nyoh ah oh-ree-nahr, deh-beh poh-nehr lah oh-ree-nah ehn ehl reh-see-pee-ehn-the
Excuse me!	¡Perdón/Excús eme/Con permiso!	Pehr-dohn/ Ehx-koo-seh-meh/Kohn pher mee-soh
Extend your arm.	Extiende tu brazo.	Ehx-tee-ehn-deh too brah-soh
Extend your leg and foot.	Extiende tu pierna y pie.	Ehx-tee-ehn-deh too pee-her-nah ee pee-eh
Extend your wrist.	Extiende tu muñeca.	Ehx-tee-ehn-deh too moo-nyeh-kah
First, I want to brush your teeth.	Primero, quiero limpiarle los dientes.	Pree-meh-roh kee-eh-roh leem-pee-ahr-leh lohs dee-ehn-tehs
Five o'clock.	Las cinco	Lahs seen-koh
Five o'clock (mil).	Las diecisiete horas	Lahs dee-ehs-ee-see-eh-teh oh-rahs
Four o'clock.	Las cuatro	Lahs koo-ah-troh
Four o'clock (mil).	Las dieciséis horas	Lahs dee-ehs-ee-seh-ees oh-rahs

English	Spanish	Pronunciation
Good afternoon!	¡Buenas tardes!	Boo-eh-nahs tahr-dehs
Good morning!	¡Buenos días!	Boo-eh-nohs dee-ahs
Has the pain gotten worse or gotten better?	¿Se ha puesto el dolor peor o mejor?	Seh ah poo-ehs-toh ehl doh-lohr peh-ohr oh meh-hohr
Have you been a patient before?	¿Ha sido paciente antes?	Ah see-doh pah-see-ehn-the ahn-tehs
Have you eaten?	¿Ha comido?	Ah koh-mee-doh
Hello. I need to take your temperature and blood pressure.	Hola. Necesito tomarle la temperatura y la presión de la sangre.	Oh-lah. Neh-seh-see-toh toh-mahr-leh lah tehm-peh-rah-too-rah ee lah preh-see-ohn deh lah sahn-greh
Here is the bell.	Aquí está la campana.	Ah-kee ehs-tah lah kahm-pah-nah
How are you today?	¿Como está hoy?	Koh-moh ehs-tah oh-ee
How often do you feed the baby?	¿Qué tan a menudo alimenta al bebé?	Keh tahn ah meh-noo-doh ah-lee-mehn-tah ahl beh-beh
How often do you urinate?	¿Cuántas veces orina?	Koo-ahn-tahs beh-sehs oh-ree-nah
How old are you?	¿Cuántos años tiene?	Koo-ahn-tohs ah-nyohs tee-eh-neh
How severe is the pain?	¿Qué tan severo es el dolor?	Keh tahn seh-beh-roh ehs ehl doh-lohr
I also need a urine sample.	También necesito una muestra de orina.	Tahm-bee-ehn neh-seh-see-toh oo-nah moo-ehs-trah deh oh-ree-nah

English	Spanish	Pronunciation	English	Spanish	Pronunciation
I am going to check the oxygen tank.	Voy a checar el tanque de oxígeno.	Boh-ee ah cheh-kahr ehl tahn-keh deh ohx-ee-heh-noh	I am here to help you with exercises.	Estoy aquí para ayudarlo con ejercicios.	Ehs-toh-ee ah-kee pah-rah ah-yoo-dahr-loh kohn eh-hehr-see-see-ohs
I am going to collect a stool sample.	Voy a recoger una muestra de excre-mento.	Boh-ee ah reh-koh-hehr oo-nah moo-ehs-trah deh ehx-kreh-mehn-toh	I am the nurse (female).	Yo soy la enfermera.	Yoh soh-ee lah ehn-fehr-meh-rah
			I am the nurse (male).	Yo soy el enfermero.	Yoh soh-ee ehl ehn-fehr-meh-roh
I am going to cover you with a sheet.	Voy a cubrirlo con una sábana.	Boh-ee ah koo-breer-loh kohn oo-nah sah-bah-nah	I have the bedpan.	Tengo el bacín/ pato.	Tehn-goh ehl bah-seen/ pah-toh
I am going to cover you.	Lo voy a cubrir.	Loh boh-ee ah koo-breer	I need to take your temper-ature and blood pressure.	Necesito tomarle la temperatura y la presión de la sangre.	Neh-seh-see-toh toh-mahr-leh lah tehm-peh-rah-too-rah ee lah preh-see-ohn deh lah sahn-greh
I am going to explain the collection of urine.	Le voy a ex-plicar la colección de orina.	Leh boh-ee ah ehx-plee-kahr lah koh-lehk-see-ohn deh oh-ree-nah			
			I want to help you stand up.	Quiero ayu-darlo a s entarse.	Kee-eh-roh ah-yoo-dahr-loh ah sehn-tahr-seh
I am going to get a wheel-chair.	Voy a traer una silla de ruedas.	Boh-ee ah trah-her oo-nah see-yah deh roo-eh-dahs	I want you to use a cane.	Quiero que use un bastón.	Kee-eh-roh keh oo-seh oon bahs-tohn
I am going to help you lie on the stretcher.	Voy a ayudarlo a acostarse en la camilla.	Boh-ee ah ah-yoo-dahr-loh ah ah-kohs-tahr-seh ehn lah kah-mee-yah	I will give you a bath.	Voy a bañarlo.	Boh-ee ah bah-nyahr-loh
			I will help you sit.	Le ayudaré a sentarse.	Leh ah-yoo-dah-reh ah sehn-tahr-seh
I am going to help you.	Voy a ayu-darlo.	Boh-ee ah ah-yoo-dahr-loh	I will show you your room.	Le mostraré su cuarto.	Leh mohs-trah-reh soo koo-ahr-toh
I am going to insert your dentures.	Voy a ponerle la den-tadura.	Boh-ee ah poh-nehr-leh lah dehn-tah-doo-rah	I will start by taking vital signs.	Voy a empezar por tomar los signos vitals.	Boh-ee ah ehm-peh-sahr pohr toh-mahr lohs seeg-nohs bee-tah-lehs
I am going to take the ra-dial pulse.	Voy a tomar tu pulso radial.	Boh-ee ah toh-mahr too pool-soh rah-dee-ahl			
I am going to take your blood pres-sure and pulse.	Voy a tomar la presión y el pulso.	Boh-ee ah toh-mahr lah preh-see-ohn ee ehl pool-soh	I will start by taking vital signs.	Empezaré por tomar los signos vitales.	Ehm-peh-sah-reh pohr toh-mahr lohs seeg-nohs bee-tah-lehs

English	Spanish	Pronunciation	English	Spanish	Pronunciation
I will take your blood pressure.	Tomaré tu presión de sangre.	Toh-mah-reh too preh-see-ohn deh sahn-greh	Keep the side rails up at night.	Mantenga los barandales levantados durante la noche.	Mahn-tehn-gah lohs bah-rahn-dah-lehs leh-bahn-tah-dohs doo-rahn-the lah noh-cheh
If it hurts, tell me.	Si duele, avísame.	See doo-eh-leh, ah-bee-sah-meh			
If you have questions, please let me know.	Si tiene preguntas, por favor avíseme.	See tee-eh-neh preh-goon-tahs, pohr fah-bohr ah-bee-seh-meh	Keep your feet together.	Mantenga los pies juntos.	Mahn-tehn-gah lah pee-ehr-nah eh-leh-bah-dah
If you need more sheets, call the assistant.	Si necesita más sábanas, llame a la/al asistente.	See neh-seh-see-tah mahs sah-bah-nahs, yah-meh ah lah/ahl ah-sees-tehn-teh	Keep your leg elevated.	Mantenga la pierna elevada.	Mahn-tehn-gah lah pee-ehr-nah eh-leh-bah-dah
			Left . . .	Izquierdo . . .	Ees-kee-ehr-doh
Is that enough?	¿Es suficiente?	Ehs soo-fee-see-ehn-teh	Let me know how you feel.	Dígame cómo se siente.	Dee-gah-meh koh-moh seh see-ehn-teh
Is that too much?	¿Es mucho?	Ehs moo-choh	Let's walk.	Vamos a caminar.	Bah-mohs ah kah-mee-nahr
Is the pain there all the time, or does it come and go?	¿Está el dolor allí todo el tiempo, o va y viene?	Ehs-tah ehl doh-lohr ah-yee toh-doh ehl tee-ehm-poh, oh bah ee bee-ehn-eh?	Lie down (please)!	¡Acuéstese (por favor)!	Ah-koo-ehs-teh-seh (pohr fah-bohr)
			Lift the foot.	Levante el pie.	Leh-bahn-teh ehl pee-eh
Is there any pain?	¿Tiene algún dolor?	Tee-eh-neh ahl-goon doh-lohr	Lift your arm(s).	Levanta tu/los brazo(s).	Leh bahn-tah too/ lohs brah-soh(s)
Is there anything else bothering you?	¿Hay otra cosa que le moleste?	Ah-ee oh-trah koh-sah keh leh moh-lehs-teh	Lift your hand.	Levanta tu mano.	Leh bahn-tah too mah-noh
Is your appetite bad?	¿Tiene mal apetito?	Tee-eh-neh mahl ah-peh-tee-toh	Lift your head.	Levanta la cabeza.	Leh bahn-tah lah kah-beh-sah
Keep moving.	Siga moviéndose.	See-gah moh-bee-ehn-doh-seh	Lift your leg.	Levanta la pierna.	Leh bahn-tah lah pee-her-nah
Keep the leg straight.	Antenga la pierna derecha.	Mahn-tehn-gah lah pee-her-nah deh-reh-chah	Lift your right arm.	Levente el brazo derecho.	Leh-bahn-teh ehl brah-soh deh-reh-choh
			Lift your right foot.	Levante el pie derecho.	Leh-bahn-teh ehl pee-eh deh-reh-choh

English	Spanish	Pronunciation	English	Spanish	Pronunciation
Look straight ahead.	Mira hacia adelante.	Mee-rah ah-see-ah ah-deh-lahn-teh	Open your mouth.	Abra la boca.	Ah-brah lah boh-kah
Lower the foot.	Baja el pie.	Bah-hah ehl pee-eh	Open your mouth, please.	Abra la boca, por favor.	Ah-brah lah boh-kah, pohr fah-bohr
Lower your head.	Baja la cabeza.	Bah-hah lah kah-beh-sah	Place the urine in the brown plastic bottle.	Ponga la orina en la botella de plástico café.	Pohn-gah lah oh-ree-nah ehn lah boh-teh-yah deh plahs-tee-koh kah-feh
Lower your legs.	Baje las piernas.	Bah-heh lahs pee-ehr-nahs			
Make a fist!	¡Cierre la mano/Haga un puñto!	See-eh-reh lah mah-noh/ Ah-gah oon poo-nyoh	Please, swallow.	Traga, por favor.	Trah-gah pohr fah-bohr
May I help you?	¿Puedo ayu-darlo?	¿Poo-eh-doh ah-yoo-dahr-loh?	Pull the cord in the bathroom.	Jale el cordón en el baño.	Hah-leh ehl kohr-dohn ehn ehl bah-nyoh
Move it side to side.	Muévela de lado a lando.	Moo-eh-beh-lah deh lah-doh ah lah-doh	Put the spoon in your mouth.	Ponga la cuchara en la boca.	Pohn-gah lah koo-chah-rah ehn lah boh-kah
Nine o'clock.	Las nueve.	Lahs noo-eh-beh	Rest.	Descanse.	Des-kahn-seh
Nine o'clock (mil).	Las veintiuna horas.	Lahs beh-een-tee-oo-nah oh-rahs	Seven o'clock.	Las siete.	Lahs see-eh-teh
Noon/midnight.	Las doce.	Lahs doh-seh	Seven o'clock (mil)	Las diecinueve horas.	Lahs dee-ehs-ee-noo-eh-beh oh-rahs
Noon/midnight (mil).	Las cero horas.	Lahs seh-roh oh-rahs	Sit down, please.	Siéntese, por favor.	See-ehn-teh-seh pohr fah-bohr
Now, stand up and walk.	Ahora, levántese y camine.	Ah-oh-rah, leh-bahn-teh-seh ee kah-mee-neh	Sit in the chair.	Siéntese en la silla.	See-ehn-teh-seh ehn lah see-yah
Nursing care of the patient.	Cuidados del paciente.	Koo-ee-dah-dohs dehl pah-see-ehn-teh	Six o'clock.	Las seis	Lahs seh-ees
			Six o'clock (mil).	Las dieciocho horas	Lahs dee-ehs-ee-oh-choh oh-rahs
On a scale from 1 (insignificant) to 10 (unbearable):	En una escala del uno (insignificante) al diez (intolerable):	Ehn oo-nah ehs-kah-lah dehl oo-noh (een-seeg-nee-fee-kahn-the) ahl dee-ehs (een-toh-leh-rah-bleh)	Something to drink?	Algo de tomar/ beber?	Ahl-goh deh toh-mahr/ beh-behr
			Stay sitting.	Quédese sentado.	Keh-deh-seh sehn-tah-doh
			Taking formula?	¿Tomando fórmula?	Toh-mahn-doh fohr-moo-lah
One o'clock.	La una	Lah oo-nah	Ten o'clock.	Las diez.	Lahs dee-ehs
One o'clock (mil).	Las trece horas	Lahs treh-seh oh-rahs	Ten o'clock (mil).	Las veintidós horas.	Lahs beh-een-tee-dohs oh-rahs
			Thank you!	¡Gracias!	Grah-see-ahs

English	Spanish	Pronunciation	English	Spanish	Pronunciation
The bell will sound.	La campana sonará.	Lah kahm-pah-nah soh-nah-rah	Tomorrow you are going to have your surgery.	Mañana le van a hacer la cirugía.	Mah-nyah-nah leh bahn ah ah-sehr lah see-roo-hee-ah
The bladder.	La vejiga.	Lah beh-hee-gah			
The doctor.	El doctor.	Ehl dohk-tohr	Try to calm down.	Trate de cal-marse.	Trah-teh deh kahl-mahr-seh
The hospital.	El hospital.	Ehl ohs-pee-tahl			
The meals are served at 7 AM.	Los alimentos se sirven a las siete de la mañana.	Lohs ah-lee-mehn-tohs seh seer-behn ah lahs see-eh-teh deh lah mah-nyah-nah	Twice a day.	Dos veces al día.	Dohs beh-sehs ahl dee-ah
			Two o' clock.	Las dos.	Lahs dohs
			Two o' clock (mil).	Las catorce horas.	Lahs kah-tohr-seh oh-rahs
The nurse.	El/la enfer-mero(a).	Ehl/lah ehn-fehr-meh-roh[ah]	Void a little, then put urine in this cup.	Orine un poco, luego ponga la orina en esta taza.	Oh-ree-neh oon poh-koh, loo-eh-goh pohn-gah lah oh-ree-nah ehn ehs-tah tah-sah
The salt and pepper are in these packets.	La sal y la pimienta es-tán en estos paquetes.	Lah sahl ee lah pee-mee-ehn-tah ehs-tahn ehn ehs-tohs pah-keh-tehs			
			Wait!	¡Espere!	Ehs-peh-reh
			Wash your face!	¡Lávese la cara!	Lah-beh-seh lah kah-rah
The water is in the glass/ pitcher.	El agua está en el vaso/la jarra.	Ehl ah-goo-ah ehs-tah ehn ehl bah-soh/ lah-hah-rah	Watch his navel.	Vigile su ombligo.	Bee-hee-leh soo ohm-blee-goh
The water is warm. Can you feel?	El agua está tibia. ¿Puede sentir?	Ehl ah-goo-ah ehs-tah tee-bee-ah. Poo-eh-deh sehn-teer	What can I help you with?	¿En que puedo ayu-darlo?	Ehn keh poo-eh-doh ah-yoo-dahr-loh
			What caused the pain?	¿Qué causó el dolor?	Keh kah-oo-soh ehl doh-lohr
There is an emergency light.	Hay una luz para emer-gencias.	Ah-ee oo-nah loos pah-rah eh-mehr-hehn-see-ahs	What did you eat?	¿Qué comió?	Keh koh-mee-oh
			What do you do?	¿Qué hace usted?	Keh ah-seh oos-tehd
			What foods do you dislike?	¿Qué alimen-tos le dis-gustan?	Keh ah-lee-mehn-tohs leh dees-goos-tahn
This is the call bell/buzzer.	Esta es la campana/el timbre.	Ehs-tah ehs lah kahm-pah-nah/ehl teem-breh	What foods do you like?	¿Qué alimen-tos le gustan?	Keh ah-lee-mehn-tohs leh goos-tahn
Three o'clock.	Las tres	Lahs trehs			
Three o'clock (mil).	Las quince horas	Lahs keen-seh oh-rahs			
Three times a day.	Tres veces al día.	Trehs beh-sehs ahl dee-ah	What formula does he take?	¿Qué fórmula toma?	Keh fohr-moo-lah toh-mah

English	Spanish	Pronunciation	English	Spanish	Pronunciation
What is the color of the urine?	¿Cuál era el color de la orina?	Koo-ahl eh-rah ehl koh-lohr deh lah oh-ree-nah	You can drink water.	Puede tomar agua.	Poo-eh-deh toh-mahr ah-goo-ah
What is the pain like?	¿Qué tipo de dolor tiene?	Keh tee-poh deh doh-lohr tee-eh-neh	You can smoke on the patio.	Puede fumar en el patio.	Poo-eh-deh foo-mahr ehn ehl pah-tee-oh
What is this?	¿Qué es esto?	Keh ehs ehs-toh	You cannot smoke here.	No puede fumar aquí.	Noh poo-eh-deh foo-mahr ah-kee
What is wrong?	¿Qué pasa?	Keh pah-sah	You have false teeth.	Tiene dentaduras postizas.	Tee-eh-neh dehn-tah-doo-rahs pohs-tee-sahs
What is your name?	¿Cómo se llama?	Koh-moh seh yah-mah			
What makes the pain better?	¿Qué hace mejorar el dolor?	Keh ah-seh meh-hoh-rahr ehl d oh-lohr	You need to be admitted.	Necesita internarse al hospital.	Neh-seh-see-tah een-tehr-nahr-she ahl ohs-pee-tahl
When was the last time you used the toilet?	¿Cuándo fue la última vez que hizo del baño/ que obró?	Koo-ahn-doh foo-eh lah ool-tee-mah behs keh ee-soh dehl bah-nyoh/ keh oh-broh	You need to drink water.	Necesita tomar agua.	Neh-seh-see-tah toh-mahr ah-goo-ah
			You will be all right!	¡Va a estar bien!	Bah ah ehs-tahr bee-ehn
Where do you work?	¿Dónde trabaja?	Dohn-deh trah-bah-hah	Your appetite is good?	¿Tiene buen apetito?	Tee-eh-neh boo-ehn ah-peh-tee-toh
Where does it hurt?	¿Dónde le duele?	Don-deh leh doo-eh-leh			
You ate well.	Comió bien.	Koh-mee-oh bee-ehn	Your clothes go in the closet.	Su ropa va en el closet/ ropero.	Soo roh-pah bah ehn ehl kloh-seht/ roh-peh-roh
You can also ask for snacks.	También puede pedir aperitivos.	Tahm-bee-ehn poo-eh-deh peh-deer ah-peh-ree-tee-bohs			

Translations taken from Joyce EV, Villanueva ME: *Say it in Spanish: a guide for health care professionals,* ed 2, Philadelphia, 2000, WB Saunders.

GLOSSARY

Abrasion. A rubbing on the surface of the skin. Chapter 23

Abuse. Hurting a person physically, emotionally, or financially. Chapter 2

Active listening. A way of communicating with another person that shows you are interested in the conversation. Chapter 3

Activity therapist. Plans and directs social and recreational activities. Usually works in long-term care settings. Chapter 1

Acute. Short-term or sudden. Chapters 8, 29

Acute care. Care provided during a short-term illness or injury. Chapter 1

Adipose tissue. Fat tissue. Chapter 7

Admission. The official entry of a person into a health care facility. Chapter 22

Advance directives. Information regarding patients' wishes about medical care when they are no longer able to give that information. Chapter 31

Alzheimer's disease (AD). A disease of the brain cells that control memory, thinking, judgment, language, behavior, and personality. It is the most common form of dementia. Chapter 30

AMA (against medical advice) discharge. When the patient leaves the facility without the doctor's permission or against medical advice. Chapter 22

Ambulation. Walking. Chapter 12

Anal. Pertaining to the opening at the end of the anal canal, the end portion of the large intestine. Chapter 24

Anesthesiologist. A doctor who specializes in providing medications (anesthesia) during surgery. Chapter 28

Anti-embolism stockings. Elastic stockings worn to prevent the formation of blood clots (embolism). Chapter 28

Apnea. Not breathing. Chapter 31

Arterial. Related to the arteries, the blood vessels that carry blood away from the heart. Chapter 23

Arthritis. Inflammation of the joints. Chapter 12

Ascites. A buildup of fluid in the abdomen. Chapter 8

Aspiration. Taking in, such as aspirating fluids into the lungs. Chapter 19

Assessment. Getting information about the patient's condition. Chapter 22

Atrophy. Decrease in muscle size. Chapter 12

Aural temperature. Temperature taken in the ear, same as tympanic membrane temperature. Chapter 13

Axilla/axillary temperature. Temperature taken under the arm or in the armpit. Chapter 13

Bacteria. Very small living things, some of which cause illness or disease; germs. Chapters 8, 9

Bedpan. A container made of metal or plastic used by a bedridden person to collect stool and/or urine. Chapter 20

Bedside commode. A chair with an opening for a bedpan or a container. Chapter 20

Biohazardous waste. Items that are soiled with blood or body fluids and may be harmful to others. Chapter 9

Bladder. A muscular sac that stores urine. Chapter 20

Blister. A swelling on the skin filled with watery matter. Chapter 23

Blood pressure. The pressure of blood in an artery. Chapter 13

Body alignment. The correct positioning of the head, back, neck, and limbs. Chapter 11

Body systems. Organs that work together to perform a specific function. Chapter 7

Body temperature. A measurement of the amount of heat in the body. Chapter 13

Bradycardia. A heart rate below 60 beats per minute. Chapter 13

Bronchitis. Inflammation of the bronchi. Chapter 8

Care plan. The directions for the care needed by a patient. Chapter 3

Catastrophic reaction. When people with dementia are unable to control their behavior and react to the frustration they feel by showing too much emotion in a situation. During a catastrophic reaction people may try to hit people because they are angry or afraid. Chapter 30

Cell. The basic unit of body structure. Chapter 7

Centigrade or Celsius (C). A scale used for measuring temperature. Chapter 13

Cerumen. Earwax. Chapter 7

Ceruminous gland. Specialized sweat gland in the ear that secretes cerumen. Chapter 7

Cesarean section (C-section). A surgical procedure in which the baby is delivered through an incision in the abdomen rather than through the vagina, or birth canal. Chapter 32

Cheyne-Stokes respiration. An irregular breathing pattern with slowing of respiration with periods of not breathing. Chapter 31

Chronic. Long-lasting or ongoing. Chapters 8, 29

Closed bed. A bed that is made with the covers pulled up. Made after a room has been cleaned and is available for another patient or in a long-term care center where the resident stays out of bed for the day-time hours. Chapter 14

Cognitive. The intellectual (thinking) functions of the brain. Chapters 6, 30

Communication. Sending and receiving information between two or more people. Chapter 3

Condom catheter. An external device applied to a male patient's penis and attached to a drainage bag. Chapter 20

Confidential. Keeping patient information private. Chapter 3

Conflict. A disagreement or a difference of opinions. Chapter 3

Confusion. A mental state in which people do not know who the people around them are, where they are, or what time period they are in. Both memory and thinking are affected. Chapters 6, 30

Consent. Giving permission for care or treatment. Chapter 2

Constipation. Difficulty passing hard dry stools out of the body. Chapter 21

Constrict. To reduce in size, to close. Chapter 24

Contagious. Refers to a disease that can be spread from one person to another, such as a cold or the flu. Chapter 8

Continent. In control of bowel and/or bladder functioning. Chapter 15

Contractures. Joints that do not have a normal shape, which is caused by shortening of the muscle. Chapters 12, 29

Coroner. A person with the legal power to pronounce the patient dead. Chapter 31

Cradle (overbed cradle). A frame placed at the foot of the bed to prevent bed linens from resting on the feet and lower legs. Chapter 14

Crater. A cup-shaped opening. Chapter 23

Culture. Set of values, beliefs, and customs of a group of people. Chapter 4

Cyanosis. Change from the usual color to a bluish color. Chapter 27

Cytobrush. A small brush used to obtain a specimen for a Pap smear. Chapter 26

Dangling. Allowing the patient to sit on the side of the bed for 1 to 2 minutes to adjust to the change from a lying to a sitting position. Chapter 11

Defecation. A bowel movement (BM). Chapter 21

Dehydration. Excessive loss of fluids from the body tissues. Chapter 19

Delirium. Confusion that is temporary and can come on suddenly. Delirium is likely to be the side effect of a medication, an illness, or an infection. Chapter 30

Dementia. Confusion caused by an injury to the brain or a long-term lack of blood flow to the brain. The confusion starts slowly, gets worse over time, and is permanent. Chapters 6, 30

Dermis. The layer of tissue under the epidermis. Chapter 7

Development. Changes in psychological and social functioning; how people act or behave at different ages of their life. Chapters 5, 33

Developmental task. Also known as a **conflict** or **identity crisis.** Set of behaviors or actions a person is able to do during a stage of life. Chapter 5

Diabetes. A chronic disease caused by not enough production or use of insulin by the body. Chapter 23

Diarrhea. Frequent passage of liquid stools. Chapter 21

Diastolic pressure. The lower (or bottom) number of a blood pressure reading obtained while the heart muscle is relaxed and the pressure in the artery is lower. Chapter 13

Dilate. To enlarge or to widen. Chapter 24

Disability. A lost physical or mental function. Chapter 29

Discharge. The patient's release from the health care facility. Chapter 22

DNR ("Do Not Resuscitate") order. An order written by the doctor when the patient does not want any life-prolonging treatment such as cardiopulmonary resuscitation (CPR). Chapter 31

Drawsheet. A small sheet placed sideways across the bed to cover the area of the bed between the patient's shoulders and thighs. Can be changed if it becomes dirty or may be used to reposition the patient in the bed. Sometimes called a lift sheet. Chapter 14

Dysuria. Painful or difficult urination. Chapter 20

ECG or EKG (electrocardiogram). A recording of the electrical activity of the heart. Chapter 28

Edema. Swelling, buildup of fluid in the tissues. Chapters 19, 23

8 Stages of psychosocial development. Theory described by psychologist Erik Erikson about how a person grows and develops throughout life. Chapter 5

Elective. Done by choice. Chapter 22

Emergency. An event that calls for immediate action; a situation that is unplanned and threatens the life of the patient. Chapters 22, 34

Emotional neglect. Not giving care and attention. Chapter 2

Employee evaluation. A review of the employee's work. Chapter 35

Employment agency. An agency that helps job seekers find employers. Chapter 35

Enema. Putting a liquid solution into the rectum. Chapter 21

Enteral nutrition. Giving nutrients through the digestive tract using a tube. Chapter 19

Epidermis. The outer layer of the skin. Chapter 7

Episiotomy. A surgical incision made to enlarge the vaginal opening for delivery. Chapter 32

Ethics. A person's beliefs about what is right and wrong. Chapter 2

Expiration. The act of breathing out. Chapters 7, 27

Fahrenheit (F). A scale used for measuring temperature. Chapter 13

Fainting. Short-term loss of consciousness. Chapter 34

Feces. Semisolid mass of waste products from the intestine. Chapter 21

First aid. Care given to an injured or ill person until professional help arrives. Chapter 34

Flatulence. Excessive amounts of air or gas in the stomach and intestines. Chapter 21

Foot board. A frame placed at the foot of the bed to prevent bedclothes from resting on the feet and lower legs. Chapter 14

Force. Strength of the pulse. Chapter 13

Fowler's position/semi-Fowler's position. The head of the bed is raised 60 to 90 degrees for Fowler's position and 30 to 60 degrees for semi-Fowler's position. The patient's knees are elevated just a little to avoid pressure on the back of the legs. Chapter 11

Fracture. Broken bone. Chapter 12

Frequency. Urinating at frequent intervals. Chapter 20

Fundus. The top of the uterus. Chapter 32

Gangrene. A condition in which the tissue dies. Chapter 8

Geriatrics. Health care specialty for the care of older adults. Chapter 6

Gerontology. Study of the changes that occur with aging. Chapter 6

Goal. Outcome or result that patients and their caregivers want. Chapter 3

Graphic forms. Forms in the medical record used for recording vital signs. Chapter 13

Growth. Series of physical changes that occur as a person ages. Chapters 5, 33

Halitosis. Bad breath. Chapter 16

Hallucinations. Seeing, hearing, or feeling something that is not real. Chapter 30

Harassment. Action, statement, or behavior that offends another person. Chapter 3

Health Insurance Portability and Accountability Act of 1996 (HIPAA). A law that protects people who might suffer discrimination in health coverage based on a factor that relates to a person's health. Chapter 3

Heart rate. The number of pulse beats, or heartbeats, that are counted in 1 minute. Chapter 13

Height. How tall the patient is, usually in feet and inches. Chapter 22

Hematuria. Blood in the urine. Chapter 20

Hemiplegia. Paralysis on one side of the body. Chapter 8

Hemorrhage. A large amount of sudden uncontrolled bleeding. Chapters 10, 34

Hepatitis. Inflammation of the liver. Chapter 8

Hierarchy of needs. Model of basic human needs developed by psychologist Abraham Maslow. Chapter 4

Holistic. Term meaning "whole." Chapter 4

Hormones. Substances secreted by the endocrine glands into the bloodstream. Chapter 7

Hospice. A type of care that provides support for the patient and family during the dying process. Chapter 31

Hospital gown. A thin cotton garment provided to patients that ties behind the neck and waist to secure an open back seam. Chapter 18

Hyperglycemia. High blood sugar. Chapter 8

Hypertension (high blood pressure). Blood pressure reading above 140/90 mm Hg. Chapter 13

Hypoglycemia. Low blood sugar. Chapter 8

Hypotension (low blood pressure). Blood pressure reading below 100/60 mm Hg. Chapter 13

Hypoxia. A condition in which the cells do not get enough oxygen. Chapter 27

ID band. Identification band applied to the patient's wrist that gives information that may include the patient's name, room number, patient number, doctor, and age. Chapter 22

Immune system. The body system that protects us from infections. Chapter 9

Impaction. A buildup of feces in the rectum. Chapter 21

Incentive spirometer. A device that measures the amount of air a person is able to take into the lungs. Chapter 27

Incident. Any unexpected situation that can cause harm to a person. Chapters 8, 10, 21

Incontinence. Inability to control the release of urine from the bladder or stool through the rectum. Chapters 8, 20, 21

Incontinent. Not in control of bowel and/or bladder functioning. Chapter 15

Indwelling catheter. A tube inserted into the bladder and attached to a drainage bag. Chapter 20

Infection. An illness that occurs when a disease-producing germ enters the body. Chapter 9

Infection control. A facility program that helps you to avoid spreading infections. Chapter 9

Inpatient care. Care provided to the patient who is in the hospital and stays there overnight. Chapter 1

Inspiration. The act of breathing in. Chapters 7, 27

Intensive care unit. A hospital unit that gives care to patients who need to be watched closely. Chapter 22

Interview. A meeting between 2 or more people. Chapter 35

Irregular pulse. The heart is beating in an uneven way, with different amounts of time between heartbeats. Chapter 13

IV (intravenous). A needle inserted into a vein to allow medications or fluids to be given to a patient. Chapter 18

Jaundice. A yellowish discoloration of the skin. Chapter 8

Joint. The union where two or more bones come together. Chapter 7

Kidneys. Bean-shaped urinary organs that filter the blood. Chapter 20

Lawsuit. Legal charges by someone who says he was injured or hurt by another person. Chapter 2

Lice. Tiny white insects that attach to the hair strands. Chapter 17

Licensed practical nurse (LPN)/ licensed vocational nurse (LVN). Licensed nurse who gives patient care, drugs, and treatments. Works under the supervision of a registered nurse. Chapter 1

Lift sheet. A small sheet placed sideways across the bed to cover the area of the bed between the patient's shoulders and thighs. Can be changed if it becomes dirty or may be used to reposition the patient in the bed. Sometimes called a drawsheet. Chapter 14

Lochia. Discharge that flows from the vagina after childbirth. Chapter 32

Malpractice. Professionals, such as a nurse, doctor, or dentist, not doing something that they are responsible for so that the patient is hurt. Chapter 2

Managed care. Ways insurance companies try to control health care costs. Chapter 1

Mattress pad. A pad placed between the mattress and the bottom sheet that absorbs moisture and keeps the patient from perspiring if the mattress is covered with plastic. Chapter 14

Medicaid. State-managed health care plan that covers health care services for people with low income. Sometimes covers older, blind, and disabled people. Chapter 1

Medical record (chart). Written record containing medical information about a patient. Chapter 3

Medicare. Federal government health care plan that pays for health care services for people over age 65. Chapter 1

Metastasize. To spread. Chapter 8

Microorganisms. Tiny living objects, sometimes called germs. Chapter 9

Minimum data set (MDS). Patient assessment and screening tool used in long-term care. Required by the Omnibus Budget Reconciliation Act of 1987 (OBRA). Chapter 3

Mitered corner. A method of folding the sheets at the corners at a right angle that has a neat appearance. Chapter 14

Nasal cannula. A small plastic tube with curved pieces that fits into the opening of the nose to provide oxygen. Chapter 27

Need. Something that is required for a person's survival or well-being. Chapter 4

Neglect. Not giving food, clothing, personal care, or medical care and treatment. Chapter 2

Negligence. An action that harms a person because of someone not being careful. Chapter 2

Nephrons. Filter unit of the kidney. Chapter 20

Networking. An informal way to find out about job openings. Chapter 35

Nocturia. Frequent urination at night. Chapter 20

Nonverbal communication. Type of communication that uses gestures, posture, facial expressions, and eye contact. Chapter 3

Nosocomial infection. An infection people get while they are a patient in the hospital or resident in a nursing home. Chapter 9

NPO. The abbreviation for "nothing by mouth." Chapter 28

Nursing assistant. Person who gives hands-on patient care such as bathing and feeding. Works under the supervision of a registered nurse and in some states a licensed practical nurse/licensed vocational nurse. Chapter 1

Nursing assistant registry. Record of information about nursing assistants licensed or certified in a state. Chapter 2

Nursing process. The process of getting information, identifying problems, planning care, giving care, and evaluating the care given. Chapter 3

Nutrients. Substances in food that support life. Chapter 19

Objective information. Observations you make about things that you can see, hear, feel, or smell. Chapter 3

Observation. Information you obtain by using your eyes, ears, nose, and sense of touch. Chapter 3

Occupational therapist (OT)/occupational therapy assistant (OTA). Helps patients to learn the skills they need to resume activities of daily living such as dressing and grooming. Focuses on small (fine) motor skills. Chapter 1

Occupied bed. A bed that is made while the patient is in it. Chapter 14

Oliguria. Less than 500 ml of urine in a 24-hour period. Chapter 20

Omnibus Budget Reconciliation Act of 1987 (OBRA). Laws passed by Congress to improve the quality of care for nursing home residents. Chapter 2

Open bed. A bed that is made with the covers fanfolded to the foot of the bed in preparation for a new admission or a patient who will return to the bed after the linens are changed. Chapter 14

Ophthalmoscope. An instrument used to look at the eye. Chapter 26

Oral temperature. Temperature taken in the mouth. Chapter 13

Organs. Group of tissues that perform a specialized function, such as the lungs. Chapter 7

Orthostatic hypotension. A rapid drop in blood pressure that occurs with a change in position. Chapters 11, 12

Ostomy. A surgical procedure in which an opening is made to allow the passage of urine from the bladder or intestinal contents from the bowel to exit the body through an opening in the abdomen called a stoma. Chapter 21

Otoscope. An instrument used to look at the inside of the ear canal. Chapter 26

Outpatient care. Health care services for a person who is not hospitalized. Chapter 1

Palliative care. When the goal of medical and nursing care is to keep the person as comfortable as possible rather than to cure the disease. Chapter 31

Paralysis (paralyzed). Inability to move. Chapter 8

Paraplegia. Paralysis from the waist down. Chapter 8

Parenteral nutrition. Giving nutrients through a tube that does not enter the digestive system such as intravenous (IV) fluids. Chapter 19

Pathogens. Disease-causing organisms. Chapter 7

Pediatric patient. A child 18 years old or under. Chapter 33

Percussion hammer. An instrument used to test reflexes. Chapter 26

Perineal. Pertaining to the part of the body between the pubic bone and the coccyx (tailbone). Chapter 24

Peristalsis. Wavelike movement. Chapter 21

Personnel policies. A set of rules for employees. Chapter 35

Perspiration. Sweat. Chapter 7

Pharmacist. Fills prescription orders. Teaches and advises patients, caregivers, and health care team members about drugs. Chapter 1

Physical therapist (PT)/physical therapy assistant (PTA). Help patients relearn skills such as getting out of bed and using things such as crutches and walkers. Focuses on improving large-muscle skills. Chapter 1

Pneumonia. Inflammation/infection of the lungs. Chapters 12, 27, 29

Podiatrist. Foot doctor. Chapter 17

Poison. Any substance that causes illness or death when taken into the body. Chapter 34

Polyuria. Abnormally large amounts of urine. Chapter 20

Postmortem care. Care of the person after death. Chapter 31

Postpartum care. Care of the new mother and her baby for 6 weeks after delivery. Chapter 32

Pressure ulcer. An inflammation or sore that develops over areas where the skin and tissue underneath are injured due to a lack of blood flow and oxygen supply as a result of constant pressure. Chapters 12, 14, 23

Private health insurance. A plan that pays for the cost of health care. Each insurance plan has its own rules. Not paid for by state or federal money. Chapter 1

Private room. A room that has only 1 patient in it. Chapter 22

Prone position. The patient is on the abdomen. Chapter 11

Protective pad. An absorbent pad that is placed over the bottom sheet or the drawsheet to give additional protection. Pads are cloth or disposable. Frequently used with patients who are incontinent, vomiting, or bleeding. Sometimes called an underpad. Chapter 14

Pulse. The throbbing felt over the artery as the heart beats. Chapter 13

Pulse oximeter. A device that measures the amount of oxygen in the blood through the skin. Chapter 27

Quadriplegia. Total paralysis from the neck down. Chapter 8

Reality orientation. Helping people to know and remember people around them and the place and time they are in. Chapter 30

Rectal temperature. Temperature taken in the rectum. Chapter 13

Rectal tube. A tube inserted about 4 inches into the patient's rectum to relieve flatulence and abdominal bloating or distention. Chapter 21

Reference. A statement about your abilities given by another person, usually a previous employer. Chapter 35

Registered dietitian (RD). Looks at a patient's nutritional needs. Supervises meal planning and preparation. Teaches patients and caregivers about nutrition and diets. Chapter 1

Registered nurse (RN). Licensed nurse who plans, coordinates, and supervises patient care and carries out doctors' orders. Supervises LPNs/LVNs and nursing assistants. Chapter 1

Regular pulse. The heart is beating in an even, steady way. Chapter 13

Rehabilitation. Health care to help people maintain or return to their highest level of normal activity after an illness or injury. Also known as restorative care. Chapter 1

Report. Process by which patient information and care needs are given to the nurse or the next shift of caregivers. Chapter 3

Resident assessment protocols (RAPs). Guidelines that help nurses develop a care plan for a long-term care resident. Required by OBRA. Chapter 3

Respiration. The cycle of breathing in and out. Chapters 7, 13, 27

Respiratory therapist. Performs breathing treatments and procedures. Chapter 1

Restraint. Any manual or chemical item or device that restricts a person's freedom of movement or body access. Chapter 10

Résumé. A summary of your education and work experience. Chapter 35

Rhythm. Pattern of the pulse, described as regular or irregular. Chapter 13

Rigor mortis. A temporary stiffening of the muscles after death, which occurs shortly after death. Chapter 31

Saliva. Liquid in the mouth secreted by the salivary glands, sometimes called "spit." Chapter 7

Seizure (convulsion). Sudden uncontrolled muscle contraction resulting from abnormal brain activity. Chapters 8, 10, 34

Self-actualization. Term that relates to people's need to be creative and fulfill their potential. Chapter 4

Self-esteem. What people think about themselves. Chapter 4

Semi-private room. A room that is shared with at least 1 other patient. Chapter 22

Shearing. Pressure against the skin as tissues slide in the opposite direction from the underlying bones, such as when a patient slides down in bed. Chapter 23

Shock. Abnormal condition of the body in which there is not enough blood supply to the body's tissues. Chapter 34

Sims' position. The patient begins in a side-lying position and is turned toward the abdomen. Chapter 11

Skin tear. A break in the skin that occurs when the top layer of the skin is separated from the underlying layers. Chapter 23

Social worker. Helps organize services to provide patient care, especially after a patient leaves the hospital or nursing home. Plans transfers to other facilities for patients who cannot return home. Chapter 1

Speech language pathologist/ speech therapist. Assists patients who have speaking and swallowing disorders. Chapter 1

Sphygmomanometer. An instrument used to measure blood pressure. Chapters 13, 26

Sputum. Mucus from the respiratory system that is spit or forced out of the mouth. Chapter 25

Staffing agency. An agency that hires health care workers and provides staff to facilities that need help on a temporary basis. Chapter 35

Standard Precautions. Precautions that protect you from patients with known infections and from patients who have infections that they are not aware of. Chapter 9

Stethoscope. An instrument that has two earpieces attached by flexible tubing to a diaphragm that is placed against the patient's skin to hear heart and lung sounds. Chapters 13, 26

Stoma. Opening. Chapter 21

Subcutaneous. Tissue beneath the dermis that contains the fat layer. Chapter 7

Subjective information (symptoms). Information patients tell you about how they feel. Chapter 3

Sundowning. Behavior problems that get worse in the late afternoon or evening as the sun goes down. Chapter 30

Supine position. The patient rests on the back with the arms and legs straight down at sides. Chapter 11

Suppository. A medication put into the rectum. Chapter 21

Surgical bed. A bed that is made with the covers fanfolded to the side so that the transfer from a stretcher to the bed is easier. Chapter 14

Sutures. A type of immovable joint in between the bones in the skull. Chapter 7

Systolic pressure. The higher (or top) number of a blood pressure reading obtained while the heart muscle is contracting and the pressure in the artery rises. Chapter 13

Tachycardia. A heart rate above 100 beats per minute. Chapter 13

Tissue. Groups of cells that perform a specialized function. Chapter 7

Toe pleat. A 3- to 4-inch fold in the top covers across the foot of the bed that allows patients to freely move their feet under the top covers. Chapter 14

Transfer. To move a patient from one place to another in the facility. Chapter 22

Trapeze. A bar hung above the patient's bed to assist the person with moving in the bed. Chapter 11

Tuning fork. A metal instrument used to test bone and air conduction of sound. Chapter 26

Tympanic membrane temperature. Temperature taken in the ear, same as aural temperature. Chapter 13

Underpad. An absorbent pad that is placed over the bottom sheet or the drawsheet to provide additional protection. Pads are cloth or disposable. Frequently used with patients who are incontinent, vomiting, or bleeding. Sometimes called a protective pad. Chapter 14

Universal Precautions. Precautions designed to protect health care workers from diseases carried in the blood such as human immunodeficiency virus (HIV), acquired immunodeficiency syndrome (AIDS), and hepatitis. Chapter 9

Unoccupied bed. A bed that is made while the patient is out of the bed. Chapter 14

Ureters. Small tubes that connect the kidney to the urinary bladder. Chapter 20

Urethra. A small tube that drains urine from the bladder. Chapter 20

Urgency. The need to urinate right away. Chapter 20

Urinal. A plastic container used by men to urinate. Chapter 20

Vaginal speculum. A metal or plastic instrument used in an exam of the female genitalia. Chapter 26

Validation therapy. A method of talking with someone that allows confused people to talk about their thoughts and feel safe and accepted. Chapter 30

Venous. Related to the veins, the blood vessels that carry blood towards the heart. Chapter 23

Verbal communication. Type of communication that uses words, tone of voice, and rate of speech. Chapter 3

Virus. One-celled microorganism that is much smaller than a bacterium. Chapter 9

Vital signs. Temperature, pulse, respiration, and blood pressure. Chapters 13, 22

Void. To urinate. Chapter 20

Weight. How much a patient weighs in pounds or kilograms. Chapter 22

Wound. Any physical injury involving a break in the skin. Chapter 23

Chapter 1

1. Doctors office/clinics
   Hospitals
   Nursing homes and rehabilitation facilities
   Home care
2. She will be moved to a nursing home and rehabilitation facility.
3. A home care agency will best be able to help the family.
4. The patient and/or the patient's family are the most important members of the health care team.
5. Most health care is paid for by Medicare, Medicaid, private health insurance.
6. d. Social worker
7. a. RN

Chapter 2

1. Give basic daily care, including bathing, feeding, and dressing
   Take a person's temperature, pulse, and respirations
   Give range-of-motion exercises
   Measure height and weight
   Admit, transfer, and discharge patients
   Apply heat and cold treatments
   Collect specimens
   Assist with oxygen therapy
   Prepare a patient for surgery
   Care for a dying person
   Care for new mothers and their babies
   Lift and transfer patients
2. Training program, competency evaluation, nursing assistant registry, and ongoing in-service education program guidelines
3. The nursing assistant registry is a record of everyone who is licensed or certified in that state.
4. The person and/or person's clothing are dirty and unkempt.
   The person has lost weight and/or is dehydrated.
   Medications are not given properly, or the person is overmedicated.
   The person has many injuries that are hard to explain.
   The person has many visits to the emergency department.
   The person has unexplained fractures or broken bones.
   The person has new and old bruises.
   The person has unexplained marks on the body such as welts, bite marks, or burns.
   The person is nervous and upset, afraid, anxious, or very quiet and refuses to talk or answer questions.
   The person lives in dirty, unsafe living conditions.
   The person is kept alone in a small space for long periods of time.
   Caregivers do not allow the patient to have a private conversation with another person.
   The person may not have a doctor or may see many doctors.
   The person has bleeding or bruising of the genitals.
   The person has blood or stains on underwear.
5. Report your observations to your charge nurse. If you are worried about the safety and well-being of your patient, report and discuss your concerns immediately with your supervising nurse.
6. c. Improving quality of care for nursing home residents
7. d. All of the above
8. b. Arriving at work on time
9. b. Carrying out assigned tasks on time
10. a. Respecting others' personal and cultural differences
11. d. All of the above
12. d. Respect each person as an individual.
13. a. Dropping and breaking a patient's glasses while cleaning them

14. b. Making false statements about a person verbally
15. a. Physical, emotional, or financial harm

Chapter 3

1. Communication is sending and receiving information.
2. Gestures, posture, eye contact, facial expression
3. The care plan is simply the directions for the care needed by a patient.
4. A goal is an outcome or result that patients and their caregivers can work toward. A goal helps patients work toward their highest level of function, independence, or rehabilitation possible.
5. Minimum data sets (MDSs), resident assessment protocols (RAPs), interdisciplinary care planning (ICP) conferences
6. Your facility will have a list of approved abbreviations that you may use.
7. M. Jones, CNA
8. a. Nonverbal communication
9. c. Ask the nurse if she could speak with him privately, then state her concerns factually, using a calm voice.
10. c. Verbal
11. a. Confidentiality
12. c. Objective data
13. d. Subjective data
14. b. Graphic record
15. c. Draw one line through the misspelling. Write "mistaken entry" and your initials above the mistake, then rewrite the word correctly.

Chapter 4

1. A "need" is something that is required for a person's survival or well-being.
2. This term refers to a set of values, beliefs, and customs practiced by a group of people.
3. You respond that you cannot share that information. You then refer the person to the supervising nurse.

4. b. Holistic
5. b. Physical
6. c. Safety and security
7. a. Cultural
8. b. "You are welcome to stay. Children need their parents when they feel scared."
9. d. The right to refuse treatment

Chapter 5

1. Growth
2. Development
3. d. All of the above
4. c. Toilet training
5. c. Independence and self-reliance
6. c. Childhood
7. b. Adolescence
8. c. Sense of identity
9. b. Young adulthood
10. c. Middle adulthood
11. d. Late adulthood

Chapter 6

1. Geriatrics
2. Older adults may experience reduced ability of the body to fight infection.
3. If people have few friends outside work, retirement may make them feel lonely and isolated. If people have not developed other hobbies and interests, they may feel they are not doing anything important. The income of people who retire is often about half of their work earnings. Insurance benefits may be less, and people may be spending more on health care expenses.
4. Focus on improving the quality of life, health, and safety of residents in long-term care facilities
5. d. Thinner, more fragile tissue
6. a. Less bone and muscle mass
7. c. Reduced blood flow to the brain
8. a. Arteries are narrowed and stiff; circulation decreases.
9. Capacity is decreased.
10. d. All of the above

11. b. Memory loss and slower response time
12. c. Privacy and confidentiality
13. c. Maintain personal choice

Chapter 7

1. Ball-and-socket joint
2. Tendons
3. Respiratory system
4. Digestive system
5. Endocrine system
6. Pancreas
7. a. Cell
8. a. Integumentary
9. d. Musculoskeletal
10. a. Nervous system
11. c. Cardiovascular system
12. a. Urinary system
13. d. Reproductive system
14. d. Immune system
15. a. The skin becomes drier and more fragile.
16. c. The urine is less concentrated.

Chapter 8

1. Diabetes occurs when the body cannot produce enough insulin to metabolize the food that the person eats.
2. Direct contact, indirect contact, airborne, vehicle contamination, and vector
3. b. Athlete's foot
4. a. Gout
5. a. Cataract
6. b. Hypertension
7. d. It is an infection/inflammation of the lungs.
8. c. Gallstones
9. a. They are more common in women than in men.
10. c. Gonorrhea
11. b. An abnormally fast metabolism
12. d. Measles

Chapter 9

1. Infections are caused by microorganisms. An infection occurs when the body is invaded by a disease-producing microorganism.
2. Fever or chills, pain, redness, swelling, drainage, fatigue, nausea, disorientation (this is more commonly seen in the elderly)
3. The chain of infection is the manner in which infections can live and be spread.
4. The Centers of Disease Control (CDC) guidelines for health care workers that protect you from patients with known infections and patients who have infections that they are not aware of
5. c. To keep the facility as germ-free as possible
6. d. All of the above
7. a. Airborne

Chapter 10

1. Know the safety policies and procedures at your facility.
   Think about safety each day.
   Use only equipment you have been properly trained to use.
   Do only those jobs for which you have been trained.
   Be aware of what is going on around you.
2. Do not try to stop the fall. Ease the person to the floor as gently as you can, and call for help. Stay with the patient until the charge nurse arrives. Do not try to lift a resident who has fallen until the nurse has checked for injuries.
3. If a patient is having a seizure, call for help. Position the patient on her side if she is on the floor or in bed. If the patient is standing, ease her to the floor gently so she is not injured. Clear the area around the patient, and put a pillow or blanket under her head. Stay with the patient until the seizure has ended or until the charge nurse arrives. Make a mental note of the time the seizure started and report the length of the seizure to the charge nurse.

4. **R**—Rescue any patients in danger by moving them away from the fire.
   A—Activate the alarm system.
   C—Contain the fire by closing doors and windows.
   E—Extinguish the fire if it is small.
5. In the event of a tornado, move all patients away from windows. Remove any heavy objects, such as plants, from windowsills. Close the drapes or blinds, and pull the privacy curtains around any patients who remain in their beds. If you are involved in a tornado, stay calm and follow the directions of your supervisor.
6. If you receive this type of call, make note of the exact time of the call. Be calm and courteous; do not interrupt the caller. Pay special attention to any noises in the background such as music, machinery, or other voices. Write down exactly what the caller says, and notify your supervisor as soon as the caller hangs up. Always take a bomb threat seriously.
7. Try to park in a well-lit area. If you have to walk to your car in the dark, use the buddy system. Keep the building safe by reporting any unauthorized visitors or suspicious activity. Promptly report any violent or threatening incidents to your supervisor. Be sensitive to racial and cultural differences, and treat others with respect.
8. Any manual or chemical item or device that is attached to or next to the person's body that restricts the person's freedom of movement or body access that the person cannot easily remove
9. d. All employees
10. b. Hemorrhage
11. d. All of the above

Chapter 11

1. Using good body mechanics:
   Protects you from injury when moving patients or objects
   Reduces fatigue and strain on your back
   Makes your muscles work with you to maximize strength
   Makes lifting, transferring, and moving objects and patients easier
   Provides you with balance and stability when lifting
2. It makes the patient more comfortable.
   It improves blood flow.
   It prevents contractures and respiratory problems.
   It relieves pressure over bony areas such as the hips and heels.
3. c. To decrease rubbing against the patient's skin
4. a. At least every 1½ to 2 hours if they are in bed and every 20 to 30 minutes if they are sitting in a chair
5. b. Back
6. c. Position the chair on his right side
7. False

Chapter 12

1. Proper rest and sleep are important to good health. They are even more important to a person who is recovering from an injury or illness. A person who is well rested can deal with pain better and has a better response to pain medications.
2. Pneumonia, muscle atrophy, contractures, orthostatic hypotension, constipation, pressure ulcers, and/or blood clots
3. Active ROM means that patients participates in the exercises or are able to do them on their own or with your help. Passive ROM means that they need you to do the exercises for them.
4. a. 5 to 10 hours
5. c. To prevent contractures
6. c. Instruct the patient to step forward with the weaker foot first.
7. c. Step behind the patient, pulling the patient close to your body, and slowly lower the patient to the floor.
8. Back rub

Chapter 13

1. Temperature, pulse, respiration, and blood pressure
2. Vital sign readings should be reported to the nurse when a result is above or below the normal range or is changed from a previous measurement.
3. Ear, mouth, and axilla
4. 60 to 100 beats per minute
5. This reading indicates hypotension and should be reported to the charge nurse.
6. 138 is the systolic, and 82 is the diastolic.
7. The systolic measures the force of the blood in the artery when the heart is pumping, and the diastolic measures the force of the blood in the artery when the heart is at rest.
8. Height and weight are measured when a person is admitted to a health care facility.
   When a person is examined at a doctor's office
   When an infant or child is examined during a well-child examination
9. d. All of the above
10. a. It is within the normal range.
11. b. Axillary
12. c. Mr. Thompson has tachycardia.
13. a. Report these findings to the nurse.
14. b. Theses readings indicate hypertension.

Chapter 14

1. Wrinkles are uncomfortable and can lead to the development of pressure sores.
2. Place the pillowcase in the dirty linen hamper, and obtain a clean one.
3. Mattress pad, bottom sheet, drawsheet or lift sheet, underpad/protective pad, top sheet, pillowcase, blanket and/or bedspread
4. c. Mattress pad
5. b. In a linen closet with the door kept closed
6. d. In the dirty linen hamper
7. d. As often as needed to keep the bed clean and dry
8. a. A bed that is made while the patient is in it

9. c. Linens on special mattresses are changed according to the manufacturer's instructions.
10. b. For patients who have had foot surgery
11. True

Chapter 15

1. Bathing:
   Cleanses the skin of dirt and waste products
   Makes the patient more comfortable
   Stimulates circulation to the skin
   Gives the nurse assistant an opportunity to look at the condition of the patient's skin
2. A partial bed bath involves washing the face, hands, underarms, and the genital/perineal area
3. Patients who are continent are in control of the bladder and bowel functions. Patients are incontinent when they are not in control of their bowel or bladder functions.
4. a. 105° F
5. c. Each morning with grooming and after each bowel movement (BM)
6. Drying, itching

Chapter 16

1. Mouth care removes food particles, stimulates circulation to the gums, and prevents halitosis (bad breath). Mouth care also helps to prevent cavities in the teeth and mouth infections.
2. Mouth care is usually given in the early morning before breakfast, and before bedtime.
3. Loose or broken teeth; red or swollen gums; dry, cracked or coated tongue; sores or white patches in the mouth or on the tongue; black or brown areas on the teeth, which could be signs of tooth decay; poorly fitting dentures
4. d. In cool water in a denture cup

5. b. Every 2 hours
6. False

Chapter 17

1. Hair should be combed or brushed each morning and throughout the day as needed to maintain a neat appearance.
2. Disposable razors should be placed in a sharps container.
3. Eyeglasses should be stored in an eyeglass case in the nightstand when not in use.
4. Hearing aids should be cleaned daily according to the manufacturer's instructions and stored in their protective case when not in use.
5. c. Allow the beauty shop to wash her hair
6. c. 105° F
7. a. Notify the charge nurse.
8. d. Foot doctor
9. Infections

Chapter 18

1. In a nursing home or long-term care facility, the resident usually dresses in street clothes each day. Appropriate daytime dress depends upon the time of year and the resident's plans for the day. The resident should be dressed in clothes that are clean and in good condition.
2. Because the elderly have less body fat, many elderly patients feel cold when the nursing assistant does not.
3. c. When it is dirty or after bathing
4. b. Provide privacy for the patient
5. a. Remove the gown from the arm without the IV first
6. d. Guide each arm out of the garment, then slip it over the patient's head.

Chapter 19

1. A well-balanced diet provides energy and helps you resist illnesses. A good diet is also important to help your body grow and to repair injured tissues.
2. Carbohydrates—cereals, breads, pastas, rice, potatoes, fruits, vegetables, and sugars
   Proteins—meat, eggs, fish, poultry, dairy products, nuts, and beans
   Fats—butter, oils, salad dressings, whole milk, fish, and nuts
   Vitamins—A, B, C, D, E, and K
   Minerals—calcium, potassium, and iron
3. In addition to nutrients, your body needs fluid and fiber to keep it going.
4. Bread, cereal, rice, and pasta
   Vegetables
   Fruit
   Milk, yogurt, and cheese
   Meat, poultry, fish, dried beans, eggs, and nuts
   Fats, oils, and sweets
5. Enteral nutrition is giving nutrients through the digestive tract using a tube.
6. Thirst; constipation; decreased urination; low blood pressure; weak, rapid pulse; confusion or disorientation; dry lips and mucous membranes; rapid weight loss
7. 390 ml
8. b. Dehydration
9. d. No concentrated sweets
10. a. Ice cream
11. d. 2000 to 3000 ml
12. d. Patients should be fed using a spoon.

Chapter 20

1. Kidneys, ureters, bladder, and urethra
2. Urine is stored in the urinary bladder
3. Age, diseases, amount and kinds of liquids taken in, body temperature, drugs, amount of salt in the diet
4. Follow the person's normal voiding routine and habits.
   Provide for privacy when using the bathroom.
   Allow enough time for the person to urinate; do not rush the person.

Provide 2000 to 3000 ml of fluid per day unless instructed otherwise by the charge nurse.

Answer the signal light promptly.

5. Regaining control of bladder function makes people feel better about themselves and increases their quality of life.
6. Bedside commode, bedpan, or urinal
7. A condom catheter may be used for incontinent male patients. It is sometimes called an external catheter, Texas catheter, or urinary sheath. A condom catheter slides over the penis and is secured to the skin with an elastic type of tape that comes with the catheter. A condom catheter can be attached to either a leg bag or a drainage bag.
8. b. 1000 to 2000ml
9. c. Hematuria
10. a. Nocturia
11. a. Notify the charge nurse before emptying the container.
12. d. Clean the catheter washing from the body toward the bag.

Chapter 21

1. *Constipation*—difficulty passing hard dry stools. This may be caused by a diet lacking in fiber or fluids, drugs, aging, inactivity, and some diseases.

   Diarrhea—frequent passage of liquid stools. This may be caused by infections, drugs, some foods, and germs in food or water.

   Flatulence—excessive amounts of air or gas in the stomach and intestines.

   Impaction—a buildup of feces in the rectum. A fecal impaction can occur from untreated constipation. The person may have liquid stools that pass around the impaction.

   Incontinence—inability to control the release of stool through the anus.
2. Follow the person's normal bowel routine and habits.

Provide for privacy when using the bathroom.

Allow enough time for the person to defecate; do not rush him.

Provide 2000 to 3000 ml of fluid per day unless instructed otherwise by the charge nurse.

Encourage a diet with adequate fiber such as fresh fruit and vegetables.

Encourage activity such as walking to increase peristalsis.

3. Bowel training programs can help people with fecal incontinence get control of their bowel function again. Some people need bowel training after an illness or injury. Regaining control of bowel function makes the person feel better about himself and increases his quality of life. Bowel retraining also helps the person to develop a regular bowel elimination routine and helps to avoid constipation and impaction.
4. An enema is the introduction of a liquid solution into the rectum. Enemas remove feces from the colon, relieve constipation or flatulence, and help remove an impaction. Enemas are also given to clean the bowel before surgery or diagnostic tests.
5. Clamp the tube if the person complains of abdominal cramping, expels the solutions, or is unable to hold the solution. Unclamp the tubing, and complete the administration when the symptoms subside.
6. A rectal tube is used to relieve flatulence and abdominal bloating or distention.
7. A rectal tube is left in place for the amount of time requested by the charge nurse but no more than 30 minutes.
8. Bags are usually changed 1 to 2 times a week or as desired by the person. Some people change their pouch or bag each day.
9. c. Peristalsis
10. c. Soapsuds enema
11. a. 105° F
12. d. With warm water and soap

Chapter 22

1. It is decided between the nurse on the unit the patient is transferring from and the nurse on the unit the patient is transferring to.
2. Make sure the room is clean and odor free. Make sure the bed is made according to your facility's policy.
   Place clean towels and washcloths in the bathroom.
   Provide an admission kit if used by your facility.
3. An ID band is used to identify patients for all procedures while they are in the hospital.
4. When the patient is in the car with the door closed
5. a. Admission
6. d. All of the above
7. a. Height, weight, and vital signs
8. b. Transfer
9. c. Hand it to the nurse on the new unit
10. c. Discharge
11. c. Notify the nurse

Chapter 23

1. Patients who are at risk for pressure ulcers are those who:
   Are unable to move because of paralysis, weakness, or coma
   Are unwilling to move because of severe pain, depression, or confusion
   Are unable to control bowel or bladder function
   Have poor food or fluid intake, are dehydrated
   Have poor circulation, especially patients with diabetes
   Are elderly, obese, or very thin
   Have casts, braces, or splints
2. Stage I
3. A back rub makes the patient more relaxed, eases muscle tension, and increases circulation. During a back rub, the nursing assistant has a chance to look at the skin for signs of redness or breakdown.

4. Poor venous or arterial blood flow
5. To improve circulation in the lower legs
6. Redness; swelling; warmth; pain or tenderness; drainage, especially yellow, green, or brown; foul odor; increased body temperature
7. To support the wound and hold dressings in place
8. a. Pressure ulcer
9. b. Skin tear
10. a. Good nutrition
11. c. Pull toward the wound

Chapter 24

1. Doctors order heat and cold applications for comfort and to help with healing.
2. Ask the charge nurse for directions.
3. d. Decrease swelling
4. c. Decrease bleeding
5. b. An elderly patient
6. b. All heat and cold applications require a doctor's order.
7. a. Every 5 minutes
8. c. Fill the bag $\frac{1}{2}$ to $\frac{2}{3}$ full of crushed ice
9. Aquathermia pad

Chapter 25

1. Laboratory testing of urine gives information about how the urinary system is working. Urine also gives information about nutritional status and other diseases.
2. Laboratory testing of stool gives information about how the gastrointestinal system is working. The tests give information about infections, internal bleeding, and digestive problems.
3. Laboratory testing of sputum provides information about medical problems in the respiratory system. Information about infections such as tuberculosis and other diseases such as lung cancer can be obtained.
4. a. Keep the collection bottle cold in the refrigerator or by placing it on ice in a basin in the bathroom.

5. False
6. Gloves

Chapter 26

1. A physical exam is performed as a routine procedure each year. It may also be done when applying for an insurance policy or before starting a new job. A physical exam is also done when a person is admitted to the hospital or nursing home.

2.

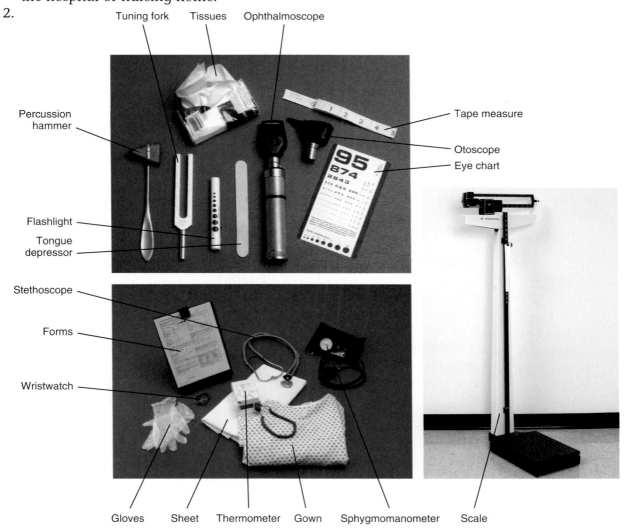

Tuning fork Tissues Ophthalmoscope

Percussion hammer

Tape measure

Otoscope

Eye chart

Flashlight

Tongue depressor

Stethoscope

Forms

Wristwatch

Gloves Sheet Thermometer Gown Sphygmomanometer Scale

3. b. The nursing assistant should ask the patient if he needs to use the bathroom and obtain a stool or urine specimen if needed.
4. a. Sitting
5. a. Make sure the patient is comfortable and warm

Chapter 27

1. Breathing
2. *Age*—The elderly have weaker respiratory muscles, and lung tissue is not as elastic. This makes coughing more difficult and can lead to pneumonia, or an inflammation/infection of the lungs.
   Smoking—Smoking damages the lungs and can lead to lung disease.
   Diseases—Emphysema, lung cancer, asthma, and allergies are diseases that can affect respiratory functioning.
   Drugs—Some medicines, especially pain medications, affect the part of the brain that controls respiration and can even cause a person to stop breathing.
   Pain, fever, exercise—All of these increase the body's need for oxygen, so respiratory function is affected.
3. Restlessness
   Confusion
   Dizziness
   Feeling tired
   Behavior changes
   Personality changes
   Nervousness
   Increased pulse rate
   Fast or difficult breathing
   Cyanosis
4. A nasal cannula consists of a small plastic tube with short, curved prongs that fit into the opening of the nose about $\frac{1}{4}$ inch to provide oxygen. The cannula is held in place by looping it over the ears and securing it under the person's chin.
5. c. 12 to 20
6. b. Coughing
7. d. Sitting
8. a. Flowmeter
9. False

Chapter 28

1. Taking the patient's vital signs
   Measuring height and weight
   Assisting the person with undressing and putting on a hospital gown
   Applying the identification bracelet
   Obtaining a urine specimen if needed
2. NPO means nothing by mouth.
3. It is important that the patient's stomach be empty during surgery to prevent nausea and vomiting during the procedure.
4. A surgical skin prep is performed to help prevent infections
5. IV pole, thermometer, stethoscope and sphygmomanometer, emesis basis, tissues
6. While each institution has its own routine, vital signs are usually taken every 15 minutes for the first hour, every 30 minutes for 2 hours, and then every hour for 4 hours. If vital signs are within normal limits, they are taken every 4 hours for the next 1 to 3 days, depending on the type of surgery performed.
7. Anti-embolism stockings should be removed each shift to check for skin breakdown or redness.
8. d. All of the above

Chapter 29

1. It is the process of helping injured or ill people return to their highest possible level of wellness. It also refers to care that helps a person regain health, independence, and strength after an injury or illness.
2. To maintain present function
   To restore or regain lost function after illness, injury, or surgery
   To prevent complications of immobility such as contractures, pneumonia, and blood clots
3. The resident or patient is the most important member of the rehabilitation team.
4. Following the care plan to help people achieve their goals
   Providing emotional support and encouragement
   Focusing on the people's abilities, not their disabilities
   Treating the person with dignity and respect

Trying to understand people's feelings if they are discouraged or sad

Allowing as much time as the person needs to complete activities of daily living such as bathing, dressing, and grooming

Providing assistive devices as indicated on the care plan and assisting the person with using them correctly.

5. a. Acute
6. a. Occupational therapy

Chapter 30

1. Confusion refers to a mental state in which people do not know who the people around them are, where they are, or what time period they are in. Both memory and thinking are affected.
2. Dehydration, infections, constipation in an elderly person, medications, hearing or vision loss, depression, new surroundings
3. Follow the person's care plan so that the care is the same from day to day.

   Call the person by name and identify yourself.

   Explain what you are doing and why as you assist with care.

   Provide a clock, calendar, and familiar objects to help the person become reoriented to the surroundings.

   Maintain a calm, quiet environment free from noise and confusion.
4. Dementia is confusion that is caused by an injury to the brain or a long-term lack of blood flow to the brain. The confusion starts slowly, gets worse over time, and is permanent.
5. Alzheimer's disease
6. Stage I
7. A hallucination is seeing, hearing, or feeling something that is not real.

8. When people with dementia are unable to control their behavior and react to the frustration they feel by showing too much emotion in a situation. During a catastrophic reaction people may try to hit people because they are angry or afraid.
9. Look for signs that the person is getting upset.

   Treat the person with respect; do not argue with the person.

   Speak calmly and quietly.

   Speak to the person in short simple sentences.

   Know people as individuals, including their likes and dislikes.

   Provide rest periods throughout the day.

   Assist the person with using the bathroom at least every 2 to 3 hours.

   Maintain a constant routine from day to day.

   Maintain a calm, quiet environment free from noise and confusion.

   Provide a safe area for the person to wander freely.
10. e. All of the above
11. c. Phobic disorder
12. a. Anxiety disorder
13. Delirium

Chapter 31

1. Personal experiences, culture, religion, and the age of the person who is dead or dying
2. Advance directives give information about the patients' wishes about medical care when they are no longer able to give that information.
3. Denial, anger, bargaining, depression, and acceptance

4. Hospice is a type of care that provides support for the patient and family during the dying process. It is provided to a person who has a life expectancy of 6 months or less. The idea behind hospice care is that death is a natural part of the life cycle. Hospice care encourages the patient to make each day the best it can be. Hospice care can be provided in a hospital, nursing home, or the patient's home because it is a way of providing care, not a place.

5. Decreased urine output and/or incontinence may occur.
   Decreased blood pressure may occur.
   Skin may become cool, pale, or gray.
   An irregular breathing pattern with slowing of respiration with periods of not breathing (apnea) called Cheyne-Stokes respirations may occur.
   Body temperature may rise even though the arms and legs are cool to the touch.
   Pulse is fast, weak, and irregular.
   Mucous may collect in the back of the throat, causing a "death rattle."

6. Postmortem care is care of the person after death.

7. d. Allow for frequent rest periods.

Chapter 32

1. The term *postpartum care* is used to describe the care of the new mother and her baby for 6 weeks after delivery. During this time the mother returns to her pre-pregnant state.

2. The uterus returns to its normal size in about 5 to 6 weeks.

3. Lochia is discharge that flows from the vagina after childbirth.

4. An episiotomy is a surgical incision made to enlarge the vaginal opening for delivery.

5. A cesarean section is a surgical procedure in which the baby is delivered through an incision in the abdomen rather than through the vagina or birth canal.

6. At the time of delivery identification bands with matching numbers are placed on each mother and her infant. The bands contain the name of the mother and the doctor, as well as the baby's sex. When taking a baby to his mother, the staff member checks the numbers on the baby's ID band with those on the mother. This ensures that each woman receives the correct infant.

7. d. All of the above

8. c. 110 to 150 beats per minute

9. Back or side

Chapter 33

1. People's culture is different from their race or ethnic background. A culture is made of people with similar values, beliefs, language, dress, diet, and acceptable behaviors.

2. One of the most important things you can do to help your young patient feel secure is to involve the parent/guardian as much as possible in the child's care.

3. The single most important emotional need of children is to feel loved and accepted by the people who are important in their lives.

4. She is in the early childhood developmental phase, more specifically toddler phase.

5. This is normal; she is trying to become more independent.

6. False

7. False

Chapter 34

1. An emergency is an event that calls for immediate action

2. In most areas across the United States, EMS can be activated by dialing 911 on a telephone. This will put you in contact with an EMS operator who will send the police, fire department, and paramedics. In some rural areas it may be necessary to contact the service you need by dialing directly.

3. The phone number and address you are calling from, the type of assistance that is needed, and the number and types of injuries involved

4. Fainting is a short-term loss of consciousness.

5. Low blood sugar, anemia or lack of iron in the blood, any condition in which there is a rapid loss of blood, heart and circulatory problems such as heart attack or stroke, prolonged exposure to extreme heat, a sudden change in body position such as standing up too quickly (postural hypotension), severe pain, sudden emotional stress, fright or anxiety, taking medications

6. A hemorrhage is sudden uncontrolled bleeding.

7. Heart attack, sudden blood loss, blood poisoning from major infection, exposure to extreme heat or cold for too long, fractures of a large bone, a severe allergic reaction, very low blood sugar such as occurs with diabetes, drug overdose

8. Infants, small children, and the elderly are most likely to die from burn injuries.

9. These symptoms may happen right after a person is bitten or stung or within 30 to 60 minutes.

10. A poison is any substance that causes illness or death when taken into the body.

11. Severe allergic reactions; face, head, nose or lung injuries; carbon monoxide poisoning; choking; drug overdose; poisoning; respiratory diseases such as asthma, emphysema, or pneumonia; congestive heart failure; heart attack; blood clot in a lung

12. Irregular heart beat, heart attack, heart failure, electrocution, medications

13. a. Rest, cold compresses, and elevating the area

14. c. Seizure

Chapter 35

1. Networking, classified advertisements, employment agencies, staffing agencies, and the Internet

2. The job you are interested in and the reason you are interested in working for the facility, why you should be considered for the position, and a request for an interview, making sure your address and phone number are included in the letter

3. Social security card, state picture ID or driver's license; a copy of your nursing assistant certification or proof of enrollment in the nursing assistant training program at your school; name and location of all schools attended, including dates of attendance; name, title, address, and phone number for at least three references; employment information for at least the last 5 years, including phone numbers, addresses, and supervisors' names; a copy of your résumé, a pen

4. d. A summary of your education and work experience

5. a. A pair of dark colored dress pants and a nice blouse or shirt with a collar

6. d. Smoking a cigarette immediately before the interview

7. c. 12 hours per year

8. b. Complete a competency evaluation before returning to work

9. 2 weeks

ILLUSTRATION CREDITS

Chapter 1

1-1, from Potter, P.A., & Perry, A.G. (2003). *Basic nursing: a critical thinking approach* (5th ed.). St. Louis: Mosby. **1-2,** from Elkin, M.K., Perry, A.G., & Potter, P.A. (2003). *Nursing interventions and clinical skills* (3rd ed.). St. Louis: Mosby. **1-4,** from Birchenall, J., & Streight, E. (2002). *Mosby's textbook for the home care aide* (2nd ed.). St. Louis: Mosby.

Chapter 2

2-1, A; 2-4, from deWit, S. (2000). *Fundamental concepts and skills for nursing* (1st ed.). Philadelphia: W.B. Saunders. **2-2,** reprinted with permission of the National Council of State Boards of Nursing, Chicago, Ill. Copyright © November, 2001 by Promissor, Inc. Reproduced from the candidate handbook and the Promissor Website. Copyright © 2002, with the permission of Promissor, Inc. **2-5,** modified from Medical Consultants Network, Inc., Englewood, Calif. **2-6, A,** from Birchenall, J., & Streight, E. (2002). *Mosby's textbook for the home care aide* (2nd ed.). St. Louis: Mosby. **2-7,** from Elkin, M.K., Perry, A.G., & Potter, P.A. (2003). *Nursing interventions and clinical skills* (3rd ed.). St. Louis: Mosby.

Chapter 3

3-1, redrawn from deWit, S. (2000). *Fundamental concepts and skills for nursing* (1st ed.). Philadelphia: W.B. Saunders. **3-2; 3-10, A; 3-10, C,** from deWit, S. (2000). *Fundamental concepts and skills for nursing* (1st ed.). Philadelphia: W.B. Saunders. **3-3, 3-12, 3-13,** from Elkin, M.K., Perry, A.G., & Potter, P.A. (2003). *Nursing interventions and clinical skills* (3rd ed.). St. Louis: Mosby. **3-7,** courtesy Delmar Gardens Enterprises, St. Louis. **3-8; 3-10, C,** courtesy Marian Medical Center, CHW, Santa Maria, Calif. **3-9; 3-10, B,** courtesy SSM, St. Louis. **3-11,** Courtesy Centers for Medicare & Medicaid Services.

Chapter 4

4-1, from Maslow, A.H. (1987). *Motivation and personality.* Upper Saddle River, NJ: Prentice Hall. **4-3,** from deWit, S. (2000). *Fundamental concepts and skills for nursing* (1st ed.). Philadelphia: W.B. Saunders.

Chapter 5

Unn. 5-1, Unn. 5-2, Unn. 5-4, from Wong, D.L., and others (1999). *Whaley and Wong's nursing care of infants and children* (6th ed.). St. Louis: Mosby. **Unn. 5-3, Unn. 5-6, Unn. 5-8,** from deWit, S. (2000). *Fundamental concepts and skills for nursing* (1st ed.). Philadelphia: W.B. Saunders. **Unn. 5-5,** from Bowden, V.R., Dickey, S.B., & Greenberg, C.S. (1998). *Children and their families* (1st ed.). Philadelphia: W.B. Saunders. **Unn. 5-7,** from Lewis, S.M., and others (2000). *Medical-surgical nursing* (5th ed.). St. Louis: Mosby. **Table 5-1,** data from Bowden, V.R., Dickey, S.B., & Greenberg, C.S. (1998). *Children and their families* (1st ed.). Philadelphia: W.B. Saunders; and from Wong D.L., and others (1999). *Whaley and Wong's nursing care of infants and children* (6th ed.). St. Louis: Mosby. **5-1, 5-2, 5-3, 5-4, 5-5, 5-6,** from Birchenall, J., & Streight, E. (2002). *Mosby's textbook for the home care aide* (2nd ed.). St. Louis: Mosby. **5-8,** from Potter, P., & Perry, A. (2005). *Fundamentals of nursing* (6th ed.). St. Louis: Mosby.

Chapter 6

6-2, B, from James, S., Ashwill, J., & Droske, S. (2002). *Nursing care of children: principles and practice* (2nd ed.). Philadelphia: W.B. Saunders. **6-5,** from Christensen, B., & Kockrow, E. (2002). *Foundations of nursing* (4th ed.). St. Louis: Mosby.

Chapter 7

7-2; 7-3; 7-4, A, B; 7-6; 7-8; 7-9; 7-10; 7-11; 7-12; 7-13; 7-17; 7-18; 7-19; 7-20, A, B; 7-21; 7-22; 7-23; 7-24; 7-25; 7-26; 7-27; 7-28; 7-29; 7-30, from Herlihy, B., & Maebius, N. (2002). *The human body in health and illness* (soft cover) (2nd ed.). Philadelphia: W.B. Saunders. **7-5, 7-7,** modified from Herlihy, B., & Maebius, N. (2002). *The human body in health and illness* (soft cover) (2nd ed.). Philadelphia: W.B. Saunders.

Chapter 8

Box 8-1, Source: American Heart Association. **8-1; 8-2; 8-3; 8-4; 8-8; 8-9; 8-20; 8-21, A, B; 8-33; 8-34; 8-36,** from Mir, A. (1995). *Atlas of clinical diagnosis* (1st ed.). London: Baillière Tindall. **8-5,** from Belcher, A. (1992). *Mosby's clinical nursing series: cancer nursing.* St. Louis: Mosby. **8-6, 8-14, 8-17,** from Phipps, W., Sands, J.K., & Marek, J.F. (1999). *Medical-surgical nursing: concepts and clinical practice.* St. Louis: Mosby. **8-7,** from Auerbach, P. (2001). *Wilderness medicine* (4th ed.). St. Louis: Mosby. **8-10, A, B; 8-11; 8-12; 8-26,** from Thibodeau, G.A., & Patton, K.T. (2002). *Anatomy and physiology* (5th ed.). St. Louis: Mosby. **8-16,** courtesy Siemens Hearing Instrument, Piscataway, N.J. **8-19, 8-23,** from Lewis, S.M., and others (2000). *Medical-surgical nursing* (5th ed.). St. Louis: Mosby. **8-25,** from Forbes, C.D., & Jackson, W.F. (1993). *A color at-las and text of clinical medicine* (2nd ed.). London: Mosby. **8-22, 8-27, 8-28, 8-29, 8-30, 8-31,** from Herlihy, B., & Maebius, N. (2002). *The human body in health and illness* (soft cover) (2nd ed.). Philadelphia: W.B. Saunders. **8-32, A, B,** courtesy U.S. Public Health Service. **8-35, A, B,** from Moschella, S., & Hurley, H.J. (1992). *Dermatology* (3rd ed.). Philadelphia: W.B. Saunders.

Chapter 9

9-1, from Kumar, V., Cotrane, R., & Robbins, S. (2002). *Basic pathology* (7th ed.). Philadelphia: W.B. Saunders. **9-6, 9-7, 9-8, 9-9, 9-10, 9-12, 9-13, 9-14, 9-15, 9-16, 9-21, 9-22, B,** from deWit, S. (2000). *Fundamental concepts and skills for nursing* (1st ed.). Philadelphia: W.B. Saunders. **9-2, 9-19, 9-20,** from Potter, P., & Perry, A. (2005). *Fundamentals of nursing* (6th ed.). St. Louis: Mosby. **9-11, 9-17, 9-18,** from Elkin, M.K., Perry, A.G., & Potter, P.A. (2003). *Nursing interventions and clinical skills* (3rd ed.). St. Louis: Mosby. **9-22, A,** from Gerin, J. (2003). *Health careers today* (3rd ed.). Philadelphia: Mosby.

Chapter 10

10-3, 10-9, from Birchenall, J., & Streight, E. (2002). *Mosby's textbook for the home care aide* (2nd ed.). St. Louis: Mosby. **10-4, 10-28,** from Elkin, M.K., Perry, A.G., & Potter, P.A. (2003). *Nursing interventions and clinical skills* (3rd ed.). St. Louis: Mosby. **10-10, 10-17,** from Potter, P., & Perry, A. (2005). *Fundamentals of nursing* (6th ed.). St. Louis: Mosby. **10-15, 10-16,** from Bonewit, K. (2003). *Clinical procedures for med-ical assistants* (6th ed.). Philadelphia: W.B. Saunders. **10-18, 10-19, 10-20, 10-21, 10-23, 10-24, 10-25, 10-26, 10-27, 10-29, 10-30,** Courtesy J.T. Posey Co., Arcadia, Calif.

Chapter 11

11-1; 11-2; 11-3; 11-4, A; 11-5; 11-7; 11-8; 11-10; 11-11; 11-12; 11-13; 11-14; 11-15; 11-18; 11-19; 11-20; 11-21; 11-22; 11-23, from deWit, S. (2000). *Fundamental concepts and skills for nursing* (1st ed.). Philadelphia: W.B. Saunders. **11-4, B; 11-6; 11-16; 11-17; 11-24; 11-25; 11-26,** from Elkin, M.K., Perry, A.G., & Potter, P.A. (2003). *Nursing interventions and clinical skills* (3rd ed.). St. Louis: Mosby. **11-9,** from Potter, P., & Perry, A. (2005). *Fundamentals of nursing* (6th ed.). St. Louis: Mosby.

Chapter 12

12-1, 12-5, 12-7, 12-8, 12-9, 12-10, 12-11, 12-12, 12-13, 12-14, 12-15, 12-16, 12-17, 12-18, 12-20, from deWit, S. (2000). *Fundamental concepts and skills for nursing* (1st ed.). Philadelphia: W.B. Saunders. **12-2,** from Wong D.L, and others (2001). *Wong's essentials of pediatric nursing* (6th ed.). St. Louis: Mosby. **12-6,** from Potter, P., & Perry, A. (2000). *Fundamentals of nursing* (5th ed.). St. Louis: Mosby. **12-19, 12-23, 12-24,** from Elkin, M.K., Perry, A.G., & Potter, P.A. (2003). *Nursing interventions and clinical skills* (3rd ed.). St. Louis: Mosby. **12-21,** from Birchenall, J., & Streight, E. (2002). *Mosby's textbook for the home care aide* (2nd ed.) St. Louis: Mosby.

Chapter 13

13-1, courtesy Great Plains Regional Medical Center, North Platte, Neb. **13-2; 13-4; 13-5; 13-6; 13-9; 13-10; 13-11; 13-23; 13-30; 13-31, C; 13-36; 13-45, A; Table 13-1,** from deWit, S. (2000). *Fundamental concepts and skills for nursing* (1st ed.). Philadelphia: W.B. Saunders. **13-3, 13-12, 13-13, 13-14, 13-22, 13-28,** from Birchenall, J., & Streight, E. (2002). *Mosby's textbook for the home care aide* (2nd ed.). St. Louis: Mosby. **13-7,** from Potter, P., & Perry, A. (2005). *Fundamentals of nursing* (6th ed.). St. Louis: Mosby. **13-16; 13-21; 13-29; 13-31, A; 13-34; 13-35; 13-37; 13-38; 13-39; 13-40; 13-41; 13-45, B,** from Potter, P.A., & Perry, A.G. (2003). *Basic nursing: a critical thinking approach* (5th ed.). St. Louis: Mosby. **13-18, 13-20, 13-27, 13-46, 13-47, 13-48, 13-49,** from Elkin, M.K., Perry, A.G., & Potter, P.A. (2003). *Nursing interventions and clinical skills* (3rd ed.). St. Louis: Mosby. **13-25, 13-26, Table 13-7,** from Christensen, B., & Kockrow, E. (2002). *Foundations of nursing* (4th ed.). St. Louis: Mosby. **13-31, B,** courtesy Critickon, Inc.

Chapter 14

14-2, 14-3, 14-24, from Birchenall, J., & Streight, E. (2002). *Mosby's textbook for the home care aide* (2nd ed.). St. Louis: Mosby. **14-4,** from Christensen, B., & Kockrow, E. (2002). *Foundations of nursing* (4th ed.). St. Louis: Mosby. **14-6, 14-9, 4-14, 14-15, 14-16, 14-18, 14-19,** from deWit, S. (2000). *Fundamental concepts and skills for nursing* (1st ed.). Philadelphia: W.B. Saunders. **14-7, 14-11, 14-12,** from Elkin, M.K., Perry, A.G., & Potter, P.A. (2003). *Nursing interventions and clinical skills* (3rd ed.). St. Louis: Mosby. **14-23, A, B, D,** courtesy Hill-Rom. **14-23, C,** courtesy KCI.

Chapter 15

15-1, from Elkin, M.K., Perry, A.G., & Potter, P.A. (2003). *Nursing interventions and clinical skills* (3rd ed.). St. Louis: Mosby. **15-3,** from deWit, S. (2000). *Fundamental concepts and skills for nursing* (1st ed.). Philadelphia: W.B. Saunders. **15-4, 15-5, 15-7, 15-8, 15-9, 15-11, 15-31, 15-32, 15-33, 15-34, 15-35,** from Birchenall, J., & Streight, E. (2002). *Mosby's textbook for the home care aide* (2nd ed.). St. Louis: Mosby. **15-24,** from Potter, P.A., & Perry, A.G. (2003). *Basic nursing: a critical thinking approach* (5th ed.). St. Louis: Mosby.

Chapter 16

16-1, 16-2, 16-3, 16-4, 16-7, from Birchenall, J., & Streight, E. (2002). *Mosby's textbook for the home care aide* (2nd ed.). St. Louis: Mosby. **16-9,** from deWit, S. (2000). *Fundamental concepts and skills for nursing* (1st ed.). Philadelphia: W.B. Saunders. **16-10,** from Potter, P.A., & Perry, A.G. (2003). *Basic nursing: a critical thinking approach* (5 ed.). St. Louis: Mosby.

Chapter 17

17-13, 17-27, 17-30, from deWit, S. (2000). *Fundamental concepts and skills for nursing* (1st ed.). Philadelphia: W.B. Saunders. **17-21,** from Potter, P.A., & Perry, A.G. (2003). *Basic nursing: a critical thinking approach* (5th ed.). St. Louis: Mosby. **17-28,** from Elkin, M.K., Perry, A.G., & Potter, P.A. (2003). *Nursing interventions and clinical skills* (3rd ed.). St. Louis: Mosby. **17-29,** courtesy CLG Photographics, Inc.

Chapter 18

18-1, 18-2, 18-6, 18-7, 18-8, 18-9, 18-13, 18-14, from Birchenall, J., & Streight, E. (2002). *Mosby's textbook for the home care aide* (2nd ed.). St. Louis: Mosby.

Chapter 19

19-1, Wardlaw, G. (1994). *Contemporary nutrition* (2nd ed.). New York: McGraw-Hill. **19-2, Box 19-1, Table 19-1,** from Birchenall, J., & Streight, E. (2002). *Mosby's textbook for the home care aide* (2nd ed.). St. Louis: Mosby. **19-3,** courtesy U.S. Department of Agriculture, Washington, D.C. **19-4, 19-5, 19-9, 19-10, 19-13, 19-15, Box 19-2,** from Elkin, M.K., Perry, A.G., & Potter, P.A. (2003). *Nursing interventions and clinical skills* (3rd ed.). St. Louis:

Mosby. **19-7, 19-12, 19-17, Table 19-3,** from deWit, S. (2000). *Fundamental concepts and skills for nursing* (1st ed.). Philadelphia: W.B. Saunders.

Chapter 20

20-1, 20-2, 20-3, 20-7, 20-26, from Birchenall, J., & Streight, E. (2002). *Mosby's textbook for the home care aide* (2nd ed.). St. Louis: Mosby. **20-4, 20-6, 20-15,** from Christensen, B., & Kockrow, E. (2002). *Foundations of nursing* (4th ed.). St. Louis: Mosby. **20-5, 20-8, 20-9, 20-10, 20-11, 20-13, 20-14, 20-25, 20-32,** from Elkin, M.K., Perry, A.G., & Potter, P.A. (2003). *Nursing interventions and clinical skills* (3rd ed.). St. Louis: Mosby. **20-12, 20-16, 20-33,** from deWit, S. (2000). *Fundamental concepts and skills for nursing* (1st ed.). Philadelphia: W.B. Saunders. **20-17, 20-19, 20-20, 20-21, 20-22, 20-23, 20-24, 20-30, 20-31, 20-34,** from Potter, P.A., & Perry, A.G. (2003). *Basic nursing: a critical thinking approach* (5th ed.). St. Louis: Mosby.

Chapter 21

21-2, courtesy C.B. Fleet Company, Lynchburg, Va. **21-3, 21-4, 21-5, 21-6, 21-13, 21-16, 21-17, 21-21,** from deWit, S. (2000). *Fundamental concepts and skills for nursing* (1st ed.). Philadelphia: W.B. Saunders. **21-7, 21-11, 21-19,** from Potter, P.A., & Perry, A.G. (2003). *Basic nursing: a critical thinking approach* (5th ed.). St. Louis: Mosby. **21-8,** from Christensen, B., & Kockrow, E. (2002). *Foundations of nursing* (4th ed.). St. Louis: Mosby. **21-9, 21-14, 21-22,** from Elkin, M.K., Perry, A.G., & Potter, P.A. (2003). *Nursing interventions and clinical skills* (3rd ed.). St. Louis: Mosby. **21-15, 21-18,** courtesy Hollister, Inc., Libertyville, Ill. **21-20,** courtesy ConvaTec, Princeton, N.J. **Table 21-1,** from Lewis, S.M., Collier, I.C., & Heitkemper, M.M. (1996). *Medical-surgical nursing* (4th ed.). St. Louis: Mosby.

Chapter 22

22-1, 22-3, from deWit, S. (2000). *Fundamental concepts and skills for nursing* (1st ed.). Philadelphia: W.B. Saunders. **22-2,** from Bonewit, K. (2003). *Clinical procedures for medical assistants* (6th ed). Philadelphia: W.B. Saunders. **22-4,** courtesy Ashland Community Hospital, Ashland, Ore. **22-5,** reprinted with permission of Briggs Corporation, Des Moines, Iowa, 50306, (800) 247-2343. **22-6,** courtesy Barnes-Jewish Hospital, St. Louis. **22-7,** courtesy Marian Medical Center, Santa Monica, Calif.

Chapter 23

23-1, 23-13, Unn. 23-1, Unn. 23-2, Unn. 23-3, Unn. 23-4, Unn. 23-5, Unn. 23-6, Unn. 23-7, Unn. 23-8, from Elkin, M.K., Perry, A.G., & Potter, P.A. (2003). *Nursing interventions and clinical skills* (3rd ed.). St. Louis: Mosby. **23-2, 23-19, 23-20, 23-21,** from deWit, S. (2000). *Fundamental concepts and skills for nursing* (1st ed.). Philadelphia: W.B. Saunders. **23-3,** courtesy Dr. Barbara Braden. **23-4, 23-5, 23-6,** courtesy Sammons Preston Rolyan. **23-8, 23-9, 23-11, 23-23,** from Christensen, B., & Kockrow, E. (2002). *Foundations of nursing* (4th ed.). St. Louis: Mosby. **23-12,** from Bloom and Ireland (1992). St. Louis: Mosby. **23-14,** from Belch, J., and others (1996). *Color atlas of peripheral vascular diseases* (2nd ed.). St. Louis: Mosby. **23-15, 23-16, 23-17,** from Birchenall, J., & Streight, E. (2002). *Mosby's textbook for the home care aide* (2nd ed.). St. Louis: Mosby. **23-18, 23-22,** from Potter, P.A., & Perry, A.G. (2003). *Basic nursing: a critical thinking approach* (5th ed.). St. Louis: Mosby.

Chapter 24

24-2, 24-5, 24-9, 24-16, 24-18, from Elkin, M.K., Perry, A.G., & Potter, P.A. (2003). *Nursing interventions and clinical skills* (3rd ed.). St. Louis: Mosby. **24-3,** from Christensen, B., & Kockrow, E. (2002). *Foundations of nursing* (4th ed.). St. Louis: Mosby. **24-4, 24-15,** from Birchenall, J., & Streight, E. (2002). *Mosby's textbook for the home care aide* (2nd ed.). St. Louis: Mosby. **24-6, 24-17, 24-19,** from Bonewit, K. (2003). *Clinical procedures for medical assistants* (6th ed). Philadelphia: W.B. Saunders. **24-11,** courtesy Arizant Healthcare, Inc. **24-13,** courtesy Andermac, Inc., Yuba City, Calif.

Chapter 25

25-2, from Wong, D.L. and others (2002). *Maternal-child nursing care* (2nd ed.). St. Louis: Mosby. **25-4, 25-8, 25-13, 25-14, 25-17,** from Elkin, M.K., Perry, A.G., & Potter, P.A. (2003). *Nursing interventions and clinical skills* (3rd ed.). St. Louis: Mosby. **25-5, 25-6, 25-7, 25-12, 25-15, 25-16,** from Birchenall, J., & Streight, E. (2002). *Mosby's textbook for the home care aide* (2nd ed.) St. Louis: Mosby. **25-9, 25-10, 25-11,** from Grimes, D. (1991). *Infectious diseases* (1st ed.). St. Louis: Mosby.

Chapter 26

Unn. 26-1, Unn. 26-2, Unn. 26-3, Unn. 26-4, Unn. 26-5, Unn. 26-6, Unn. 26-7, Unn. 26-8, Table 26-1, from Potter, P.A., & Perry, A.G. (2003). *Basic nursing: a critical thinking approach* (5th ed.). St. Louis: Mosby.

Chapter 27

27-2, 27-3, 27-11, from Birchenall, J., & Streight, E. (2002). *Mosby's textbook for the home care aide* (2nd ed.). St. Louis: Mosby. **27-4, 27-5, 27-8, 27-13, 27-14,** from Elkin, M.K., Perry, A.G., & Potter, P.A. (2003). *Nursing interventions and clinical skills* (3rd ed.). St. Louis: Mosby. **27-6, 27-7, 27-9, 27-10, 27-12, 27-15, 27-16, 27-18, 27-21,** from deWit, S. (2000). *Fundamental concepts and skills for nursing* (1st ed.). Philadelphia: W.B. Saunders. **27-17,** courtesy Dale Medical Products, Plainville, Md. **27-19,** courtesy Nellcor Puritan Bennett. **27-20,** reprinted with permission of Teleflex Medical.

Chapter 28

28-1, 28-2, 28-3, 28-4, 28-5, 28-7, 28-8, from deWit, S. (2000). *Fundamental concepts and skills for nursing* (1st ed.). Philadelphia: W.B. Saunders.

Chapter 29

29-2, 29-4, 29-5, 29-6, 29-7, 29-9, courtesy Northcoast Medical, Inc. **29-3,** courtesy Sammons, Preston, Ability One. **29-8,** Ability One Corporation.

Chapter 30

30-1, from Birchenall, J., & Streight, E. (2002). *Mosby's textbook for the home care aide* (2nd ed.). St. Louis: Mosby. **30-3,** courtesy Alzheimer's Association. **30-4,** from deWit, S. (2000). *Fundamental concepts and skills for nursing* (1st ed.). Philadelphia: W.B. Saunders.

Chapter 31

31-1, 31-2, from deWit, S. (2000). *Fundamental concepts and skills for nursing* (1st ed.). Philadelphia: W.B. Saunders.

Chapter 32

32-1; 32-4; 32-5, B, C, D; 32-7, B, C, D, courtesy Marjorie Pyle, RNC, Lifecircle, Costa Mesa, Calif. **32-2, 32-6, 32-8, 32-9,** from Lowdermilk, D., & Perry, S. (1999). *Maternity nursing* (5th ed.). St. Louis: Mosby. **32-3,** from Herlihy, B., & Maebius, N. (2002). *The human body in health and illness* (soft cover) (2nd ed.). Philadelphia: W.B. Saunders. **32-5, A; 32-7, A,** courtesy Kim Molloy, San Jose, Calif.

Chapter 33

33-1, courtesy Tina Kult. **33-2, 33-3, 33-4, 33-5, Box 33-1, Box 33-2,** from Wong, D.L., and others (1998). *Whaley & Wong's nursing care of infants and children* (6th ed.). St. Louis: Mosby. **Table 33-1,** courtesy Mark Graber, MD, University of Iowa/Mosby.

Chapter 34

34-1, 34-7, 34-8, 34-11, 34-12, from Birchenall, J., & Streight, E. (2002). *Mosby's textbook for the home care aide* (2nd ed.). St. Louis: Mosby. **34-4,** from Ignatavicius, D. (2002). *Medical-surgical nursing: critical thinking for collaborative care* (4th ed.). St. Louis: W.B. Saunders. **34-5, 34-6,** from Sanders, M. (1994). *Mosby's paramedic textbook* (1st ed.). St. Louis: Mosby. **34-9, 34-10,** from deWit, S. (2000). *Fundamental concepts and skills for nursing* (1st ed.). Philadelphia: W.B. Saunders.

Chapter 35

35-3, 35-4, 35-7, 35-8, 35-9, from Birchenall, J., & Streight, E. (2002). *Mosby's textbook for the home care aide* (2nd ed.). St. Louis: Mosby. **35-6,** reprinted with permission of Briggs Corporation, Des Moines, Iowa, 50306, (800) 247-2343.

Appendix A

Courtesy Centers for Medicare & Medicaid Services.

Appendix B

Courtesy NANDA International: *NANDA nursing diagnoses: definitions and classification 2003-3004.* Philadelphia: NANDA, Copyright 2002.

Appendix C

Translations from Joyce, E.V., & Villanueva, M.E. (2000). *Say it in Spanish: a guide for health care professionals* (2nd ed.). Philadelphia: W.B. Saunders.

INDEX

The letter *b* indicates box, *f* indicates figure, and *t* indicates table.